AMINO ACID COMPOSITION AND BIOLOGICAL VALUE OF CEREAL PROTEINS

AMINO ACID COMPOSITION AND BIOLOGICAL VALUE OF CEREAL PROTEINS

Proceedings of the International Association for Cereal Chemistry Symposium on Amino Acid Composition and Biological Value of Cereal Proteins

Budapest, Hungary, May 31–June 1, 1983
with supplemental invited contributions

Edited by

RADOMIR LÁSZTITY and MÁTÉ HIDVÉGI

Department of Biochemistry and Food Technology,
Technical University of Budapest, Hungary

D. Reidel Publishing Company

A MEMBER OF THE KLUWER ACADEMIC PUBLISHERS GROUP

Dordrecht / Boston / Lancaster

Library of Congress Cataloging in Publication Data

International Association for Cereal Chemistry Symposium on Amino Acid Composition and Biological Value of Cereal Proteins (1983 : Budapest, Hungary)
Amino acid composition and biological value of cereal proteins.

Includes index.
1. Grain—Congresses. 2. Grain—Composition—Congresses. 3. Amino acids—Congresses. 4. Plant proteins—Congresses. 5. Cereals as food—Congresses. 6. Grain as feed—Congresses. I. Lásztity, Radomír. II. Hidvégi, Máté, 1955— . III. International Association for Cereal Chemistry. IV. Title.
SB188.2.I576 1983 641.3'31 84-29827

ISBN-13: 978-94-010-8844-2 e-ISBN-13: 978-94-009-5307-9
DOI: 10.1007/978-94-009-5307-9

Distributors for the U.S.A. and Canada
Kluwer Academic Publishers,
190 Old Derby Street, Hungham, MA 02043, U.S.A.

Distributors for Albania, Bulgaria, Chinese People's Republic, Cuba, Czechoslovakia, German Democratic Republic, Hungary, Korean People's Republic, Mongolia, Poland, Romania, the U.S.S.R., Vietnam, and Yugoslavia
Kultura Hungarian Foreign Trading Company
P.O.B. 149
H-1389 Budapest 62, Hungary

Distributors for all remaining countries
Kluwer Academic Publishers Group,
P.O.Box 322, 3300 AH Dordrecht, Holland

Joint edition published by D. Reidel Publishing Company, Dordrecht, Holland
and
Akadémiai Kiadó, Budapest, Hungary

Softcover reprint of the hardcover 1st edition 1985

PREFACE

Cereals belong to the most important elements in the history of mankind. From the beginning of agriculture, cereals have been by far the most important staple food in the world. Although the cereal consumption decreased to a low level in the developed countries in Europe and North America, in the developing countries over two-thirds of the calorie and protein intake is based on cereals. A substantial quantity of cereals goes indirectly into food via feed to animals.

Generally, cereal proteins are classified as proteins of lower biological value because of shortage in lysine and some other essential amino acids. Recent developments in the determination and evaluation of the biological value of proteins and protein mixtures suggest that the oversimplified earlier evaluation of cereal proteins must be reviewed.

This book contains the edited proceedings of the International Symposium on "Amino Acid Composition and Biological Value of Cereal Proteins", held in Budapest, Hungary, May 31-June 1, 1983, under the sponsorship of the International Association for Cereal Chemistry, Hungarian Scientific Society for Food Industry and Grain Trust, Hungary, with supplemental invited contributions.

Scientists (biologist, plant breeders, farmers, chemists, biochemists, engineers, food technologists and nutritionists) from 17 countries presented and reviewed, along with participants from 20 countries, the recent methodology and trends in the determination of the biological value of cereal proteins, the amino acid composition of cereal proteins and factors influencing the composition and the role of cereal proteins in nutrition and animal feeding.

The editors hope that the contribution of well known specialists, working in the different fields related to cereal science and technology, make the Proceedings a valuable source of information for agronomists, food scientists and technologists, nutritionists and decision makers interested in the more effective and widespread use of cereals, cereal proteins and protein preparations, and in the improvement of the biological value of cereal proteins, foods and feeds containing cereal proteins.

The editors are particularly grateful to the staff of the Akadémiai Kiadó, Budapest, Hungary and D. Reidel Publishing Company, Dordrecht, Holland for the excellent preparation of this book.

Professor Radomir Lásztity

CONTENTS

PART 5

CEREALS IN FOOD AND FEED

INTRODUCTION

PROGRESS OF GRAIN CULTIVATION AND RESEARCH IN HUNGARY

The temperate climate of Hungary, its soil and its relief ensure favourable conditions for growing cereals. These basic fundamentals together with our economic policy made the dynamic development of our cultivation of grain crops possible. Up to the seventies, the yield of wheat crops increased by more than a factor of 2.5 as compared to the yield in the sixties. In 1982 it was 4400 kg/ha, but the record yield achieved in 1980 was 4760 kg/ha. In the period 1976-1980, Hungary took 8-th place among the wheat-growing countries of the world, or for average yield 6-th place when considering only the countries growing wheat on fields above 200 000 ha.

The considerable increase in the yield of wheat in Hungary is both a result of growing new species with a rich yield, and of the complex mechanization of agriculture.

The yield of our most important cultivated plant, corn, was also doubled in the above period of time. Similar results have been achieved for corn.

The increase in yields in obviously not a unique phenomenon restricted to Hungary. The change in conditions for growing wheat can be found all over the world, as is shown by the increase of the average yields. In the opinion of geneticists, this is not yet the end of this significant increase; the biological potential does promise even greater results. It seems that the yield will be restricted rather by economic arguments than biological considerations.

Wheat is a very important basic material in food production. In the years preceding the Second World War, about half of the everyday energy requirement of humans was provided by food on flour basis, and about one-third of it by animal nutrients. Nowadays this ratio is reversed, food of flour basis forming about 1/3 of the necessary energy, and animal nutrients 40-45%. This change has occurred in all parts of the world well-provided with food. Consequently, there has been a decrease in the usage of grain crops as basic nutrition.

A characteristic picture of the state of agriculture in Hungary can be obtained by comparing the total dry residue of agricultural products. It is apparent from this that wheat contributes 25%; a similar amount is provided by corn. The amounts of rough fodder and cereal fodder are also significant, and the remaining 14% includes all the other main agricultural products, such as grapes, fruit, sugar, etc.

Thus the subject of today's symposium, "Amino acid composition and biological value of cereal proteins", is very important in Hungary,let alone the fact that in countries not so well-provided with food the major part of food consumed consists of cereal nutrients. That is, in several countries the amount of animal nutrient available is catastrophically low, therefore a very important role is played there by the quality, quantity and distribution of crops. In this light, the role of growing grain crops has another significance. The wheat grown in Hungary serves primarily to satisfy the demands of the population with flour, about 1.6 million tons being used for this purpose. The export is also significant: it forms about 20-25% of the harvest, but the amount used for forage is also very high, being nearly 50%. On studying these numbers we can conclude that Hungary is relatively rich in wheat, and also in other fodders, so that besides the significant extent of wheat export, we also have an indirect export, i.e. the wheat used for feeding is exported in the form of animal nutrients. Statistics show that, in addition to the almost 11 million Hungarian people, we provide nutrients for a further 8-9 million people at a similarly high level. From this it follows that the quality and quantity of animal breeding also depends on crop growing. This means that the dynamic development of Hungarian food production is based on the results of crop-growing.

In Hungary, there are two famous research institutes dealing with the improvement of wheat: in Martonvásár and in Szeged. In recent decades they have increased the number of species considerably, developing wheat and corn species equivalent to the best foreign species, or even better under domestic conditions, the breed of which are now in progress. As I mentioned earlier, our conditions are favourable for growing high quality wheat, but the increase in demand and the potential for wheat export makes continued research work on the improvement of yield and quality imperative. In Hungary, the agrotechnical branch of agricultural research is very important. It encompasses studies into the effective utility of green crops, the mode of cultivation, various types of dunging, pesticides and irrigation. Of equal importance is the research aimed at the determination of the optimum time for fertilizing, or at clarifying the role of the individual components of fertilizers. In the opinion of researchers, the genetic potential of the new species is utilized only in about 70%. The results of top state farms support this statement convincingly. Further research work is done on increasing the yield and improving the quality, and an ever increasing role in this is played by the state farms. Outstanding results are obtained by there farms. These production systems work with up-to date agrochemistry, special systems of machines, programmed plant protection, and soil conservation, because the value of a given wheat species can only assert itself under optimum agrotechnical conditions. The exploitation of the genetic productivity of the new crop species with a rich yield and a high quality is only possible by the practical application of the most recent scientific results.

Numerous Hungarian researchers are also dealing with the nutritive value of crop proteins, as it is demonstrated by the lectures in this symposium. The research work in Hungary concerning cereals is coordinated in two great projects. One of them is the governmental research programme "Development of grain crop cultivation" in progress at the two above mentioned institutions, and the other one is the branch research programme "Development of products and production of cereal-based food" led by the Research Institute for Milling and Baking Industry. These projects comprehend the whole field of grain crops from the improvement to the production of different crop-based foods.

In Hungary there are old traditions for the improvement, processing and industrial utilization of wheat; it is enough to refer to the improvement experiments at the end of the last century, or to the appearence of the new, improved species at the beginning of this century, or to the scientific methods developed for studying flour. This last event recently had its 50-th anniversary. However, the Hungarian inventors of the chill-casted crushing cylinder providing the basis for an up-to-date milling industry, and of the plansifter could also be mentioned in this context.

Hungarian experts also take part in the work of the International Association for Cereal Chemistry. One of the main fields of activity of ICC is concerned with the unifying of experimental methods, i.e. with international standardization. Those who keep track of the Hungarian standards find numerous signs of well grounded investigations based on international comparisons of the different workshops of ICC. The forums of ICC are suitable for lectures of international standard delivered by Hungarian experts in cereals, today's opportunity also being one of them. The Hungarian researchers take an active part in the workshops of ICC, thereby enriching international scientific life with domestic results. We have also acquired new knowledge by hearing about the identification of wheat species by biochemical procedures, the application of up-to-date instruments such as NIR spectroscopy or atomic absorption spectroscopy in the rapid determination of the composition of crops, etc.

In addition to our activity in the workshops, we also take part in documentation, as a result of which valuable pieces of information can be exchanged. In connection with the 50-th anniversary mentioned earlier, in 1978 a working committee of the group dealing with documentation was organized. ICC provides a good opportunity for deepening the connections between researchers of different countries and the exchange of information. The atmosphere of the Commission is determined by the common interest in the investigation of cereals, particularly in their chemistry.

The book is a significant landmark in this work, and I hope that the researchers will learn by this more about each others' work; at the same time, they will get an overview of the successful work on cereal research and production in Hungary.

Professor Lajos Lénárt,
General Manager,
Grain Trust, Hungary

PART 1

GENERAL PROBLEMS

Proc. Int. Assoc. Cereal Chem. Symp. Amino Acid Compn and Biol. Value of Cereal Proteins .Budapest, Hungary 1983, R. Lásztity, M. Hidvégi, eds

CEREAL PROTEINS - PAST, PRESENT, FUTURE

RADOMIR LÁSZTITY

Department of Biochemistry and Food Technology,
Technical University of Budapest, H-1111 Budapest,
Müegyetem rkp. 3, Hungary

ABSTRACT

Since the beginning of agricultural production in the prehistoric time, cereals have been the main agricultural products in most parts of the world playing an important role in nutrition generally, and in the protein supply. Although the amino acid composition of the cereal proteins and the role of essential amino acids were not known, the mixed diet containing different proteins was characteristic of the greatest part of the population.

At present, the knowledge of the amino acid composition, the development in the science of nutrition, the new methods of the determination of the biological value of proteins and their mixtures opened the possibility for the realization of optimal nutrition from the point of view of protein needs. This optimal protein supply is well realized in the feeding of animals in the up-to-date animal husbandry. Unfortunately, the different economical, political and other problems have not allowed till now the optimal protein supply for the world's millions.

The new achievments in plant physiology and genetics, the new methods of genetic manipulation open new ways for the use of cereal proteins. Increased yields, higher protein content and also improving of the biological value may increase the role of cereal proteins in nutrition and also the direct use of cereal protein preparations in food processing and production.

INTRODUCTION

Since the beginning of agricultural production in the prehistoric time, the cereals /wheat, rice, maize, rye, barley, sorghum, millet, etc./ were the main agricultural products in most parts of the world playing an important role in the nutrition generally and also in the protein supply. Although most amino acid composition of the cereal proteins and the role of essential amino acids were not known, the mixed diet containing different proteins was characteristic of the greatest part of population allowing a compensation of the effects of the unsatisfactory content of some essential amino acids in cereal proteins. Later the steady growth of the population and the limited increase of agricultural production /especially animal husbandry/ changed this situation. In many countries the mixed protein diet changed to a diet based on the overhelming consumption of cereals resp. cereal products representing 80-90% of the total energy and protein supply. The latter fact is connected with an inadequate essential amino acids resp. protein supply representing one of the biggest problems in developing countries to be solved.

In last decades an oversimplified estimation of cereal proteins /low lysine content, deficiency in some other essential amino acids, relatively low biological value/ was accepted by the majority of experts. This fact connected with some others /high starch and energy content of cereals, non-digestible crude fiber content, etc./ led to a rapid decrease of cereal consumption in industrial countries. The low cereal consumption /lower than optimal according the experts of nutrition/ caused also some problems.

The facts mentioned above and also the growing importance of cereals in feeding and industrial uses stimulated and stimulate the research on cereal proteins. Some results of this work and future trends will be discussed in this paper bearing in mind first of all the nutritional problems.

GENERAL CHARACTERIZATION OF CEREAL PROTEINS

According to the data of FAO /1981/ the world production of cereals was estimated at 1663 million metric tons / see Table 1 /. In the last period the area under cereals and also the production increased. The most marked increase was observed in the production of wheat, maize, rice and barley. A decreasing tendency was characteristic for oats and rye.

The greatest part of the produced cereals is used for human consumption. From the other forms of use animal feed, industrial uses and seed-corn are the most important. The total protein consumption of the world population is estimated at more than 100 million metric tons. The proportion of the cereal proteins is more than the half of the total protein production of the world. If we consider that the production of milk and meat is also based on feed-containing cereals, it is clear that in the covering of the needs in protein the cereal proteins play the most important role.

The chemical composition of cereals is characterized by a high content of starch, relatively important protein content and relatively low lipid content. The differences

Table 1.

World production of the cereals [a] /10^6 metric tons/

Sort of cereal	Year 1976	1977	1978	1979	1980	1981
Total cereals	1479	1470	1600	1553	1561	1663
Wheat	425	387	451	428	444	458
Rice /paddy/	350	371	386	377	397	413
Maize	350	370	392	418	394	451
Barley	172	160	179	157	154	158
Rye	30	28	27	23	26	24
Oats	50	51	47	43	43	44
Sorghum	55	61	53	65	56	72
Millet	33	35	28	27	28	30
Triticale	0,4[x]	0,4[x]	0,4[x]	0,5[x]	0,6[x]	0,6[x]

[x]Estimated data

[a]from FAO Production Yearbook 1981

between different cereal grains are significant, also between different varieties of the same cereal. The average chemical composition of the cereals is demonstrated in Table 2. /Lásztity 1984/.

Table 2.

Average gross composition of cereal grains /% dry weight basis/

Cereal grains	Protein	Fat	Starch	Fiber	Ash
Wheat	12.2	1.9	71.9	1.9	1.7
Rye	11.6	1.7	71.9	1.9	2.0
Barley	10.9	2.3	73.5	4.3	2.4
Oats	11.3	5.8	55.5	10.9	3.2
Maize	10.2	4.6	79.5	2.3	1.3
Millet	10.3	4.5	58.9	8.7	4.7
Sorghum	11.0	3.5	65.0	4.9	2.6
Rice	8.1	1.2	75.8	0.5	1.4
Buckwheat	11.0	2.4	64.0	11.0	1.8

According to the comprehensive studies of Osborne the wheat proteins were divided into four classes on the basis of solubility: albumins soluble in water; globulins, soluble in salt solutions / 10 % NaCl solution was frequently used/, but insoluble in water; gliadins, soluble in 70-90 % ethanol; and glutenins, insoluble in neutral aqueous solutions, saline solutions or alcohol. The terms gliadin and glutenin are usually reserved for preparations from wheat. Osborne suggested the generic names, prolamin and glutelin, for the equivalent protein fractions of other cereal grains.

The fractionation of the cereal proteins on the basis of solubility has retained its importance to the present time. Nevertheless, on the basis of the recent results of biochemistry from the scientific point of view, the classification according to the biological function is, the most acceptable. On the basis of biological functions, the proteins of the cereal grains were divided into two classes: metabolically active or cytoplasmic proteins and storage proteins. This classification of the proteins is now well established. The former correspond roughly to the group of albumins and globulins /according to Osborne's classification/, and the latter comprise the prolamins and glutelins. However, some overlapping of the properties and the function is possible.

On the basis of the morphology of cereal grains,the proteins may be divided into three groups: endosperm proteins, proteins of the aleurone layer and proteins of the embryo /or germ/. The different possibilities of the classification are summarized in Table 3. To the group of the cytoplasmic proteins belong the enzymes as most important metabolically active proteins, the membrane proteins, non-enzymic regulatory proteins, proteins of organelles,etc. Storage proteins are typically endosperm proteins, nevertheless,smaller amounts of storage proteins may be found also in the aleurone layer and in the embryo.

From the chemical point of view the existence of complex proteins is also interesting. In Osborne's classification the complex proteins were not taken into account. The newer investigations show that the protein-lipid and protein-carbohydrate interactions,resp. the lipo- and glycoproteins play a very important role in forming the properties and technological value of different cereals.

Cytoplasmic and storage proteins differ considerably in physical properties and amino acid composition. Generally, the cytoplasmic proteins are easily soluble in water or salt buffer-solutions, their molecular weight is relatively small and the molecules have globular form. The storage proteins of the endosperm are generally insoluble in water and salt solutions. It is characteristic for the endosperm storage proteins that they include two types of proteins: a low

Table 3.

Possibilities of the classification of cereal proteins

On the basis of morphology	On the basis of biological function	According to solubility /Osborne/	On the basis of chemical composition
Endosperm proteins	Metabolically active /cytoplasmic proteins	Albumins	Simple proteins
Proteins of the aleurone layer	- enzymes	Globulins	Complex proteins
Proteins of the embryo	- membrane proteins	Prolamins	- lipoproteins
	- proteins of ribosomes	Glutelins	- glycoproteins
	- regulatory proteins		- nucleoproteins
	- other proteins		etc
	Storage proteins		
	- low molecular weight proteins		
	- high molecular weight proteins		

molecular weight protein consisting of one polypeptide chain and having only intramolecular disulfide bonds and a high molecular weight protein consisting from many polypeptide chains cross-linked by intermolecular disulfide bonds.

Concerning the distribution of metabolically active and storage proteins, it can be stated that the proteins of the aleurone layer and germ belong mainly to the group of metabolically active proteins and the storage proteins are presumably located in the endosperm. Modern milling procedures allow to achieve a comparatively clean separation of the embryo /or germ/, pericarp-aleurone layer /or bran/, and endosperm /or flour/.

The protein concentration in the different morphological

parts /endosperm, aleurone layer, embryo/ of the cereal grains shows big variations.

The protein content of the germs is the highest /about 30%/; relatively high concentration /about 20%/ may be observed in the aleurone layer, and the lowest protein concentration belongs to the endosperm. The ultrastructure of the endosperm of different cereal grains is similar. The storage proteins form a matrix or/and protein granules surrounding the starch granules. It was observed by many research workers that the protein concentration varies from the inner to the outer endosperm parts. Finally, the total content of essential amino acids depends on the mass ratio of the main morphological parts of the grain. The more developed aleurone layer, the greater germ at, represent a higher content in protein and essential amino acids.

AMINO ACID COMPOSITION

As a result of increased interest and also wide use of new techniques of determination of amino acid composition of proteins now we have a more adequate picture about the essential amino acid content of cereal proteins and also of their fractions and subfractions.

Wheat, rye and triticale proteins.

The total wheat protein and especially the storage proteins of endosperm are poor in lysine /see Table 4 / and therefore their biological value is relatively low. Nevertheless, because in mixed diets /feed mixtures/ the wheat protein may be easily completed with proteins having complementary amino acid composition /higher lysine content and lower amount of sulfur-containing amino acids/ the real value of the wheat protein in nutrition /feeding/ is higher than it may be calculated from the amino acid composition. Discussing the nutritional value of gluten proteins, it must be mentioned that a small part of the population is sensitive to particular gliadin components of wheat. The disease – called coeliac disease or gluten sensitive enteropathy – is characterized by malabsorption of nutrients as a consequence of damage to the absorptive epithelial cells that line the small intestine.

The cytoplasmic proteins of wheat have generally a better amino acid composition from the point of view of nutritional value, because their lysine content is higher and the glutamic acid /glutamine/ content lower than that of the gluten proteins. Some of the albumin components in wheat have special amino acid composition. For example albumins 13A and 13B isolated by Feillet and Nimmo /1970/ contain practically no phenylalanine /see Table 4 /. Probably such protein preparations may be used in special diets for people having inherited disorder in amino acid metabolism.

Table 4.
Amino acid composition of some proteins of wheat /mol/10^5 g protein/

Amino acid	Albumin[a] 13 A	Albumin[a] 13 B	Gliadin	Glutenin
Lysine	23	48	5	13
Histidine	14	1	15	13
Arginine	56	53	15	20
Threonine	25	24	18	26
Serine	56	66	38	50
Aspartic acid	55	70	20	23
Glutamic acid	106	95	317	278
Glycine	75	75	25	78
Alanine	26	76	25	34
Valine	72	101	43	41
Leucine	74	68	62	57
Isoleucine	23	16	37	28
Proline	69	88	138	114
Tyrosine	36	29	16	25
Phenylalanine	16	-	38	27
Tryptophan	16	35	5	8
Cystine	66	54	10	10
Methionine	21	17	12	12

a = from Feillet and Nimmo /1970/

The rye proteins are characterized by a relatively higher lysine content relating to wheat /see Table 5/. The properties of triticale proteins are generally intermediate of those of the parents. The differences between storage and cytoplasmic proteins concerning amino acid composition are of the same character as by wheat proteins.

Maize proteins

The amino acid composition of the total protein of maize kernel is characterized by a low content of lysine and tryptophan /see Table 6 /. Especially some storage proteins

Table 5.

Amino acid composition of wheat, and rye grain resp.glutenin /g amino acid/100 g protein/

Amino acid	Rye[a] grain	Rye[a] glutenin	Wheat grain	Wheat glutenin
Lysine	3.42	3.98	2.52	2.1
Histidine	2.20	2.42	2.20	1.9
Ammonia	n.d.	3.39	n.d.	n.d.
Arginine	4.93	5.06	4.61	3.8
Aspartic acid	6.82	6.32	4.71	4.8
Threonine	3.26	3.58	2.87	3.8
Serine	4.11	5.24	4.53	5.2
Glutamic acid	30.51	29.23	31.52	39.7
Proline	12.29	12.24	10.44	12.6
Glycine	3.82	4.98	3.89	5.3
Alanine	4.06	4.29	3.40	3.9
Valine	5.21	5.19	4.22	4.8
Methionine	1.68	1.66	2.11	1.5
Isoleucine	4.26	3.66	3.59	3.9
Leucine	6.68	7.37	6.79	8.1
Tyrosine	3.27	3.86	3.20	3.8
Phenylalanine	4.82	4.96	4.75	4.4
Tryptophan	1.13	0.90	1.32	1.1
Cystine	1.90	2.50	2.24	2.7

a = from Bushuk /1974/

are very poor in these amino acids. Since discovery of high-lysine opaque-2 corn /Mertz et al. 1964/ considerable research effort has been expanded to develop hybrids with high quality proteins.

The higher lysine content of the opaque-2 mutants is connected with the fact that in these mutants the synthesis of zein /the protein fraction with the lowest lysine content/ is suppressed. As a result of the lower zein content the amino acid composition of high-lysine mutants is different of that of normal maize /see Table 6 /. The high-lysine mutants have not only higher lysine content but also a lower glutamic acid and proline content.

Table 6.
Amino acid composition of maize kernel proteins and their fractions / g/100 g protein/

Amino acid	Total grain /normal/[a]	Total grain /High lysine W22/[b]	Maize albumin[c]	Maize globulin[c]	Zein[c]	Glutelin[c]
Lysine	2.6	3.8	6.9	6.6	0.5	3.0
Histidine	2.8	4.1	3.4	4.1	0.9	2.5
Arginine	3.8	5.2	8.5	11.1	2.4	4.1
Aspartic acid	7.3	9.4	8.4	9.5	5.5	7.1
Threonine	3.6	4.4	4.8	5.1	2.4	3.4
Serine	4.8	5.6	4.2	5.3	6.3	5.9
Glutamic acid	23.6	20.9	14.3	15.4	25.7	20.0
Proline	8.3	11.0	7.8	5.8	10.2	10.9
Glycine	3.4	5.2	6.4	6.8	1.7	4.5
Alanine	7.9	7.9	6.6	4.4	10.9	6.2
Valine	5.3	6.7	5.5	6.0	3.1	5.1
Methionine	1.8	3.2	1.7	2.1	1.8	2.4
Cysteine	1.1	1.9	n.d.	n.d.	0.3	3.4
Isoleucine	3.7	4.3	4.0	2.7	3.5	3.2
Leucine	13.6	12.5	6.9	4.6	17.3	12.0
Tyrosine	4.4	5.2	4.0	2.6	3.1	4.6
Phenylalanine	5.1	6.0	3.6	3.4	5.3	4.9
Tryptophan	0.7	0.8	3.1	4.4	0.6	0.8

a from Baudet et al. /1966/
b from Misra et al. /1972/
c from El Kady /1983/

The nutritive value of total maize protein and especially of zein is relatively low because of the poor lysine and tryptophan content of these proteins. The biological value of maize proteins calculated on the basis of different chemical indices varies between 30-47. Nevertheless, maize proteins may be supplemented well by proteins containing more lysine and tryptophan and poor in amino acids containing sulfur. Casein or proteins of legumes including soya are suitable for these purposes. Also a combination of wheat and maize flours may be advantageous. The germ proteins and also germ protein isolates have a more convenient amino acid composition and higher biological value. High-lysine mutants, have a higher biological value.

The proteins of barley and oats

The amino acid composition of the total protein of barley is similar to the other cereal grains.

High glutamic acid /glutamine/ and proline content, relatively low amount of basic amino acids and considerable cystine content characterize the barley proteins. Some data about the amino acid composition of barley proteins are shown in Table 7. The amino acid composition of the total protein shows some changes depending on the level of nitrogen fertilization and total protein content. Several authors reported that increases in the nitrogen content of barley seed, resulting from increased nitrogen fertilization, lead to a decrease in the relative lysine content of the grain proteins. It was concluded that the decreased relative lysine content of the whole grain is due to the increased synthesis of hordein. The latter protein fraction is poor in lysine /see Table 7 /. Selection of cereal varieties of improved protein quality, based on a screening programme for elevated grain lysine levels, has led to the recognition of the high-lysine barley mutant, Hyproly. The investigation of the ultrastructure of the high-lysine barley and also the study of the distribution of the protein between different fractions revealed that the higher lysine content is connected with a lower hordein content in the barley seeds.

The nutritive /feeding/ value of barley proteins may be generally characterized similarily to other cereal proteins. From the point of view of biological value, the LMW-storage proteins are of poorest quality because of their very low content in lysine. As by other cereals the cytoplasmic proteins are more rich in essential amino acids than the storage proteins. The better total protein composition of high lysine mutants is connected with higher nutritive value. Oat protein has some unique features in comparison with other cereal grain proteins. The average amino acid composition of the oat proteins is more advantageous from the point of view of nutritional value. This fact is connected probably with the substantially differing distribution of the classical protein fractions /albumins, globulins, prolamins and glutelins according to Osborne/ in oats and other cereal grains. The proportion of albumins and globulins is much higher.

Table 7.

Amino acid composition of the barley proteins /g/16 g nitrogen/

Amino acid	Normal[a] barley	Hordein[b]	Glutelin[b]	Albumin[b]	High-[c] -lysine mutant 1508	Globulin[b]
Lysine	3.5	0.5	2.2	5.1	5.35	5.3
Histidine	2.1	1.0	1.9	1.9	2.77	1.7
Arginine	4.4	2.0	3.2	3.8	7.05	5.5
Aspartic acid	6.1	1.6	4.2	10.4	8.29	8.1
Threonine	3.5	2.0	3.8	4.6	4.33	4.4
Serine	4.2	4.2	5.7	5.4	4.77	5.4
Glutamic acid	24.6	34.7	25.9	14.5	17.02	15.5
Proline	10.9	23.0	14.1	7.3	7.25	9.3
Glycine	4.2	2.5	6.3	8.9	5.63	9.6
Alanine	4.1	2.4	5.1	10.6	5.08	7.9
Cystine	2.5	1.6	0.5	0.5	2.07	0
Valine	5.4	4.6	6.5	7.2	5.77	7.6
Methionine	1.6	0.9	1.3	1.9	2.16	1.8
Isoleucine	3.8	3.8	4.2	4.1	3.57	3.8
Leucine	6.9	6.9	8.2	7.9	6.91	7.9
Tyrosine	2.5	2.4	2.7	2.4	3.70	2.8
Phenylalanine	5.1	5.9	4.3	3.7	4.38	3.6
Tryptophan	1.4	0.9	1.1	2.5	1.61	2.1

[a]Tkachuk and Irvine /1969/

[b]Brandt /1976/

[c]Martens and Knudsen /1980/

The lysine content of oats is higher than that of other cereal proteins and the glutamic acid /glutamine/ and proline content is relatively lower. The differences between endosperm storage proteins and cytoplasmic proteins are also observed in oats but they are not so extensively expressed as in other cereals /see Table 8 /.

Table 8.

Average amino acid composition of the different protein fracitons isolated from oats grown in Hungary /g amino acid/100 g protein/

Amino acid	Total protein	Albumins	Globulins	Prolamins	Glutelins
Lysine	4.5	8.3	4.9	3.1	5.2
Histidine	2.3	3.1	3.3	1.6	3.1
Arginine	7.4	5.3	8.5	5.0	9.1
Aspartic acid	8.9	12.5	9.8	4.2	10.8
Threonine	3.7	5.5	3.8	2.3	4.8
Serine	5.1	6.3	4.3	3.2	4.7
Glutamic acid	21.0	15.1	19.5	36.1	19.1
Proline	5.3	5.8	5.4	11.3	8.1
Glycine	5.3	6.5	5.8	3.0	4.0
Alanine	5.2	7.1	6.5	3.8	4.1
Cystine	1.9	1.7	1.8	3.1	1.4
Valine	5.3	7.3	5.1	5.5	4.4
Methionine	1.9	2.2	1.9	3.3	1.5
Isoleucine	3.9	4.1	4.7	3.8	4.3
Leucine	7.7	8.9	7.0	10.3	7.1
Tyrosine	3.3	2.6	2.4	2.1	4.8
Phenylalanine	5.1	7.8	6.1	7.5	7.1
Tryptophan	1.7	1.7	1.4	1.6	1.9

Proteins of rice, millet and sorghum

The amino acid composition of the total protein of the rice grain is generally characterized by a higher lysine content and lower glutamic acid /glutamine/ content in comparison with other cereals. The varietal differences in the gros amino acid composition are probably connected with the different solubility fraction distribution. The differences between the brown rice and the milled rice are also connected with the changes in the distribution of protein fractions. Some data are summarized in Table 9. Due to the differences in the protein fraction distribution, the amino acid composition of the different morphological parts of the rice grain and also that of the milling products are also different. All the by--products of the rice milling have higher levels of lysine and lower content of glutamic acid than milled rice. The gross amino acid composition of the rice protein changes very slightly if proteins of waxy and normal rice grains are investigated. Some differences were observed between the gross amino acid composition of the total protein of low- and high-protein cultivars. A negative correlation was found between the protein content and lysine level.

Table 9.
Amino acid composition of rice, sorghum and millet

Amino acid	Milled rice[a]	Rice germ[b]	Rice bran[b]	Sorghum[c]	Millet[d]
Lysine	3.9	4.5	4.3	2.3	1.2
Histidine	2.0	1.6	1.4	2.3	2.2
Arginine	8.7	6.6	6.1	3.6	2.6
Aspartic acid	10.0	9.5	9.6	6.6	5.6
Glutamic acid	20.7	15.3	16.8	21.2	17.1
Serine	5.6	5.2	5.2	4.4	5.1
Threonine	3.9	3.7	3.3	3.2	2.9
Cystine	2.1	1.2	1.2		1.2
Methionine	2.3	3.0	2.7	1.3	1.7
Glycine	4.7	4.5	4.1	3.4	2.3
Alanine	6.1	5.5	7.1	8.5	8.0
Valine	5.0	5.5	5.6	4.8	4.2
Isoleucine	3.6	3.7	4.9	3.8	3.5
Leucine	9.3	8.1	9.2	12.2	8.5
Phenylalanine	4.7	5.2	6.1	5.3	4.1
Proline	5.0	8.1	5.2	6.2	4.9
Tyrosine	4.3	4.9	5.0	4.5	2.8
Tryptophan	1.5	1.5	1.4	n.d.	n.d.

a from Hussein /1978/
b from Ronda Lain and Soto Rodriguez /1965/
c from Jones and Beckwith /1970/
d from Nesterin and Skurichin /1979/

The amino acid composition of sorghum proteins is similar to that of maize proteins. Sorghum is usually high in glutamic acid, leucine, alanine, proline and aspartic acid. The lysine content of the sorghum proteins is relatively low. The gross amino acid composition of the sorghum protein is depending on the total protein content. Glutamic acid, alanine and leucine are highly positively correlated with the protein content. Oppositely,lysine and glycine are highly negatively correlated with the protein content.

The amino acid composition of millet is generally characterized by low level of lysine, tryptophan, threonine and sulphur containing amino acids. Certain lines show higher values for lysine similarly to opaque-2 mutants of the corn. The differences in amino acid composition between the different morphological parts of the kernel have similar character as in other cereal grains. The endosperm /flour/ is lower in lysine, arginine and glycine and higher in methionine than the whole grain.

ENZYME INHIBITORS IN CEREALS

It was found first by Kneen and Sandstedt /1943/ that the albumin fraction of wheat contains α-amylase inhibitor proteins. Due to the growing of our knowledge in biochemistry, to the efforts to increase the efficacy of feeding and protein consumption in the last two decades,intensive research work was done in this field. As a result of these investigations it was found that the occurrence of natural enzyme inhibitors is a general phenomenon in all cereals,especially in germs,but also in endosperm.Petrucci et al. /1974/ using gel filtration chromatography separated three groups /families/ of α-amylase inhibitors in wheat. The molecular weights of the families were 12000, 24000 and 60000. The principal inhibitors of the 12000 and 24000 family have relative electrophoretic mobilities of 0.28 and 0.19 and are frequently referred to by these codes. Reviews covering the molecular properties, the biology /including genetics/, and the possible nutritional signifiance of wheat α-amylase inhibitors were published by Marshall /1975/ and Buoconore et al. /1977/.

The α-amylase inhibitors from wheat do not inhibit the α- and β-amylases from wheat or other cereals but inhibit in various degrees the α-amylases from various animal species, insects and bacteria. It may be supposed that the protein α- amylase inhibitors were developed in wheat to provide the plant with protection against insect predators. The low α- amylase activity of mature kernels may be caused by an inhibitor-enzyme complex which dissociates on germination.

Probably these inhibitors may be used in the control of the α-amylase activity in flours and doughs prepared from germinated wheat.

Protease inhibitors were found first in wheat germ by Hochstrasser and Werle /1969/. They separated two trypsin inhibitors having molecular weights of about 12000 and 17000. Later other research workers found also protease inhibitors in wheat germ and in endosperm, too. The trypsin inhibitors separated by gel filtration chromatography are basic proteins with molecular weight between 10 and 24 kilodaltons. Most of the components showing inhibitory effect are not homogeneous, they could be separated into more components by gel electrophoresis.

Later trypsin inhibitors were found also in other cereals. The trypsin and chimotrypsin inhibitors of rye and triticale /Tsen 1974/ are also basic proteins with low molecular weight.

The trypsin inhibitors are characterized by high thermostablility. Heating in boiling water for 1 hour could not fully destroy them. The barley seeds contain two types of trypsin inhibitors /Boisen and Djurtoft 1982/. Two isoinhibitors were isolated and the amino acid compositons and approximate molecular weights were determined. The same was reported also about the trypsin inhibitors of maize /Melville and Scandalios 1972/ and rice /Tashiro and Maki 1978, Maki et. al 1980/.

Recently, Jones and Meredith /1982/ reported about the inactivation of α-amylase by purothionins. The amounts of purothionin used in these experiments were greater than that normally extractable from flour used as amylase source. However, they postulated, that if the purothionins are compartmentalized in the seeds, the effective concentration of purothionin in this small area might be comparable to that used in the experiments.

FUTURE TRENDS

In the last years - after a long period of decrease - a stagnation /in some countries a slight increase/ of cereal consumption was observed. This tendency is in accordance with the views of nutritionists recognizing the importance of cereals in human nutrition, especially the beneficial effect of dietary fiber on the physiology of nutrition. It can be stated also that the role of cereals as most important feeds components remained unchanged. The further trends in uses of cereals for food and feed depend mainly on two factors:

- new achievements in the plant breeding and practical use of genetic engineering;
- development of new types of food products on cereal basis and new forms of use of cereal protein preparations.

For a long time one of the main purposes in cereal breeding is the increase of protein content and improving of its quality. Although some very valuable and interesting results were achieved and many high-protein and high-lysine cultivars are known, it is from day to day clearer that a faster and more effective development could be achieved only by practical realization of the knowledge collected in molecular biology. The history and example of high-lysine mutants shows that for the application of genetic engineering in cereal breeding an exact knowledge of genes controlling protein synthesis and the mechanism of protein synthesis is necessary.

Concerning the mechanism of protein synthesis many experimental data were collected.

An excellent review on the protein synthesis in the developing wheat endosperm has been published by Kasarda et al. /1976/. Concerning the storage proteins of barley, the review of Cameron-Mills et al. /1980/ may be mentioned.

The results of the research work on the biosynthesis of storage proteins of maize were summarized by Mossé and Landry /1980/. Some work concerning other cereals is reviewed by Simmonds /1978/.

On the basis of the observations made on wheat during the different stages of the development of the endosperm, three mechanisms of the protein biosynthesis appear to be operating. These three mechanisms which may be observed or postulated at different stages of the development by electronmicroscopy, are:

- synthesis on polyribosomes which are abundant in the cytoplasm surrounding the large central vacuole;
- synthesis on ribosomes bound to, or associated with, protein bodies, which may be seen developing whithin the vacuoles between 12-20 days post anthesis /p.a./. In all alternative mechanism, the protein may be synthetized in the cytoplasm and transported to the vacuole either through the lumen of the endoplasmatic reticulum, or by a process akin to pinocytosis;
- synthesis on the endoplasmatic reticulum-bond ribosomes and accumulation whithin the lumen of this organelle.

The results of the investigation of other cereals show that probably these statements may be generalized for all cereal grains.

Concerning the biosynthesis of the different classes of proteins, several studies were made by research workers. On the basis of these investigations it can be generally stated that the metabolically active /cytoplasmic/ proteins /belonging to the group of albumins and globulins/ are synthetized rapidly in the early stage of kernel development. It is likely that this takes place on the polysomal aggregates present in the cytoplasm. The results show that the cytoplasmic proteins are present in a significant amount even at the earliest stages at which the material could be analysed. On the basis of the observation that high protein wheats have a greater proportion of their total protein as acetic acid soluble or storage protein, it was suggested that after the developing wheat kernel has satisfied its requirements for cytoplasmic proteins, any additional nitrogen is channeled into the synthesis of storage proteins. The results of other investigations agree with these findings.

With application of new techniques of DNA investigation our knowledge concerning genes coding cereal proteins was enlarged. As example some results relating to barley protein synthesis will be shown.

As a first step towards analysis of the hordein structural genes, hordein polypeptides have been synthetized in vitro with barley polyribosomes /Brandt and Ingversen 1977, 1978./. A cell free protein synthetizing system is employed containing ribosomal subunits and transfer RNA, with all the additional factors essential for the protein synthesis provided by a wheat-germ extract or a rabbit reticulocyte lysate. The newly synthetized hordein polypeptids are detected by inclusion of 35S-labeled methionine in the cell free system and autoradiography of the translation products on SDS-polyacrylamide gel.

The mRNA fraction from membrane-bound polyribosomes coding for hordein polypeptides has been isolated and purified using poly-U-Sepharose 4 B affinity chromatography and sucrose density centrifugation. The purified mRNA showed an increased template activity for all the major hordein polypeptides synthetized in vitro.

The second stage in these studies has involved the production of cDNA probes complementary to hordein mRNA, which can be used to localize the hordein structural genes. Single stranded cDNA was synthetized from a template of purified hordein mRNA employing reverse transcriptase. The second strand was synthetized using E. coli DNA polymerase I., giving a double stranded cDNA molecule. This double stranded cDNA is cloned by insertion into the bacterial plasmic vector. The details of a DNA cloning technology for the study of barley storage proteins are summarized in the review paper of Cameron-Mills et al. /1980/. Localization of the structural genes for hordein polypeptides among the barley chromosomes may now be attempted using the cloned cDNA as probe. The fine structure of the Hor-2 locus on chromosome 5, which codes for the hordein-2 group, may now be explored and the number and distribution of its component genes determined. These investigations, and similar investigations with other cereals /maize, wheat/, combined with a further understanding of the genetic regulation of the hordein genes, will provide an important basis for future breeding strategies aimed at producing high-yielding, high-lysine barley, maize and wheat varieties.

Due to the increasing shortage of food proteins and efforts to produce new types of cheaper, but biologically acceptable foods, using new protein sources, the demand for vegetable proteins with satisfactory amino açid composition and especially good functional praperties has grown rapidly in last time. Parallely also the industrial production of different protein products /protein concentrates/ has a growing tendency.

The advantages of the production and use of vegetable food protein concentrates may be summarized as follows:

- in many cases the protein-containing raw material could not be directly used as food;
- the raw material may contain other, from point of view of nutrition harmful, components /enzyme inhibitors, plant toxins, etc./;
- using protein concentrates the forms of application may be more wide and different protein foods of new type may be produced;
- in some technological processes protein rich by-products are formed which may be used for food purposes;
- the protein content of some plant raw materials is too low and so they are not an adequate source of protein;
- the separation of proteins from waste-waters reduce the pollution;
- the costs of storage and transport of protein concentrates is much lower.

One of the most known cereal protein concentrates is the vital gluten produced in many countries of the world. Total production of vital gluten was estimated to about 120 thousand tons per year /Sarkki 1980/. The largest utilizer of vital gluten is the baking industry, but it is also used in breakfast foods, pet foods, meat analogues, processed meat and other foods. The quality of vital gluten is mostly characterized by protein content /normally 75-80 %/, by water absorption /vital gluten of good quality absorbs 1.5-2 times its own weight and this absorption remains constant under any conditions/, the velocity of swelling /during 20-60 s the maximal water absorption and swelling must be achieved/. The production of other protein preparations from wheat is not yet significant.

The procedures used for the production of protein preparations from wheat may be generally classified as follows:

- air /dry/ processing;

- wet processing using water or water solutions;
- procedures using not aqueous solvents.

The air classification of flours based on the density differences of starch and storage wheat protein particles is widely used and permits the production of preparations enriched in protein content by 20-25% amount of proteins. The wet processes are mostly connected with the starch production. Generally, wheat flour dough is produced and the starch and gluten are separated by washing. The remaining wet gluten is dried under mild conditions. In the old processes the water soluble proteins were lost and great amount of waste-water was formed. The newer procedures /Raisio-process, Farmaco--process, etc./ try to save all the protein and other components of wheat producing not only starch and vital gluten, but also other protein preparations /germ, soluble proteins/ and fiber.

The production of wheat protein concentrates using flotation methods with organic solvents is at this time only in experimental stage, no industrial uses are known.

Among the chemically modified gluten preparations the succinylated and acylated products may have an importance because of the better solubility and higher swelling and water absorbing capacity.

The enzymatically degraded gluten preparations /hidrolysed gluten/ may be also used in the production of some special foods, and also in the production of meat flavors.

The germ of maize is potentially a copious source of protein for human uses. It can be used directly or in defatted form in the baking industry or in the form of protein preparations /protein concentrates/ also for protein enrichment or protein substitution in different food products.

The demand for low-cost vegetable protein supplements to increase the nutritional value of cereals and other foods encouraged research into improved products from maize germ.

The chemical and nutritional problems of the cereal germs used in bakery products were recently reviewed by Tsen /1980/. The functional properties of the germ protein isolate /extracted by 70 % ethanol and diluted sodium hydroxide/ were studied by Restani et al. /1980/. It was found that the water sorption of germ proteins is extremely high and the sorption-desorption process is reversible. Emulsifying properties were also good, with a sharp minimum at pH 5.5. Fat absorption was quite high as compared to other food proteins.

Current industrial dry milling processes using complex system of grinding, sieving, aspiration and air flotation give possibility to produce germ preparations and protein enriched flours. Air classification process - generally used as a means of producing high protein fractions from cereal flours - results in maize flour fractions with moderately increased protein content. The goal of the wet milling process is separation of highly pure starch from protein and other constituents of maize. However, important feeds and other products are derived in large quantities from protein-rich by-products. An essential initial step in the wet milling process is steeping the maize in 0.1-0.2 % SO_2 solution. As the effect of this treatment and also an increased proteolytic activity results in a lot of soluble proteins and N-containing compounds which are collected in the steep waters. Condensed fermented maize extractives contain 24.8 % of protein. The maize germ meal produced in wet milling process contains more than 20 % protein. One of the most valuable products of wet milling is the gluten meal containing about 60 % of protein. The protein is composed mainly of zein and maize glutelin, in consequence low in lysine and tryptophan but relatively rich in sulphur-containing amino acids. The feed gluten meal has a strong odor and flavor and a tendency to develop rancidity due to the high content of unsaturated fatty acids. To upgrade the gluten meal for human use,it is necessary to extract the oil, pigments and typical flavor. A process resulting in maize protein concentrate suitable for human consumption is described by Sternberg et al. /1980/. It was also reported that this protein concentrate has good water-binding capacity and also fat emulsifying properties. The essential amino acid content of the different products of the wet milling process are summarized in Table 10.

The zein of the maize has been one of the industrially produced proteins since longer time. The world production is estimated to 500 t/year. In the current production process the zein is extracted by 88 % isopropylalcohol containing 0.25 % sodium hydroxide at 60 °C. After clarification the solution is chilled to -15 °C to precipitate zein. The normal commercial product contains 3-4 % oil and about 500 mg/kg xanthophyl. The possibility of improving the nutritional quality of zein using plastein reaction was investigated by Arai et al. /1975/. This reaction permits after hydrolysis of the zein to introduce essential amino acids into the polypeptide chain. During the plastein reaction not only new essential amino acids are incorporated but also a condensation of the peptides occurs. Zein is currently used primarily as a coating agent in pharmaceutical or food applications. For nuts, zein coatings retard rancidity; and for candies, it restricts moisture access and provides glaze. The greatest potential for zein was perceived in its use in textile fibers.

Fermentation of the cereal grains to make alcohol produces a protein-rich material /spent grain stillage/ after alcohol is distilled.Most of the spent grain stillage is recovered in different forms as a dryed feed ingredient.

Table 10.
Essential amino acid content of some products of wet milling process of maize

Amino acid	Maize germ meal[a]	Maize gluten protein concent-rate[b]	Maize gluten feed[a]	Soya concen-trate[b]
Lysine	4.2	1.7	2.9	6.3
Methionine + cystine	4.5	5.4	4.3	2.8
Threonine	5.0	3.6	4.1	4.3
Leucine	8.0	15.4	8.6	7.9
Isoleucine	3.3	3.6	2.9	4.6
Phenylalanine + Tyrosine	7.1	11.1	6.2	8.9
Valine	5.5	4.7	4.8	4.8
Tryptophan	0.8	0.7	0.4	1.5

a from Reiners et al. /1973/
b from Sternberg et al. /1980/

NUTRITIVE VALUE, PROTEIN CONCENTRATES

As it was mentioned at the characterizing of oat proteins, their amino acid composition is more advantageous from the point of view of nutrition than that of other cereal grain proteins. This is in first line connected with the higher lysine and also basic amino acid content. In addition some results of the studies reported recently /Gould 1980/ suggest that oats possess some physiological properties which may have implications to man and appear to be unique to oats among the cereal grains.

It was reported /Eppendorfer 1977/ that oats with increased protein concentration that results from higher nitrogen fertility, has a higher digestibility in rat feeding experiments. The biological value of the total protein declines only slightly, so that increase in digestibility is nearly parallel with the increase of net protein utilization.

Due to the good nutritional quality of oat proteins, efforts were made to develop oat protein concentrates. The procedures used for the production of concentrates are diffe-rent. The air classification procedure may be used with high effectivity. Although in the case of flours of other cereals the protein rich fractions obtained by this procedure contain maximally 25 % protein, the air classification of oat flours resulted in an amount of 5 % concentrate with 85 % protein concentration. Wet processes are also known using alkaline solutions for the solubilization of the proteins.

The numerous examples of production of different cereal protein preparations demonstrate the great possibilities of production. Probably the newer results in breeding /protein quality improving/ the application of plastein reaction /resynthesis of proteins from amino acids and peptides by enzymes/ could be the basis of production of "tailor made" cereal proteins and new types of vegetable protein foods.

REFERENCES

Arai, S., Yamasita, M. and Fujimaki, M. /1975/. Plastein reaction and its applications. Cereal Foods World 20, 107.

Baudet, T., Mossé, J., Landry, J. and Moureaux, T. /1966/. Etudes sur les protein du mais I. Composition en acides aminées des fractions azotés du grain. Ann. Physiol. Veg. 8, 321-329.

Boisen, S. and Djurtoft, R. /1982/. Protease inhibitor from barley embryo inhibiting trypsin and trypsin-like microbial proteases. Purification and characterisation of two isoforms. J.Sc.Fd.Agric. 33, 431-440.

Brandt, A. /1976/. Endosperm protein formation during kernel development of wild type and high-lysine barley mutant. Cereal Chem. 53, 890-901.

Brandt, A. and Ingversen, J. /1977/. In vitro synthesis of barley endosperm proteins on wild type and mutant templates. Carlsberg Res.Commun. 41, 311.

Brandt, A. and Ingversen, J. /1978/. Isolation and translation of hordein messenger RNA-s from wild type and mutant endosperm in barley. Carlsberg Res.Commun. 43, 351.

Buoconore, V., Petrucci, T. and Silano, V. /1977/. Wheat protein inhibitors of α-amylase. Phytochem. 16, 811.

Bushuk, W. /1974/. Proteins of triticale. Chemical and physical characteristics. In: Triticale: first man-made cereal, C.C. Tsen /ed./ AACC, St. Paul, Minn., pp. 128.

Cameron-Mills, V., Brandt, A. and Ingversen, J. /1980/. The molecular biology of barley storage protein synthesis. In: Cereals for food and beverages - Recent progress in cereal chemistry, G.E. Inglett and L. Munck /eds./ Academic Press, New York, pp. 339-364.

El Kady, A. /1983/. Investigation of the maize proteins and their biological value. Ph.D. Thesis. Technical University Budapest.

Eppendorfer, W. H. /1977/. Nutritive value of oat and rye grain protein as influenced by nitrogen and amino acid composition. J.Sc.Fd.Agric. 28, 152-156.

FAO /1981/. Statistical production yearbook. FAO, Rome.

Feillet, P. and Nimmo, C.C. /1970/. Soluble protein of wheat III. Isolation and characterization of two albumins, Alb. 13A and Alb. 13B from flour. Cereal Chem. 47, 447-464.

Gould, R.M. /1980/. Biofunctional properties of oats. In: Cereals for food and beverages - Recent progress in cereal chemistry, G.E. Inglett and L. Munck /eds./ Academic Press, New York, pp. 447-460.

Hochstrasser, K. and Werle, E. /1969/. Purification of trypsin inhibitors from germ of wheat and rye seeds, localization of the active centers. Z. Physiol. Chem. 359, 249-254.

Hussein, H.A. (1978). Plant proteins and their role in the solving of hte ARE's protein crisis. Thesis D.Sc. Technical University of Budapest.

Jones, B. L. and Meredith, P. /1982/. Inactivation of alpha-amylase activity by purothionins. Cereal Chem. 59, 321.

Jones, R.W. and Beckwith, A.C. /1970/. Proximate composition and proteins of three grain sorghum hybrids and their dry mill fractions. J.Agr.Fd. Chem. 18, 33-36.

Kasarda, D.D., Bernardin, J.E. and Nimmo, C.C. /1976/. Wheat proteins: In: Advances in cereal science and technology, Vol. 1., Y. Pomeranz /ed./ AACC, St. Paul, Minn., pp. 158-236.

Kneen, E. and Sandstedt, R.M. /1943/. An amylase inhibitor from certain cereals. J.Amer.Chem.Soc. 65, 1247.

Lásztity, R. /1984/. The chemistry of cereal proteins. CRC Press, Boca Raton, Fl.

Lásztity, R., Berndorfer-Kraszner, E. and Huszár, M. /1980/. On the presence and distribution of some bioactive agents in oat varieties. In: Cereals for food and beverages- Recent progress in cereal chemistry, G.E. Inglett and L. Munck /eds./ Academic Press, New York, pp. 429-445.

Maki, Z., Tashiro, M., Sugihara, N. and Kanamosi, M. /1980/. Double-headed nature of trypsin inhibitor from rice bran. Agr. Biol. Chem. /Japan/ 44, 953-955.

Marshall, J.J. /1975/. α-Amylase inhibitors from plants. Am. Chem.Soc. Symp.Ser. 15, 244.

Martens, H. and Knudsen, K.E. /1980/. Fractioning barley proteins by computer factor analysis. Cereal Chem. 57, 97-106.

Melville, J.G. and Scandalios, J.G. /1972/. Maize endopeptidase: genetic control, chemical characterization and relationship to an endogeneous trypsin inhibitor. Biochem.Genet. 7, 15-31.

Mertz, E., and Bates, L.S. Nelson, O.E. /1964/. Mutant gene that changes composition and increase lysine content of maize endosperm. Science 145, 279-280.

Misra, P.S., Jambunathan, R., Mertz, E.T., Glover, P.V., Barbosa, H.M. and McWhirter, K.S. /1972/. Endosperm protein synthesis in maize mutants with increased lysine content. Science 176, 1425-1427.

Mossé, J. and Landry, J. /1980/. Recent research in major maize proteins, zeins and glutelins. In: Cereals for food and beverages - Recent progress in cereal chemistry, G.E. Inglett and L. Munck /eds./ Academic Press, New York, pp. 255-273.

Nesterin, M.F. and Skurichin, I.M. /1979/. Chimitcheskij sostav pishtchevych produktov. /Chemical composition of food products./Pişhtchevaya Prom., Publ., Moscow.

Petrucci, T., Tomasi, M., Cantagalli, P. and Silano, V. /1974./ Comparison of wheat albumin inhibitors of α-amylase and trypsin. Phytochem. 13, 2487-2495.

Reiners, R.A., Wall, J.S. and Inglett, G.E. /1973/. Corn proteins: potential for their industrial use. In: Industrial uses of cereals, Y. Pomeranz /ed./ AACC, St. Paul, Minn., pp. 285-301.

Restani, P., Riccardi, A. and Cerletti, P. /1980/. Functional properties of corn germ protein related to the interaction with water and with fats. Ann.Technol.Agric.Aliment. 29, 409-414.

Ronda Lain, E. and Soto Rodriguez, E. /1965/. Subproductos del arroz I-III. Rev.Nutr. /Madrid/ 3, 92.

Sarkki, M.L. /1980/. Wheat gluten. In: Cereals for food and beverages - Progress in cereal chemistry, G.E. Inglett and L.Munck /eds./ Academic Press, New York, pp. 155-169.

Simmonds, H. /1978/. Structure, composition and biochemistry of cereal grains. In: Cereals 78'- Better nutrition for worlds millions, Y. Pomeranz /ed./ AACC, Winnipeg, pp. 105-137.

Sternberg, M., Phillips, R.D. and Daley, L.H. /1980/. Maize protein concentrate. In: Cereals for food and beverages - Recent progress in cereal chamistry, G.E. Inglett and L. Munck /eds./ Academic Press, New York, pp. 275-285.

Tashiro, M. and Maki, Z. /1978/. Partial purification and some properties of a trypsin inhibitor from rice bran. Agr. Biol.Chem. /Japan/ 42, 1119.

Tkachuk, R. and Irvine, G.N. /1969/. Amino acid composition of cereal and oilseed meals. Cereal Chem. 46, 206-218.

Tsen, C.C. /ed./ /1974/. Triticale: first man-made cereal. AACC, St. Paul Minn.

Tsen, C.C. /1980/. Cereal germs used in bakery products: chemistry and nutrition. In: Cereals for food and beverages - Recent progress in cereal chemistry, G.E. Inglett and L. Munck /eds./ Academic Press, New York, pp. 245-253.

Proc. Int. Assoc. Cereal Chem. Symp. Amino Acid Compn and Biol. Value of Cereal Proteins
Budapest, Hungary 1983, R. Lásztity, M. Hidvégi, eds

CEREAL UTILIZATION IN WEST AFRICA

D.Y. DAKO

Department of Nutrition and Food Science, University of Ghana, Legon, Ghana

Abstract

Cereals provide over 50% of the calorie and a substantial portion of the daily protein intakes of West-Africans. Cereals generally follow the same initial processing steps before they are utilized and traditional recipes with few exceptions are similar in the whole region. Cereals in West-Africa are normally consumed with legumes and fish. Among the legumes cowpeas and groundnuts are the commonest and most popular. It is concluded that provided sufficient legumes are available, the traditional cereal-legume diets provide adequate protein of good quality for the people.

INTRODUCTION

There are a variety of staple foods consumed in West Africa. These include cereals and the starchy roots and fruits. While the consumption of starchy roots and fruits are limited to certain geographical areas, cereals are consumed in the whole region.

Cereals contribute in several countries in West Africa about 50% of the total energy intake of the people. In many communities their contribution to the energy intake may be higher than 50% and may exceed 70% of the total energy intake.

Cereals also contribute substantially to the protein intakes of the people in the region. Protein contribution from cereals may average about 50% of total protein. The main use of cereals in the region is for human consumption including beverages.

Among the cereals consumed in West Africa are Finger millet (Eleusine coracana), bullrush millet (Pennisetum typhoides), maize (Zea mays), sorghum (Sorghum spp.), wheat (Triticum vulgare), and rice (Oryza sativa). Millets and sorghum according to Annegers (1973) were established in West Africa before 500 BC. These grains are found mainly in the Sudanic, Subsudanic and Southern Sahelian zones of West Africa i.e. Niger, Mali, Upper Volta, Senegal, Gambia and the northern parts of Nigeria, Ghana, Togo and Benin. These cereals were important along the Ghana - Benin coastal plains during the 16th Century. Muller (1676) noted the presence of these grains in the dry coastal region. However the grains are not grown in these areas today as they have been replaced by other cereals. In Accra, Ghana, a small plot of millet is maintained by fetish priests and used only in connection with a traditional celebration marking the end of the hungry season. It has however been observed that during severe droughts which occur periodically in West Africa, millets are grown in the Ghana - Benin region.

Maize is grown mainly in the subguinean and sub-sudanic zone and along the Ghana-Benin coastal plains. Maize has become a dominant crop since its introduction in Ghana, Togo, Benin, Ivory Coast, Guinea as well as parts of southern Nigeria.

The cultivation of rice is gaining popularity in most countries in West Africa. The main rice growing areas are however the West Guinean zone of Sierra Leone, Liberia and Senegal, with considerable quantities also being grown in the Ivory Coast, Guinea and Nigeria.

Wheat is the most recent addition to cereals in West Africa, but its use is increasing and large sums of foreign exchange are spent yearly in importing this commodity which is hardly grown in Weat Africa. The object of this paper is to discuss the place of cereal grains in the diet of West Africans.

PRODUCTION

Production estimates are given in Table 1. These have been compiled from the FAO Production Year Book (FAO 1981).

In terms of area and total tonnage of production, sorghum and millet are by far the most important cereals in West Africa. Oke (1976) stated that sorghum is by far the largest cultivated crop in Nigeria. In 1981, 7,065,000 metric tonnes of millet and sorghum were produced in Nigeria. As shown in Table 1, in the Upper Volta, of the total area of 2,240,000 hectares under cereal cultivation in 1981, only 140,000 hectares was not under the cultivation of millet and sorghum. Total quantity of millet and sorghum produced in that year was 1,150,000 metric tonnes as compared to only 129,000 metric tonnes for maize and rice. In Ghana, about the same size of land, 440,000 hectares, was under sorghum/millet production as was under production of all other cereals in 1981.

The total land under sorghum cultivation in Senegal in 1981 was 850,000 hectares compared with 80,000 hectares for rice and 49,000 hectares for maize. A total of 750,000 metric tonnes of millet was produced as compared with 120,000 and 55,000 metric tonnes for rice and maize, respectively.

These are only a few examples selected to demonstrate the importance of millet and sorghum in West Africa. In view of the persistent droughts in West Africa in the past few years, it is believed that more attention would be given to these crops which can be introduced into non traditional areas.

As can be seen from Table 1, rice could be said to be the only cereal cultivated in Liberia and Sierra Leone, which produced 216,000 and

TABLE 1

Estimates of Cereal Production in West Africa 1981

Country	Sorghum		Millets		Maize		Rice	
	1	2	1	2	1	2	1	2
Benin	80	100	11	23	349	427	161	12
Gambia	-	-	38	35	12	13	33	40
Ghàna	142	210	73	230	420	350	79	83
Guinea	15	7	-	-	63	55	330	380
Ivory Coast	35	53	48	82	300	615	550	475
Liberia	-	-	-	-	-	-	216	180
Mali	-	-	930	1420	80	90	142	172
Niger	273	982	1117	303	9	12	38	23
Nigeria	3835	6025	3230	5050	1580	1746	1241	600
Senegal	-	-	750	850	55	49	120	80
Sierra Leone	11	7	9	9	14	13	400	400
Togo	-	-	107	170	137	120	20	21
Upper Volta	750	1200	400	900	100	100	29	40

1 = Production x 1000 MT

2 = Area under cultivation x 1000 HA

400,000 metric tonnes, respectively. No other estimates of cereals apart from rice was given for Liberia in the FAO estimates of 1981. Similarly, Sierra Leone, has only very small areas of land under cereal production apart from rice. A mere total of 29,000 hectares was reported for millets, sorghum and maize as compared with 400,000 hectares for rice. Other countries which produced relatively large quantities of rice in West Africa in 1981 were Senegal, Ivory Coast, Guinea and Nigeria. The main maize producing countries in West Africa are Benin, Guinea, Ghana, Ivory Coast, Nigeria, and Togo. As will be shown later, these countries are among the maize eating countries in West Africa.

CONSUMPTION AND CONTRIBUTION OF CEREALS TO THE ENERGY AND PROTEIN INTAKE OF WEST AFRICANS

In discussing cereal consumption in West Africa one might observe that countries and the people can be classified into three groups, according to whether their major staple is rice, millet/sorghum or maize. Apart from these groups, there are countries which have two or more cereal staples in their diets, although the two cereals may not be eaten by all people in these countries. Rice is eaten in moderate amounts in all West Africa. However, the main rice eating countries are Liberia and Sierra Leone, which consumed 277g and 297g per head per day respectively in 1977. These countries as indicated are the only countries which produced hardly any other cereals apart from rice. Gambia, Senegal, Ivory Coast, Guinea and Mali are rice eating countries which have other staples as well as rice, e.g: in the Ivory Coast and Guinea, maize is the other main staple, while in Senegal, Gambia and Mali, millet is the other main staple. The consumption pattern of cereals is shown in Table 2.

According to Table 2, the main maize eating countries are Benin, Ivory Coast, Togo, Guinea and Ghana.

In 1977, consumption of maize was highest in Benin, where the average intake per head per day was 145g and the country consuming least among the group was Ivory Coast, where the consumption per head per day was 67g. It should be noted that Ivory Coast and Guinea in this group consumed daily about 108g and 157g of rice respectively in 1977.

Millet/sorghum eating countries in West Africa are Niger, Upper Volta, Mali, Nigeria, Senegal, Gambia and Togo. The people of Niger seem to consume more millet/sorghum per head than any country in the region, a total of 369g per head per day. In Mali, 323g per head per day of millet was consumed in 1977.

Wheat consumption in general is on the increase in the whole region, with Senegal and Ivory Coast being the highest consumers of wheat. The Senagalese and Ivorians consumed 50g and 32.2g per head per day in 1977 respectively.

The contribution of cereals to the energy and protein intakes of West Africans is given in Table 3, and was compiled from FAO Food Balance sheets (FAO 1980).

As can be inferred from Table 3, the daily energy intake of Nigerians

TABLE 2

Consumption of Cereals in West Africa g/caput/day (FAO 1981)

Country	Sorghum	Millet	Rice	Maize	Wheat
Benin	40.3	6.4	17.5	145.0	13.6
Gambia	14.4	106.3	225.5	23.0	13.8
Ghana	23.1	18.1	14.6	75.1	24.1
Guinea	2.1	-	157.3	114.7	11.5
Ivory Coast	7.8	8.6	108.8	67.8	32.7
Liberia	-	-	277.0	-	15.4
Mali	-	323.5	63.7	32.7	11.6
Niger	96.7	273.2	10.0	7.3	5.0
Nigeria	108.1	81.5	18.6	38.5	17.9
Senegal	-	171.5	134.7	25.2	49.7
Sierra Leone	4.5	4.7	297.7	7.9	18.2
Togo	-	37.9	20.7	11.6	10.0
Upper Volta	225.4	136.5	16.3	30.0	6.2

TABLE 3

Contribution of Cereals to Daily Energy and Protein Intakes of West Africans (FAO 1981)

Country	Total Energy Cals	Total Protein (g)	Energy-Cals derived from	Protein (g) Cereals
Benin	2246	50.8	858	22.8
Gambia	2326	55.0	1474	33.4
Ghana	1986	45.1	549	14.6
Guinea	1943	42.6	1128	27.4
Ivory Coast	2495	53.9	863	20.8
Liberia	2421	44.3	1067	21.3
Mali	2117	55.7	1594	35.7
Niger	2138	63.3	1434	32.3
Nigeria	2257	51.5	964	26.4
Senegal	2272	65.5	1412	38.2
Sierra Leone	2088	44.8	1220	24.6
Togo	2066	47.6	808	21.6
Upper Volta	1990	63.6	1432	40.5

was 2257 calories and out of this total 964 calories was derived from cereals. The major cereal in the diet was millet/sorghum which provided 66% of the energy obtained from cereals. Table 3 also shows that cereals provided 26.4g protein daily which amounted to 50% of the daily protein consumed by Nigerians.

In Niger, the highest millet/sorghum consuming country, millet/sorghum provided in 1977 93% of the calories obtained from cereals.

Protein derived from cereals accounted for 51% of the total protein intake.

In these maize eating countries the starchy roots and fruits are important and provide significant amounts of energy and protein in the diet of the people.

In Ghana, e.g. starchy roots and fruits provided in 1977 36% of the daily energy and 18% of the daily protein intake.

PROCESSING

Vogel and Graham (1979) observed that with few exceptions, the basic recipes for traditional sorghum/millet foods of different countries were similar. This observation is generally true also for other cereals. In general the initial processing step in cereal utilization in West Africa can be one of the following; soaking, grinding, dehulling, roasting and germination. These are followed by various steps summarized below in Figs 1 and 2 (Sefa-Dedeh personal communication 1983).

The products prepared from the cereals have been given number designations as follows:

1	=	porridge
2	=	solid snack food
3	=	dumpling
4	=	solid mash
5	=	agglomerated cereal
6	=	beverage

A letter designation denotes that the same raw material has been used for the product e.g. 1B is koko or ogi porridge prepared from maize, and 3B is a product kenkey prepared also from maize. It should be noted that all these three products follow the same processing line although they have different rheological properties.

Muller (1970) suggested a rheological classification for traditional Ghanian and Nigerian cereal foods. This classification has been extended to include foods from some other West African countries (Table 4).

Although the list of foods in Mullers adapted table does not cover the whole region, it tends to confirm that traditional recipes are similar, e.g. Tô in the Upper Volta is the same food as Tuwo and Tuo in Nigeria and Ghana respectively. Also Nigerian foods, ogi, kamu and akamu are similar to koko in Ghana.

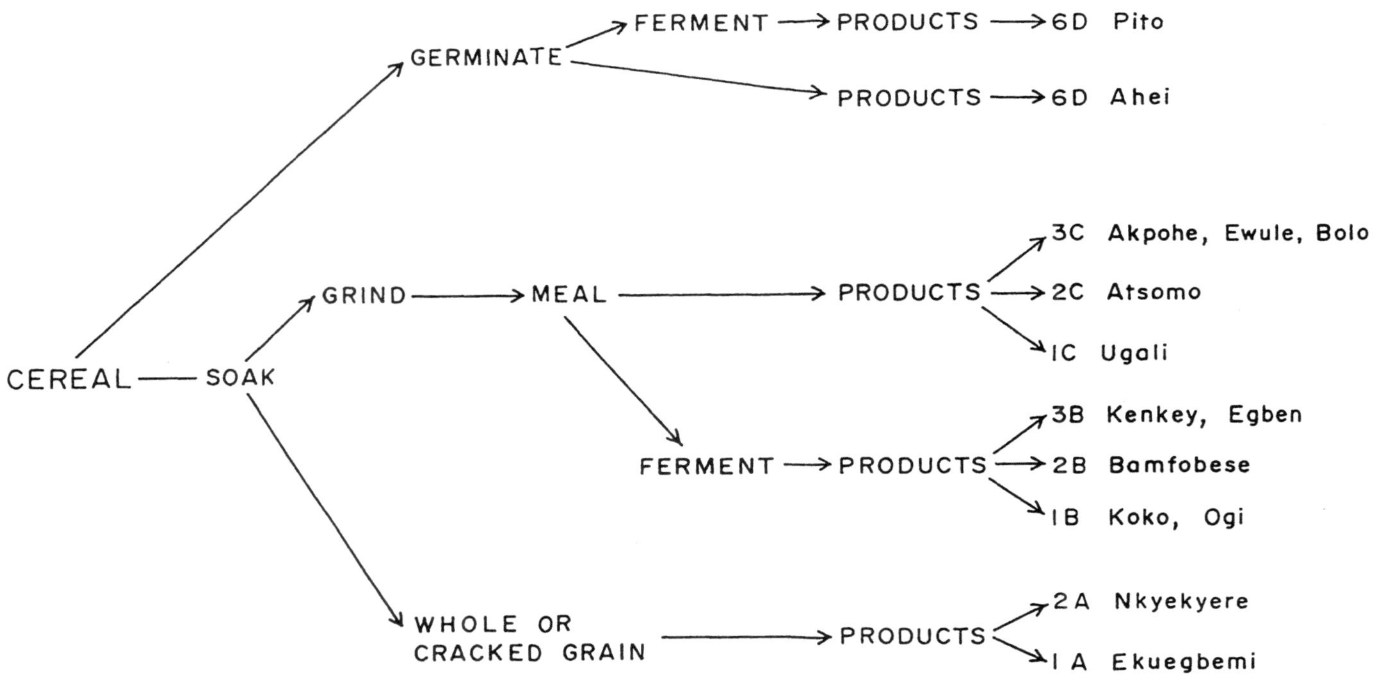

Fig. 1 Cereal Processing Steps in West Africa

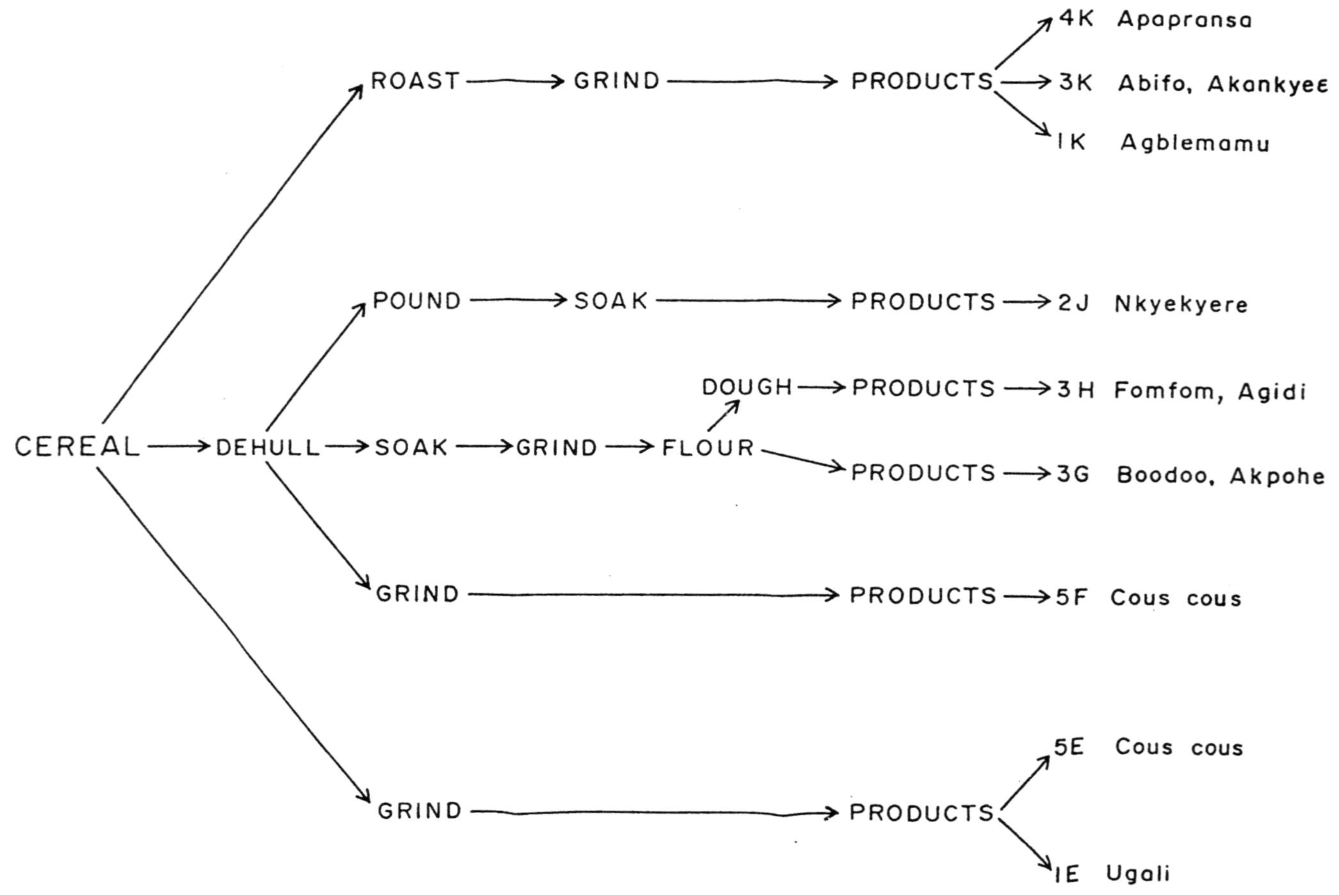

Fig. 2. Cereal Processing Steps in West Africa

Traditional processes summarized in Figs 1 and 2 are generally time consuming and tedious operations. Further, the actual time spent in the preparation of foods can be very considerable. The laborious nature of these processes might partially explain the drift away from traditional cereals in favour of processed imported cereals. In a recent study Dako (1981 unpublished) found that villagers preferred wheat grains to maize. This preference may be due to convenience and cost. Imported wheat grains provided as food aid is normally cheaper than maize and also needs no processing before cooking.

PROTEIN VALUES OF CEREAL DIETS IN WEST AFRICA

Cereal proteins, generally, are deficient in lysine. Tryptophan and threonine are other amino acids which may be deficient in some cereals. The protein quality of cereals is largely dependent on these essential amino acids. Fortunately cereals are seldom eaten alone, they are normally eaten with other foods.

In the areas where millet and sorghum are the main staples they are usually eaten with a legume. According to the IDRC-MR 13 (1980) the first choice of a cereal in certain rural areas in Senegal is millet, and first choice for a legume to combine with the cereal in these areas is groundnut followed by cowpeas. In Nigeria, Oke (1976) reported that about 18g cowpeas and 11g of groundnuts are eaten daily alongside various staples.

In Niger 69.6g cowpeas and 8.7g of groundnuts are eaten daily with millet. Similarly in Mali 14.6g of pulses (unspecified) and 13.1g groundnuts are eaten daily (FAO 1980). According to Da et al. (1981) "Tô" prepared from sorghum in the Upper Volta is eaten with a sauce made from tomatoes, okra or gumbo, chillies, cowpeas and leaves. Tô has different spellings in West Africa, but essentially it is the same food preparation; e.g. Tuo prepared in Ghana from millet, sorghum maize or rice as well as Tuwo prepared from the same cereals in Nigeria Tô (Tuo, tuwo) is normally eaten with a legume sauce.

Fish is another protein supplement in the diet of West Africans. Rice and fish is the national dish in Senegal (IDRC-MR 13 1980). In Ghana and Togo, when fish is available, considerable quantities are eaten. Kenkey (Ghana), kon (Togo), prepared from fermented maize is eaten with fish. This is a common food among the coastal inhabitants. Couscous which is prepared from millet in Senegal but sometimes prepared from sorghum and maize is served with meat (IDRC-MR 13 1980). However the use of meat is not widespread and in many areas couscous is eaten with a vegetable sauce, which may include a legume.

In West Africa therefore apart from cereals, a considerable amount of daily protein requirement is obtained from legumes, mainly cowpeas and groundnuts. Fish is the most important animal protein in most countries in West Africa especially in the coastal areas. The essential amino acids content of cereals consumed in West Africa is given in

TABLE 4

Classification of Cereal Foods in West Africa according to Muller (1970)

Food	Cereal	Country	Properties
Hura	Millet	Nigeria	Moisture content 65-80%
Eko (boiled and gelatinized ogi)	Maize	Nigeria	
Agidi (boiled koko dough)	Maize	Ghana	
Banku (boiled koko dough)	Maize	Ghana	
Akple (boiled maize dough)	Maize	Ghana/Togo	
Fula	Millet	Ghana/Nigeria	
Mutu	Sorghum/ Millet	Togo	
Kenkey (fermented maize dough)	Maize	Ghana	
Kon (fermented maize dough)	Maize	Togo	
Nsihu	Maize	Ghana	
Abolo (baked sweetened maize dough)	Maize	Togo/Ghana	
Abolo (steamed sweetened maize dough)	Maize	Togo/Ghana	
Baked or fried products			Moisture content below 50%
Bread	Wheat	all W.Africa	
Atshomo (fried sweet wheat flow pastry)	Wheat	Ghana	
Togbei (fried sweet wheat flour pastry)	Wheat	Ghana	
Bamfobese (fried sweet corn dough)	Maize	Ghana	
Beverages			
Pito (Hausa beer drunk warm)	Sorghum/ Millet	Nigeria, Ghana, Upper Volta	Low viscosity liquids

Table 4 continued

Food	Cereal	Country	Properties
Brukutu (beer-lquid decanted)	Sorghum/ Millet	Ghana	Water content exceeding 94%
Kunnu Tsakie (beer sedimented stirred before drinking	Sorghum/ Millet	Ghana	
Aliha (coloured with caramel sweetened, unfermented non alcoholic)	Maize	Ghana/Togo	
Iced Kenkey	Maize	Ghana	
<u>Porridges</u>			
Ogi, Kamu, Akamu	Maize, Sorghum Millet	Nigeria	Moisture content about 90%
Koko	Maize, Sorghum Millet	Nigeria, Ghana	
Ablemamu, Akasa (similar to Koko but prepared from roasted maize flour)	Maize	Togo/Ghana	

Table 5 which also gives the essential amino acid content of cowpeas, groundnuts and fish. The Table confirms that sorghum, millet, rice and wheat are deficient in lysine while maize is equally limiting in lysine and tryptophan. From the Table it can also be seen, that while the legumes are deficient in the sulphur containing amino acids, fish protein is limiting in tryptophan. The cereals have however relatively high amounts of sulphur containing amino acids limiting in the legumes, while the legumes have relatively high amounts of lysine limiting in the cereals. Thus legume proteins complement cereals proteins when eaten together. The protein value of a cereal-legume combination is better than the protein value of the individual components alone. It is possible that the age old practice of consumption of cereal legume diets has been the result of observations and experience gained centuries ago.

TABLE 5

Amino Acid Composition of Cereals and some Protein Foods consumed in West Africa (FAO 1970)

Amino Acid	Maize	Millet	Rice	Sorghum	Wheat	Cowpea	Ground-nut	Fresh Fish all types	Hens Eggs whole
			mg/gN						
Isoleucine	230	256	238	245	204	236	211	299	393
Leucine	783	598	514	832	417	440	400	480	551
Lysine	167	214	237	126	179	427	221	569	436
Methionine/cystine	120/97	154/148	145/67	87/94	94/159	73/68	72/78	179/73	210/152
Phenylalanine	305	301	322	306	282	323	311	245	358
Tyrosine	239	203	218	167	187	163	244	229	260
Threonine	225	241	244	189	183	225	163	286	320
Tryptophan	44	122	78	76	68	68	65	-	-
Valine	303	345	344	313	276	283	261	382	428

Several publications have appeared in the literature about the supplementary value of different proteins. In this paper, the supplementary value of cereal/legume diets in West Africa is discussed by making references to a few of the relevant publications.

Oke (1975) suggested a method for assessing optimum supplementations of cereal based diets with grain legumes by plotting the amino acid score of the limiting amino acid of a mixed cereal legume diet against the ratio of the mixture. The intercept indicates the ratio of the mixture that will provide optimal protein value. Oke's results show that the optimum combination ratio for maize/cowpea diet is 75:25, for millet/cowpea 75:25, for sorghum/cowpea 70:30, and for rice/cowpea 95:5. These findings agree with Bressani and Scrimshaw (1961), who demonstrated the value of combining maize and cowpea proteins. They established that a combination of proteins in the ratio of 50:50 cowpea to maize gave the highest Protein Efficiency Ratio (PER). The PER obtained was 1.84 for this ratio. Other combinations gave less PER values than the 50:50 ratio.

Similar results were obtained by Dako (1966) when he fed rats a 50:50 protein ratio of maize and blackeyed peas, or cowpeas from Nigeria. A summary of his results are given in Table 6.

TABLE 6

Effect of Legume supplementation on the PER of Maize

Ratio of protein	Maize	Blackeyed pea	Cowpea	Casein
100:0	1.74	1.77	1.41	3.55
Maize legume 50:50	-	2.41	2.39	-

It can be seen from Table 6 that the addition of blackeyed pea or cowpea to maize increased the PER value significantly from 1.74 to 2.41 and 2.39 for blackeyed peas and cowpeas respectively. In Nigeria "ewa" and in Ghana "aprapansa" and "asebutu" are prepared from cowpea/blackeyed pea-maize combinations. Dako (1966) suggests that the protein value of these foods could be improved by adopting the desired combinations as provided by laboratory results.

Jansen (1974) calculated the amino acid scores for lysine, threonine, tryptophan and methiomine and cystine against whole egg protein for sorghum, ragi millet, maize and rice, supplemented with protein concentrates including fish meal and groundnut flour. Table 7 presents the amino acid scores at levels of 0 to 32 parts of supplement per 100 parts of cereal. Jansen considers these amino acids as of practical

TABLE 7

Amino Acid Scores of 4 Amino Acids in Cereals Supplemented with Groundnut Flour and Fish Meal (Jansen 1974)

Cereal Amino Acid	Amino acid score (a) Parts supplement/100 parts cereal by weight				
Ragi millet + fishmeal	0	4	8	16	32
Lysine	38	63	78	95	111
Threonine	78	84	88	93	97
Methionine + cystine	94	92	91	90	89
Tryptophan	164	144	133	119	105
Ragi millet + groundnut flour					
Lysine	38	46	51	57	64
Threonine	78	78	79	79	79
Methionine + cystine	94	89	86	81	77
Tryptophan	164	155	149	141	132
Maize + fishmeal					
Lysine	49	71	84	100	115
Threonine	90	93	95	98	100
Methionine + cystine	76	79	80	82	84
Tryptophan	60	66	69	72	76
Maize + groundnut flour					
Lysine	49	54	58	63	68
Threonine	90	88	87	85	84
Methionine + cystine	76	74	73	71	70
Tryptophan	60	69	75	83	91
Sorghum + groundnut flour					
Lysine	38	45	50	56	64
Threonine	78	78	78	79	79
Methionine + cystine	66	71	74	77	81
Tryptophan	107	108	108	109	109
Sorghum + fishmeal					
Lysine	38	62	77	95	111
Threonine	78	84	88	93	97
Methionine + cystine	66	71	74	77	81
Tryptophan	107	101	98	93	89
Rice + Fishmeal					
Lysine	69	92	103	115	125
Threonine	87	92	95	98	101
Methionine + cystine	85	85	86	86	86
Tryptophan	121	109	103	96	90
Rice + Groundnut flour					
Lysine	69	72	73	75	77
Threonine	87	85	84	83	82
Methionine + cystine	85	81	78	75	71
Tryptophan	121	119	118	116	114

$$\text{Chemical Score} = \frac{\text{mg amino acid/g essential amino acid/nitrogen x 100}}{\text{mg amino acid in whole egg/g essential amino acid/nitrogen in whole egg}}$$

importance when cereal based diets are being improved by supplementation. The data of the amino acid composition and nitrogen content of the cereals and protein foods were obtained from FAO (1970). Jansen's calculations show that fish is a very effective supplement to ragi millet, the amino acid score of the mixture is raised progressively from 38 to 111 by the increasing proportions of fish. In contrast, the addition of groundnut to ragi millet is at all levels unable to raise the amino acid score of lysine satisfactorily. Fish is also better than groundnut as a supplement to maize because the low lysine content of groundnut does not improve the lysine content of the groundnut maize mixture (Table 7). Sorghum can also effectively be supplemented by fishmeal. Fishmeal raises the lysine content, but has little effect on the sulphur containing amino acids. Groundnut is not a very good supplement to sorghum according to Jansen's calculations since the amino acid scores of both lysine and the sulphur amino acids do not change to any satisfactory level.

Rice as can be seen from Table 7 is well supplemented by fish, as fish raises the threonine and lysine content of the mixture. Groundnut is an ineffective supplement to rice because of low levels of lysine and threonine.

Jansen's work therefore shows that groundnut is not a very effective supplement to cereals although Oke (1976) claimed its suitability.

An improved groundnut supplement can be found in many places in West Africa in the form of a groundnut sauce/soup containing fish or meat, e.g. rice and groundnut sauce of soup plus fish found in Ghana and Togo.

Based on the above discussion, it would seem that the protein value of cereal based diets in West Africa are reasonably good, providing that the traditional way of consuming cereals with legumes and in most areas, also with fish is maintained. This obviously depends on increased production and use of legumes, which in the past has not always matched efforts put into cereals by many West African States.

FUTURE OF CEREAL BASED DIETS

In the past, especially during the 1960's, many attempts were made in preparing and manufacturing weaning foods based on cereal-legume combinations. These foods, which were nutritionally good did not market well due to many reasons including the expense, the technology used, as well as the acceptability of the products to those for whom they were meant.

In our department at the University of Ghana, Legon, a product is being tested, which is based on maize and cowpea. The development of the product has been based on a well-known traditional process of preparing 'gari' (a fermented cassava product). The Legon maize-cowpea product has the same functional characteristics as 'gari' which is a widely used convenience food in Nigeria, Togo, Benin and Ghana. This new product, in addition to being highly nutritious, is a food which is familiar to the people in the region. It is convenient and the technology required for its preparation is available and known at the village level. It can also be produced on a large scale for urban populations. This product and similar ones, it is hoped, will go a long way in providing much needed convenience foods of good quality which will be available to the whole family.

REFERENCES

Annegers, J.F. 1973 Ecology of dietary patterns and nutritional status in West Africa Ecology of Food and Nutr. 2, 107-119.

Bressani, R. and Scrimshaw, N.S. 1961 The development of InCAP vegetable mixtures
1. Basic animal studies.
In: Meeting protein needs of infants and pre-school children. Proceedings of an International Conference. Wahsington DC. National Research council Publication 843, 35.

Da S., Akigbala J.O., Rooner, L.W., Scherring, J.F. and Miller, F.R. 1981 Evaluation of Tô quality in a sorghum breeding program. International Symposium on sorghum grain quality ICRISAT Patanchery, India 11-23.

Dako, D.Y. 1966 Der Proteinwert afrikanischer Leguminosen in Abhangigkeit von der Vorbehandlung und Kombination mit anderen Nahrungs-mittein. Thesis Landwirtsch. Fak. Justus Liebig Univ. Giessen, W. Germany.

Dako, D.Y. 1981 (Unpublished) Poverty and Nutritional status in Ghana, ISSER, Lehon, Ghana.

FAO Rome, Italy. 1970 Amino acid composition of foods.

FAO Rome, Italy, 1980 Food Balance Sheets.

FAO Rome, Italy, 1981 Production Year Book No. 15.

IDRC-MR 13, 1980 Post-Harvest Technology in Senegal-Current Practises and Future Needs, Ed. Yaciuk G. and Yaciuk A.N., International Development Research Centre, Box 8500, Ottawa, Canada K19 3119.

Jansen, G.R. 1974 The amino acid fortification of cereals.
In: New Protein Foods
Edited by Althschul, A.M., Vol. 1A.
Technology 39-120.

Muller, H.G. 1970 Traditional cereal processing in Nigeria and Ghana, Ghana Jnl. Agric. Sci. 3., 187-195.

Muller, J.W. 1676 — Die Africanische Landschaft, FETU. Reprinted - akademische Druck - und Verlags - gesellschaft Graz - Austria 1968.

Oke, O.L. ,1975 — A method for assessing optimum supplementation of a cereal based diet with grain legumes. Nutr. Rep. Inter. 11, 313-321.

Oke, O.L. 1976 — The potential of millet and sorghum as food in Nigeria.
In: proceedings of a Symposium on Sorghum and Millets for Human Food. Ed. Dendy D.A. v 121-124.

Sefa-Dedeh. 1983 — Personal Communication - Cereal Processing in West-Africa. University of Ghana, Legon.

Vogel, S. and Graham M. 1979 — Sorghum and Millet: Food Production and Use. Report of Workshop held in Nairobi, Kenya 4 - 7 July, 1978. IDRC-123e. International Development Research Centre, Box 8500, Ottawa, Canada KIG 3119.

Proc. Int. Assoc. Cereal Chem. Symp. Amino Acid Compn and Biol. Value of Cereal Proteins Budapest, Hungary 1983, R. Lásztity, M. Hidvégi, eds

THE ROLE OF CEREAL AND PLANT PROTEINS IN THE WORLD FOOD SUPPLY

GYÖRGY KÁRPÁTI, BRWA M. SAEED*

Faculty of Agriculture, University of Agricultural Sciences, H-9200 Mosonmagyaróvár, Lucsony 15-17, Hungary
*Central Food Research Institute H-1022 Budapest, Herman Ottó 15, Hungary

ABSTRACT

FAO reports /1982/ showed clearly a very wide range of variations in food supply among countries of different parts of the world. The range of difference is between 40.6 to 119 g protein per day, from which vegetable proteins represent 87 to 20 % of the total supply respectively. This proves that the proteins of plant origin hold a prominent role.

The production conditions, transformation energy and protein loss highly limit the productivity of animals and their efficiency as a protein source. Moreover, animal productivity is dependent on the plant production which is originally climate dependent.

Therefore, it is the duty of food scientists to find ways for producing acceptable plant products with the highest nutritional value by complementation and supplementation to meet the ever increasing need for accessible protein of good quality.

INTRODUCTION

One of the complex problems of over-population is the shortage of food supplies, especially proteins. The rapid increase of human population has caused many serious problems. More than two-thirds of the world's population do not receive adequate nourishment.

In many parts of the world, particularly in developing countries, imbalances in animal protein food are more and more prevalent. Today these foods are filling a greater proportion of the world's food requirement. One solution to the problem of protein malnutrition is the replacement of expensive animal proteins in high-carbohydrate foods such as pasta and bread, without creating imbalances in the essential amino acids. This includes for example the replacement of egg and milk proteins by legumes.

Table 1 shows that the protein consumption in the USA is 106.7 g/day, 70 % of which is of animal origin. While in Bangladesh 40.6 g/day is consumed, only 13 % of it is of animal origin.

Table 1. The food supply in some countries in 1978-1980

Country	Food energy MJ/man/day			Protein g/man/day		
	Total	Vegetable origin	Animal origin	Total	Vegetable origin	Animal origin
Hungary	14,485.3	9,327.5	5,157.8	104.3	56.0	38.3
German Dem. Republic	14,501.7	8,860.1	5,641.6	90.4	33.2	67.2
Ireland	15,440.6	9,991.7	5,453.0	109.0	45.1	63.8
U.S.A.	14,973.2	9,520.2	5,457.1	106.7	34.7	72.0
Brazil	10,319.7	8,663.3	1,656.4	59.3	36.8	22.6
Irak	10,836.3	9,991.7	844.6	66.8	52.7	14.1
India	8,191.8	7,826.9	364.9	48.5	43.9	4.6
Bangladesh	7,695.7	7,421.0	274.7	40.6	35.3	5.3

The minimum safe limit of protein consumption for maintainance of health is 29-46 g/day. According to data from different countries, the average chemical score of the wholeday protein consumed could be summarized as below:

developed countries 80 %
developing countries 70 %
underdeveloped countries 60 %.

The climatic conditions, geographical situation, agricultural and technical development, in addition to the social and religeous habits of a given country determine the quantity and quality of its food production /Tables 2, 3/.

The production of meat and wheat /kg/head/ differs widely from one part of the world to another /Table 3.a/.

The production cost of meat is the highest one. The productivity of an animal is limited by many factors: The transformation energy and protein loss are high. There is high risk of depending on agricultural production as a feed stuff which is affected by climate and diseases, in addition to the difficulties of storage and transportation. Besides that the animal proteins are not uniformly of high nutritive value.

Table 2. World production of protein bearing plants

Plant	Total production /1000 tons/						
	World	Africa	U.S.A.	South America	Asia	Europe	Oceania
grains/total	1 663,828	76,329	414,473	74,725	661,439	245,356	24,201
wheat	458,195	8,584	103,781	11,743	137,371	91,942	16,773
rice	413,785	8,562	10,736	13,258	376,232	1,808	789
barley	158,488	3,197	24,358	806	17,216	66,215	3,636
maize	451,704	32,860	231,937	38,406	86,570	63,627	304
rye	24,473	10	1,437	231	1,561	12,717	17
millet	29,653	10,282	-	238	17,588	32	13
soybeans	87,941	319	56,605	19,575	10,320	552	70
dry beans	14,053	1,353	3,328	2,984	5,672	643	2
dry peas	8,215	327	251	111	2,764	628	136
potatoes	256,978	5,127	18,938	10,531	37,929	111,270	1,182

Table 3. The world's meat production in 1981

	Production /1000 tons/						
	World	Africa	U.S.A.	South America	Asia	Europe	Oceania
Total	142,303	6,740	30,328	11,942	35,373	38,674	3,879
Beef	45,548	2,870	12,546	7,124	3,952	10,373	1,993
Buffalo	1,304	121			1,167	16	
Mutton	5,984	731	181	262	1,679	1,121	1,193
Goat	2,049	561	30	65	1,258	92	2
Pork	55,195	374	8,754	1,762	20,102	18,650	303
Hourse	569	60	157	87	115	150	1
Poultry	28,696	1,241	8,400	2,526	6,514	7,372	343

Table 3.a. World production of meat and wheat

Continent	Production /kg/head/	
	meat	wheat
Oceania	168	100
U.S.A.	79	1,050
Europe	79	500
Asia	13	275
Africa	14	158
Average	25-26	350-360

DISCUSSION

Protein content and its quality

The importance of mixed nutrition is a well-known fact. The results of the research works of the last decades in this field have proved this fact /Kofrányi, 1973/. These results show that a 100 % utilization could be obtained - on N-balance basis - even if one or two of the proteins are of lower quality. Kofrányi /1973/ showed that a 1:1 mixture of maize and peas could result in a biological value of 98 %, while separately their biological values are 76 and 72 % respectively. He showed also that not only an egg and potato mixture could give a biological value above 100 %, but this could be reached by a mixture of rice, maize and wheat mixture as well, if it is supplemented by egg or milk proteins.

Experimental interpretation

Bread and other food products made from wheat flour, represent the most important food source almost all over the world. From the nutritive point of view, generally the grain proteins are of low value. Therefore a great need exists for improving the biological value of such proteins, especially in the developing countries.

Similarly, rice which represents another main food source in Asia and the Middle East, should be taken into consideration Rice protein has a fairly good balance of essential amino acids, although the proportions are not ideally balanced and the total protein content is low /Satterlee et al., 1979/. Polished rice, for example, contains about 6 % protein. New varieties of rice containing as much as 11 % have been developed. But these are not grown, because of the inverse relationship between yield and protein content /Clifford, 1979/.

The amino acid analysis of nine milled rices showed that the limiting essential amino acids of rice protein are lysine and threonine /Bressani et al., 1971, Bressani, 1981/. Hegsted and Juliano /1974/ found that the lysine content ranged from

3.19 to 4.07 g/16 g N with corresponding chemical scores of 58-74 %. The reinforcing of rice with 0.1 % lysine and 0.2 % threonine increased its biological value, its NPU with a chemical score of 100 % /Hegsted and Juliano, 1979/.

In this work, the complementation of wheat and rice flours were studied. As it is known, supplementation with the limiting amino acids improves the protein quality but does not increase the quantity, while by complementation both protein content and nutritive value are increased. The rate of complementation depends on the quantity and quality of the proteins. Ionescu and Dutescu /1978/ produced pasta of high protein content /25 %/ by complementation, while Niesen et al. /1980/ used peas flour and peas protein concentrates.

Tables 4, 5 and 6 show the composition of the raw materials used in this study. Different rates of combinations were used /Table 7/. The amino acid composition increased significantly by the supplementation by peas or soy-bean flour.

The changes in the biological value by different rates of complementation are shown in Figs 1, 2 and 3. The determination of in vitro digestibility of the mixtures showed values of 91-95 %. These results prove that a mixture with 14-20 % protein content could be prepared with reasonably high biological value, whithout using a protein of animal origin.

With the aid of a programmable computer, the prices of different mixtures, containing raw materials locally available in Hungary, were calculated. The following points were taken into consideration:

maximum PV	141 %
energy value	10 MJ
protein content	12-18 %
fat content	25-45 %
carbohydrates	40-60 %.

Taking the above factors into consideration, a daily diet modell containing proteins of animal origin with 12 % protein, 28 % fat, 60 % carbohydrates with a production cost of 27.2 Ft for an adult's daily requirement, while a diet model with similar nutritive and energy value based on proteins from vegetable origin costs only 14,5 Ft.

It is interesting to mention that without the knowledge of chemical indexes Evens /1908/ suggested the daily food requirement from the following:

1 l	milk
500 g	bread
125 g	cheese
125 g	legumes
500 g	potatoes
50 g	fat.

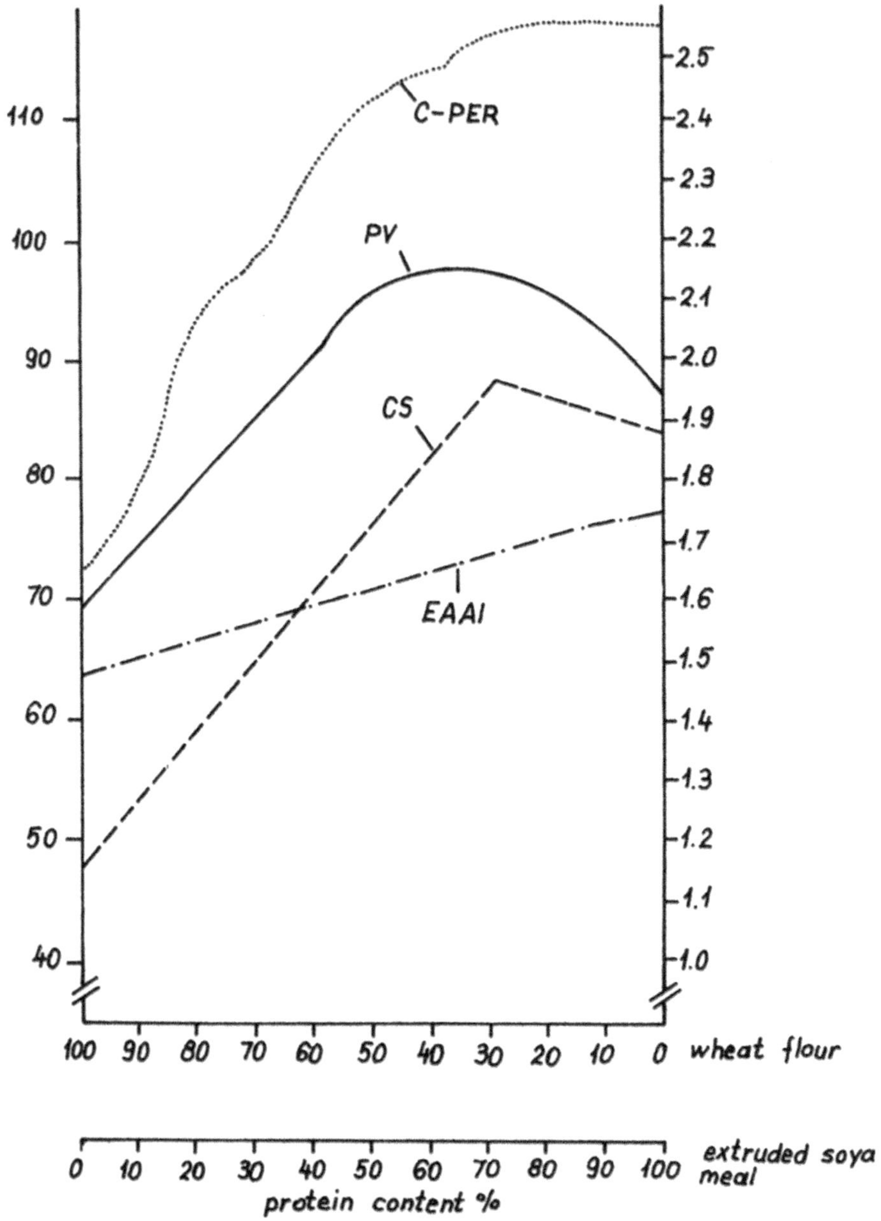

Fig. 1. Diagram showing the changes in the chemical indexes of the mixtures by changing the mixing ratios

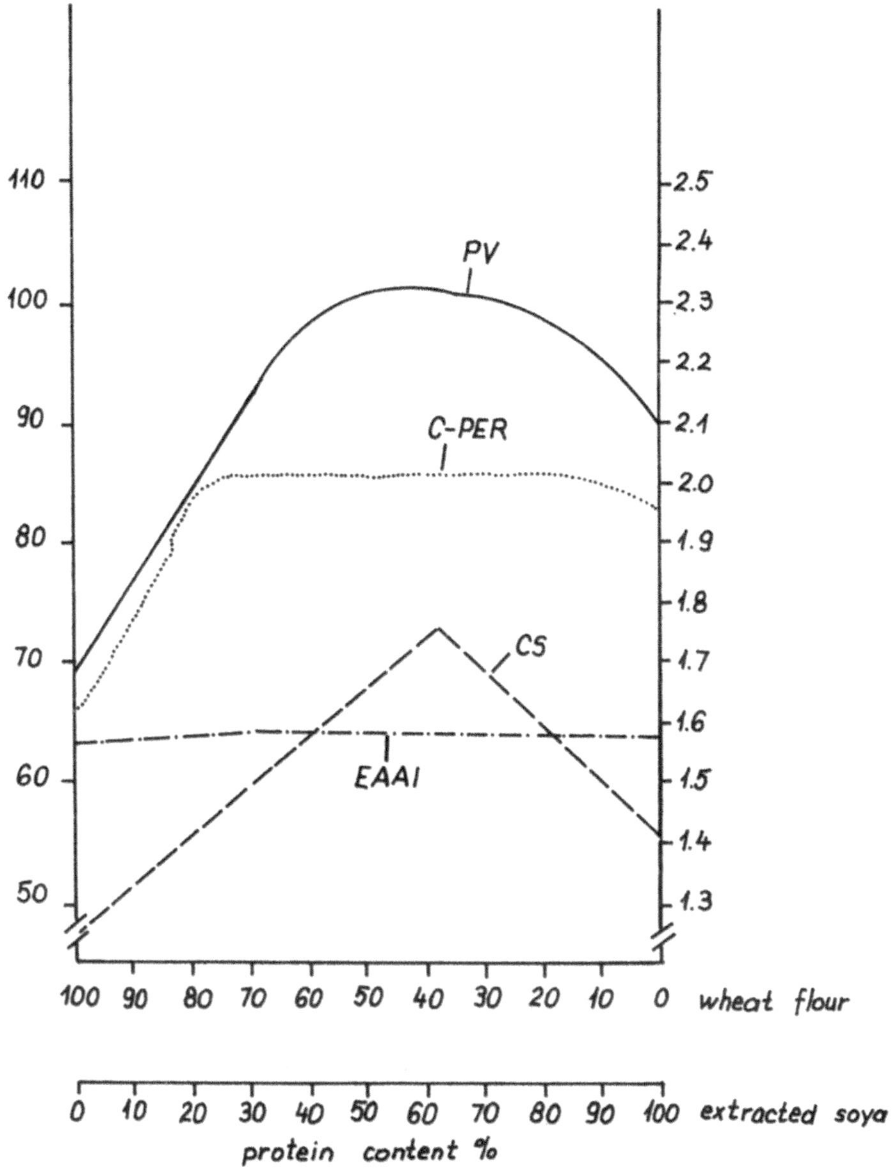

Fig. 2. The changes in the chemical indexes by changing the mixing ratios of wheat flour and extracted soya

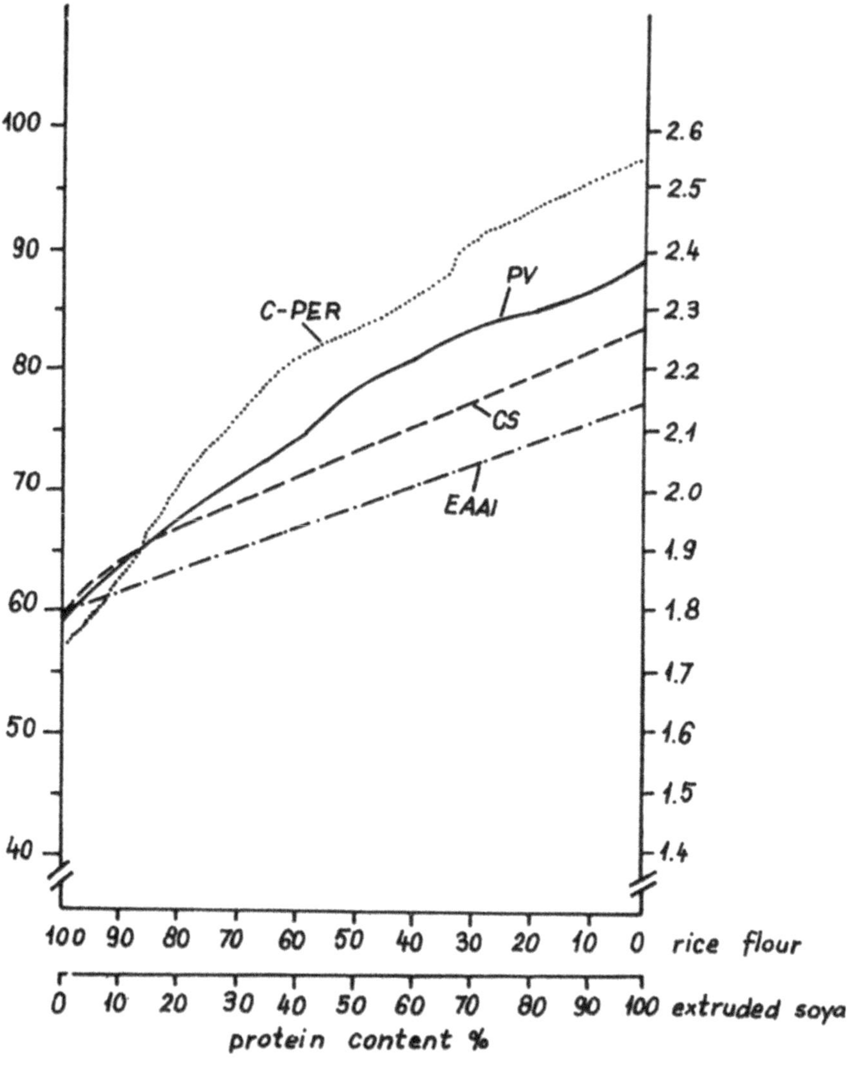

Fig. 3. The changes in the chemical indexes by changing the mixing ratio of rice flour and extruded soya flour meal

Table 4. Chemical composition of the raw materials /g/100 g matter/

	moisture	protein	fat	carbohydrate /calculated/	ash	energy /KJ/100 g material/
whole-fat extruded soya meal	5.20±0.04	41.60±0.06	21.49±0.98	26.90	4.81±0.01	1,963.12
extracted soya meal	8.68±0.06	47.26±0.06	0.58±0.01	37.30	6.18±0.02	1,442.52
yellow peas flour	8.03±0.12	27.16±0.06	1.32±0.04	60.49	3.00±0.02	1,522.40
rice flour	12.56±0.07	6.90±0.06	0.59±0.02	79.39	0.56±0.01	1,471.97
wheat flour BL 55	9.36±0.13	12.30±0.04	1.26±0.12	76.56	0.52±0.02	1,540.48

Table 5. The essential amino acid composition of the raw materials /g/16 g^{-1} N/

	Lys	Thr	Met Cys	Val	Ile	Leu	Arom	Trp
extruded soya	5.87	4.33	2.96	5.55	4.33	6.47	8.03	1.23
extracted soya	4.93	3.34	1.99	4.08	3.94	6.45	6.69	1.06
yellow peas	4.68	2.98	1.36	3.50	2.43	5.23	2.27	1.84
rice flour	3.33	3.48	2.17	5.07	2.61	6.38	5.22	1.30
wheat flour	2.60	3.57	3.50	3.98	3.98	7.40	6.26	0.98

According to their chemical composition, they supply:

145 g	protein
93 g	fat
465 g	carbohydrates.

However, all data mentioned above show that the protein of vegetable origin represents a very important source of protein for the ever growing population all over the world.

This work was aimed to show the importance of using wheat and other plant proteins in the preparation and technology of food products.

Table 6. The chemical indexes of raw materials

	chemical score	EAA index	calculated PER	predicted value
extruded soya	84.57 sulph.	77.27	2.5577	88.96
extracted soya	86.86 sulph.	63.52	1.9674	90.62
yellow peas	38.85 sulph.	49.72	0.8650	26.01
rice flour	60.54 lys.	59.57	1.7384	60.61
wheat flour	47.27 lys.	63.28	1.6276	69.85

Table 7. The ratio of mixing of the raw materials with the moisture and protein content of the different mixtures

materials	mixing ratio	protein content %	moisture content %
wheat flour-extruded soya meal	92:8	15	9.68
wheat flour-extruded soya meal	67:33	22	7.97
wheat flour-yellow peas flour	88:12	14	8.80
wheat flour-yellow peas flour	48:52	20	8.30
extruded soya-rice flour	23:77	15	10.64
extruded soya-rice flour	52:48	25	9.02
wheat flour	100	12.3	9.30

REFERENCES

Bressani, R. /1981/. The role of soybeans in food systems. JAOCS, 53 /3/, 392-400.

Bressani, R., Elias, L.G. and Juliano, B.O. /1971/. Evaluation of protein quality. J. Agr. Food Chem. 19, 1028-1036.

Clifford, M.H. /1979/. Conditions and trends in the world protein economy. JAOCS, 56, 173-177.

FAO/WHO /1973/. AdHoc Expert Committee, Energy Group. Protein requirements. WHO technical report series No. 522. Roma. Italy.

FAO/WHO /1975/. Informal Gathering of Experts. Food and Nutrition. 1, 11-12.

FAO /1982/. Production yearbook 1981. Vol. 35. Roma.

FAO /1982/. Trade yearbook 1981. Vol. 35. Roma.

Hegsted, D.M. and Juliano, B.O. /1974/. Difficulties in assessing the nutritional quality of rice protein. J. Nutr., 104 /6/, 772-781.

Hegsted, D.M. and Juliano, B.O./1979/. Determination of the relative nutritive value of proteins. J. Agric. Food Chem., 16, 190-195.

Ionescu, N. and Dutescu, F. /1978/. New methods for manufacture of high protein pasta. Industric Si. Chimic Alimentura 13, 115-122.

Kofrányi, E. /1973/. Evalution of traditional hypothesis on the biological value of protein. Nutrition Reports Internation, 7 /1/, 45-50.

Nielsen, A., Sumner, A.K. and Whalley, L.L. /1980/. Fortification of pasta with pea flour and airclassified pea protein concentrate. Cereal Chem., 57 /3/, 203-206.

Evens, C. /1908/. Die deutsche Bäckerei.

Satterlee, L.D., Marshall, H.F. and Tennyson, J.M. /1979/. JAOCS, 56, 103-110.

Proc. Int. Assoc. Cereal Chem. Symp. Amino Acid Compn and Biol. Value of Cereal Proteins Budapest, Hungary 1983, R. Lásztity, M. Hidvégi, eds

AMINO ACID PROBLEM OF CEREALS AT DAILY MEALS

F. VANÍČEK, B. TUREK

Regional Centre of Hygiene, Skrétova St. 15, 303 22 Plzen, Czechoslovakia, Cooperation: Research Institute of Food Industry, Na Belidle 21, 150 38 Prague 5, Bakery Works, Plzen Industry of Milk Nutrition, Novy Bydzov

ABSTRACT

The utilization of food proteins for biosyntheses and activities of the active tissue mass is dependent upon the energy of carbohydrates. If the ratio of carbohydrates to proteins consumed at a daily meal is low, proteins themselves are used as a source of energy, which is an unwholesome loss of the building blocks and can become a health hazard in case both proteins and carbohydrates are scanty or less suitable. Therefore, gluconeogenesis ought to be limited only to emergency cases, and, to abate its incidence, the presented study suggests to consume, with every daily meal, a slice of about 50 g of industrially and in accordance with the state norms produced bread, or a piece of roll, pastry, or any cereal product, enriched quantitatively with sodium caseinate and whey proteins.

INTRODUCTION

Metabolic pathways and functions of food proteins and carbohydrates

Food proteins are the only exogenous source of amino acids, which form the building blocks of all the nitrogen-containing tissues and biocatalysts in the body. All biosyntheses and activities of amino acids are energy-consuming procedures, using the macroergic phosphate ~P (derived from ATP) as the only source of chemical energy. The energy-carrying nucleotides ATP obtain their ~P predominantly by oxidative reactions of glucose, which is most frequently a metabolic product of carbohydrates consumed at daily meals, less frequently a metabolic product of glucogenic amino acids.

As described in approved textbooks of physiology for students (Wright 1967, Ganong 1976, Harper 1977, Trojan 1982, and others), the molecules of glucose, galactose and fructose, and of all the amino acids, set free by hydrolytic processes from carbohydrates and proteins in the gastrointestinal tract, are absorbed by enterocytes of the small intestine and delivered into the blood flow of the portal vein, which carries them to the liver and outpours them into the sinuses of the liver acini. Therefrom they permeate through a one-row layer of endothelial cells to get into contact with the hepatocytes that perform the greatest deal of all carbohydrate- and amino acid-metabolic procedures in the body, changing also galactose and fructose into glucose, producing large amounts of ATP, glycogen, ribose, deoxyribose, NAD^+, $NADP^+$ and heat energy, and at the same time also a great number of proteosyntheses not only of the liver- but almost of all the serum proteins, except immunoglobulins. Every molecule of glucose as well as of each single amino acid must be activated by ATP before entering into any reaction. An immense number of glucose oxidations in hepatocytes demand also large amounts of oxygen, which is supplied by the hepatic artery, in addition to the portal vein. The rest of glucose and the amino acid molecules that were not withdrawn by the liver continues its course with the blood flow to other tissues. This same big catabolic and anabolic process is repeated after every daily meal.

Fats consumed with daily meals, predominantly triacylglycerols, do not take part in these procedures because they are not transported by the portal vein; only the water-like short-chain fatty acids (occurring merely in the milk fat and constituting about 10% of all the fatty acids in butter) follow the course of the portal vein and get utilized in the liver. The consumed triacylglycerols are not transportable by the blood flow because of their voluminous low-density- and water-insoluble mass. They are split up into di- and monoglycerides, fatty acids, and glycerol, absorbed and reesterified to triacylglycerols in enterocytes of the small intestine, and conglomerated with cholesterols, phospholipides, and apoproteins into transportable forms of chylomicrons. These flow on in lymph vessels via the <u>ductus thoracicus</u> into the blood system to be split up in adipose tissues by lipoprotein-lipase into glycerol, which flows to liver, and into fatty acids, which are absorbed and deposited in adipose tissues as long-chain fatty acids, or reesterified by the glycerol that is synthesized within the adipose cells themselves, the reesterified triacylglycerols being deposited therein as well. The remnants of chylomicrons, devoid of triacylglycerols, continue then their circulation in the course of which their single components are withdrawn by other tissues, or incorporated by the liver into the plasmatic lipoproteins VLDL, LDL, or HDL. The circulation of chylomicrons lasts only a few minutes. Therefore, the triacylglycerols consumed with daily meals do not come into contact with the liver, and hence do not play any role in the normal proteosynthetic activities.

Recommended rations of proteins and carbohydrates

The daily rations of proteins per person have been established on the basis of indirect calorimetry and nitrogen balance in the urine with sufficient accuracy regarding the quantification of protein foods for consumers of different groups as to age, sex, weight, height, physical activity, and gynecological condition.

On the other hand, the ration of carbohydrates per person per day has not been distinctly delimitated from that of fats. Consequently, the ration of fats is most often set up too high at the expense of carbohydrates on the false assumption that fat, and especially fat meats, are better sources of energy than carbohydrates.

However, as we have shown in the foregoing paragraphs, fats can by no means replace carbohydrates in the biosyntheses and activities of the active tissue mass for the very reason that they follow quite another course of circulation than amino acids do, and likewise for the reason, as we are going to explain below, that their long-chain fatty acids are incompletely utilized in the liver, which results in the formation of ketone bodies there, as well as for the reason that in some other tissues (e.g. in erythrocytes and potentially in CNS, too) their utilization either does not occur at all, or proves conditionally limited.

It follows from the afore-said that food proteins do create with carbohydrates an operational unit. Its carbohydrates are not replaceable by fat seeing that the fat runs a different metabolic course from that of amino acids and glucose. It is, therefore, clear that carbohydrates as the only source of energy in biosyntheses must always be consumed whenever proteins are consumed, that means with every meal.

The requirement for carbohydrates is materially much higher than that for proteins because carbohydrates supply energy not only for the protein metabolism, but largely also for all the metabolic, kinetic, and thermal needs of the body. Moreover, glucose itself takes part in many energy-consuming biosynthetic procedures, either alone or jointly with the nitrogen compounds, particularly with nucleotides and nucleic acids, or with vitamins and mineral substances. Furthermore, the rate of proteosyntheses extends also upon the endogenous amino acids that get free in the unceasing processes of reconstructions of all existing body proteins.

In the daily dietary recommendations of the WHO and in most official nutritional norms, the optimum daily ration of carbohydrates is set up to 52-56% of the daily energy, and that of proteins to 12-16%. The lower limit of both nutrients is more obligatory than the upper, the upper protein limit being usually tolerated up to 20%, and that of carbohydrates up to 60-65%. In ČSSR the recommended average daily ration is 56% for carbohydrates and 16% for proteins, which means the weight- (as well as energetic-) ratio of 3.5:1.

<u>Metabolic half-times of glucose- and amino acid molecules</u>

The circulation of glucose in the blood lasts about 1-4 hours following the intake. The digestion of proteins is slower, the absorption of amino acids starts later on, but is also rapid. The tissues withdraw single molecules in the number they need. Biosyntheses never set in before the whole ATP energy and all the required amino acids are gathered within the cell. Is any amino acid missing, the synthesis does not go off. All the components that have not been used up within 4-6 hours after the last food intake are quickly oxidized to CO_2 and H_2O under release of heat, or they are metabolized and deposited as fat. Thus, incorrect mutual ratios of carbohydrates to proteins can just as well contribute to obesity as surpluses of energetic foods do.

Factors triggering off gluconeogenesis

If the influx of glucose into the blood is not prolonged within about 4 hours by another food intake, the level of glucose in the blood begins to sink. The liver reacts immediately by releasing adequate amounts of glucose from its glycogen reserves. These are, however, very limited (less than 100 g) and never get quite exhausted seeing that, in a very short time afterwards, the liver cells start off a compensatory glucose production from non-carbohydrate sources, most frequently out of the amino acids, derived from the consumed proteins. If these are not available, amino acids of the living tissues, particularly those of muscles, liver, and red blood cells, get unbound and deaminated to substitute the lacking glucose.

The frequency of gluconeogenesis

Gluconeogenesis is undoubtedly a very frequent event coming round currently in a mild degree almost daily, whereas in more severe degrees it occurs at the weight reduction attempts, in states of hunger and starvation, in cases of imbalanced carbohydrate-protein ratios at daily meals, in most cases of the excess meat- and low cereal consumption, in cases of young boys and girls beginning a hard work or training without an adequate food adjustment (anemia of the beginning sportsmen), in cases of long between-meal intervals, in all cases of a low glucose tolerance, or of a considerable lack of insulin receptors on the cell membranes, or of the defective insulin-binding capacity of the receptors, i.e. in all cases of diabetes. Hence, gluconeogenesis can always set in whenever carbohydrates are not available, or not utilizable in the ratio of about 3.5-4.0 of carbohydrates to 1.0 of proteins, and whenever the long-chain fatty acid oxidations prevail over the glucose oxidations.

Health hazards of gluconeogenesis

The change of amino acids into glucose is always wasteful because the amino acids that take part in gluconeogenesis lose their amino group, and thereby fail to be any more utilizable in biosyntheses of nitrogen compounds. Moreover, the detoxication and the removal of ammonia, which arises from the liberated amino groups, requires a high degree of energy (3 mols ATP against 1 mol NH_3).

In addition to this, the lack of carbohydrates, calling forth gluconeogenesis, induces also mobilization of the free long-chain fatty acids deposited in adipose tissues, offering them in return for glucose. Unfortunately, the liver is a bad recipient of long-chain fatty acids. It is capable of oxidizing the 2-carbon acetyl CoA, not, however, the 4-carbon ketone bodies (acetacetates), which appear in large quantities in the course of long-chain fatty acid oxidations in the liver. The liver cells pass on the ketone bodies to other tissues that do utilize them, but the liver cells under these conditions starve, the unexploited fats accumulate, and the biosynthetic activities of the liver deteriorate.

A low-degree gluconeogenesis is a harmless process provided it occurs exceptionally during an else well-balanced carbohydrate-protein nutrition. However, very frequent and long-lasting cases of gluconeogenesis, as may occur in the above enumerated situations, can result in a deep and rather general upset of the carbohydrate-protein nutrition, and hence should be avoided.

Preventive measures

The liver is capable of a considerable regeneration, if the intake of carbohydrates improves and the harmful fats get removed. The liver is the main producer of bipolar phospholipides, which, as components of chylomicrons and plasmatic lipoproteins, mediate the transport of fats in extracellular fluids, and likewise, as components of the cell- and other bio-membranes mediate also the transport of fatty acid molecules through the bio-membranes. Moreover, the liver produces another kind of phospholipides, the lecithins, that remove from it superfluous fats, which can cause steatosis. The active component of these lecithins, the choline, is synthesized in the liver from the amino acid serine- and 3 labile methyl groups, supplied by the amino acid methionine. Hence, a well-balanced protein-carbohydrate meal not only protects from, but also cures, steatosis of the liver.

As pointed out before, carbohydrates should always be consumed simultaneously with proteins. This postulate had been raised more than a hundred years ago, yet the mechanisms substantiating it were not explained until the metabolic pathways of food proteins and carbohydrates in the body as well as the half-times of their metabolites were elucidated. Albanese and Orto in the fourth (1968) and the fifth (1973) editions of the "Modern Nutrition" expressed this postulate as follows: "The nitrogen-sparing action of carbohydrates is most effective when the carbohydrate is consumed simultaneously with protein. This timing seems to be very important, because, when glucose is fed more than 4 hours before or after the protein meal, it loses its maximum protein-sparing action."

MATERIALS AND METHODS

In order to secure the optimum ratios of suitable carbohydrates and proteins for all consumers at all daily meals, it is desirable to supply both adequate amounts of suitable carbohydrates and high quality proteins, containing also all the necessary vitamins and minerals.

To secure sufficient amounts of suitable carbohydrates and proteins, we have to make the most of our own inland resources. Our rich resources of carbohydrates are cereals and sugar, of proteins milk and meat.

Sugar is not acceptable as a main component of any fit carbohydrate-protein food owing to its entire lack of proteins, mineral substances, and vitamins. Neither its high sweetness, rapid hydrolysis, and liability to stimulate the fat and cholesterol formation in the body make it in the least recommendable.

On the other hand, cereals, in our conditions especially wheat and rye, are very convenient for such a purpose because of their high content of suitable carbohydrates as well as their easily supplementable amount of proteins, mineral substances, and vitamins, which promises not only high rates of ATP production, but also high rates of biosyntheses. Therefore, cereals contribute less to the fat formation, yet by far more to physiologic activities, than both pure sugars and pure starch do.

Milk is an acceptable source of high quality proteins but their share in it is rather low. However, all proteins of milk are easily separable from the undesirable water and fat, and therefore prove very fit for supplementing the cereal products.

Meats are almost entirely devoid of carbohydrates but rich in proteins and fats. Nevertheless, the biological value of their proteins is much lower than that of the whole milk proteins. Apart from that, it is rather difficult to separate the pure meat proteins. The fats contained in meats are very poor sources of glucose (only their glycerol moiety is glucogenic), so there can be no doubt that the meat proteins very often undergo wasting due to a frequent occurrence of gluconeogenesis. Moreover, the long-chain fatty acids of the meat fats are dissimilated in the liver to the ketone bodies, which are not utilizable as a source of energy by the liver cells. In addition, meat fats introduce considerable amounts of cholesterol into the body. Therefore, meats have proven unfit for developing a special supplementary carbohydrate-protein product. Still, as a main course of meals they may be quite recommendable in well-balanced combinations with rich sources of carbohydrates.

In order to improve the carbohydrate-protein balance of meals, reviving the help-yourself-service (bread, or bread and butter, or bread with jam, ready-prepared on the table) at any daily meals is to be recommended providing the cereal component of the bread were adequately enriched.

RESULTS OF OUR ATTEMPTS TO PRODUCE THE PROTEIN-ENRICHED EVERYDAY BREAD

Out of our contemporary cereal products, rye-wheat bread, wheat-rye bread, and wheat daily rolls are most capable of forming the basis of an everyday well-balanced complementary product. Any one of the above nutrients is produced industrially according to the national standards, and consumed almost generally, at least with 2 or 3 daily meals, in a qantity of about 50-100 grams. However, the protein content of these cereal products is somewhat lower than 1:3.5 and becomes still lower owing to the losses on digestion and absorption, which range from 20 to 30% with respect to the flour milling degree. Moreover, there appears also a considerable lysine-, and a slight threonine- and valine deficiency.

Table 1. Amino acid values per gram protein in the standard- and the caseinate/whey protein-enriched bread and rolls. (Assessed by the Research Institute of Food Industry, Prague)

Amino acids	Standard bread %	Enriched bread %	Standard rolls %	Enriched rolls %
Lys	3.20	4.65	2.56	4.18
His	2.11	2.11	2.06	2.15
Arg	4.08	3.50	3.32	3.51
Cys	2.26	1.80	2.18	1.70
Asp	5.68	7.14	4.85	5.96
Met	1.69	2.24	1.73	1.79
Thr	2.94	3.74	2.94	3.49
Ser	4.07	4.43	4.55	4.77
Glu	30.81	27.04	33.55	28.92
Pro	11.34	11.19	12.25	11.12
Gly	3.84	3.04	3.42	3.12
Ala	3.99	3.80	3.30	3.63
Val	4.79	5.11	4.31	4.79
Ileu	3.84	4.20	3.82	4.27
Leu	7.22	7.90	7.29	7.99
Trp	2.67	2.98	2.62	3.35
Phe	5.46	5.11	5.24	5.27

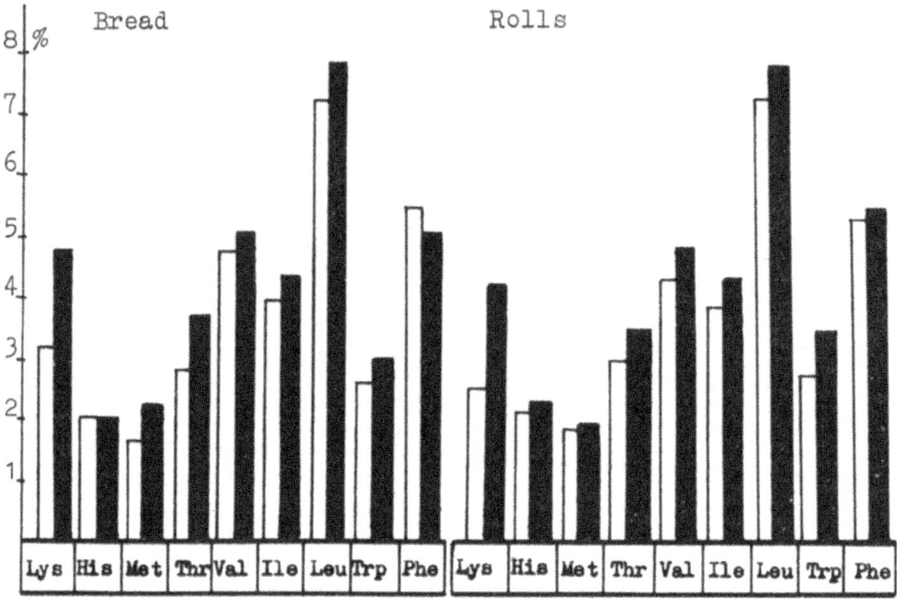

Fig. 1. Percentage of the single amino acids per 1 g of protein in the standard- (white column) and the caseinate/whey protein-enriched (black column) bread and rolls

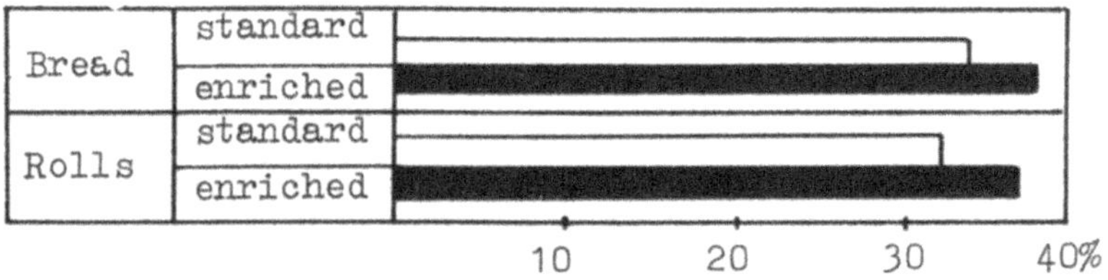

Fig. 2. Percentage of total essential amino acids (incl. His) in proteins of the standard- (white) and the caseinate/whey protein-enriched (black) bread and rolls

Still, by adding 5% of dehydrated casein and 2.5% of dehydrated whey proteins to the bread flour mixture (55% of wheat and 45% of rye flour) we raised the protein-carbohydrate weight ratio in the bread up to 1:3.5 . The content of the essential amino acids rose to 35%, and the content of lysine from 31.5 mg up to 47 mg/g protein. The rolls enriched with the same quantities of casein- and whey proteins gave similar levels. Thus the highest daily ration of 250 g of the enriched bread or rolls supplied approximately 1600 mg of lysine, which is considerably more than ever do require the National Academy of Sciences of the U.S.A. (1974), and the Lebensmittel-Lexikon of the GDR (1979).

The objective won by enrichment of these cereal products was, therefore, fairly positive, nevertheless, the increase in the total protein content was a little below the expected level, evidently due to a slow solubility of casein.

In order to raise the solubility, we adopted the promptly soluble dehydrated sodium caseinate instead of casein, preserving the same proportions in the mixture of caseinate with the dehydrated whey proteins (5% and 2.5% respectively). However, in the meantime the standard for the bread flour mixture was changed to 60% of rye- and 40% of wheat flour, whereas the wheat flour ingredient in rolls remained unchanged. The subsequent results are given in Table 1 and graphically in Figures 1 and 2.

Hence, the total protein content has risen by 6%, which is by 1.5% more than it was previously achieved by pure casein, and, consequently, also the volume of the essential amino acids has increased (by 37-38%, including histidine). The lysine level rose to 1697-1890 mg within the all-day 250-gram bread ration, which is approximately by one third more then the standard levels require. It follows therefrom that adding the mixture of dry sodium caseinate and whey proteins in a total amount of about 5% would be quite satisfactory. A slice of this bread or a part of roll weighing round 50 g, eaten at any daily meal either alone or with butter, or with any sort of spread, or with tea, or as a supplement to any meal, will guarantee a safe carbohydrate-protein balance to start any kinds of proteosyntheses along with the active tissue mass activities.

The bread and the rolls enriched by adding 4% of dry sodium caseinate and 1% of dehydrated whey proteins have fairly good physical and taste qualities, not disturbing in the least the palatability of any food. The quantity of milk, spent on this kind of cereal protein supplementation, amounts to less than 200 ml per person per day, leaving, at that, the milk fat and the milk sugar for further processing.

DISCUSSION

Food proteins and carbohydrates run the same metabolic pathways and supplement each other in biosyntheses, and unilaterally also in energetic functions. The physiological course of their metabolism and activities give evidence that carbohydrates and proteins ought to be supplied simultaneously in due qualities and quantities at every daily meal.

The metabolic pathways of food fats follow quite a different course, and play a different role in human bioenergetics than the carbohydrates do. This is why not only the question of any carbohydrate-protein rationing, but also the question of any fat rationing in the human nutrition should be treated from its specific physiological aspect.

Our study tends to demonstrate the importance of a critical confrontation of the common boarding practice with the increasing knowledge of physiology so that further discrepancies and health hazards involved in today's nutrition may be revealed and removed.

REFERENCES

Albanese, A.A. and Orto, L.A. (1968). The proteins and amino acids. In: Modern nutrition in health and disease. 4th ed., M.G. Wohl and R.S. Goodhart (ed.), pp. 95-255. Ditto as 5th ed., (1973). R.S. Goodhart and M.E. Shils (ed.) Lea and Febiger, Philadelphia, pp. 28-88.

Autorenkollektiv (1979). Lebensmittel-Lexikon. VEB Fachbuchverlag, Leipzig.

Ganong, W.F. (1976). Review of medical physiology (in Czech). 1st ed., Avicenum, Prague.

Harper, H.A. (1977). Review of physiological chemistry (in Czech). 1st ed., Avicenum, Prague.

National Academy of Sciences (1974). Recommended dietary allowances: a report of the Food and Nutrition Board. 8th ed., Washington D.C.

Trojan, S. et al. (1982). Physiology for medical faculties I-IV (in Czech). Charles University, Pedagogical State Publishing House, Prague.

Wright, S. (1967). Applied physiology (in Czech). Health Service State Publishing House, Prague.

Proc. Int. Assoc. Cereal Chem. Symp. Amino Acid Compn and Biol. Value of Cereal Proteins Budapest, Hungary 1983, R. Lásztity, M. Hidvégi, eds

NUTRITIONAL FUNCTIONS OF CEREALS

J. RIGÓ

National Institute of Dietetics, H-1085 Budapest, Makarenko 24, Hungary

Quite a big number of researches are dealing with the physiological function, the more efficient utilization of grain-proteins, which are of major importance in the nutrition of humanity. Despite the decreasing consumption of cereals in the higly developed industrial countries, the daily 150 - 500 g of bread-consumption, falling to the share of one person, is in itself already demonstrating the importance of the researches.

The biological value of grain-proteins, as compared to ovalbumin, can be found between 50 - 60, corresponding to mediocre value. These facts render intelligible, why such a big number of researches and researchers are dealing with the problem, how to use more efficiently, how to affect the most advantageously the nutritive value of grain-proteins.

The biological value of proteins in general, hence also that of grain-proteins, is fundamentally determined by the ratio between the essential amino acids to be found in the cereals and the requirement of essential amino acids of the living creature, consuming protein. However, this ratio can be affected, modified by numerous factors. Between these factors there may be some derivatives of nitrogen, not bound to protein, the characteristic amino acids, preliminary materials of amino acid, which are to be considered as nitrogen-sources. Here may be ranked also some other nutritive materials and metabolites, having a function in the metabolism of proteins. For this reason in some cases results given by biological and chemical values can disjoin. Even being conscious of this, the most important way of raising the biological value and the most frequent possibility, besides the purification by development, are given by the technique of complementation. Békés and Zsigmond /1980/ have raised considerably the biological value of the products of baking industry, complementing them by means of applying a one-purpose-function. Some of their results are shown in Table 1.

Table 1.

Changes in biological value /Békés and Zsigmond 1980/

Product	Biological value	
	Starting point of the value	Value after complementation
White bread	75.3	111.4
Watery cake	61.8	118.1
Milky cake	90.9	122.3
Potato cake	59.1	126.4

In the course of the last few years some examinations have been carried out in our country for improving the biological value resp.the amino acid composition of the grain-proteins, in case of noodles by adding complementary protein-sources /skim milkpowder, protein-concentrate decomposed by means of enzymes, soya flour, vital gluten, egg/. Such examinations were and are in course in the Research Institute of the Baking Industry, in the Central Food Research Institute and similar researches are carried out by the investigators of the National Institute of Dietetics, too. The products contain generally 18, 28 or 38 % protein . The working team of the Central Food Research Institute complemented the lack of lysine by mixture of 70 g wheat flour with 30 g soya flour. A pease flour of 24 % or a milk protein concentrate of 14 % optimal mixing rates have also been achieved with. Protein rates used by us for enriching are shown in Table 2.

Table 2.

Protein rates used for enriching cakes of various protein-contents in %

Food	% of protein		
	18	28	38
Milk-powder	3.7	-	-
Milk-protein concentrate decomposed by means of enzymes	-	8	10
Extruded soya-flour	-	3	5
Gluten	-	6	12
Egg	1.5	2	2

Composition of nutritive materials and energy-contents of noodles are indicated in Table 3.

Table 3.

Nutritive materials' composition of noodles

Nutritive material	Noodle	Noodles rich in protein		
		1	2	3
Protein	12.9	18.2	28.4	39.3
Fats	1.8	2.6	3.3	4.4
Carbohydrate	75.8	68.8	56.4	42.7
Water	9.1	10.2	10.0	10.1
Ash	0.4	0.6	2.2	3.5
Energy	1553 kJ	1555 kJ	1544 kJ	1522 kJ

Carbohydrate content of noodles of different protein-composition is decreasing proportionally with the raising of protein-content and the cooking-time is decreasing too. Noodles of bigger protein-content, having at the same time a decreased carbohydrate-content, are recommended for the diet of patients suffering from diabetes and of others suffering from lack of protein.

Besides examining nutritive materials we also performed tasting examinations for determining the savour- and enjoyment value. Evaluation was carried out by means of the triangular and so-called not-structured scale. The examinators could indicate the enjoyment-value of the various kinds of cakes on a determined scale "from bad to excellent", resp. "from 0 to 100". The examinations proved unambiguously the high enjoyment-value of cakes with a protein-content of 18 %, reminding the literary observation as regards considerable changes in the cake's structural and physico-chemical features after having increased the protein by more than 5 %.

Among the materials used for enrichment I would like to call the attention to the milk-protein concentrate, decomposed by means of enzymes, having a protein-content of 84 %, produced by the Central Food Research Institute. Due to the treatment by enzymes its digestibility is about 30-35 % higher than that of a concentrate, not treated by enzyme. This way the quotient of digestibility of farinaceous products is also improving. The concentrate treated by enzymes can be advantageously applied also in the diet of patients suffering from resorbtive disorders. Observations of récent years call the attention to the necessity of bearing more and more in mind, in case of damaged absorbtion, the absorbtion of the oligopeptides. It was proved that the absorbtion of amino acid is better in case of oligopeptides, than in case when the diet consists of free amino acids. The peptic diet came into being, the advantageous effect of which is explained by the more resistant carrier-system of the oligopeptides /Matthews 1976/.

By means of the adequate hydrolysis of vital gluten various hydrolysates of peptic-, resp. amino acid content can be obtained. The gluten products, decomposed by enzymes, can enlarge considerably the physiological and dietotherapeutic application of wheat proteins. These hydrolysates may count upon a wide-spread application in absorbtive disorders, in diseases of gastroenteritis and for burning lesions, due to the high requirement of protein and proline.

Partial hydrolysates may constitute a basis of starting the peptic diet, whereas the entire hydrolysates that of the elementary diet, resp. of various flavourings.

Among the proteins, isolated in more or less clean state, fractions poor in phenylalanine of the endosperm wheat proteins may count upon special interest, which may be efficient basic materials for foods, or food preparations in a from of the enzymopathies, the phenylketonuria, developing in lack of phenylalanine-hydroxylase.

It is here, that I mention another form of enzymopathies: the gluten-enteropathy, when the gliadin is injoring the intestinal mycodern. Among the cereals, application of foods with rice- and corn-protein content is offering a possibility for carrying out the patient's diet, destined for all his life.

Ammonia occurring during desammonifying the amino acids is participating in forming carbamides /sorts of urea/. It is during the examination of the biscuit Amolett proposed for slimming cure, that we took note of the fact, that the serum carbamide /urea/ level was decreasing when consuming the product enriched with methylcellulose. In the table the converted methylcellulose values are figuring that were given in the course of our research work. We stated, that the serum carbamide level of the rats was significantly decreasing due to the effect of the biscuit enriched with methylcellulose. Results are shown in Table 4.

Table 4.

Effect of methylcellulose on the change of the serum carbamide-nitrogen

Diet	Number of animals	mg/100 ml and st-deviation	p
Checking	20	13 ± 3.3	
Methylcellulose of 4 %	40	11 ± 4.2	$p < 0.05$
Methylcellulose of 8 %	40	7 ± 1.5	$p < 0.001$

Visek /1978/ reported the interaction between the dietary fibre and the decrease of ammonia. According to Visek's data 3.5 -- 4.0 g of ammonia are hydrolyzed by bacterial urease/s/ in the gastrointestinal tract, in the case of consuming daily 100 g protein, in fixation of one part of it the dietary fibre has a role.

When performing examinations together with my colaborator Tulok, we experienced the decrease of ammonia level, after having added glutamic acid and aspartic acid among experimental circumstances. Presumably the relatively high glutamic acid and aspartic acid content of wheat flour had also a certain role in reaching this effect.

By all means, the high /54 %/ dietary fibre content of wheat bran, containing cellulose in 21 % and its relatively high aspartic acid content of 1.55 % and glutamic acid content of 2.58 % are drawing the attention to new possibilities of researching the mechanism of affecting the metabolism of proteins.

When making observations we examined the quantity of indigestible protein, constituting one of the components of the dietary fibre-complex. The difference between the raw- and digestible proteins to be found in cereals is significant. Complex components of dietary fibre are shown in Fig. 1.

Difference between the raw- and digestible proteins was experienced by us also during the research of the dietary fibre. After pepsinic and pancreatinic digestion by hydrochloric acid the components of non digestible protein can be traced.

Lásztity /1981/ called the attention to the more difficult digestibility of native globular proteins, being in connection with the spheric impediment, issuing from the tertiary structure. There remains frequently a nucleus, which is inaccessible for larger enzymes.

The trend of raw- and digestible protein content of the studied cereals is shown in Table 5.

Table 5.

Protein content of cereals g/100 g

Food	Raw-protein	Digestible-protein
Wheat bran for meal	13	10.9
Wheat germ for meal	25.2	23.6
Corn-groats	7.4	6.05
Corn-flour	7.8	6.7
Rye-flour	6.1	6.6
Product enriched with gluten	14.0	11.4

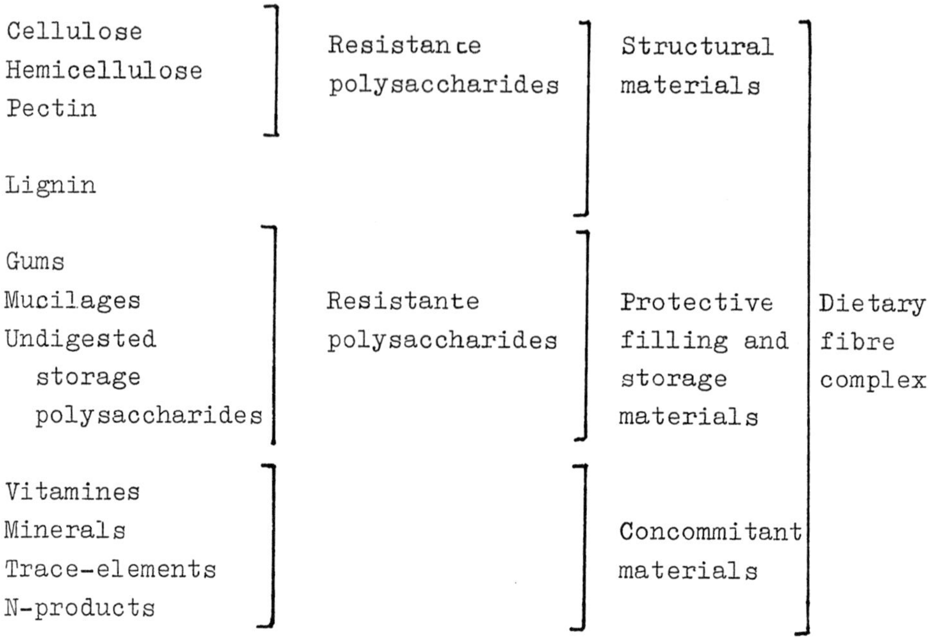

Figure 1. Components of the dietary fibre

Proteins to be found in the dietary fibre complex give certainly an answer to the question, why secretion of nitrogen is increasing in the stool after having consumed a diet rich in dietary fibres.

Physiological significance of dietary fibres is multilateral. Owing to their physico-chemical features they are absorb water, are well-swelling, possess a property of changing cations, they are absorbing organic molecules, biliou and sebabic acids. By all these properties they are decreasing the intraluminary pressure in the large bowel and the transit time, and can be of use in the prophylaxis and therapy of numerous diseases peculiar to civilized communities, like diverticulosis and other diseases of the large bowel. The favourable effect of cereals' dietary fibre content is known and used more and more frequently in the case of hypercholesterionaemy, adiposity, diabetes mellitus, large bowel's diseases, obstipation, diverticulosis. To these fibres are joining the proteins in the frame of the "dietary fibre complex".

Cereals of major dietary fibre content as well as the quantities of indigestible proteins are shown in Table 6.

Table 6.

Dietary fibre and indigestible protein content of cereals g/100g

Product	Dietary fibre	Indigestible protein
Wheat bran	54	2.9
Corn-groats	23	1.3
Wheat germ	22.3	1.6
Corn-flour	5.5	1.3

We determined the content of water-soluble and insoluble dietary fibre as well as the total dietary fibre in cereals according to Hellendoorn et al. /1975/, Elchazly and Thomas /1976/, Schweizer and Würsch/1979/ and Horváth et al./1983/. The results are shown in Table 7.

Table 7.

The dietary fibre content of cereals

	Water-soluble	Water-insoluble	Total
Wheat bran	49	5.0	54.0
Graham flour	18.9	4.6	23.5
Wheat germ	17.2	5.1	22.3
Rye flour	14.6	5.5	20.1
Brown bread /rich in fibre/	10.0	6.5	16.5

Scanning electron micrograph of the water-soluble and water-insoluble dietary fibre from wheat bran are shown in Fig. 2., Fig. 3.

With dietary fibre special dietotherapical aims can be achieved due to the physico-chemical characteristics of the cellulose such as binding of ammonia and decreasing of serum carbamid level. The pectin has an influence on fat metabolism /Kay and Truswell, 1977, Rigó et al. 1983/. The pentose content of hemicellulose is important in increasing the quantity of stool /Cummings et al. 1978/. The lignin has a connection with binding of certain toxical materials and with the bacterial degradation of dietary fibre /Hartley, 1978/. So the aspects for the future are the investigation of the components of dietary fibre and the production of food based on this investigation. The physico-chemical characteristics of the components of dietary fibre can be summed up as follows:

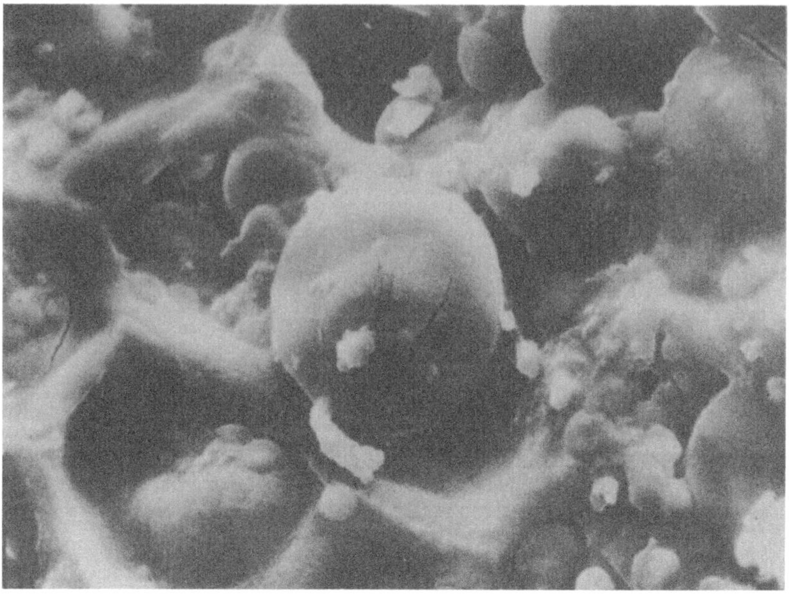

Figure 2. Scanning electron micrograph of water-soluble and water-insoluble dietary fibre from wheat bran/x8050

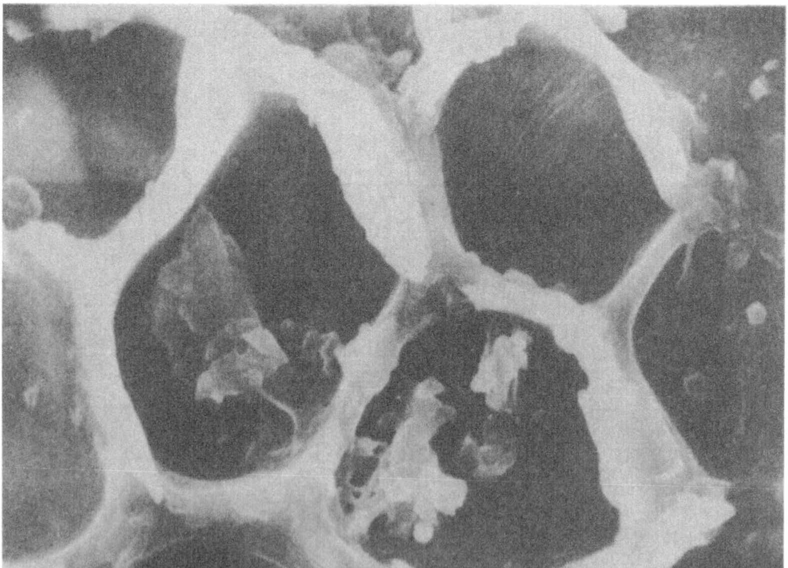

Figure 3. Scanning electron micrograph of water-insoluble dietary fibre from wheat bran /x8050/

Cellulose: water-holding property
decrease of intraluminal pressure
decrease of ammonia
decrease of urea content
inhibition of activity of digestive enzymes
inhibition of absorption

Hemicellulose: water-holding property
decrease of intraluminal pressure
increase of fecal bulk
decrease of transit time
cation exchange
inhibition of intestinal absorption

Pectin: water-holding property
gel-formation
bile-acid adsorption
decrease of serum cholesterol
increase of fecal steroids
inhibition of carbohydrate absorption
toxic materials adsorption

Lignin: bile-acid adsorption
antioxidant property
inhibition of degradation of dietary fibre by bacteria
inhibition of absorption of iron
toxic materials adsorption

The wheat bran and especially the wheat germ for meal, rich in fibres, which are used for human alimentation in an ever growing scope for increasing the fibre content of different products, possess a favourable composition also as regards supply of amino acid. Composition of amino acid in wheat bran and wheat germ is shown in Table 8.

Lysine content of wheat germ is remarkable, which may have a role in complementing the amino acid of bakery products. Its trypsin-impeding, antinutritive effect is decreasing during thermal treatment.

Particular attention is called to the mineral substances, first of all magnesium content, necessary for the integration of proteins. Magnesiums connected to the pectine and lignine fractions get an essential role in incorporating the proteins.

Menaker and Kleiner /1952, 1954/, as well as Carrillo /1961/ reported about three decades ago, that lack of magnesium entailed harmful consequences to building-up proteins. It was proved empirically that animals held on a diet of higher protein, but low magnesium content were building-up less protein and growing less, than animals consuming less protein, but more magnesium. It is Colbi and Frye /1951/, who reported that a bigger protein-input was creating in rats such a state that even in case of a normal input of magnesium development of a state of lack in magnesium could be counted upon.

Table 8.

Amino acid content of wheat bran and wheat germ for meal /in % of the dry-material content/

Amino acids	Wheat germ	Wheat bran
Aspartic acid	2.98	1.55
Threonine	1.20	0.49
Serine	1.30	0.62
Glutamic acid	4.71	2.58
Proline	1.38	0.87
Glycine	1.47	0.78
Alanine	1.66	0.69
Cystine	0.26	0.30
Valine	1.43	0.68
Methionine	0.34	0.20
Isoleucine	0.84	0.37
Leucine	1.63	0.80
Tyrosine	0.43	0.24
Phenylalanine	0.91	0.52
Histidine	0.62	0.40
Lysine	1.46	0.55
Arginine	1.80	0.91

Content of mineral substances in cereals is shown in Table 9.

Table 9.

Content of mineral substances in cereals g/100 g

Food	Mg^+	K^+	Ca^{++}	Na^+
Wheat bran for meal	0.49	1.88	0.34	0.019
Wheat germ for meal	0.23	0.94	0.23	0.013
Corn groats	0.06	0.20	0.10	0.03
Corn flour	0.12	0.27	0.01	0.01
Rice flour	0.04	0.12	0.02	0.01

Ratio of mineral substances can be of special interest, which can get an important role not only in building-up proteins, but also in improving the grade of supply of popular nutrition with mineral substances.
This ratio is shown in Fig. 4.

1. Physiological requirement:

$$\frac{Na^+ + Ca^{++}}{K^+ + Mg^{++}} = 1$$

2. Consumption of Hungary, day/person:

$$\frac{Na^+ + Ca^{++}}{K^+ + Mg^{++}} = 2.3$$

3. Wheat bran:

$$\frac{Na^+ + Ca^{++}}{K^+ + Mg^{++}} = \frac{1.9 + 340}{1088 + 490} = 0.3$$

4. Wheat germ:

$$\frac{Na^+ + Ca^{++}}{K^+ + Mg^{++}} = \frac{13 + 230}{940 + 230} = 0.2$$

Figure 4. Ratio of mineral substances in wheat bran and wheat germ

The intermediary metabolism of proteins is also affected by some vitamins. In this respect riboflavin B_2, pyridoxine B_6 and tocopherol, as vitamins promoting the anabolism have a function. These vitamin quantities are shown in Table 10.

Table 10.

Vitamins affecting the metabolism of protein mg/100 g

Foodstuff	Vitamin		
	Riboflavin	Pyridoxine	Tocopherol
Potato for meal	0.4-0.6	1.2-1.6	1.7
Wheat germ	0.5-0.8	-	17.6
Corn groats	0.1-0.2	0.4-0.6	2.0
Corn flour	0.1-0.3	0.4-0.5	2.2
Rice flour	1.9-2.0	0.1-0.3	1.4

I wished to cast a light on the nutrition-physiological and dietotherapeutic aspects of judging the nutritive values of cereals and grain proteins, used recently in human nutrition, in broader context.

It is known that the biological value of proteins obtained by complementation techniques is higher than the value of the various components. Exploitation of grain proteins is promoted by the complementing materials consumed in the course of mixed alimentation, further by the mineral substances, vitamins helping their incorporation.

When determining the nutritive value, it is a problem for the moment that nowadays we are determining at the most 50-60 nutritive materials, while several hundreds of metabolites are consumed. The effect of these metabolites is at present not yet or hardly known. With the new metabolite effects arising from the speedy development of agrochemistry, neither the science of nutrition, nor the experts dealing with foodstuff chemistry can keep pace for the time being. Nevertheless, it can be stated by now that dynamic studies based on chemical determinations, dealing with the components in correlation with functioning of the organism, can entail further help and progress in judging the cereals from point of view of nutrition physiology.

REFERENCES

Békés, F., Zsigmond, A. /1980/. Az in vitro kémiai indexek alkalmazása az élelmiszerek minősitésében és a nagytápértékü uj élelmiszerek technológiájának kialakitásában "Étkezési fehérje biológiai értéke" Nemzetközi Tudományos Kollokvium Budapest, 1-18.

Carrillo, B.J., Pond, W.G., Krook, L., Lovelace, F.E., Loosli, J.K. /1961/ Response of growing rats to diets varying in magnesium, potassium and protein content. Proc. Soc. Exp. Biol. Med. /N.Y./ 107, 739.

Colby, R.W., Frye, C.M. /1951/. Effect of feeding high levels of protein and calcium in rat rations on magnesium deficiency syndrome. Am.J.Physiol. 166, 408.

Cummings, J.H., Branch, W., Jenkins, D.J.A., Southgate, D.A.T., Houston, H., James, W.P.T. /1978/. Colonic response to dietary fibre from carrot, cabbage, apple, bran and guar gum. Lancet, 7, 5-8.

Elchazly, M., Thomas, B. /1976/. Über eine biochemische Methode zur Bestimmung der Ballaststoffe und ihrer Komponenten in pflanzlichen Lebensmitteln. Zeitschrift für Lebensmittel-Untersuchung und Forschung, 162, 329-340.

Hartley, R.D. /1978/. The lignin fraction of plant cell walls. Am. J. Clin. Nutr. 31, 90-93.

Hellendoorn, E. W., Noordhoff, M.G., Slagman, J. /1975/. Enzymatic Determination of the Indigestible Residue /Dietary Fibre/ Content of Human Food. J. Sci. Food. Agric. 26, 1461-1568.

Horváth-Mosonyi, M., Rigó, J., Hegedüs-Völgyesi, E. /1983/. Study of dietary fibre content and fibre components of carrots. Acta Alimentaria, 12, 199-210.

Kay, R.M., Truswell, A.S. /1977/. Effect of citrus pectin on blood lipides and fecal steroid excretion in man. Am. J. Clin. Nutr. 30, 171-175.

Lásztity, R. /1981/. Gabonafehérjék. Mezőgazdasági Kiadó, Budapest.

Matthews, D.M., Siamak, A.A. /1976/. Peptide absorption. Gastroenterology, 71, 151-156.

Menaker, W., Kleiner, I.S. /1952/. Effect of deficiency of magnesium and other minerals on protein synthesis. Proc. Soc. Exp. Biol. Med. 81, 377.

Menaker, W. /1954/. Influence of protein intake on magnesium requirement during protein synthesis. Proc. Soc. Exp. Biol. Med. /N.Y./ 85, 149.

Rigó, J., Pados, Gy., Horváth-Mosonyi, M. /1983/. The effect of wheat bran enriched with pectin on the hyperlipoproteinaemie. 16 th World Congress of the International Society for Fat Research /ISF/ Budapest.

Schweizer, T.F., Würsch, P. /1979/. Analysis of Dietary Fibre. J. Sci. Food. Agric. 30, 613-619.

Visek, W.J. /1978/. Diet and cell growth modulation by ammonia. Am. J. Clin. Nutr. 31, 216-220.

Proc. Int. Assoc. Cereal Chem. Symp. Amino Acid Compn and Biol. Value of Cereal Proteins Budapest, Hungary 1983, R. Lásztity, M. Hídvégi, eds

CEREAL PROTEINS IN HUMAN NUTRITION

L. R. HACKLER

Department of Home Economics, State University of New York College, Oneonta, NY 13820, USA

Cereals are usually thought of as a valuable source of calories, but they also represent an important source of protein. Cereal protein is especially valuable in our diets when we consider complementation of amino acids between various plant sources. Cereal protein represents an important component in the diets of people, roughly 16 to 45 grams per capita per day. This represents 70% of the total protein available in some areas of the world. Grains and grain legumes represent important sources of calories and protein. In fact, these two food sources represent our hope for overcoming protein calorie malnutrition in the developing countries. The consumption of cereal proteins in conjunction with food legumes results in a better balance in essential amino acids, thus higher protein quality. The complementary effects of various cereal:legume:tuber combinations are presented. It is important to keep in mind that combinations of plant proteins can be selected to provide high quality protein, especially for adults. Hopefully, this paper will stimulate others to evaluate protein combinations for providing high quality protein.

Cereals and cereal-based food products have historically represented an important source of food for man. Cereals are usually thought of as a valuable source of calories, but they also represent an important source of protein. Cereal protein is especially valuable in our diets when we consider complementation of amino acids between various plant sources.

Several aspects of the nutritional attributes of cereals and cereal-based products in the diet of man have been discussed in some detail by numerous authors (Chen, Fox and Kies, 1967; Lee et al., 1971; Shukla, 1975; Harden et al., 1976; Lorenz and Lee, 1977; Wall and Paulis, 1978; Navarette and Bressani, 1981; and Mattern, 1984). Cereal diets with both small and large amounts of animal protein can be identified around the world. The United States represents a country that consumes large amounts of animal protein, while some of the developing countries such as Africa, China, and India consume less than 10% of their protein from animal sources (Abbott, 1973). Consequently, protein quality is a more critical issue for many people throughout the world who consume diets that contain a high proportion of protein from cereal foods with limited amounts of animal protein or even high quality legume protein.

This article is not intended to resolve protein/calorie malnutrition problems, but to serve as a guide or to encourage people to look for complementation of proteins as a means of improving their protein status. Utilization of local resources is a key to improving nutritional status. Hopefully, this article will stimulate nutritionists, dietitians, and others involved in feeding programs to evaluate food combinations that are acceptable within a population group that may provide diets in which the protein sources provide complementary amino acid mixtures.

Protein/Calorie Dilemma

Although calories have gained greater recognition during the past two decades as one of the two crucial components that must be corrected if world malnutrition is to be resolved, protein remains as the dominant factor, or consideration, by many scientists because of its unique role in nutrition and health along with its impact on economics or cost of food. Shukla (1975) referred to protein as "the very touchstone of life, of health, and of the physical and mental development of man," and "foods containing proteins . . . are seemingly the limiting factors for the fuller survival of humanity." Cereal grains represent 50-60% of the total world protein supply (Shukla, 1975). Table 1 gives representative protein contents of several cereals.

Table 1. Protein Content of Some Cereals[1]

	Protein %[2]
Barley (*Hordeum vulgare*)	10.1
Corn (*Zea mays*)	10.3
Oat (*Avena sativa*)	22.4
Rice (*Oryza sativa*)	8.5
Rye (*Secale cereale*)	13.6
Sorghum (*Sorghum vulgare*)	12.4
Triticale (*Triticosecale*)	20.2
Wheat (*Triticum aestivium*)	13.4

[1]Values were adapted from Shukla, 1975.
[2]Protein percent is expressed on the dry matter basis.

It is readily apparent that there is a wide range in protein content among the cereal grains. On a dry matter basis the values range from 8.5% protein for rice to 22.4% protein for oat. It is also interesting to note that the protein content of triticale is higher than either of its parents (20.2% vs. 13.6% for rye and 13.4% for wheat).

It seems appropriate to discuss briefly the standard method for measuring protein content of foods before addressing the main thesis of this paper, namely, the usefulness and importance of cereal proteins in human nutrition.

The publication of the classical method for determining nitrogen by Kjeldahl (1883) was a major milestone in protein nutrition research. It is one of the most dependable tests available for determining the protein content of grains. The Kjeldahl procedure measures only nitrogen (N); it does not distinguish between protein N and nonprotein N. This can lead to errors if very much of the N is nonprotein N, especially if it is something other than amino acids. For most foods, more specifically cereal grains, the nonprotein N is negligible. Furthermore, if the nonprotein N is primarily composed of amino acids, it is not a serious problem; in other words, the amino acids can be utilized.

The chemical determination of amino acids extends and supplements the total nitrogen values as measured by the Kjeldahl or some other protein procedure. Although the amino acid make-up of a protein is responsible for its usefulness in the body (Rose, 1938), there are many unresolved problems associated with the analytical procedures used for measuring amino acid contents of food proteins (Cherry, 1981; Hackler, 1971; Sarwar et al., 1983).

Since foods contain nitrogenous components other than amino acids, it is important to recognize that some food components may contain significant quantities of nitrogenous compounds other than amino acids, some of which have non-specific nutritive value as precursors of tissue protein. For example, nucleic acid may be present in single cell proteins at levels up to 12% and should not be regarded as equivalent to true protein. Thus, amino acid determinations by chemical procedures extend the usefulness of protein determinations by telling us what proportion of the protein is amino acids. The Kjeldahl nitrogen method is still the standard for comparing various other procedures for losses.

Cereal protein represents an important component in the diets of people, roughly 16 to 45 grams per capita per day (Hulse, 1981). This represents 70% of the total protein available in some areas of the world. Very little animal protein which is of higher biological value is accessible or attainable by many people. Consequently it is important that particular attention is given to complementation of amino acids from various protein foods.

Protein Needs

The amount of protein needed per day for humans has decreased with increasing knowledge. Early estimates for protein were in the 112 (Atwater, 1903)[1] to 118 g/day (Voit, 1876), while the NRC 1980 recommendation is for 56 grams protein/day for an adult man. The per capita consumption of protein in the U.S. is much closer to the original estimates of Voit and Atwater than it is to the NRC 1980 recommendation. On the other hand, in the heavily populated and developing countries protein supplies are much less than in the more highly developed countries. In this regard, it is important to note that the short-term nitrogen balance studies with adult humans suggest that protein needs can be met by smaller levels than the 56 g/day NRC recommendation. In fact, the endogenous urinary protein excretion values in several studies indicate that 11 to 17 grams of protein would be excreted by a 70 kg man (24 to 38 mg N/kg body weight) (Irwin and Hegsted, 1971). Hegsted et al. in 1946 found the minimum protein requirement to be about 18 grams protein/square meter (m^2) with an all-plant protein diet, while Phansalkar and Patwardhan (1956) found a slightly higher need of 22 grams protein/m^2 on an all-plant protein diet. Young and Scrimshaw (1968) and Calloway and Margen (1971) have reported the metabolic fecal protein (MFP) loss in studies with men eating a protein-free diet to be about one gram, while a somewhat lower value has been reported by other investigators (Hegsted et al., 1946). Using the higher MFP value, it can be seen that about 23 grams protein are necessary to meet maintenance needs without taking into account needs related to skin, lung, hair, and sweat losses as well as various stresses. Therefore, a somewhat larger intake is needed to account for other avenues of loss of protein (Costa et al., 1968; Calloway et al., 1966).

It has been well documented that diets which provide eight grams of nitrogen (8 x 6.25 = 50 g protein) or even as little as four grams of nitrogen which would equal 25 g protein (Calloway et al., 1966; Costa et al., 1968; Clark, Kollenkark and Halvorson, 1978) will keep most individuals in positive nitrogen balance based on short-term laboratory studies. However, consumption of less than eight grams of nitrogen might be ill-advised if the protein is predominately from cereal foods with minimal protein intakes from animal or high quality legumes. Fifty grams of protein represents a level that will allow for some biological variation among individuals. Although numerous investigators have supported short-term laboratory studies (Bricker et al., 1949; Kies, 1979; Scrimshaw and Young, 1979; Bressani et al., 1979) integumental losses may not be adequately met, nor losses due to other stresses associated with vari_us illnesses.

Amino Acid Mixtures (complementation)

The amino acid composition of some cereals, legumes, and tubers is presented in Tables 2, 3, and 4, respectively. These tables do not represent a complete listing of cereals, legumes, or tubers, but will serve the purposes of this article, namely, to emphasize the potential complementary effects of combining cereals with legumes or tubers. Generally speaking, the cereals are somewhat deficient in lysine, while the legumes are high in lysine with the exception of groundnuts. On the other hand, the cereals are higher in the sulfur amino acids than are the legumes. Tubers are some better in lysine than the cereals but are low in the sulfur amino acids.

In Table 5, one can compare the FAO 1973 amino acid pattern with that of NRC 1980 and Mitchell's pattern of 1954 which is based on the amino acid composition of whole egg. It is readily apparent that there are differences in the three patterns. It is not the intent of this article to discuss the logic behind each of the patterns, but it is well to note that whole egg is higher for each of the amino acids and

Table 2. Amino Acid Composition of Some Cereals,[1] gm/16 gm nitrogen

	Barley	Corn (Zea Mays)	Oats	Rice (brown)	Rice (polished)	Rye	Sorghum	Wheat (whole grain)	Wheat (flour 70-80%)	Triticale
Lysine	3.46	2.67	3.71	3.79	3.62	3.39	2.02	2.86	2.08	3.1
Isoleucine	3.58	3.68	3.78	3.81	4.19	3.50	3.92	3.26	3.65	3.2
Leucine	6.67	12.5	7.26	8.22	8.22	6.16	13.3	6.67	7.04	6.0
Valine	5.04	4.85	5.10	5.50	5.78	4.75	5.01	4.42	4.13	2.9
Phenylalanine	5.14	4.88	5.01	5.15	4.85	4.42	4.90	4.51	4.86	3.9
Tyrosine	3.10	3.82	3.30	3.49	3.20	1.92	2.67	2.99	2.32	1.5
Total aromatic	8.24	8.70	8.30	8.64	8.05	6.34	7.57	7.50	7.18	5.4
Methionine	1.66	1.92	1.68	2.32	2.13	1.46	1.39	1.50	1.46	4.5
Cystine	2.27	1.55	2.67	1.07	1.54	1.90	1.50	2.54	2.54	1.8
Met & Cys	3.94	3.47	4.35	3.39	3.66	3.36	2.90	4.05	4.00	6.3
Tryptophan	1.54*	.70	1.26*	1.25*	1.34*	.74*	1.22	1.09*	1.07*	1.7
Threonine	3.31	3.60	3.31	3.90	3.31	3.34	3.02	2.93	2.69	3.1
Histidine	2.11	2.72	2.10	2.50	2.34	2.21	2.14	2.29	2.08	2.2
Arginine	4.72	4.19	6.29	8.26	7.57	4.58	3.07	4.61	3.54	5.5

[1]Data were compiled from FAO, 1970, except for triticale; Bider (1968) as presented by Hulse and Laing, 1974.

*Analyzed microbiologically.

Table 3. Amino Acid Compositions of Some Legumes,[1] gm/16 gm nitrogen

	Groundnut	Mung Bean	Soybean	Soya Milk	Bean
Lysine	3.54	8.06	6.38	5.57	7.20
Isoleucine	3.38	3.57	4.54	4.88	4.19
Leucine	6.40	7.06	7.78	7.95	7.62
Valine	4.18	4.14	4.80	4.70	4.59
Phenylalanine	4.98	4.90	4.94	5.01	5.22
Tyrosine	3.90	2.50	3.14	3.81	2.53
Total aromatic	8.88	7.39	8.08	8.82	7.74
Methionine	1.15	.53	1.26	1.44	1.06
Cystine	1.25	1.09	1.33	1.62	.85
Met & Cys	2.40	1.23	2.59	3.06	1.90
Tryptophan	1.04	.80*	1.28	1.36*	1.01*
Threonine	2.61	3.34	3.86	3.66	3.97
Histidine	2.37	2.91	2.53	2.40	2.83
Arginine	11.2	5.52	7.23	7.23	5.68

[1]Data were compiled from FAO, 1970.
*Analyzed microbiologically.

Table 4. Amino Acid Composition of Some Tubers,[1] gm/16 gm nitrogen

	Cassava	Potato	Sweet Potato	Yam
Lysine	4.14	4.78	3.42	4.10
Isoleucine	2.80	3.78	3.68	3.74
Leucine	3.95	6.03	5.44	6.46
Valine	3.34	4.67	4.53	4.66
Phenylalanine	2.50	4.02	3.86	4.80
Tyrosine	1.60	2.74	2.34	3.22
Total aromatic	4.10	6.75	6.19	8.02
Methionine	1.33	1.30	1.70	1.60
Cystine	1.44	.59	1.10	1.15
Met & Cys	2.77	1.89	2.80	2.75
Tryptophan	1.15	1.65*	1.71*	1.28
Threonine	2.64	3.76	3.78	3.60
Histidine	2.06	1.50	1.34	1.89
Arginine	10.9	4.98	4.91	7.63

[1]Data were compiled from FAO, 1970.
*Analyzed microbiologically.

Table 5. Comparison of Amino Acid Patterns (mg per gm nitrogen)

	Reference Patterns		Whole Egg
	FAO (1973)	NRC (1980)	Mitchell, 1954
Lysine	344	319	438
Isoleucine	250	262	481
Leucine	438	438	575
Valine	312	300	450
Phenylalanine			394
Tyrosine			281
Phe & Tyr	375	456	675
Methionine			250
Cystine			150
Met & Cys	219	162	400
Tryptophan	62	69	94
Threonine	250	219	269
Histidine	--	106	150

probably provides an excess of some of the amino acids, in particular the sulfur amino acids. Studies reported in 1959 raised questions with regard to the high level of the sulfur amino acids in some amino acid scoring procedures (Fomon, 1959; Fomon and May, 1959). The FAO and NRC patterns are quite similar; however, there are some subtle, but important, differences. The NRC pattern is lower for valine (4%), lysine (6%), threonine (12%) and methionine + cystine (26%), and higher in isoleucine (5%) and phenylalanine + tyrosine (22%). Since lysine, the sulfur amino acids, tryptophan, and threonine are most likely to be limiting in diets of poorly fed individuals, it is readily apparent that decreasing the amount of lysine, threonine, and the sulfur amino acids in the NRC pattern will make it somewhat easier to meet this pattern than it will be for the other two indices, especially the EAAI based on the amino acid composition of whole egg.

Hackler (1977a) suggested that perhaps only three or four amino acids might serve for the evaluation of a protein's usefulness for humans. Based on the FAO 1973 pattern, lysine was first limiting in approximately 50% of the foods evaluated, while methionine + cystine was first limiting in about 30% and threonine was only first limiting in one food but second limiting in almost 40% of the foods (Hackler, 1977b). Amino acid patterns for evaluation of protein quality were described in the classic paper of Block and Mitchell (1946). Mitchell (1954) suggested calculation of a geometric mean with whole egg as a reference pattern. Based on this procedure, the index value is higher than the chemical score value of the first limiting amino acid.

Amino Acid Analyses

Some other points need to be made with regard to evaluating

protein quality for humans using amino acid composition data. First of all, there is a great deal of inter- and intra-laboratory variation in amino acid analysis of food proteins (Cavins et al., 1972; Knipfel et al., 1971; Sarwar et al., 1983; and Williams et al., 1979). The hydrolysis time is one of the areas in which considerable variation has been observed (Cherry, 1981; Hackler, 1974; Hackler, 1981; Happich, Bodwell and Phillips, 1981; Moore and Stein, 1963). The sulfur amino acids along with tryptophan represent unique problem areas insofar as variability between laboratories is concerned. The most recent collaborative study found the interlaboratory coefficient of variability for tryptophan to be up to 24%, while methionine and cystine had a coefficient of variation up to 17% (Sarwar et al., 1983). The within-laboratory variation for all amino acids was less than 5% in the same study. Seligson and Mackey (1984) have also recently discussed the use of amino acid composition data of five protein sources and the variability that can be observed by the chemical scoring procedure and observed that the source of the analytical data and the reference pattern used can influence the results obtained. Thus, one must use amino acid composition data and reference patterns with some caution. Another factor that must be considered along with the problems associated with amino acid analyses is the matter of digestibility of the protein to amino acids for absorption and use within the body.

Grains/Legumes/Tubers

As mentioned previously, grains and grain legumes represent important sources of calories and protein. In fact, these two food sources represent our hope for overcoming protein calorie malnutrition in the developing countries. The consumption of cereal proteins in conjunction with food legumes results in a better balance in essential amino acids, thus higher protein quality. The complementary effects of the two proteins are readily apparent from the information in Tables 6 and 7, where amino acid scores have been computed by the modified essential amino acid index (EAAI) of Mitchell (1954), the FAO 1973 and the NRC 1980 patterns. Based on the FAO pattern, protein in cereal grains is first limiting in lysine. This is also the case for the NRC scoring procedure with the exception of triticale which indicates that valine is first limiting. The EAAI pattern indicates that lysine, isoleucine or valine may be first limiting depending on the cereal grain being tested (Table 6). Legume protein is first limiting in the sulfur amino acids (Table 7) with the exception of groundnut protein which is first limiting in lysine by both the FAO and NRC scoring procedures. Also, soya milk is borderline first limiting in valine. Generally speaking, the second limiting amino acid in the legumes is either threonine or isoleucine, depending on the amino acid pattern used. Thus, one can quickly recognize that consuming, for example, corn and soybeans together will result in a complementary effect. This is illustrated in the data presented in Table 8. The FAO score is higher for the cereal:soybean mixture (Table 8) than for the cereal (Table 6) or soybean (Table 7) when evaluated separately.

Table 9 contains a comparison of the limiting amino acids of cereal:bean mixture. Methionine + cystine is first limiting in this food combination except for triticale (valine) and wheat (threonine).

Table 6. Comparison of Limiting Amino Acids in Cereals by Using Three Different Reference Patterns[1]

Cereals	FAO Score[2]	First Limiting Amino Acid	Second Limiting Amino Acid	EAAI[3]	First Limiting Amino Acid	Second Limiting Amino Acid	NRC Score[4]	First Limiting Amino Acid	Second Limiting Amino Acid
Barley	63	Lys	Iso	69	Iso	Lys	68	Lys	Iso
Corn (Zea Mays)	48	Lys	Try	65	Lys	Try	52	Lys	Try
Oats	67	Lys	Thr	71	Iso	Lys	73	Lys	Iso
Rice (brown)	69	Lys	Iso	73	Iso	Met & Cys	74	Lys	Iso
Rice (polished)	66	Lys	Thr	73	Lys	Iso	71	Lys	Thr
Rye	62	Lys	Try	60	Iso	Lys	66	Lys	Try
Sorghum	37	Lys	Thr	63	Lys	Met & Cys	39	Lys	Thr
Triticale	56	Lys	Val	63	Val	Iso	60	Val	Lys
Wheat (whole grain)	52	Lys	Thr	63	Lys	Iso	56	Lys	Iso
Wheat (flour 70-80%)	38	Lys	Thr	60	Lys	Iso	41	Lys	Val

[1]Scores calculated by using amino acid compositions from FAO (1970) except for triticale; Triticale scores calculated by using amino acid compositions of Bider (1968) as presented by Hulse and Laing (1974).

[2]Scores calculated by using the FAO (1973) pattern as the reference pattern.

[3]Essential Amino Acid Index calculated by using whole egg as reference pattern, Mitchell (1954).

[4]Scores calculated by using the NRC (1980) pattern as the reference pattern.

Table 7. Comparison of Limiting Amino Acids in Legumes by Using Three Different Reference Patterns[1]

Legumes	FAO Score[2]	First Limiting Amino Acid	Second Limiting Amino Acid	EAAI[3]	First Limiting Amino Acid	Second Limiting Amino Acid	NRC Score[4]	First Limiting Amino Acid	Second Limiting Amino Acid
Bean	54	Met & Cys	Val	70	Met & Cys	Iso	73	Met & Cys	Try
Groundnut	64	Lys	Thr	61	Met & Cys	Iso	69	Lys	Thr
Mung Bean	35	Met & Cys	Try	60	Met & Cys	Iso	48	Met & Cys	Try
Soybean	74	Met & Cys	Thr	74	Met & Cys	Iso	100	--	--
Soya Milk	87	Met & Cys	Thr	76	Met & Cys	Iso	98	Val	--

[1]Scores calculated by using amino acid compositions from FAO (1970).

[2]Scores calculated by using the FAO (1973) pattern as the reference pattern.

[3]Essential Amino Acid Index calculated by using whole egg as reference pattern, Mitchell (1954).

[4]Scores calculated by using the NRC (1980) pattern as the reference pattern.

Table 8. Limiting Amino Acids of Cereal:Soybean (50:50) Mixture[1]

	Cereal:Soybean Mixture		
	FAO Score[2]	First Limiting Amino Acid	Second Limiting Amino Acid
Barley	90	Thr	Lys
Corn	82	Lys	Met & Cys
Oats	90	Thr	Lys
Rice (brown)	85	Met & Cys	Lys
Rice (polished)	89	Met & Cys	Thr
Rye	85	Met & Cys	Lys
Sorghum	76	Lys	Met & Cys
Triticale	77	Leu	Val
Wheat (whole grain)	84	Lys	Thr
Wheat (flour 70-80%)	77	Lys	Thr

[1]Scores calculated by using amino acid compositions from FAO (1970).
[2]Scores calculated by using FAO (1973) pattern as the reference pattern.

Table 9. Limiting Amino Acids of Cereal:Bean (50:50) Mixture

	Cereal:Bean Mixture		
	FAO Score	First Limiting Amino Acid	Second Limiting Amino Acid
Barley	83	Met & Cys	Thr
Corn	77	Met & Cys	Try
Oats	89	Met & Cys	Thr
Rice (brown)	75	Met & Cys	Thr
Rice (polished)	79	Met & Cys	Thr
Rye	75	Met & Cys	Try
Sorghum	68	Met & Cys	Lys
Triticale	75	Val	Thr
Wheat (whole grain)	85	Met & Cys	Thr
Wheat (flour 70-80%)	83	Thr	Met & Cys

Threonine is second limiting in all of the mixtures except for sorghum (lysine) and wheat (methionine + cystine).

A comparison of the limiting amino acids in tubers by three different reference patterns is presented in Table 10. The first and second limiting amino acids vary depending upon the reference pattern used. Other comparisons and various combinations are shown in Tables 11, 12, 13, and 14 in which only the FAO 1973 scoring pattern was used.

Investigations by Clark et al. (1971) and Lee et al. (1971) have demonstrated the ability of rice protein to promote positive nitrogen balance in adult humans. Howe et al. (1972) studied six combinations of rice, white wheat flour, and nonfat dry milk that provided six grams of nitrogen/day and reported that a 75:25 combination of protein from rice:wheat flour was as effective as a 50:50 protein combination from rice:milk. Chen, Fox and Kies (1967) reported that lysine is the first limiting amino acid in rice for human adults as measured by nitrogen retention. Clark et al. (1972) studied four levels of nitrogen from a combination of rice, milk, and wheat and reported that both 8.0 and 7.0 grams of dietary nitrogen from these sources would permit sufficient nitrogen retention to cover integumental losses. Therefore, diets of less than 44 grams of protein per day might be inadequate for maintaining a healthy populace.

Ashur et al. (1973) fed healthy young men and women experimental diets that supplied 8.0 grams of nitrogen from white wheat flour, bulgur, and rice with various combinations of nonfat dry milk, whey, chickpea, or sesame. Although small differences in nitrogen balance were observed, they were not statistically significant. Other research from the same laboratory suggests that combining cereal food proteins may be beneficial or superior to replacing with their constituent amino acids (Bailey and Clark, 1976). Occasionally this point is overlooked and needs to be reinforced from time to time. Briley, Miles and Longenecker (1979) have also demonstrated the beneficial aspects of combining plant proteins on protein quality. They studied the addition of 5, 10, and 15% sunflower flour in a yeast-leavened bread and found a 14, 23, and 32% increase in protein quality, respectively.

Another means of improving the protein quantity and quality of cereal proteins is through selection of superior varieties. Chavan and Duggal (1978a) reported superior amino acid contents of newly developed high-yielding varieties of rice.

Lysine is the first limiting essential amino acid in corn protein for human adults; however, the second limiting essential amino acid is influenced by level of nitrogen in the diet. At a high level (12 or 13 grams nitrogen/day) methionine is first limiting, while with a four-gram nitrogen intake, tryptophan is second (first) limiting (Kies and Fox, 1970). Lysine is still the first limiting amino acid in opaque-2 corn for human adults, but opaque-2 corn protein is superior to field corn protein (Kies and Fox, 1972).

Navarrete and Bressani (1981) observed an improvement in protein digestibility of beans by the addition of maize. Nitrogen equilibrium was reached by .114 grams nitrogen/kg body weight/day with beans alone

Table 10. Comparison of Limiting Amino Acids in Tubers by Using Three Different Reference Patterns[1]

Tubers	FAO Score[2]	First Limiting Amino Acid	Second Limiting Amino Acid	EAAI[3]	First Limiting Amino Acid	Second Limiting Amino Acid	NRC Score[4]	First Limiting Amino Acid	Second Limiting Amino Acid
Cassava	66	Thr	Val	52	Iso	Phe & Tyr	56	Phe & Tyr	Leu
Potato	54	Met & Cys	Leu	62	Met & Cys	Iso	73	Met & Cys	Leu
Sweet Potato	62	Lys	Leu	60	Met & Cys	Iso	67	Lys	Leu
Yam	74	Lys	Met & Cys	66	Met & Cys	Iso	80	Lys	Iso

[1]Scores calculated by using amino acid compositions from FAO (1970).

[2]Scores calculated by using the FAO (1973) pattern as the reference pattern.

[3]Essential Amino Acid Index calculated by using whole egg as reference pattern, Mitchell (1954).

[4]Scores calculated by using the NRC (1980) pattern as the reference pattern.

Table 11. Limiting Amino Acids of Cereal:Groundnut (50:50) Mixture

	Cereal:Groundnut Mixture		
	FAO Score[1]	First Limiting Amino Acid	Second Limiting Amino Acid
Barley	64	Lys	Thr
Corn	56	Lys	Thr
Oats	66	Lys	Thr
Rice (brown)	66	Lys	Thr
Rice (polished)	65	Lys	Thr
Rye	63	Lys	Thr
Sorghum	51	Lys	Thr
Triticale	60	Lys	Val
Wheat (whole grain)	58	Lys	Thr
Wheat (flour 70-80%)	51	Lys	Thr

[1]Scores calculated by using the FAO (1973) pattern as the reference pattern.

while 0.098 grams of nitrogen/kg of body weight/day of an 87:13 mixture of beans:maize promoted nitrogen equilibrium. Feeding studies were conducted with rats to show the beneficial aspects of combining rice with different pulses by Chavan and Duggal (1978b). Rice in combination with soybean, red gram, green gram, or black gram was found superior to rice alone; but rice and soybean or green gram appeared superior in all cases to the rice and red or black gram. Therefore, some combinations are better than others for improving protein quality.

Nicol and Phillips (1978) studied the utilization of protein and amino acids in diets containing cassava, rice, or sorghum in Nigerian men. Based on their results they agreed with the FAO 1973 committee report that the sulfur amino acids and tryptophan needs should be reduced from the FAO 1957 provisional pattern, but they did not support the increases in lysine and threonine advocated by the 1973 committee report.

The preceding has emphasized the role and the importance of cereal protein in preventing, as well as in overcoming, protein malnutrition. Before concluding this paper it should be emphasized that the position and importance of cereals in our diets can be improved by the development of improved varieties (Mattern, 1984). Attention should be given to not just yield but to nutritional value along with disease resistance and improvement in various processing and functionality characteristics. Protein is an important component with regard to the nutritional value of cereals and their complementation with other protein sources. Nitrogen intakes of 7.0 g from combinations of wheat flour (3.5 g of nitrogen) with 1.75 grams of nitrogen each with two

Table 12. Comparison of Limiting Amino Acids of Tubers and Polished Rice (50:50 mixture) to Tuber or Polished Rice Alone

	Tuber:Rice Mixture			Tuber			Polished Rice		
	FAO Score[1]	First Limiting Amino Acid	Second Limiting Amino Acid	FAO Score[1]	First Limiting Amino Acid	Second Limiting Amino Acid	FAO Score[1]	First Limiting Amino Acid	Second Limiting Amino Acid
Cassava	70	Lys	Thr	66	Thr	Val	66	Lys	Iso
Potato	76	Lys	Met & Cys	54	Met & Cys	Leu			
Sweet Potato	64	Lys	Met & Cys	62	Lys	Leu			
Yam	70	Lys	Thr	74	Lys	Met & Cys			

[1]Scores calculated by using the FAO (1973) pattern as the reference pattern.

Table 13. Limiting Amino Acids of Soybean:Cereal and Groundnut:Cereal Mixtures (25:75)

	25:75 Mixture		
	FAO Score[1]	First Limiting Amino Acid	Second Limiting Amino Acid
Soybeans +			
Barley	76	Lys	Thr
Corn	65	Lys	Thr
Oats	80	Lys	Thr
Rice (brown)	81	Lys	Met & Cys
Rice (polished)	78	Lys	Thr
Rye	75	Lys	Thr
Sorghum	57	Lys	Thr
Triticale	68	Val	Lys
Wheat (whole grain)	69	Lys	Thr
Wheat (flour 70-80%)	58	Lys	Thr
Groundnuts +			
Corn	53	Lys	Try
Oats	66	Lys	Thr
Rice (brown)	68	Lys	Met & Cys
Rice (polished)	65	Lys	Thr
Wheat (whole grain)	55	Lys	Thr
Wheat (flour 70-80%)	44	Lys	Thr

[1]Scores calculated by using the FAO (1973) pattern as the reference pattern.

other sources (beans, corn, rice, and milk) were not statistically different for adult men and women (Clark et al., 1973).

Santos et al. (1979) have also reported on the nutritional efficacy of a rice and bean diet for preschool children at various energy intakes. Nitrogen retention was the highest for a 3000 kcal diet as compared to a 2300 and 1400 kcal intake/day. All three caloric intakes promoted positive nitrogen retention.

Ganapathy et al. (1981) investigated the effect of an all-plant diet which supplied 46 grams of protein/day, primarily as bread made from white wheat flour, and observed lowered plasma albumin values, although all the young men were in positive nitrogen balance. This suggests that a somewhat higher protein intake may be desirable.

Rye is a cereal crop which makes a significant contribution to the diets of some people. Kubiczek, Molski and Rakowska (1976) reported

Table 14. Comparison of Limiting Amino Acids of Cereal:Tuber:Legume Mixtures (1:1:1)

			Mixture		
Cereal	Tuber	Legume	FAO Score[1]	First Limiting Amino Acid	Second Limiting Amino Acid
Barley	Potato	Soybean	80	Met & Cys	Lys
Oats	Potato	Soybean	84	Met & Cys	Lys
Rice (polished)	Potato	Soybean	77	Met & Cys	Lys
Wheat (whole grain)	Cassava	Soybean	79	Thr	Lys
Rye	Yam	Bean	76	Met & Cys	Lys
Sorghum	Cassava	Mung Bean	67	Met & Cys	Thr

[1]Scores calculated by using the FAO (1973) pattern as the reference pattern.

that lysine was the first limiting amino acid in most varieties of rye, with methionine and tryptophan as the next limiting amino acids.

Triticale, which was developed from a cross between wheat and rye, has been of academic interest for over 100 years; however, it has been only within the last 10 to 15 years that its potential usefulness in counteracting undernutrition in some of the developing countries has been evaluated. Triticale is a unique plant that exists as either a hexaploid or an octaploid. Zillinksy in 1973 reviewed its history. The International Maize and Wheat Improvement Center in Mexico has had primary responsibility for the development of improved lines of triticale to combat protein calorie malnutrition. The FAO scoring procedure (Table 6) indicates that lysine is first limiting followed by valine, while the NRC score and EAAL suggest that valine is first limiting with either lysine or isoleucine second limiting.

Sorghum is an economically produced grain in some parts of the world, especially on marginal soil and under poor climatic conditions than other cereals (Peo and Hudman, 1958). Sorghum is the second most important cereal feed grain grown in the United States (Anon., 1975; Rooney and Clark, 1968; Watson, 1959) and it ranked third after rice and wheat as a cereal for human consumption in Asia and second to maize in Africa (Rachie, 1969). Harden et al. (1976) identified lysine and threonine as the first and second limiting amino acids of sorghum as determined in weanling rats.

Much progress has been made in the establishment of protein and amino acid requirements in general terms, much remains to be accomplished in fine tuning needs for specific ages, the influence of sex, activity level, etc. Scrimshaw in 1976 reviewed the international efforts to establish protein requirements and safe allowances for adults using the expert-committee approach. He emphasized that such committees can and do reach inaccurate conclusions, in part due to insufficient knowledge of the relevant literature and may also lack the time to carefully study and evaluate unpublished data presented at the meetings. Also, the committee make-up may be poor. According to Scrimshaw (1976), what was considered a "safe allowance of protein" by an FAO expert-committee in 1971 is now known to be inadequate for long-term maintenance of health in young adults even when energy intakes are wholly adequate or even excessive. Keeping the preceding in mind, one is hopeful that amino acid scoring procedures developed based on amino acid needs will be more accurate than earlier procedures based on whole egg. However, it should be stressed that a single pattern for all ages may not be much better. What must be addressed in future research is the development of several amino acid patterns based on age, sex, and various stresses (both environmental and biological).

Finally, it is important to keep in mind that combinations of plant proteins can be selected to provide high quality protein, especially for adults. For younger children greater care must be taken to assure adequate high quality protein during rapid phases of growth. Hopefully, this paper will stimulate others to evaluate protein combinations for providing high quality protein.

REFERENCES

Abbott, J.C. 1973. The efficient use of world protein supplies. Protein Advisory Group (PAG) Bulletin 3(1): 25-35.

Anonymous. 1975. Research to meet U.S. and World Food Needs. Report of a Working Conference. Agricultural Research Policy Advisory Committee, Kansas City, Missouri, Volume 1, p. 141.

Ashur, S.S., Clark, H.E., Moon, W.H. and Malzer, J.L. 1973. Nitrogen retention of adult human subjects who consumed wheat and rice supplemented with chickpea, sesame, milk, or whey. Am. J. Clin. Nutr. 26: 1195-1201.

Atwater, W.O. 1903. The demands of the body for nourishment and dietary standards. 15th Ann. Rep. Storrs Agr. Exp. Sta., Storrs, Connecticut, p. 123.

Bailey, L.B. and Clark, H.E. 1976. Plasma amino acids and nitrogen retention of human subjects who consumed isonitrogenous diets containing rice and wheat or their constituent amino acids with and without additional lysine. Am. J. Clin. Nutr. 29: 1353-1358.

Block, R.J. and Mitchell, H.H. 1946. The correlation of the amino-acid composition of protein with their nutritive value. Nutr. Abstr. Rev. 16(2): 249-278.

Bressani, R., Navarette, D.A., Elias, L.G. and Braham, J.E. 1979. A critical summary of a short-term nitrogen balance index to measure protein quality in adult human subjects. In "Soy Protein and Human Nutrition," (Eds.) H.L. Wilcke, D.T. Hopskins and D.H. Waggle. Academic Press, New York.

Bricker, M.L., Shively, R.F., Smith, J.M., Mitchell, H.H. and Hamilton, T.S. 1949. The protein requirements of college women on high cereal diets with observations on the adequacy of short balance periods. J. Nutr. 37: 163-.

Briley, M.E., Miles, J. and Longenecker, J.B. 1979. High protein sunflower bread. Nutr. Reports International 19(3): 353-362.

Calloway, D.H. and Margen, S. 1971. Variation in endogenous nitrogen excretion and dietary nitrogen utilization as determinants of human protein requirement. J. Nutr. 101: 205-216.

Calloway, D.H., Colasito, J. and Matthews, R.D. 1966. Gases produced by human intestinal microflora. Nature 212: 1238.

Cavins, J.F., Kwolek, W.F., Inglett, G.E. and Cowan, J.C. 1972. Amino acid analysis of soybean meal: Interlaboratory study JOAC 55(4): 686.

Chavan, J.K. and Duggal, S.K. 1978a. Studies on the essential amino acid composition, protein fractions and biological value (BV) of some new varieties of rice. J. Sci. Fd. Agric. 29: 225-229.

Chavan, J.K. and Duggal, S.K. 1978b. Synergistic effect of different pulses on the protein quality of rice. J. Sci. Fd. Agric. 29: 230-233.

Chen, S.C., Fox, H.M. and Kies, C. 1967. Nitrogenous factors affecting the adequacy of rice to meet the protein requirements of human adults. J. Nutr. 92: 429-434.

Cherry, J.P. 1981. Progress report on topic: Amino acids. Presented at the Sixth Annual Spring Workshop of AOAC, Ottawa, Canada, May 12-14.

Clark, H.E., Howe, J.M. and Lee, C.J. 1971. Nitrogen retention of adult human subjects fed a high protein rice. Am. J. Clin. Nutr. 24: 324-328.

Clark, H.E., Howe, J.M., Magee, J.L. and Malzer, J.L. 1972. Nitrogen balances of adult human subjects who consumed four levels of nitrogen from a combination of rice, milk and wheat. J. Nutr. 102: 1647-1654.

Clark, H.E., Malzer, J.L., Onderka, H.M., Howe, J.M. and Moon, W.H. 1973. Nitrogen balances of adult human subjects fed combinations of wheat, beans, corn, milk, and rice. Am. J. Clin. Nutr. 26: 702-706.

Clark, H.E., Moon, W.H., Malzer, J.L. and Pang, R.L. 1974. Nitrogen retention of young men who consumed between sixteen and eight grams of nitrogen from a combination of rice, wheat, chicken and milk. Am. J. Clin. Nutr. 27: 1059-1064.

Clark, H.E., Moon, W.H., Bailey, L.B. and Panemangelore, M. 1976. Nitrogen retention and plasma amino acids of adults who consumed isonitrogenous diets containing rice and milk or wheat versus their constituent amino acids. Am. J. Clin. Nutr. 29: 1343-1352.

Clark, H.E., Kollenkark, M.A. and Halvorson, J.D. 1978. Ability of 6 grams of nitrogen from a combination of rice, wheat, and milk to meet protein requirements of young men for 4 weeks. Am. J. Clin. Nutr. 31: 585-591.

Costa, G., Ullrich, L., Cantor, F. and Holland, J.F. 1968. Production of elemental nitrogen by certain mammals including man. Nature 218: 546.

FAO. 1970. Amino acid content of foods and biological data on proteins. FAO Nutr. Studies No. 24, Rome, 1970.

FAO. 1973. Energy and protein requirements. Report of a joint FAO/WHO ad hoc expert committee, Rome, March 22-April 2, 1971, FAO, Rome, Italy.

Fomon, S.J. 1959. Comparative study of human milk and a soya bean formula in promoting growth and nitrogen retention by infants. Pediatrics 24: 577-584.

Fomon, S.J. and May, C.D. 1959. The adequacy of soya bean protein in promoting nitrogen retention in infancy. A.M.A.J. Dis. Child. 98: 6-10.

Ganapathy, S.N., Booker, L.K., Craven, R. and Edwards, C.H. 1981. Trace minerals, amino acids, and plasma proteins in adult men fed wheat diets. J. Am. Dietet. A. 78: 490-497.

Hackler, L.R. 1971. Methods of analyses for the sulfur amino acids. Feedstuffs 43, No. 9: 18.

Hackler, L.R. 1974. Amino acid analysis of foods with emphasis on cystine and methionine. Presented at the 34th annual IFT Meeting, New Orleans.

Hackler, L.R. 1977a. Methods of measuring protein quality. A review of bioassay procedures. Cer. Chem. 54: 984-995.

Hackler, L.R. 1977b. In Vitro Indices: Relationships to estimating protein value for the human. In Evaluation of Proteins for Humans, ed. C.E. Bodwell, The AVI Publishing Company, Inc., Westport, Connecticut, 55-67.

Hackler, L.R. 1981. Unpublished data.

Happich, M.L., Bodwell, C.E. and Phillips, J.G. 1981. Collaborative studies of amino acid analyses: A review and preliminary observations from a nine-laboratory study. In "Protein Quality in Humans: Assessment and In Vitro Estimation," (Eds.) C.E. Bodwell, J.S. Adkins and D.T. Hopkins, p. 197. AVI Publishing Company, Inc., Westport Connecticut.

Harden, M.L., Stanaland, R., Briley, M. and Yang, S.P. 1976. The nutritional quality of proteins in sorghum. J. Fd. Sci. 41: 1082-1085.

Hegsted, D.M., Tsongas, A.G., Abbott, D.B. and Stare, F.J. 1946. Protein requirements of adults. J. Lab. Clin. Med. 31: 261.

Howe, J.M., Clark, H.E., Tewell, J.E. and Senchak, M.M. 1972. Nitrogen retention of adults fed six grams of nitrogen from combinations of rice, milk, and wheat. Am. J. Clin. Nutr. 25: 559-563.

Hulse, J.H. 1981. Human implications of protein utilization. In "Utilization of Protein Resources," (Eds.) D.W. Stanley, E.D. Murray and D.H. Lees. Food and Nutrition Press, Inc., Westport, Connecticut.

Hulse, J.H. and Laing, E.M. 1974. Nutritive Value of Triticale Protein. International Development Research Centre, Ottawa, Canada.

Irwin, M.I. 1980. Nutritional Requirements of Man: A Conspectus of Research. Published by The Nutrition Foundation, Washington, D.C.

Irwin, M.I. and Hegsted, D.M. 1971. A conspectus of research on protein requirements of man. J. Nutr. 101: 385-430.

Jank, J., Kies, C. and Fox, H.M. 1981. Protein nutritional status of human subjects fed wheat and rice bran supplemented diets. Nutr. Reports International 24(3): 581-589.

Kies, C. 1979. Comparison of human and animal studies at Nebraska. In "Soy Protein and Human Nutrition," (Eds.) H.L. Wilcke, D.T. Hopkins and D.H. Waggle. Academic Press, New York.

Kies, C., Fox, H.M. and Williams, E.R. 1967. Effect of nonspecific nitrogen supplementation on minimum corn protein requirement and first-limiting amino acid for adult men. J. Nutr. 92: 377-383.

Kies, C. and Fox, H.M. 1970. Effect of level of total nitrogen intake on second limiting amino acid in corn for humans. J. Nutr. 100: 1275-1286.

Kies, C. and Fox, H.M. 1972. Protein nutritional value of opaque-2 corn grain for human adults. J. Nutr. 102: 757-766.

Kjeldahl, J. 1883. Z. Analyt. Chem. 22: 366-382.

Knipfel, J.E., Aitken, J.R., Hill, D.C., McDonald, B.E. and Owen, B.D. 1971. Amino acid composition of food proteins: Inter- and intra-laboratory variation. J. Assoc. Offic. Agr. Chem. 54: 777.

Kubiczek, R., Molski, B. and Rakowska, M. 1976. Amino acids limiting the nutritional value of rye grain protein. FSTA 8(10): 127.

Lee, C.J., Howe, J.M., Carlson, K. and Clark, H.E. 1971. Nitrogen retention of young men fed rice with or without supplementary chicken. Am. J. Clin. Nutr. 24: 318-323.

Lorenz, K. and Lee, V.A. 1977. The nutritional and physiological impact of cereal products in human nutrition. CRC Crit. Rev. Food Sci. Nutr. March, 1977, pp. 383-456.

Maclean, W.C., Jr., Lopez de Romana, G. and Graham, G.G. 1976. Protein quality of high protein wheats in infants and children. J. Nutr. 106: 362-370.

Mattern, P.J. 1984. Role of plant breeders in improving food supplies. Cereal Foods World 29(4): 243-245.

Mitchell, H.H. 1954. The dependence of the biological value of food proteins upon their content of essential amino acids. Wiss. Abhandl. Deut. Akad. Landwirtschaftwiss. Berlin. Band V/2: 279.

Moore, S. and Stein, W.H. 1963. Chromatographic determination of amino acids by the use of automatic recording equipment. In "Methods in Enzymology," Vol. 6, (Eds.) S.P. Colowick and N.O. Kaplan. Academic Press, New York.

NRC. 1980. Recommended Dietary Allowances. Ninth Revised Edition. Nutrition Research Council, National Academy of Sciences, Washington, D.C.

Navarette, D.A. and Bressani, R. 1981. Protein digestibility and protein quality of common beans (Phaseolus vulgaris) fed alone and with maize, in adult humans using a short-term nitrogen balance assay. Am. J. Clin. Nutr. 34: 1893-1898.

Nicol, B.M. and Phillips, P.G. 1978. The utilization of proteins and amino acids in diets based on cassava (Manihot utilissima), rice or sorghum (Sorghum sativa) by young Nigerian men of low income. Br. J. Nutr. 39(2): 271-287.

Obizoba, I.C., Ezekwe, M.O. and Akaigwe, B.N. 1979. Utilization of sorghum, wheat, and navy beans by human adults: protein metabolism. Nutr. Reports International 20(3): 291-301.

Obizoba, I.C. 1980. Comparative evaluation of nitrogen, mineral and vitamin utilization of human adults fed mixed protein diets supplemented with waxy and nonwaxy sorghum. Nutr. Reports International 22(4): 529-538.

Peo, E.R. and Hudman, D.B. 1958. Grain sorghum for growing-finishing swine. J. An. Sci. 17: 813-818.

Phansalkar, S.V. and Patwardhan, V.N. 1956. Utilization of animal and vegetable proteins. Nitrogen balances of marginal protein intakes and the determination of minimum protein requirements for maintenance in young Indian men. Ind. J. Med. Res. 44: 1.

Rachie, K.O. 1969. Sorghum grain: It's worldwide significance and potential. Cereal Sci. Today 14(8): 271-276.

Rooney, L.W. and Clark, L.E. 1968. The chemistry and processing of sorghum grain. Cereal Sci. Today 13(7): 258.

Rose, W.C. 1938. The nutritive significance of the amino acids. Physiol. Rev. 18: 109.

Santos, J.E.D., Howe, J.M., Duarte, F.A.M. and Oliveira, J.E.D. de. 1979. Relationship between the nutritional efficacy of a rice and bean diet and energy intake in preschool children. Am. J. Clin. Nutr. 32: 1541-1544.

Sarwar, G., Christensen, D.A., Finlayson, A.J., Friedmen, M., Hackler, L.R., Mackenzie, S.L., Pellitt, P.L. and Tkachuk, R. 1983. Inter- and Intra-Laboratory variation in amino acid analysis of food proteins. J. Food Sci. 48: 526-531.

Scrimshaw, N.S. 1976a. Shattuck Lecture--Strengths and weaknesses of the committee approach. An analysis of past and present recommended dietary allowances for protein in health and disease. N. Engl. J. Med. 294(3): 136-142.

Scrimshaw, N.S. 1976b. Shattuck Lecture--Strengths and weaknesses of the committee approach. An analysis of past and present recommended dietary allowances for protein in health and disease. N. Engl. J. Med. 294(4): 198-203.

Scrimshaw, N.S. and Young, V.R. 1979. Soy protein in adult human nutrition: A review with new data. In "Soy Protein and Human Nutrition," (Eds.) H.L. Wilcke, D.T. Hopkins, and D.H. Waggle. Academic Press, New York.

Seligson, F.H. and Mackey, L.N. 1984. Variable predictions of protein quality by chemical score due to amino acid analysis and reference pattern. J. Nutr. 114: 682-691.

Shukla, T.P. 1975. Cereal proteins: Chemistry and food applications. Crit. Rev. Food Sci. Nutr. 6: 1-75.

Tamura, E., Nishihara, A., Isobe, S. and Matsuno, N. 1958. Studies on the determination of amino acids (Report 1) on the hydrolysis-time of protein and the effect of carbohydrate and changes of the hydrosylate during storage. In Annual Report of the National Institute of Nutrition, Toyanako, Tokyo.

Unver, B., Kies, C. and Fox, H.M. 1981. Niacin/pantothenic acid/protein interrelationships affecting the nutritive values of winter wheat for humans. Nutr. Reports International 23(5): 841-852.

Voit, C. 1876. Uber die Kost in offentlichen Anstalten. Z. Biol. 12: 1.

Wall, J.S. and Paulis, J.W. 1978. Corn and sorghum grain proteins. Advances in Cereal Science and Technology 2: 135-219.

Watson, S.A. 1959. Grain sorghums. Cereal Sci. Today 4(8): 230-233.

Williams, A.P., Hewitt, D. and Cockburn, J.E. 1979. A collaborative study on the determination of cyst(e)ine in feedingstuffs. J. Sci. Fd. Agric. 30: 469-474.

Wu, V.Y. 1982. Lysine content of triticale protein increased by germination. J. Agric. Fd. Chem. 30: 820-823.

Young, V.R. and Scrimshaw, N.S. 1968. Endogenous nitrogen metabolism and plasma free amino acids in young adults given a "protein-free" diet. Brit. J. Nutr. 22: 9.

Zillinsky, F.J. 1973. Triticale breeding and research at CIMMYT. Research Bulletin No. 24. Centro Internacional de Mejoramiento de Maiz y Trigo, Mexico 6.

NOTE

[1]Many investigators, according to Atwater (1903), have misrepresented his data and have listed 125 grams as the daily need for protein as the value comparable to Voit's 118 g/day and this has continued in articles on protein needs since 1903.

PART 2

METHODOLOGY OF PROTEIN QUALITY EVALUATION

Proc. Int. Assoc. Cereal Chem. Symp. Amino Acid Compn and Biol. Value of Cereal Proteins
Budapest, Hungary 1983, R. Lásztity, M. Hidvégi, eds

PROTEIN NUTRITIONAL QUALITY: A MODELING APPROACH

L. PRESTON MERCER, J. M. GUSTAFSON, S. J. DODDS

Department of Biochemistry, School of Medicine, Oral Roberts University, Tulsa, OK 74133, USA

ABSTRACT

The protein efficiency ratio (PER) is the official method for protein quality evaluation in the United States and Canada. Two other widely used indices of evaluation are the slope ratio (SR) and net protein ratio (NPR) methods. Each of these methods has problems associated with its calculation and interpretation. In this paper, a new index, actual protein utilization (APU), is discussed and its relationship to the other indices is examined. Each of the indices of protein quality evaluation is given a theoretical basis by relating it to the four parameter mathematical model for physiological responses. The derivation of the four parameter model is given, along with its mathematical and physiological significance. To compare the indices, growth bioassays were carried out using male rats (40g, 60g, 115g) consuming three different proteins, casein, lactalbumin, and soy and an amino acid mixture. Dose-response curves were generated for each diet, and the indices PER, NPR, SLOPE, and APU were calculated. APU was shown to have ~~certain~~ characteristics which make it superior to the other methods of protein quality evaluation, i.e., it closely approximates the growth response curve and it incorporates a term for the protein intake required for maintenance.

TABLE OF CONTENTS

Section VI	Protein Efficiency Ratio (PER), Net Protein Ratio (NPR), Slope Ratio and Their Maxima as Defined by the Four Parameter Model
Section VII	A New Protein Quality Index - Actual Protein Utilization (APU)
Section VIII	A Comparative Analysis of APU, PER, NPR, and Slope Ratio
Section IX	Conclusion

I. Introduction to protein quality evaluation

The ability to assess the nutritional quality of proteins has been a challenging one. The lack of consensus on protocol for an accurate and practical method has produced a number of various methods in the last ninety years. A sample of protein quality evaluation methods is shown in Table 1.

The criteria of a valid protein quality bioassay involve precision, reproducibility, proportionality to protein quality, low cost and simplicity to perform. The great number of methods and indices that exist are all attempts at fulfilling these criteria. Some methods fit these criteria better than others, but there is no general consensus as to which method is the most useful indicator of protein quality. Discussions of the strengths and weaknesses of many of these methods are found in numerous papers and symposia on proteins (Hegsted, 1965; McLaughlan, 1980; Elliott, 1983; Bender, 1982; McLaughlan, 1971; Hegsted, 1971; Scrimshaw, 1971).

Our objectives are to provide a biological model with a theoretical basis which can be used to unify existing methods of protein quality evaluation, and to suggest a new method which will more closely fit the criteria of a valid bioassay. One problem with many of the current attempts to determine the quality of a protein is that they lack a conceptual framework relating physiological responses to nutrients in the diet. The relationship between growth response (for example) and the concentration of nutrient in the diet is complex. It involves the three factors (or dimensions) of time (t), weight gain (dW/dt) and food intake (dF/dt). These three dimensions combine to describe an organism's "growth phase plane" (Parks, 1982). It is difficult to define a specific location on an organism's "growth phase plane" with a single observation. However, that is what many protein quality evaluation procedures attempt to do. PER is an example of a single point measurement in which the total weight gain of an organism is divided (at a specified t) by its protein intake, to give an efficiency ratio. The slope ratio method, which is the linear regression of weight gain as a function of dietary protein concentration, approximates the growth phase plane with a straight line. However, we have shown that a sigmoidal curve gives a better representation of the relationship between physiological response and dietary nutrient concentration (Fig. 1).

TABLE 1

A sample of protein quality evaluation indices

Index	Method
PER "protein efficiency ratio": (Osborne et al., 1919)	The weight gain divided by the protein intake.
NPR "net protein ratio": (Bender and Doell, 1957)	The weight gain of test group plus the weight loss of non-protein group divided by the protein consumed.
BV "biological value": (Thomas, 1909) (Mitchell and Carmen, 1929)	The percent of absorbed nitrogen retained. The biological value is equal to the nitrogen retained divided by the nitrogen absorbed.
Slope-ratio assay "relative growth index": (Hegsted and Chang, 1965)	The slope of the regression between the percent of the protein in the diet and the weight gain as a percentage of the slope obtained with a protein of maximal nutritive value.
NGI "nitrogen growth index"" (Allison, 1959)	This method is based on the difference in growth at two protein levels divided by the difference in the amount of protein consumed.
NBI "nitrogen balance index": (Allison and Anderson, 1945)	Tangent of the curve relating the N balance to the absorbed N.
NU "nitrogen utilization value": (McLaughlan, 1976)	The weight change in 14 days plus 10 percent of initial and final weights to allow for maintenance of nitrogen.
RNU "relative nitrogen utilization value": (McLaughlan, 1976)	NU expressed as a percentage of lactalbumin.
RNPR "relative net protein ratio": (McLaughlan et al., 1980)	NPR compared to a reference protein, usually the protein with the highest biological value.
RPV "relative protein value": (Samonds and Hegsted, 1977)	Regression line of dose vs. response for test protein compared with reference protein omitting zero protein level.

This paper will examine the most widely used indices, PER, NPR and Slope Ratio and will suggest a new index, Actual Protein Utilization (APU).

II. A model for quantitative nutrient-response relationships

Equation (1) gives the mathematical relationship for the four parameter mathematical model for physiological relationships.

$$r = \frac{b(K.5)^n + Rmax(I)^n}{(K.5)^n + (I)^n} \qquad \text{Equation (1)}$$

Where:

r = physiological response
I = nutrient intake or concentration in the diet
b = intercept on the r axis
Rmax = maximum response
n = apparent kinetic order
K.5 = intake for ½(Rmax+b)

This equation, which we have applied to quantitative nutrient response relationships, has evolved in numerous steps from the work of Gulderg and Waage in 1863. Guldberg and Waage established that chemical equilibrium is a dynamic--not static--condition. In the "Law of Mass Action," they state that the rate of the forward reaction is proportional to the concentrations of reactants (1867). Arrhenius contributed the idea of an "active mass" or active complex in 1889. This "active mass" concept was applied to the equilibrium of chemical reactions in solution and the study of rates (1889). O'Sullivan and Tompson in 1890 confirmed the theory that enzymes follow the law of mass action. A further advance in understanding the rates of biological systems came from Brown in 1902 when he proposed the concept of an (Enzyme-Substrate) intermediate. Brown states, "High levels of substrate will cause no further increase in the rate of formation of products" (1902).

With the mechanisms proposed and the available data that existed, Henri, in 1903, took the qualitative explanation of the course of enzyme reactions and presented a rate equation (1903).

$$Vo = \frac{Ks(So)}{Ks + (So)} \qquad \text{Equation (2)}$$

Henri established that the velocity (Vo) is proportional to the enzyme concentration and that initial velocities increase up to a point, but not proportionally to the substrate concentration (So), and then level off.

An extension of Henri's work came from Michaelis and Menten in 1913. Michaelis and Menten equated the total enzyme concentration times rate of the forward reaction with Vmax and were able to determine that K_s = So at vo = ½ Vmax. The rate equation took on the form of:

$$Vo = \frac{Vmax[So]}{Ks + [So]} \qquad \text{Equation (3)}$$

In 1925 Briggs and Haldane derived the same equation by assuming a steady state condition rather than equilibrium (1925). This verified the use of Vmax for the limiting velocity and K_s for the substrate concentration at half maximal velocity.

To use enzyme kinetics for the purpose of describing a physiological response of the whole organism, two other parameters (besides Vmax and K_s) had to be developed in order for the model to accurately represent the data. The first consideration was that not all enzyme kinetic studies are conducted under conditions in which the enzymic sites are independent from each other. In an integrated physiological process they will probably be dependent on each other. This interdependence has been investigated by Hill. In 1952 Hill proposed a simplified velocity equation for allosteric enzymes with multiple substrate sites.

$$\frac{v}{Vmax} = \frac{S^n}{Ks + S^n} \qquad \text{Equation (4)}$$

With the addition of n to the rate equation, the model had the freedom to vary sigmoidally in response to any selected physiological parameter that may be used. The second consideration involved the origin of the response. In an organism, one does not start with zero substrate and zero enzyme concentration. Therefore, it becomes necessary to use a rate equation that can be directed by the nature of the response to zero nutrient at some fixed time, i.e., a constant must be added to the rate equation which allows the model to fit any range of responses that would occur at zero nutrient concentration (Mercer, 1975). This factor is "b" as defined in Equation (1). The foundation of the proposed model is based on the theory that physiological responses to nutrients are governed by enzyme kinetics.

It follows that enzymes or receptor sites that behave allosterically and which involve mass action, active complexes, and enzyme-nutrient intermediates will control the intact organism in the same way. Rates associated with the enzyme-nutrient-macromolecular interactions of the digestive, absorption, distribution, metabolic and excretory systems can be said to contribute to the kinetics of the physiological response. All of these interactions exist in discrete, steady-states of growth. Therefore, enzyme-mediated growth responses will be governed by the allosteric interactions of multiple, interdependent enzyme-substrate site systems, which can be followed by the rates determined by the four parameter model.

III. The biological basis of the four-parameter model

Almost every aspect of nutrient utilization is mediated by specific interaction with a macromolecule such as an enzyme. If one assumes that there is a rate-limiting step in a sequence of enzymatically-mediated reactions, then the appearance of response would be a function of the rate-limiting step. Such a rate-limiting step has been postulated by Almquist (1970).

The interaction of the nutrient with a specific site on the macromolecule (receptor) would give rise to a physiological response and the magnitude of the response would be directly proportional to the number of receptors occupied by nutrient. This concept allows one to apply the law of mass action to the system and derive an appropriate equation governing the quantitative relationship between nutrient and response.

In the following example, a nutrient, I, combines with a receptor, M, to yield the complex MI which produces the physiological response pr in a manner proportional to concentration of MI.

$$I + M \underset{k_2}{\overset{k_1}{\rightleftharpoons}} MI$$

$$pr = K_3[MI]$$

(where k_1, k_2, and k_3 are constants and [ ] denotes concentration).

Then at equilibrium,

$$\frac{[M][I]}{[MI]} = \frac{k_2}{k_1} = K_I$$

(where K_I is also a constant)

Next, we define M_T as the total receptor concentration so that $[M_T] = [M] + [MI]$, then

$$\frac{[M_T - MI][I]}{[MI]} = K_I$$

Rearrangement gives

$$\frac{[MI]}{[M_T]} = \frac{[I]}{K_I + [I]}$$

If PRmax is the maximal physiological response of the system when all receptors are occupied

$$PRmax = K_3[M_T]$$

then

$$\frac{pr}{PRmax} = \frac{[MI]}{[M_T]}$$

and

$$pr = \frac{PRmax[I]}{K_I + [I]}$$

This equation is identical to the Michaelis-Menten equation and it meets the criteria of observed phenomena; that is, continuous response to graded levels of nutrient intake and the Law of Diminishing Returns.

However, the equation has two limitations as discussed earlier which do not coincide with observed responses. First, the equation only describes a hyperbola, while many responses are found experimentally to be sigmoidal in nature (Mercer, 1980a). This problem may be overcome by adding a new parameter to the equation, n.

$$pr = \frac{PRmax[I]^n}{K_I + [I]^n}$$

This allows the equation to vary from a hyperbola to a sigmoid as n increases above 1.

The second limitation is that the equation describes a curve which passes through the point (0,0) of a coordinate system. This would not allow the prediction of responses such as weight loss, etc. Adding one parameter, b, removes this restriction.

$$pr = \frac{PRmax[I]^n}{K_I + [I]^n} + b$$

Rearrangement gives

$$pr = \frac{PRmax[I]^n + bK_I + bI^n}{K_I + [I]^n}$$

If we let (PRmax + b) = Rmax and simplify pr to r, we have the four-parameter mathematical model for physiological responses (Mercer, 1982).

$$r = \frac{bK_I + Rmax[I]^n}{K_I + [I]^n} \qquad \text{Equation (5)}$$

This can be more conveniently written in the form of Equation (1). This formulation does away with K_I which is only equal to K.5 when n = 1 and otherwise has no physical meaning. The extent of perturbation of the system is given, not by Rmax, but (Rmax-b).

Equation (1), based on nutrient-macromolecular interactions, is sufficient to describe the complete range of response to a nutrient as long as the rate-limiting step does not change. It also becomes possible to calculate the slope of the response curve and the efficiency of the response at any intake level. However, two particular intake levels of interest are the intake at maximum slope (Ims) and the intake of maximum efficiency (Ime).

$$Ime = K.5(n - 1)^{1/n} \qquad \text{Equation (6)}$$

$$Ims = K.5\left(\frac{n - 1}{n + 1}\right)^{1/n} \qquad \text{Equation (7)}$$

These two intakes represent the point at which the organism is operating most efficiently in terms of production of response (Ime) and the point at which the organism is most sensitive to the nutrient and changes in its intake (Ims). Both intakes depend on K.5 and n and are independent of b or Rmax. If n is < 1, there is no maximum slope or efficiency. Calculation of these two intake levels also allows calculation of the responses at these intakes r(Ime) and r(Ims).

One other useful parameter which can be calculated is the intake of zero response, Iro. Of course, this is only possible if $b < 0$.

$$\text{Iro} = \text{K.5}\left(\frac{-b}{\text{Rmax}}\right)^{1/n} \qquad \text{Equation (8)}$$

The four-parameter mathematical model derived from molecular interactions taking place in the framework of a theoretical model discussed earlier in the paper assumes that the organism in an open system (thermodynamically) and is in a dynamic steady-state equilibrium. Problems may arise if the system is in a growing steady state (Grainger, 1966). For example, catalyzed reactions can slow down or become inhibited if the catalyst-to-reactant ratio is raised (Kon, 1978). This is possible during the growth of an organism or induction of an enzyme system. However, the successful application of the four-parameter model would indicate that these problems are not serious in many instances.

As stated earlier, there are actually three variables in a typical nutrition experiment which must be taken into account. These are intake level, response, and time course. A two-dimensional relationship, therefore, requires that one of these variables be held constant. The four-parameter model assumes a constant time at which responses are measured. This is a very important consideration when parameters are compared from experiment to experiment. Thus, quantitation is meaningful only when the time element is specified. The variation of the four parameters with time has been discussed in previously published work (Mercer, 1981).

A quantitative mathematical relationship produces numerical indices of characterization which give new insight into the utilization of a nutrient. For example, establishing a minimum response (b) and maximum response (Rmax) is useful in a time of nutritional extremism such as high protein diets, low carbohydrate diets, and megavitamin therapy. These parameters establish limits on the efficacy of a nutrient in promoting a desired response. The predicted curve also promotes a uniform approach to quantitation of need, by specifying (for example) an intake level which produces a response of 95% Rmax. K.5 is the parameter which directly relates intake to response and is characteristic of the reacting system for a particular nutrient. Since K.5 is the intake of one-half maximum response, it indicates exactly where the degree of saturation of the reacting lies. Even if intake were increased to 100 times K.5, response could do no more than double. Each of these parameters is useful in characterizing the nutrient-response relationship.

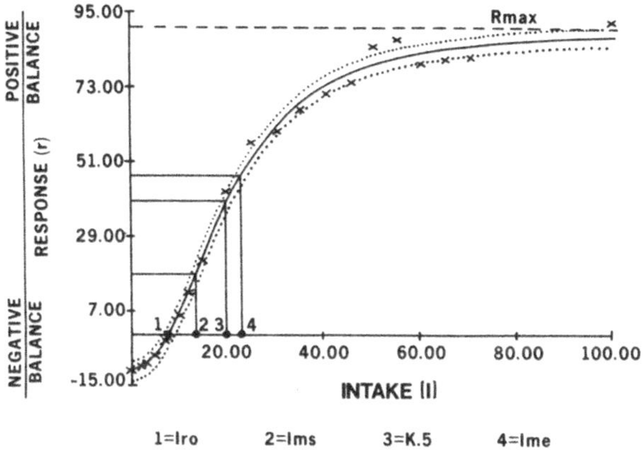

Fig. 1 Idealized nutrient-response curve generated by the four parameter mathematical model for physiological responses (Equation 1). Parameters from the curve are given in Table 2.

An idealized nutrient-response curve is shown in Figure 1. This figure demonstrates the general characteristics of the nutrient-response relationship. The four parameters (and therefore the shape of the curve) would vary for each nutrient-response relationship, but each would have K.5, Ims, etc. Figure 1 shows the computer-fit data for a curve in which Rmax = 90, K.5 = 20, n = 2.5, and b = -10. Each response arbitrarily had ±5% added by random to show average variance around the curve. Use of a weighted regression would show larger limits around Rmax and smaller limits around b. Each "x" represents one observation and the dotted lines are the 95% confidence limits.

Each observation ("x") on the curve represents a steady state equilibrium achieved by the animal based on the limiting nutrient represented by "I." All "x's" above the I axis are in positive balance with the environment and all "x's" below the I axis are in negative balance, based on the initial conditions of the experiments. For example, if r is weight change/day, I>Iro promotes positive balance or weight gain while I<Iro promotes negative balance or weight loss.

As the response approaches Rmax, the concentration of nutrient causing that response becomes less limiting until any limitation on response passes to some other nutrient or to some non-nutritional source such as the organism's genetic potential. Of course, nutritional responses are multifactorial in their cause, but experiments may be designed to test one component at a time (Mercer, 1980a).

Although several non-linear curve-fitting programs are available and satisfactory for fitting the four-parameter model, we have used a Gauss-Newton method based on the BMDX 85 program of the UCLA computer center.

This procedure gives rapid convergence when there are good starting estimates available for the four parameters (program available from author).

The results of fitting the idealized data to the model are shown in Table 2 and Figure 1.

TABLE 2
Parameters[1] calculated from intake-response curve (Fig. 1)

Parameter	Value ± SD
Rmax	90.27 ± 2.52
K.5	20.10 ± 0.79
n	2.34 ± 0.19
b	-10.39 ± 1.74
Iro	7.99
[2]RSQ	99.45
Ims	13.62
[3]r(Ims)	18.45
[4]Slope (Ims)	3.54
Ime	22.79
[3]r(Ime)	47.29
[4]Efficiency (Ime)	2.53

[1]Parameters are defined in text. [2] RSQ = sum of squares (regression)/sum of squares (total). [3]Calculated response at Ims and Ime. [4]Calculated slope and efficiency at Ims and Ime.

IV. Amino acid data: description of the four-parameter model

Forty-eight male, weanling Sprague-Dawley rats were divided into seven groups of six rats each with mean weights of 40 ± 2g. Rats were individually housed in suspended, wire-bottom cages with food and deionized water available ad libitum and 12-hour cycles of light and dark. Rats were fed a diet described in Table 3. The amino acid mixture used was the formulation described by Rogers and Harper (1965). The groups received the following amounts of amino acid mix: Group 1, 0%; Group 2, 2%; Group 3, 5%; Group 4, 10%; Group 5, 15%; Group 6, 20%; Group 7, 25%; Group 8, 30%.

Since reagent grade amino acids were used, nitrogen was not measured. Weight gains were measured every other day for 21 days. Daily weight gains were calculated as previously described (Mercer, 1979). At the end of the experiment, rats were killed by anesthetization with diethyl ether followed by exsanguination through the abdominal aorta. Liver, spleen, heart, and lung were removed and weighed. We have previously reported a comprehensive study of organ weights (Mercer, 1980a).

Results were analyzed by use of the four parameter mathematical model for physiological responses. Groups were placed on diets so that good estimates of the extremes of the response curve could be made (i.e., zero dose, "plateau" dose, and doses on the ascending part of the curve). Since we are using a four-parameter model, at least five doses must be used for statistical analysis. We have found that six or seven strategically chosen doses will suffice to give good definition to the theoretical curve.

Table 4 shows the results of the feeding experiment. Each response listed could be predicted as a systemic, continuous response to graded levels of amino acids in the diet. Each curve reflects the "Law of Diminishing Returns" and is similar to the idealized curve shown in Figure 1. Each response curve can be reconstructed using the four parameters which characterize it.

The K.5 values for these responses are very close (7.04 ± 0.37%). In a previous paper (Mercer, 1980b), we showed that liver remained a constant proportion of body weight, spleen increased, and heart and lung decreased their proportion of body weight in a similar experiment. Even though these organs vary in their relationship to the total body weight, the similarities in K.5 indicate in a single rate limiting step in their growth.

TABLE 3
Composition of the diets - Experiment 1

Component	%
Mineral mix	4.00
Cottonseed oil	8.80
Vitamin mix	2.20
Cellulose	2.00
Cornstarch + protein or Amino Acid mix	83.00

TABLE 4
Parameters calculated from feeding rats graded levels of amino acids

Parameter	Wt gains	Liver	Spleen	Heart	Lung
Rmax, g	7.95	10.55	0.66	1.04	1.47
K_5, %	7.07	6.80	7.68	6.95	6.73
n	3.87	3.71	3.32	3.24	3.44
b, g	-0.08	2.53	0.12	0.33	0.52
Iro,. %	2.15	----	----	----	----
RSQ	99.44	97.67	99.77	97.94	98.85
Ims, %	6.17	5.86	6.35	5.71	3.65
r(lms)	2.90	5.46	0.31	0.57	0.86
Slope (Ims)	1.18	1.18	0.06	0.09	0.13
Ime, %	9.28	8.90	9.86	8.92	8.72
r(Ime)	5.88	8.39	0.49	0.82	1.19
Efficiency (Ime)	0.64	0.66	0.04	0.05	0.08

[1]Parameters are defined in the text.

V. Protein data used for theoretical discussion of the protein quality indices

Experiment 1. Forty-two male Sprague-Dawley rats were divided into seven groups of six each weighing 115 ± 6g. Rats were fed graded levels of casein (%, N x 6.25): Group 1, 0.0%; group 2, 1.6; group 3, 4.0; group 4, 8.0; group 5, 12.0; group 6, 16.8; group 7, 22.4. Casein was added at the expense of cornstarch. The remainder of the diets were added as described in Table 3. Rats were individually housed in suspended, wire-bottom cages with food and water (reverse osmosis) available ad libitum. Light cycles were 12 hours on and 12 hours off. Weight gains and food intakes were measured every other day for three weeks.

Experiment 2. Forty-eight male Sprague-Dawley rats were divided into eight groups of six each, weighing 60 ± 3g. Rats were fed graded levels of an amino acid mixture described by Rogers and Harper (1965): group 1, 0%; group 2, 2; group 3, 5; group 4, 10; group 5, 15; group 6, 20; group 7, 25; group 8, 30. Amino acids were added at the expense of cornstarch. Other components of the diet were added as described in Table 3. The rats were housed and monitored as described in Experiment 1.

Experiment 3. One hundred eighty male, weanling (21 day) Sprague-Dawley rats (Charles River) were divided into groups of six weighing 40 ± 2g. Ten groups were fed graded levels of soy protein (%, N x 6.25): group 1, 1.44%; group 2, 2.88; group 3, 4.32; group 4, 7.20; group 5, 10.08; group 6, 12.24; group 7, 14.40; group 8, 18.72; group 9, 24.48; group 10, 28.8. Nine groups were fed graded levels of casein: group 1, 1.63%; group 2, 3.26; group 3, 4.88; group 4, 8.14; group 5, 9.77; group 6, 11.82; group 7, 14.65; group 8, 17.09; group 9, 22.79. Ten groups were fed graded levels of lactalbumin: group 1, .744%; group 2, 1.86; group 3, 2.98; group 4, 4.46; group 5, 6.32; group 6, 8.93; group 7, 11.90; group 8, 14.88; group 9, 17.85; group 10, 20.83. The remainder of the diets were formulated as shown in Table 3. One group was fed zero protein. All protein was added at the expense of cornstarch. Rats were housed and monitored as described in Experiment 1.

Data analysis. Daily weight gain rates (dW/dt) and food intake rates (dF/dt) were calculated as follows:

$$W = (dW/dt)t + W_o$$

$$F = (dF/dt)t + F_o$$

where W is live weight and F is cumulative food intake at time t. Wo and Fo are initial conditions. The resulting values (slopes) were fitted to the four parameter mathematical model for physiological responses: dF/dt vs % protein, dW/dt vs % protein, and dW/dt vs dP/dt (daily protein intake) where dP/dt is equal to dF/dt multiplied by % protein in diet. The four parameter model is given in Equation (1).

The data from Experiment 1 is used for the following theoretical discussion and is shown in Figures 2-8.

VI. PER, NPR, slope ratio and their maxima as defined by the four parameter model

PER

Protein Efficiency Ratio is calculated as weight gain (g)/protein intake (g). Therefore, using the four parameters, a smooth theoretical PER curve can be calculated (Fig. 5). In this study, r = dW/dt and I = dP/dt so PER is given by Equation (9).

$$PER = r/I = dW/dP \qquad \text{Equation (9)}$$

PERmax (maximum value achieved by PER curve) is calculated as the tangent of the angle between the I axis and a line drawn from (0,0) to a point tangent to the response curve (Fig. 5). The intake (I) for PERmax can be calculated using the quadratic equation and is given by Equation (10).

$$IPERmax = ((-B+(B^2-4AC)^{\frac{1}{2}})/2A)^{1/n}) \qquad \text{Equation (10)}$$

where:
$A = Rmax/(K.5)^n$
$B = Rmax(1-n) + b(1+n)$
$C = b(K.5)^n$

One can then calculate the corresponding r for IPERmax (using Equation (1)). This then allows calculation of the maximum value achieved by the PER response, PERmax.

NPR

Net Protein Ratio is calculated as [weight gain (g) - weight loss on zero protein (g)]/protein intake (g). A smooth theoretical curve can be calculated for NPR (using the four parameters) by using Equation (11) (Fig. 6).

$$NPR = (r-b)/I \qquad \text{Equation (11)}$$

The formula giving the intake (I) for NPRmax can be derived from Equation (1) and is given in Equation (12). Using this value of I, one can then calculate the corresponding r and NPRmax.

$$INPRmax = K._5(n-1)^{1/n} \qquad \text{Equation (12)}$$

NPRmax is the tangent of the angle between a line drawn parallel to the I axis through b and a line from (0,b) through the point of tangency to the response curve (Fig. 6).

Slope

The slope of the growth response curve at any I can be calculated by taking the first derivative of Equation (1) (Fig. 7). This is given in Equation (13). The first derivative is a smooth curve with a maximum value at the point of inflection of the response curve (Fig. 7).

$$SLOPE = \frac{(Rmax-b)\ (n(K.5)^n\ I^{n-1})}{(K.5^n + I^n)^2} \qquad \text{Equation (13)}$$

The intake (I) for maximum slope is given by Equation 7.

The value of SLOPEmax is then solved by substituting ISLOPEmax into Equation (13), and using the four parameters derived from Equation (1).

In Experiment 1, rats larger than those accepted by Methods of Analysis - AOAC (1980) for PER determinations were used to show greater displacement (positive and negative) from maintenance, thereby giving a clearer picture of the geometry of the calculations. Figures 2 and 3 show the relationship between food intake (dF/dt), weight gain (dW/dt) and percent casein in the diet. Since PER as well as other indices are usually determined in the 5-10% protein range, this figure shows that weight gain is adversely affected in that range while food intake is approaching saturation. If the response curve reflects only the limiting amino acid as stated by Bender (1982), changes in protein level (from 5 to 10%) may reflect changes in the limiting amino acid, thereby confusing results (1982). Also, impairment of growth may reflect other conditions which complicate interpretation of results. Construction of a "dose-response" curve (% vs. response) allows one to ascertain where the rats are in their growth phase plane so that one can judge the specific limitation mentioned by Elliott and McClure, i.e., that results of a PER assay are positively correlated to food intake and weight gain (1983).

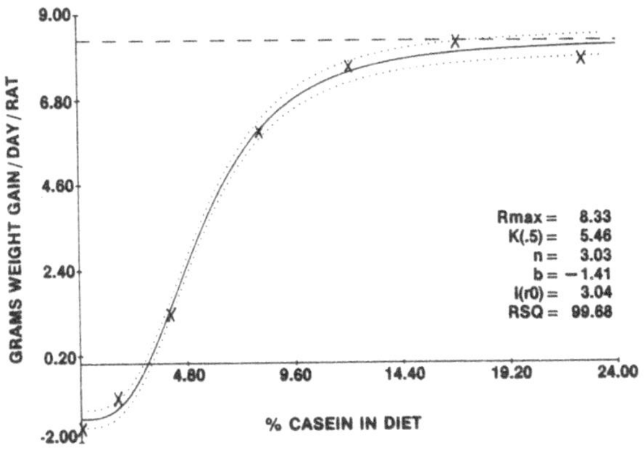

Fig. 2 Weight gain as a function of dietary casein level. Each "x" is the mean of six rats. Dotted lines are 95% confidence limits. Solid line is theoretical response curve (Experiment 1).

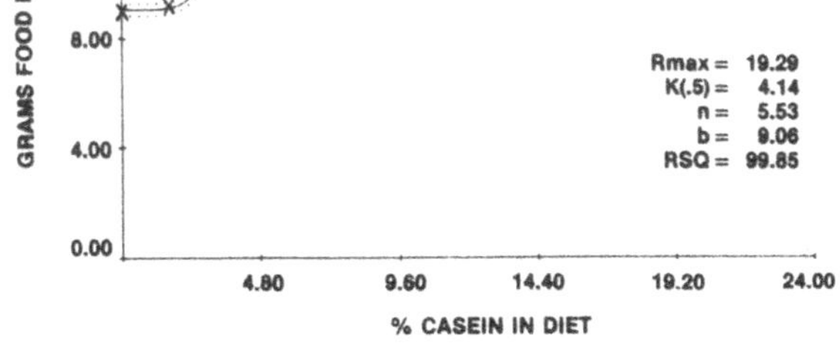

Fig. 3 Food intake as a function of dietary casein level. Each "x" is the mean of six rats. Dotted lines are 95% confidence limits. Solid line is theoretical response curve (Experiment 1).

In Figure 4 the theoretical intake-response curve is displayed by showing weight gain as a function of actual protein intake rather than concentration of protein in the diet. This curve represents the basis for protein quality evaluation indices since it represents weight gain/protein intake. To construct this curve, we used dW/dt vs dP/dt rather than Wtot/Ptot. This avoids daily fluctuations of weight and intake through utilization of a measurement that establishes a trend (slope) over the length of the experiment rather than a total weight or total protein intake measured at a single point in time. The outcome, however, gives the familiar result since dW/dt/dP/dt = dW/dP thereby producing the same units as a standard PER measurement. While there are more complex functions for dW/dt and dF/dt (Parks, 1982), the linear functions work well for short term experiments.

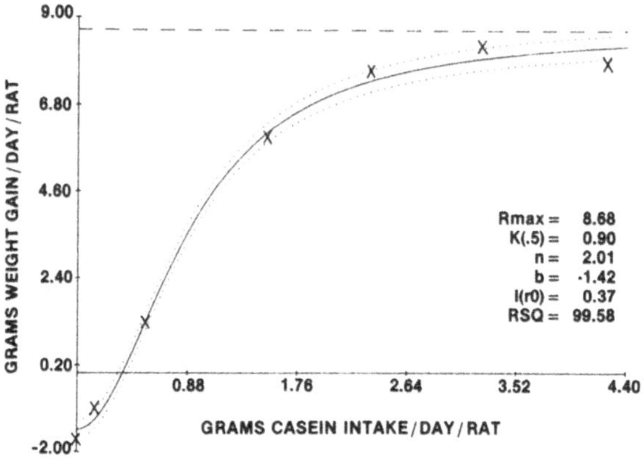

Fig. 4 Daily weight gain as a function of daily casein level. Each "x" is the mean of six rats. The solid line is the theoretical response curve. The dotted lines are the 95% confidence limits (Experiment 1).

Since the model produces a smooth, theoretical curve for weight gain vs. protein intake, it becomes possible to construct a smooth curve for PER (r/I). This is shown in Figure 5 (PER). The PER curve is positive after it crosses the intake axis at Iro. It then reaches a maximum and moves back towards zero. This is due to the fact that the original weight gain vs. protein intake curve is not linear but sigmoidal, following the Law of Diminishing Returns. Since the PER curve is not linear, a decision must be made on which PER to choose to represent a certain protein. The only unique point (greater than zero) on the PER curve is at PERmax, i.e., the intake which maximizes r/I. Intakes associated with 5-10% protein (which are usually used) are arbitrary and may give a PER near maximum for one protein but at only 50% of maximum for another protein, thereby introducing a new source of variation. Also, due to the shape of the PER curve, the same PER value could appear at two different values of intake, one on each side of PERmax. The triangle used to calculate

PERmax is shown in Figure 5 by the dotted lines, while the PER curve is shown by the dash-dot line. Since PER is simply the slope of the dotted line drawn from (0,0) to the point of tangency on the response curve, the figure shows that the numerical index is a poor approximation. This is because the actual response curve is not linear and does not go through (0,0). As the protein source being measured becomes poorer in biological value (plant source, etc.), Iro (intake or percent required for maintenance) increases. This has a tendency to make PER an even worse index of quality.

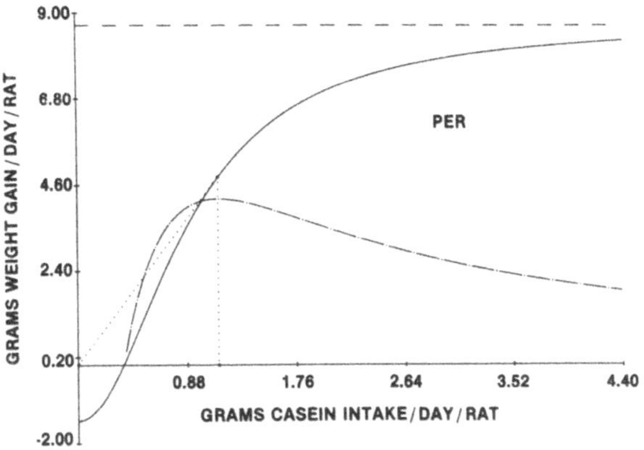

Fig. 5 PER as a function of daily casein intake. The solid line is the curve for weight gain. The dash-dot line shows the variation of PER with casein intake, and the dotted line shows the calculation of PER max.

The next index is shown in Figure 6, NPR ([r-b]/I). This index utilizes two points, i.e., the chosen response group (r) and the group on zero protein (b). NPR encompasses the full range of the response curve and is therefore superior to PER which only considers the portion above the I axis, i.e., responses > zero or maintenance. Inspection of Figure 6 (NPR) shows that the line from (0,b) to the point of tangency of the response curve is a better estimation of the "true" response curve than the PER technique. However, any increase in Iro degrades the usefulness of NPR as it does PER. NPR is also a smooth function with a maximum and intersects the I axis at (0,0). Figure 6 shows the calculation of NPRmax. The technique of adding the weight loss of rats fed a nonprotein diet to the weight gain of the test group is based on the assumption that the amount of protein required to prevent weight loss in the rat fed the nonprotein diet is equivalent to the amount of protein needed for maintenance (McLaughlan, 1980). This, of course, would only be true for a linear response in which Iro coincided with the point of intersection of the I axis and the dotted line through (0,b).

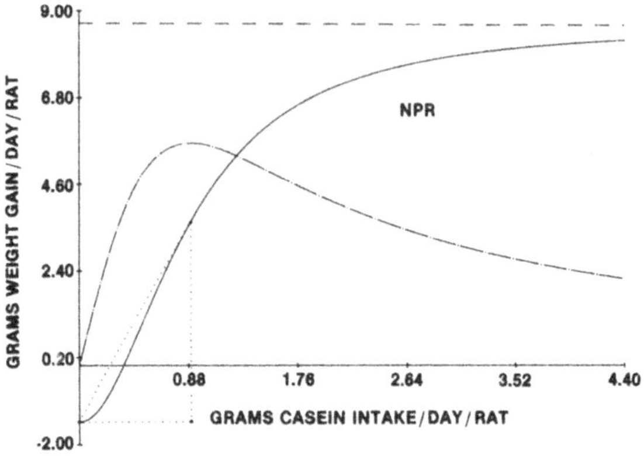

Fig. 6 NPR as a function of daily casein intake. The solid line is the curve for weight gain. The dash-dot line shows the variation of NPR with casein intake, and the dotted line shows the calculation of NPRmax.

The next case shown in Figure 7 is the one for SLOPE. The change in slope of the response curve is shown by the dash-dot line. It is a smooth function with a maximum as are NPR and PER. The point of SLOPEmax is the point at which the responding system is most sensitive to changes

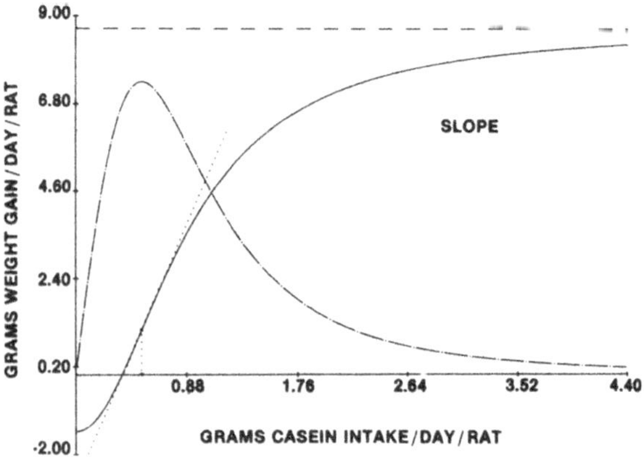

Fig. 7 Slope as a function of daily casein intake. The solid line is the curve for weight gain. The dash-dot line shows the variation of Slope with casein intake, and the dotted line shows the calculation of SLOPEmax.

in protein level or intake. It does a good job of approximating the central "linear" portion of the response curve but does not go through the point of zero intake (0,b). This has been pointed out as a deficiency of the SLOPE method but would certainly be expected in a nonlinear system.

VII. A new protein quality index-APU--actual protein utilization

Actual protein utilization is calculated as weight gain (g)/[protein intake (g) - protein intake for maintenance (g)]. The formula for this index is shown in Equation (14).

$$APU = r/(I-Iro) \qquad \text{Equation (14)}$$

where Iro is the protein intake required for maintenance and is calculated from Equation (8).

APUmax is the tangent of the angle between the intake axis and a line drawn from (Iro,0) through the point of tangency to the response curve (Fig. 8). No formula is currently available for its calculation, but it can be found easily by a simple iterative procedure using Equation (14).

The new method is shown in Figure 8 (APU). Since the four parameter model allows calculation of the level of protein intake required for maintenance (Iro), this figure can be used in a quality index without the approximation done for NPR. After one chooses the intake of interest, I, then Iro can be subtracted so that the resulting response can be divided

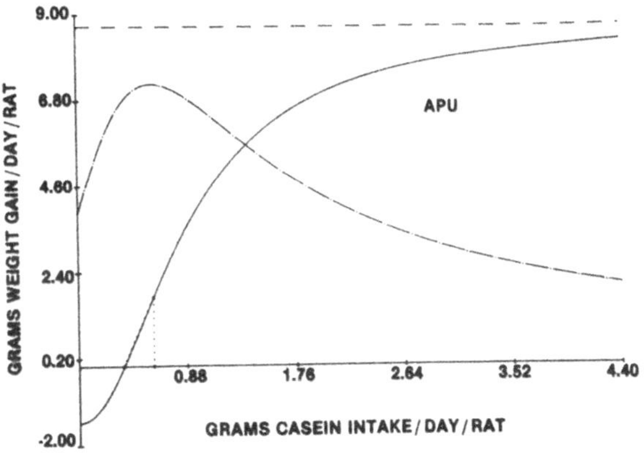

Fig. 8 APU as a function of daily casein intake. The solid line is the curve for weight gain. The dash-dot line shows the variation of APU with casein intake, and the dotted line shows the calculation of APUmax.

by the intake (I-Iro) actually required to produce it. Figure 8 (APU) shows that the dotted line drawn from Iro to the point of tangency of the response curve (APUmax) very closely coincides with the actual response curve and is therefore the best estimation of the quality of the protein. APU is a smooth curve with a maximum and intersects the r axis at the point b/-Iro. APU is therefore sensitive to variations seen in the maintenance levels of proteins with different biological values.

VIII. A comparative analysis of APU with PER, NPR and SLOPE

With the establishment of a theoretical basis, we can now make reliable correlations in describing the various methods of protein quality evaluations.

Table 5 gives the results of Experiment 1 using casein. The values for the indices are somewhat high due to the use of rats that are larger than normal for a protein quality evaluation. As Rmax increases and b decreases, the values for the indices increase. However, if one follows the AOAC protocol, this would not be a problem. Empirical observation of intakes, responses, and indices show an order that we have always observed, i.e., IPERmax > INPRmax > IAPUmax > ISLOPEmax. The order is the same for response level, but inverted for indices (SLOPEmax > APUmax > NPRmax > PERmax). Each measurement is taken at the unique point on the response curve, i.e., at the maximum value for each index, rather than a common intake or response level. This gives a uniformity to results not achieved by choosing intake-response levels at random.

TABLE 5

Maximum PER, NPR, SLOPE AND APU values (Exp. 1)

INDEX	Intake(I)	Response (r)	Value
	g/day	g/day	
PER	1.13	4.80	4.24
NPR	0.90	3.66	5.65
APU	0.61	1.75	7.21
SLOPE	0.52	1.12	7.35

The indices (actual and relative) calculated from Experiments (2) and (3) are shown in Table 6. The values agree well with the literature. PER for lactalbumin is slightly high for an undetermined reason if one assumes the theoretical maximum for PER is 4.5. The uniformity of results indicates that using INDEXmax improves the usefulness of any of the four methods, although PER seems to underestimate soy and the amino acid mixture.

If Bender is correct in saying that an index only reflects the limiting amino acid (1982), then this process could be repeated on mixtures of amino acids so that indices could be developed for each. However, diets contain proteins (not amino acid mixtures) so that other considerations (such as digestability) make studies of whole proteins valuable. The study of mixtures might be more valuable for parenteral feeding regimens, etc.

There is an interest in minimizing the time, effort, and cost required for protein quality evaluation. However, the system being analyzed is complex and a single-point evaluation may be unrealistic. The amount of information extracted from a system is proportional to the number of measurements taken. The delineation of small differences requires even more effort. One must compromise between cost and desired results, since they tend to be inversely proportional. The four parameter model requires more initial effort/cost but provides more information about the system being studied. It is a good choice for a critical study, while single-point evaluations are useful for approximations.

TABLE 6

Actual and relative PER, NPR, APU, and SLOPE for three proteins and one amino acid mixture (Exp. 2 and 3).

Index	Lactal-bumin	Casein	Soy	Amino Acid Mix
		Actual		
PER	4.91	4.35	3.16	4.40
NPR	5.35	4.69	4.08	4.82
APU	5.65	5.00	4.32	5.51
SLOPE	5.80	5.26	4.33	5.95
		[1]Relative		
PER	100	89	65	90
NPR	100	88	76	90
APU	100	88	76	98
SLOPE	100	91	75	103

[1](Test/lactalbumin) x 100

CONCLUSION

In our approach to the assessment of the nutritional quality of proteins, we have provided a theoretical framework from which the criteria of a valid protein quality bioassay can be more closely studied. We believe that the four parameter mathematical model for physiological responses provides this framework for the utilization and interpretation of protein quality evaluations. Using a modeling approach should provide a uniform comparison of results from different laboratories. This should give more reliable indices of comparisons and, hopefully, a general consensus as to which method is the most useful indicator of protein quality.

The theory that the nutrient-response relationship is sigmoidal has been verified in our laboratory with each nutrient we have investigated. The modeling of this response has proved to be a very valuable tool in a wide range of studies as well as protein quality evaluations. The use of INDEXmax may also improve the determination of protein quality by allowing each protein to be compared at its maximum response level. The model allows the calculation of a new index, Actual Protein Utilization (APU), which incorporates a term for maintenance intake levels. This should improve the comparison of proteins with low biological value.

REFERENCES

Allison, J.B. In: Protein and amino acid nutrition. Chapter 5 (ed. A. A. Albanese) London: Academic Press.

Allison, J.B. and Anderson, J.A. (1945) The relation between absorbed nitrogen, nitrogen balance and biological value of proteins in adult dogs. J. Nutr. 29, 413.

Almquist, J.H. (1970) Evaluation of nutrient requirements. New Methods of Nutr. Biochem. 4, 1-36.

Arrhenius, S. (1889) Z. Physik. Chem. 4, 226.

Bender, A.E. (1982) Evaluation of protein quality: Methodological considerations. In: Symposium on new protein sources and nucleic acid metabolism. Proc. Nutr. Soc. 41, 267-276.

Bender, A.E. and Doell, B.H. (1957) Biological evaluation of proteins: a new aspect. Br. J. Nutr., 11, 140.

Briggs, G.E. and J.B.S. Haldane. (1925) Biochem. J. 19, 383.

Brown, A. (1902) J. Chem. Soc. 81, 373.

Elliott, J.G. and F.D. McClure. (1983) Sources of variance in the bioassay of protein value. J. Assoc. Off. Anal. Chem. 66, No. 1, 46.

Grainger, J.N.R. (1966) A model of a growing steady state system. J. Theoret. Biol. 10, 387-398.

Guldberg, C.M. and P. Waage. (1867) Etudes sur les affinités chimiques. (1867) Brogger and Christic Christiania (Oslo).

Hegsted, D.M. (1971) Nitrogen requirements and utilization, p. 5. In: Nutrients in processed foods. eds. P.L. White and D.C. Fletcher. American Medical Association Publishing Sciences Group, Inc.

Hegsted, D.M. and Yet-oy Chang. (1965) Protein utilization in growing rats. I. Relative growth index as a bioassay procedure. J. Nutrition, 85.

Henri, V. (1903) "Lois générales de l'action des diastases." (1903) Herman, Paris.

Hill, A.V. (1952) J. Am. Chem. Soc. 74, 4710.

Kon, S.H. (1978) Underestimation of chronic toxicities of food additives and chemicals. (1978) Med. Hypothesis 4, 324-339.

McLaughlan, J.M. (1971) Evaluation of standard rat assays, p. 69. In: Nutrients in processed foods. eds. P.L. White and D.C. Fletcher. American Medical Association Publishing Sciences Group, Inc.

McLaughlan, J.M. (1976) J. AOAC 59, 42.

McLaughlan, J.M., Anderson, G.H., Hackler, L.R., Hill, O.C., Jansen, G.R., Keith, M.O., Sarwar, G. and Sosulski, F.W. (1980) Assessment of rat growth methods for estimating protein quality: interlaboratory study. J. Assoc. Off. Anal. Chem. 63, No. 3, 462.

Mercer, L.P., Morgan, P.H., Flodin, N.W. (1975) A theoretical model for linearization of nutrient response data. Fed. Proc. 34, 3841.

Mercer, L.P., P.H. Morgan, N.W. Flodin and A. Domm. (1979) Prediction of food intakes and growth rates in weanling rats by the four parameter model equation. Nutr. Rept. Int. 19, 1-8.

Mercer, L.P. (1980) Mathematical models in nutrition. (1980a) Nutr. Rept. Intl. 21, 189-197.

Mercer, L.P., T.B. Cole and M.R. Schweisthal. (1980b) Prediction of organ weights by the four-parameter model for nutritional responses. Nutr. Rept. Intl. 21, 595-603.

Mercer, L.P., D.F. Watson and J.S. Ramlet. (1981) Control of food intake in the rat by dietary protein concentration. J. Nutr. 111, 1117-1123.

Mercer, L.P. (1982) The quantitative nutrient-response relationship. J. Nutri. 112, 560-566.

Methods of Analysis - AOAC. (1980) 13th Ed., section 43.212, 774-775, APAC, Washington, D.C.

Mitchell, H.H. and G.G. Carmen. (1929) The biological value of the nitrogen of mixtures of patent white flour and animal foods. J. Biol. Chem. 68, 183.

Osborne, T.B., L.B. Mendel and E.L. Ferry. (1919) A method of expressing numerically the growth-promoting value of proteins. J. Biol. Chem. 37, 223.

O'Sullivan, L. and F.W. Tompson. (1890) J. Chem. Soc. 57, 834.

Parks, J.R. (1982) Introduction. In: A theory of feeding and growth in animal. 1-24, Springer-Verlag, Berlin.

Parks, J.R. (1982) In: A theory of feeding and growth in animals. 70-82, Springer-Verlag, Berlin.

Rogers, Q.R. and A.E. Harper (1965) Amino acid diets and maximal growth in the rat. J. Nutr. 87, 267-273.

Samonds, K.W. and Hegsted, D.M. (1977) In: Evaluation of proteins for humans (ed. C.E. Bodwell). Westport: Avi Publishing.

Scrimshaw, N.S. and V.R. Young. (1971) Application of assays of protein quality to human requirements for protein. 109. In: Nutrients in processed food (eds. P.L. White and D.C. Fletcher). American Medical Association Publishing Sciences Group, Inc.

Thomas, K. (1909) Ueber die biologische Wertigkeit der stickstoff-substanten in verschiedenen Nahrungsmitteln. Arch. Physiol., 219.

Proc. Int. Assoc. Cereal Chem. Symp. Amino Acid Compn and Biol. Value of Cereal Proteins
Budapest, Hungary 1983, R. Lásztity, M. Hidvégi, eds

IN VIVO METHODS IN THE EVALUATION OF THE NUTRITIONAL QUALITY OF CEREAL PROTEINS

BRIGITTA WALGER-KUNZE

Research Laboratory, College of Agriculture, H-7400 Kaposvár, Hungary

ABSTRACT

Besides the advantages of in vitro methods using the relative rapid and inexpensive estimation of amino acid (AA) concentrations in proteins, disadvantages had also been found. Problems concern the additional estimation for availability, the hydrolysis and/or the application of methods which do not correspond with AA requirements of humans or animals.

In vivo methods for prediction protein quality are much more expensive and time consuming. However, it seems to be necessary to perform in vivo tests in the future too, because the nutritive value of proteins do not only depend on the AA pattern but among others also from anti-nutritive effective attendant substances which have an adverse effect on protein metabolism.

The in vivo methods can be divided into growing tests (PER, NPR, Relative NPR, PRE, GVP, Slope Ratio Assay, Four Parameter Model Equation), nitrogen balance studies (BV, NPU, PNu%, NPV, PPW, b-Value, NBI, N-Balance Function, Isotopic studies), biochemical tests (BUN = RHW) and assays with other species than vertebrates (Tetrahymena pyr. W.).

It is recommendable to determine the protein quality of foods and feeds on humans and these species of animals destinated for. But in many instances it is not suitable to make such an agreement for technical or financial reasons. In such cases it is advantageous to design the experiments to model animals.

The advantages and disadvantages of the most used in vivo methods are described. It is established that nowadays it does not exist any in vivo method which meets all the needed requirements: to be rapid, accurate, reproducible, simple, inexpensive, applicable for most protein sources and relevant to humans and all species of animals. It seems impossible to express the nutritive quality of a protein in only one data or value. The need for an approach with more than one parameter is demonstrated by own experiments with maize samples on rats.

INTRODUCTION

The development and general application of amino acid analyses promoted our knowledge about the cause of protein quality to a large extent. Hence, it is logical and abvious to try to utilize this embracing mass of data for the evaluation of protein quality. But the total amino acid pattern and concentration itself is not always a reliable quide to the feeding value of proteins in relation to the requirement of humans and animals which are not very well established yet. There are other factors too, as the digestibility and availability of amino acids to the species concerned with. In an attempt to overcome these difficulties chemical methods were developed to determine the amounts of amino acids actually available for the nutrition of men and animals (Carpenter and Ellinger 1955, Erbersdobler 1962, Matheson 1968, Rudérus and Kihlberg 1970, Holm 1971, Pruss and Ney 1972, Hurell and Carpenter 1976, Lipton and Bodwell 1977).

The results obtained from chemical and biological assays for available lysine generally show a satisfactory correlation in most proteins of animal origin (Carpenter and Woodham 1974, Carpenter and Opstvedt 1976) but the analytical procedure is time consuming and expensive. Carpenter and Opstvedt found considerable interlaboratory differences and serious analytical problems exist for the estimation in protein sources with high carbohydrate concentration and no sufficient correlation between the results with chemical methods and nutritive value from in vivo methods could be found yet (Ostrowsky 1969, Kedenburg 1970). A review about the comparability of both on wheat was given by Bodwell (1976).

The acid hydrolysis used for most automated amino acid analyses destroys the nutritional essential amino acid tryptophan. This fact also causes problems in calculating the protein value by chemical methods. Friedman and Finley(1971) reviewed about the analytical methods for tryptophan determination and found them uncertain in response to an unknown sample (Wünsche 1969, Santarius and Belitz 1973, Matheson 1973, 1974, Gundel and Votisky 1974, Buttery and Soar 1975, Lewis et al. 1976, Steinhart and Sandmann 1977, Amaya-F et al. 1977, Steinhart 1979). So, in fact, more than one chemical method should be recommended in the interest of approximating the protein value from amino acid content. But this is tedious and expensive,too (Blohm et al. 1969).

Further difficulties in comparing the chemical and biological assays result from the fact that besides the nutritional substances above all in plant material frequently occur a number of anti-nutritive constituents which impaire the protein metabolism in humans and animals. Proteins, amino acid derivates, proteinase inhibitors, phythemaglutinins, phytooestrogenes and tannins, for instance, belong to these secondary plant substances. A review about this problem was given by Bock (1975).

These problems show it evident that the scoring methods do not adequately explain experimental observations in men and animals (Brune et al. 1968 a,b). Many factors are involved in the utilization of amino acids by vertebrates and we do not know all of them yet (Kofrányi 1973). So it is intelligible that the estimation of the protein value cannot be dispensed with in vivo methods which, not less important, should be used as control for chemical methods.

Schröder and Bock (1962) evaluated collaborative studies from several laboratories and summed up that the degree of comparability of the results from rat N-balance studies was much better than those of amino acid analyses in spite of the problems connected with the balance studies which consisted mainly in non exact N-determinations. In further investigations similar facts were found by Wünsche (1967) and Bock (1967 a,b).

The in vivo methods can be arranged in the following groups:

1. Growing tests
2. N-balance studies
3. Biochemical assays
4. Assays with other species than vertebrates

The selection which form of examination should be used depends on the aims of the experiments. It is recommendable to determine the protein quality on the species of animals destied for this, or on man. But in many cases this is not possible for technical or financial reasons. For instance, in breeding new sorts of cereals it is very often impossible to produce large samples of grain to determine their protein quality on pigs. In such cases it is advantageous to design the experiments to small animals like rats.

The comparison of the results from in vivo methods on rats and pigs is being discussed yet. Liappis et al. (1975) found large variations in the amino acid concentrations in the serum of the examined species among themselves and between man, rat, mouse, cock, rabbit, guinea pig and pig. Brune et al. (1968) obtained results from biological assays on swine and rats differing in the ratio of their requirement for lysine and methionine to a large extend but observed a very good reproducibility in the metabolism trials. Munck (1972) also found no corresponding results between swine and mouse.

On the contrary Eggum (1973) supported the use of rats because he observed a high correlation r = 0.91 between pigs and rats in digestibility and r = 0.86 in biological value mainly in grain diets.

Nutritional examinations in humans are very difficult to carry out. Nitrogen balance methods require very often long periods (Calloway 1975) and considerable differences for amino acid requirement exist between subjects regarding age, sex and size also (Hegsted 1975) Oddove and Margen 1979). Kofrányi et al. (1970) conducted long term dietary experiments with adult males and pointed out that their former measurements had shown that the biological value obtained with humans and rats were quite different. In opposite Bergen (1974) used children and growing rats for comparison and observed very similar results in the biological value of different proteins.

In spite of some caution in the interpretation of these data may be in order, this demonstrates the need for exact standardisation of any in vivo method. Only the accuracy of methods guarantees their reproducibility and comparability. A relative small error in balance studies may shift the data from a positive to a negative balance. All experimental conditions for in vivo methods must be established and kept precisely.

1. GROWTH STUDIES

1.1. Protein Efficiency Ratio (PER)

This widely used assay was developed by Osborne et al. (1919) and is the only officially accepted method in the USA and Canada. It is defined

$$PER = \frac{\text{weight gain of the test group (g)}}{\text{protein consumed (g)}}$$

Each group consists of 10 individual caged animals. The examination lasts 28 days. In case of rats the control group receives casein as protein standard, in cases of pigs Kovács and Ridly (1975 cit. in Hegedüs et al. 1981) elaborated a standard mixture with milk powder. The application of PER assay on chicks was described by Leibetseder and Hamed (1968), Stillway et al. (1972) and Buamah and Singsen (1975).

Food and water are given ad libitum. Individual PER values were calculated for each animal based on individual weight gain and consumption of diets whose protein content was previously determined.

In spite of the simple conductibility there have been many objections to the PER method for a long time. Hegsted and Worchester (1947) pointed out that the PER values go parallel to weight gain and so nothing is reached by the calculation. Bock (1965) demonstrated that the results were dependent on the quantity of protein given to the animals and from the protein quality. Bodwell (1977) took many exceptions to PER too, among them that this system does not recognize the fact that the nutritive values of low quality proteins are enhanced greatly, if they are consumed together with high quality proteins. PER also is known to underestimate the proteins with lower quality and is only suitable for proteins which permit weight gain.

Several modifications for improving the PER assay had been recommended: Different levels of protein in rations dependent on the quality of the test proteins, a fixation of the standard protein on 2.5 PER (corrected PER, relative PER) and reduction of length of experiments. Embracing examinations connected with the problems of PER methods had been undertaken by Hurt et al. (1975). Womack et al. (1975) worked out further modifications. One of the developments was done by Bender and Doell (1957): The

1.2. Net Protein Ratio (NPR)

which is very similar to PER. A protein free group is enclosed in the assay on the assumption that the loss of weight is adequate to the level of protein needed for zero weight change. So it is defined:

$$\text{NPR} = \frac{\text{weight gain of test group (g)} + \text{weight gain of protein-free group (g)}}{\text{protein consumed (g)}}$$

However, because NPR values did not turn fully suitable to Net Protein Utilization (NPU) the authors calculated the following function between the two methods and named it

1.3. Protein Retention Efficiency (PRE)

$$\text{PRE} = 3.3 + 15.5\ \text{NPR}$$

Nowadays in much cases NPR is multiplied with the factor 16 on basis of average body protein content of rats (Hegedüs et al. 1981). According to McLaughlan and Keith (1975) the main fault of the NPR assay is that it frequently overestimates the value of poor quality proteins.

Sarwar and McLaughlan (1981) tried to improve the NPR assay. They recommended the

1.4. Relative NPR value

$$\text{Relative NPR} = \frac{\text{mean NPR of test protein}}{\text{mean NPR of reference protein}} \times 100$$

Methionine supplemented casein serves as reference protein. They found that the PER for casein decreased markedly with experimental time from 3.46 at 1 week to 2.96 after 4 weeks. Corrected PER (casein = 2.5) for whole wheat bread was 70% greater at 4 weeks than at 1 week. In contrast, the Relative NPR was superior to PER because it altered very little with time.

1.5. Gross Protein Value

is a further modification of the PER method developed by Robertson et al. (1938) and Heiman et al. (1939). They defined

$$\text{GVP} = \frac{\text{g weight gain of group with test protein}}{\text{g weight gain of group with standard protein/casein}} \times 100$$

Duckworth et al. (1961) stated in embracing studies the suitability of this assay. In the GPV test the animals of each group are fed with a basis diet containing 8% protein. Casein as standard and the test protein are added as 3% to the control resp. test ration/cit. in Hegedüs et al.1981).

1.6. Slope Ratio Assay

The described growing methods are destinated to measure the protein value at one level of protein concentration in the rations. Hegsted and Chang (1965 a,b) used different levels of protein intake and extrapoled the growth response curves for standard and test proteins received in this way. They assumed the protein quality as a constant value at all levels used in the estimation of nutritive value. Yanez and McLaughlan (1970) found the slope ratio assay invalid for proteins of poor quality. The

1.7. Four-Parameter Model Equation

had been developed by Mercer et al. (1979). It works likewise with different levels of protein concentration and a control group with an N-free diet. It estimates the relation between protein concentration and daily food intake for predicting the food intake of rats based solely on the composition of their diet. The second relationship is the protein intake versus weight gain for prediction weight gain as a function of protein intake. The recommended assay should be compared with other methods.

For all these growing methods one can say that they give more or less precise informations about protein quality but do not take in consideration the causes of the different nutritive values. During growth there is not only protein accretion but also deposition of fat and water and skeletal growth. On this point of view growing tests have a limited approximation to the accurate nutritive value.

2. N-BALANCE STUDIES

The N-balance is the difference between N-uptake and N-excretion in faeces and urine:

N-Balance = N-uptake - (N in faeces + N in urine)

The basis for this method had been worked out by Thomas (1909) and Mitchell (1924 a,b) and was developed and adapted to mammals and birds by numerous studies (Schiftan 1932, Lintzel and Mangold 1935, Mangold and Columbus 1937, 1938, Mangold and Behm 1955, Nehring 1953, 1954, 1962, Hennig 1958, Nehring and Bock 1961, 1962, Nehring and Laube 1961, Wetterau 1953, 1960, Njaa 1959 a,b, 1966, Hartfiel 1961, Gebhardt 1964, Hohls 1962, 1967, Zausch 1967, Kunze 1968, Zausch and Kunze 1968, Walger-Kunze 1972, Eggum 1973).

2.1. The Biological Value (BV)

is calculated on N-balance according to Thomas and Mitchell and expresses the amount of body protein accreted from 100 g protein resorbed taking into account the N-requirement for maintenance. This requirement is estimated on animals of different body mass with N-free diets on standard conditions.

$$BV = \frac{\text{N-balance} + \text{N-requirement for maintenance}}{\text{N resorbed}} \times 100$$

The accurate determination of protein value is complicated by the fact that the N-excretions contain besides the undigestible parts of nutritive N, the so called endogen N losses which, in turn cannot be neglected. So, the basal N metabolism has to be determined with N-free diets according to Columbus (1951, 1954 a,b). He calculated the N loss with those diets to be dependent on the body mass of animals. This estimation is in discussion for a long time.

The determination of BV has to be done with precise experimental conditions. Growing rats should be of the same strain, of male sex, in the same body mass, individually housed at constant room temperature and the protein content in their diets is the threefold of their N requirement for maintenance (about 10% of the diet). The deviation for the standard diet with defatted whole egg powder is $\pm$ 4.2 BV by strictly observing the conditions. This value rises by poor quality proteins (Bock 1958, 1965, Bock et al. 1964 a,b, Horszcaruk and

Bock 1963, Arbeitskreis für Proteinbewertung 1964). The average variance for growing rats had been found by Bock to be 7.4%.

Since the BV represents the protein value of the digested protein in the endogen metabolic pathways Mitchell (1924) suggested to multiply the BV with the valid digestibility of nitrogen and named this value

2.2. Net Protein Utilization (NPU)

which represents the accreted protein in percent of intake:

$$NPU = \frac{BV \cdot N\ resorbed}{100}$$

Lintzel and Rechenberger (1940) related the N retained to N intake. They formulated

2.3. Physiologischer Nutzwert (PNu %)

(value of physiologically utilized N)

$$PNu\ \% = \frac{N\ retained}{N\ intake} \cdot 100$$

In order to circumvent the problems in connection with the dependence and constance of N requirement for maintenance per kg metabolic body weight Bender and Miller (1953b) modified the N-balance method in measuring the percentage retention of N by carcass analysis instead of from the difference between intake and output. They defined the

2.4. Net Protein Value (NPV)

in which the N content of carcasses of the test group is determined at the beginning and at the end of trials corrected by the carcass N concentration of a group with N-free diet:

$$NPV = \frac{100\ (B - B_o) - (B_k - B_o)}{J}$$

(carcass N concentration of:

B = test group at the end of trial

B_o = test group at the beginning of trial

B_k = group with N-free diet at the end of trial

J = N intake)

The N retention determined in this way is identical to the NPU estimated by the Thomas-Mitchell method (Bock 1958) but does not show up the digestibility and BV of the protein. The method is very labour consuming. A very similar method had been suggested by Müller and Hötzel (1957):

2.5. Produktiver Proteinwert (PPW) (Productive Protein Value)

They dispensed with feeding an N-free group but examined the N retained by determining the carcass N at the end and at the beginning of the test and relating the difference with N intake:

$$PPW = \frac{\text{N content of carcasses at the end of trial} - \text{N content of carcasses at the beginning of trial}}{\text{N intake}} \cdot 100$$

Kment and Leibetseder (1973) reported about the suitability of the assay on rats and pigs. But objections can be raised also because in case of negative N-balance there is no possibility for estimation of the protein value. Niess and Müller (1972) reported about an interlaboratory study for several years about the reproducibility of PPW and pointed out the importance of exact examination conditions.

The determination of protein retention is done by one level of protein in the diet and with the assumption of a constant N requirement for maintenance in relation to body weight. The level of about 10% protein in the diet is known as optimal for intensity of N retention. However, Hohls (1955) suggested to determine the maximal ability of animals for N retention which value implies the requirement for maintenance. Gebhardt (1964) formulated the

2.6. b-Wert (b-value)

He assumed that the nutritive value of proteins in growing animals is most safely determined with N balance method by Thomas Mitchell. The test conditions are fairly good to standardize excepting the level of N intake. He took into consideration the dependence of weight gain from the protein quantity given to the animal on the one side and the genetical fixed maximal ability for N retention on the other side:

$$y = A\ (1 - e^{-bx})$$

with y = N retained, x = N intake and A = max. N balance, all these per kg 0.67 live weight and in mg per day.

2.7. The Nitrogen Balance Index (NBI)

found by Allison and Anderson (1945) and Allison et al. (1946) is also determined with increasing levels of protein and then calculated by regression analysis. It is somewhat alike to the slope of b-value but much simpler and is used as a short term method for humans.

$$NBI = k \cdot N\ \text{resorbed} - N\ \text{excretion by N-free diet}$$

2.8. The true digestibility of proteins and amino acids

Some authors (Eggum 1973, Wiesemüller 1968, Uhlemann 1969, Poppe et al. 1969) suggested the true digestibility of proteins and amino acids on basis of N balance as measure. They calculated the dependence of faecal N excretion from different levels of N intake on basis of the regressive function $y = a + bx$ and found the values to agree with those of direct estimations. The method is very labour - consuming and expensive. The averaged values are summerized in amino acid tables (Bock et al. 1981). Meier and Poppe (1976) determined N balance and true digestibility of amino acids on monogatric animals, Gruhn and Raue (1974) and Schadereit et al. (1976) on chicks and Wünsche et al. (1978) on piglets.

2.9. The N-Balance Function

by Rufeger (1972) describes a method with which the quality of dietary protein can be determined independent of N intake and the N metabolism can be quantitatively analyzed without isotopes.

2.10. Isotopic Studies

The application of isotopic methods is not available for wide use yet and serves chiefly for basic research for the present. It has been shown, that some essential amino acids are highly reutilized for protein synthesis in organism. The problems connected with this method have been described by Garlick and Millward (1972). Neale and Waterlow (1974 a,b) worked with ^{14}C-labelled amino acids on rats and Hennig et al. (1977) with ^{15}N-labelled amino acids from wheat on laying hens.

3. BIOCHEMICAL ASSAYS

Numerous attempts have been made to use metabolic parameters for predicting protein value. The protein metabolism in skeletal muscles and in liver, muscle growth, cell size or weight resp. protein concentration in liver, activity of different enzymes, content and relationship of free amino acids in blood plasma, the creatinin excretion in urine should be listed up, for instance. All these parameters show more or less relations to protein intake or protein quality but they are not reliable approaches for evaluating protein quality yet (Bergner et al. 1966, Mokady et al. 1969, Kihlberg 1970, Wirthgen and Bergner 1970, Münchow and Bergner 1970, Millward and Garlick 1972, Featherstone 1972, Shannon et al. 1972, Muramatsu et al. 1973, Young et al. 1973. McLaughlan et al. 1973, Millward et al. 1974, Stewart 1974, Beecher 1974, Boehncke and Rieder 1974, Ohno and Tasaki 1976).

3.1. The Blood Urea Concentration (BUC = RHW)

is an exception between these parameters. On basis of observations by Puchal et al. (1962) that the urea concentration in blood decreases with increasing protein quality Münchow (1967) studied the relationship between the quality of different protein sources and blood urea concentration. He found a very high correlation between BV resp. NPR and the reciprocal blood urea concentration (RHW):

$$BV = 0.827 + 0.998\ RHW \qquad (r = 0.990)$$

$$NPR = -13.10 + 1.148\ RHW \qquad (r = 0.997)$$

He defined the reciprocal blood urea concentration as

$$RHW = \frac{\text{blood urea conc. (mg) 100 ml with reference protein} \quad \text{BV of reference protein}}{\text{blood urea conc. (mg/100 ml) with test protein}}$$

and worked out the examination conditions for this assay which is suitable for rats and pigs (Münchow and Bergner 1967, 1968). Eggum (1970) confirmed the applicability of this assay, Berschauer (1978) and Menke (1980) proved the method on pigs with positive results. The estimation can be done on humans too (Tayler et al. 1974, Bodwell et al. 1979).

4. ASSAYS WITH OTHER SPECIES THAN VERTEBRATES

The comparability between the different species of mammals is under discussion as above described. Much more doubtful is the comparability between insects and microorganism on the one side and mammals on the other side. Here only should be mentioned the use of yellow mealworm (Tenebrior molitor), the larvae of Red Flour Beetle (Tribolium castaneum) and Streptococcus zymogenes. Most of such tests show a lack of direct comparison because of not having proven the same diet in control animals and comparing them with values from literature only.

4.1. Assays with Tetrahymena pyriformis W.

The most used microorganism is the ciliate Tetrahymena pyr.W. Fernell and Rosen (1956) and Rosen and Fernell (1956) described the method for estimating the "Relative Nutritive Value (RNV)" of proteins:

$$\text{RNV} = \frac{\log\left(\begin{array}{l}\text{count for}\\ \text{test protein}\end{array}\right) - \log\left(\begin{array}{l}\text{count for}\\ \text{inoculum}\end{array}\right)}{\log\left(\begin{array}{l}\text{count for}\\ \text{casein}\end{array}\right) - \log\left(\begin{array}{l}\text{count for}\\ \text{inoculum}\end{array}\right)} \cdot 100$$

Stott and Smith (1966) developed this method. Baum (1966a, b) tried to estimate the protein value of foods and feeds in this way. The calculations are made by cell count or by determination of one of the cells' own biochemical substances (2-aminoethylphoshonic acid) (Maciejewicz and Antoniewicz 1978) or colorimetrically. Bergner et al. (1968) found no constant relation between BV on rats and results with Tetrahymena pyr.W. of same protein sources which is in agreement with our results under the dame conditions (Walger and Walger 1972). Rolle and Eggum (1971) stated this assay unsuitable for samples with low content of sulphur containing amino acids. In opposite Evans et al. (1977) found for meat products a correlation of r = 0.62. Hegedüs et al. (1981) showed a significant correlation between RNV and PER, but high contents of carbohydrates and meat products were difficult to determine. Problems with this assay also arise for the need of sterilization the protein sources at higher temperatures and pressures before inoculation with Tetrahymena pyr.W. which treatment destroys parts of essential amino acids.

It is doubtful whether there might be an assay that fulfil the demands in predicting protein values summerized very well by Bodwell (1977):

"An ideal rapid method should 1. be rapid, simple, reproducible, and inexpensive, 2. be applicable to a wide range of protein sources or foods currently, or foreseeably, available for meeting human needs, 3. give a linear response for proteins varying in nutritive value from low to high, 4.

provide quantitative information about the nutritional value of a protein as a single source of protein for humans and its potential value when consumed with other proteins, and 5. in application, accurately reflect as differences in protein quality only those differences that are real under practical conditions".

It is obvious that so many claims are not easy to realize with only one assay though the demands for such a method are well established by the food industry and agriculture. Many factors are involved in amino acid metabolism. Rapid methods will never give valid values for protein sources which are intended to be given aminals or humans for a long time. It is not enough to estimate a protein as low or high quality, if we are not able to show the cause. This means that a protein source which contains a high concentration of digestible essential amino acids but the animals or humans do not like to eat it because of its low palatability from anti-nutritive plant substances, is of no benefit. Low protein intake can also be observed in case of amino acid imbalance. The cause for a low intake can be determined only with several methods.

In my opinion <u>multifarious</u> methods must be applied to investigate protein value because a protein source has to be regarded as wholesome including amino acids, minerals, anti-nutritive substances, and so on. This view aggrees with Kralovánszky and Mátrai (1980) who supposed a complex approach schedule for protein sources: Estimation of the technological data, organoleptical approach (colour, palatability, smell, consistence), chemical investigation, amino acid analysis, microbiological examination, investigation for anti-nutritive substances, biological determinations, suitability for technical production, specific characteristics (solubility and so on).

The need for an approach with more than one parameter demonstrates the following comparison. (Tab. 1). We examined maize samples from 40 sorts on N content, and the daily intake, the N digestibility and BV with rats. The samples are listed in dependence of their N content. All animals were housed individually and obtained 130 mg N daily from maize protein.

Table 1

N content of maize samples and the daily N intake, N digestibility and Biological Value obtained with rats

Nr.	N x 6.25 protein %	N intake % 130 mg = 100	N digestibility %	BV	weight change g
1.	8.8	83.45	86.14	83.18	4.90
2.	8.9	69.70	85.81	71.82	- 2.25
3.	9.0	74.12	86.33	80.67	2.30
4.	9.0	61.30	81.60	64.09	- 8.70
5.	9.1	87.76	88.82	89.60	4.84
6.	9.1	97.02	89.83	76.44	8.91
7.	9.2	89.26	91.04	89.53	9.92
8.	9.2	80.72	90.71	76.85	7.50
9.	9.3	81.33	83.49	72.54	4.50
10.	9.3	70.26	84.36	76.04	1.20
11.	9.4	69.39	86.14	78.22	- 3.66
12.	9.4	47.23	90.24	77.77	- 7.58
13.	9.4	61.58	86.92	77.04	- 3.91
14.	9.4	82.62	86.03	78.00	3.55
15.	9.4	79.32	92.54	79.08	6.00
16.	9.4	72.17	90.25	73.77	3.30
17.	9.5	90.67	90.96	78.45	8.58
18.	9.5	92.16	86.80	93.11	10.90
19.	9.5	92.72	85.91	91.67	11.40
20.	9.5	73.98	86.10	76.61	- 0.33
21.	9.6	72.86	83.33	78.62	0.16
22.	9.6	78.45	85.85	75.65	0.34
23.	9.6	91.84	88.98	77.88	8.30
24.	9.8	76.72	88.40	74.74	0.42
25.	9.8	72.73	86.49	81.56	- 2.16
26.	9.9	66.33	89.30	80.54	0.90
27.	10.4	98.70	88.47	89.54	15.10
28.	10.5	82.92	90.37	73.92	0.83
29.	10.7	97.59	91.21	92.25	11.62
30.	10.8	75.82	88.76	83.87	2.92
31.	10.8	81.76	88.10	80.43	2.30
32.	10.8	70.28	88.96	82.98	- 1.00
33.	10.9	77.41	90.70	77.83	- 0.67
34.	11.0	99.03	89.71	92.84	13.33
35.	11.0	98.54	90.26	90.37	13.93
36.	11.1	70.59	91.34	82.41	- 1.17
37.	11.3	91.99	88.61	68.88	7.71
38.	11.3	85.03	89.80	75.45	2.59
39.	11.3	74.85	88.79	84.25	- 0.98
40.	11.4	74.19	90.76	79.99	2.92

We were highly surprised at the very different N intakes from the various maize types since all trials had been conducted under the same conditions and had been constantly controlled with standard proteins. We calculated the dependence of weight change from other parameters and found that only N intake and BV determined the weight change:

weight change(ge) = 0.313 mg N intake + 0.163 BV - 42.11

B = 0.884 r = 0.94

Figure 1 shows that the BV of these maize samples is dependent from N intake in a very low grade under the conditions of our standardized tests. The N intakes between 65 and 98% produce biological values between 75 and 85. But a very favourable BV is of no benefit in case of impalatibility of its protein because the N intake influences highly the weight change as can be seen in Figure 2.

It seems that N intake is not the only factor because an N intake of 70 - 80% produces weight changes from - 3 g to + 8 g. These results allow the conclusion that there are other factors too which we did not examine. If such factors are really present in maize, which is so very important for feeding domestical animals, these experiments should be verified in tests on pigs on basis of screening test results with rats.

I think this demonstration about testing the proteins from different maize types is an example for the important relevance of animal studies as a link in the chain of examinations to predict protein value.

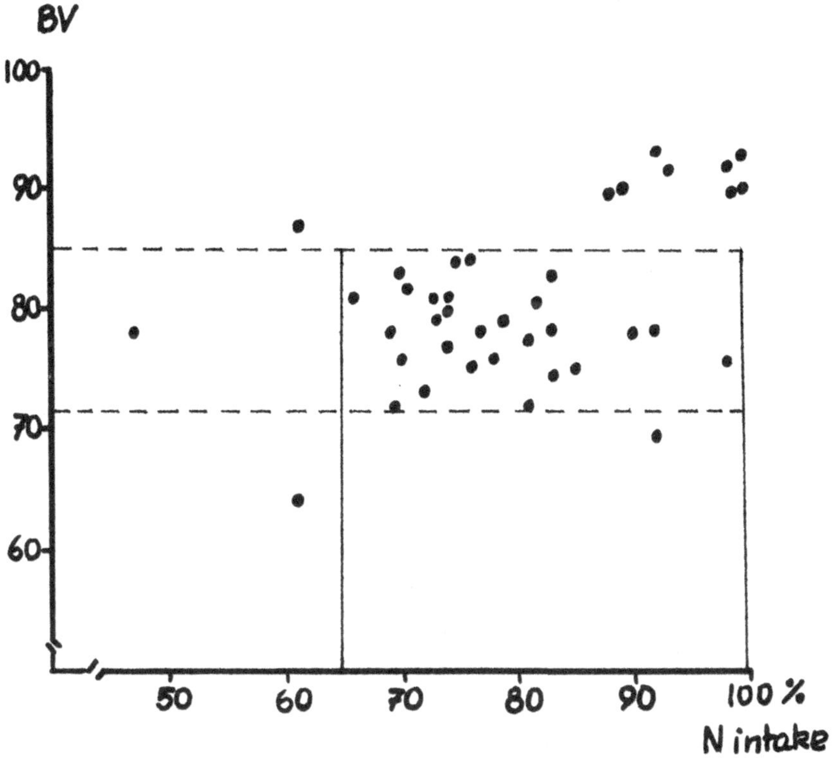

Fig. 1. N intake (%) versus BV obtained with rats

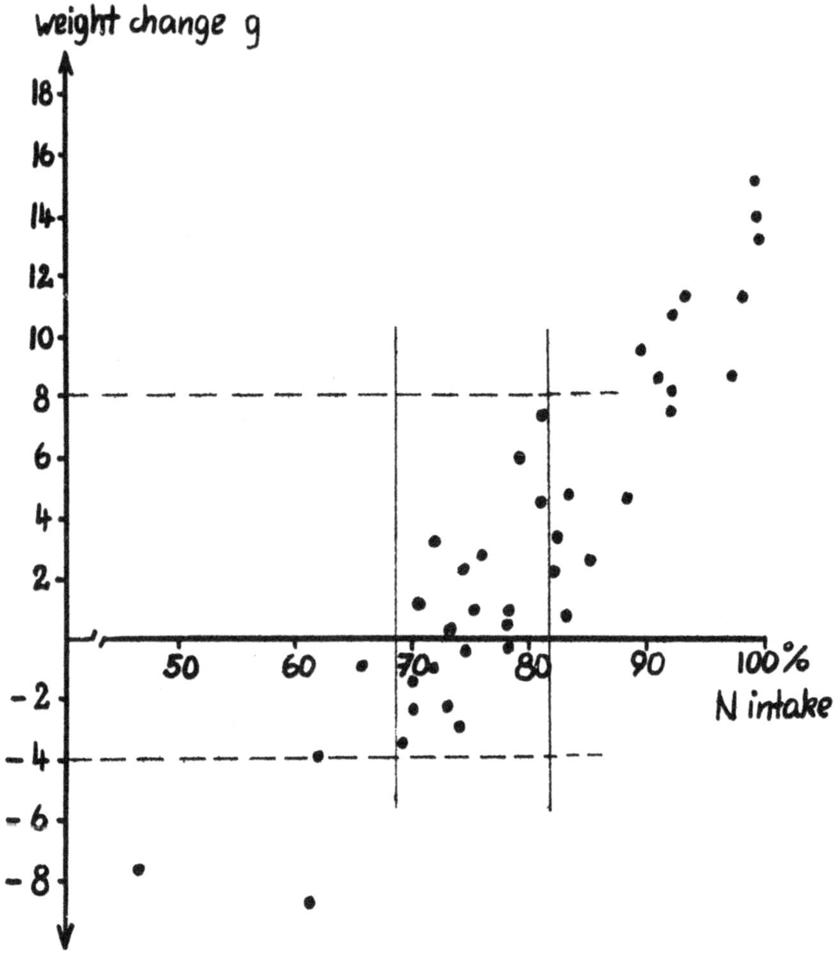

Fig. 2. The relationship of N intake to weight change of rats

REFERENCES

Allison, J.B. and J.A. Anderson 1945. The relation between absorbed nitrogen balance and biological value of proteins in adult dogs. J. Nutr. 29., 413-420.

Allison, J.B., J.A. Anderson and R.D. Seely 1946. The determination of the nitrogen balance index in normal and hypoproteinemic dogs. Ann. N.Y. Acad. Sci. 47., 245-271.

Amaya-F.J., C.T. Young and C.O. Chichester 1977. Automated determination of trypthophan in legumes and cereals. J. Agric. Food Chem. 25., 1. 139-143.

Arbeitskreis für Proteinbewertung der Gesellschaft für Ernährungsphysiologie der Haustiere 1964. Vorschrift zur Proteinbewertung in Versuchen mit Ratten Z. Tierphysiol. Tierern., 19., 257.

Baum, F. 1966. a. Über die Bestimmung des biologischen Eiweisswertes mit _Tetrahymena pyriformis W_. 2. Mitt.: Der Eiweisswert verschiedener Lebens- und Futtermittel. Nahrung 10., 6. 454-459.

Baum, F. 1966. b. Über die Bestimmung des biologischen Eiweisswertes mit _Tetrahymena pyriformis W_. 3. Mitt. Die Wirkung von Aminosäurezusätzen und Lagerdauer auf den Eiweisswert von Getreidemehlen. Nahrung 10., 7. 571-579.

Baum, F. and H. Haenel 1965. Über die Bestimmung der Biologischen Eiweisswertigkeit mit _Tetrahymena pyriformis W_. 1. Mitt.: Methodische Hinweise und Bestimmung der Wertigkeit einiger Nahrungsmittel. Nahrung 9., 5. 517-525.

Beecher, G.R. 1974. Some practical applications of protein synthesis and muscle growth. J. Anim. Sci. 38., 5. 1071-1078.

Bender, A.E. and B.H. Doell 1957. Biological evaluation of proteins: A new aspect. Brit. J. Nutr. 11., 140-148.

Bender, A.E. and D.S. Miller 1953. a. Constancy of the N/H_2O ratio of the rat and its use in the determination of the net protein value. Biochem. J. 53., VII.

Bender, A.E. and D.S. Miller 1953. b. A new brief method of estimation net protein value. Biochem. J. 53., VII.

Bergen, W.C. 1974. Protein synthesis in animal models. J. Anim. Sci. 38. 1079-1091.

Bergner, H., H. Münchow and R. Koch 1968. Untersuchungen zur Proteinbewertung von Futtermitteln 5. Mitt.: Vergleichende Eiweissqualitätsuntersuchungen im Tierversuch und auf mikrobiologischer Basis mit der Protozoe _Tetrahymena pyriformis W_. Arch. Tierernähr. 18., 3. 212-221.

Bergner, H., B. Wirthgen and H. Münchow 1966. Untersuchungen zur Proteinbewertung von Futtermitteln 1. Mitt. Die Aktivität von Glutamat-Oxalacetat-Transaminase, Glutamat-Pyruvat-Transaminase und Ornithin-Carbamoyltransferase im Serum von Schweinen nach Fütterung der Proteine aus Vollei, Gerste verschiedener Hefen oder einer eiweissfreien Diat. Arch. Tierernähr. 16., 6/7., 507-516.

Berschauer, F. 1978. Schätzung des Proteinansatzes aus der Blutharnstoffkonzentration beim Schwein. Vortr. Tagung der Gesellschaft für Tierzuchtwissenschaft, Hohenheim.

Blohm, L., P. Hendriks and J. Caris 1969. The determination of the availability of lysine via the N-dinitrophenyl-derivates, especially in carbohydrate-rich material. Wiss. Z. Univ. Rostock. Math.-Naturwiss. Reihe 18. 1/2. 183-188.

Bock, H.-D. 1958. Zur Bestimmung des N-Grundumsatzes bei wachsenden Albinoratten. Wiss. Abh. DAL, 37. 146-152.

Bock, H.-D. 1964. Über Stickstoffbilanzversuche - Problematik und Ergebnisse. Tag-ber DAL, 63., 97-109.

Bock, H.-D. 1965. Bewertung von Hahrungs- und Futterproteinen im Tierversuch unter besonderer Berücksichtigung der biologischen Wertigkeit an wachsenden Albinoratten. Habil-Schrift, Univ. Rostock, GDR.

Bock, H.-D. 1967 a. Bericht über die 2. Enquete zur Bestimmung der Stickstoff-Bilanz von Futterproteinen. Sitzungsberichte DAL XVI. 19., 39-46.

Bock, H.-D. 1967 b. Bericht über die 1. RGW-Enquete zur Bestimmung der Stickstoff-Bilanz von Futterproteinen. Int. Z. Landw. 4., 390-394.

Bock, H.-D. 1975. Methoden zur Beurteilung der Proteinqualität von Nahrungs- und Futtermitteln. Akad. Landw. DDR. Fortschr. Landw. Nahrungsgüterw. 13., 5.

Bock, H.-D. 1975. Über natürliche, antinutritiv wirkende, vorwiegend die Proteinverwertung beeinträchtigende Inhaltsstoffe pflanzlicher Futtermittel. Fortschr. Landw. Nahrungsgüttern. Akad. Landw. DDR, 13., 6.

Bock, H.-D., F. Horszcaruk and L. Angelova 1964 a. Untersuchungen über den Stickstoffumsatz im tierischen Organismus. 4. Mitt. Der Stickstoffumsatz wachsender Albinoratten bei proteinfreier. Ernährung. Arch. Tierernähr. 14., 157-165.

Bock, H.-D., K. Nehring, R. Schiemann, F. Horvorka, F. Horszcaruk and L. Angelova 1964 b. Untersuchungen über den Stickstoffumsatz im tierischen Organismus. 1. Mitt. N-Bilanzversuche an wachsenden Albinoratten. Arch. Tierernähr. 14., 13-21.

Bock, H.-D., J. Wünsche, F. Kreienbring, L. Hoffmann, W. Wiesemüller, H. Jeroch and J. Becker. Aminosäuretabellen 1981. Akad. Landwirtsch. Wiss. DDR, Forschungszentrum Tierprod. Dummerstorf-Rostock. Ber. Tierernährung.

Bodwell, C.E. 1976. Status of Chemical Methods to Determine Biologically Available Lysin in Wheat Proteins. Proceedings of the 9th National Conference on Wheat Utilization Research. Seattle, Washington 1975, Agricultural Research Service, U.S. Department of Agriculture ARS-NC-40., 181-193.

Bodwell, C.E. 1977. Problems associated with the development and application of rapid methods of assessing protein quality. Nutr. Rep. Intern. 16., 2, 163-178.

Bodwell, C.E., E.M. Kyle, E.M. Schuster, D.A. Vaughan, M. Womack, R.A. Ahrens and L.R. Hackler 1979. Biochemical indices in humans of protein nutritive value. III. Fasting plasma urea nitrogen and urinary metabolites as a low protein intake level. Nutr. Rep. Intern. 19., 5. 703-713.

Boehncke, E. and I. Rieder 1974. Untersuchungen zur Kreatininausscheidung wachsender Mastkälber. Z. Tierphysiol. Tierern. 33., 268-274.

Brune, H., E. Thier and E. Borchert 1968. a. Zur Inkongruenz der Proteinverwertung durch Ratte und Schwein und zur Variabilität ihrer Stoffwechseldaten. 108-116. Z. Tierphysiol. Tierern. 24., 1. Mitt.: Das Differenzierungsvermögen von Albinoratte und Schwein für verschiedene Futtermittel.

Brune, H., E. Thier and E. Borchert 1968. b. Variabilität der biologischen Proteinqualität verschiedener Getreidearten (Düngungs - und Standortvarianten) 3. Mitt.: Versuchsergebnisse von Stoffwechselversuchen mit Schweinen und Ratten und Vergleich mit Aminosäureindices. Z. Tierphysiol. Tierern. 24., 89-107.

Buamah, T.F. and E.P. Singsen 1975. Studies on the protein efficiency ratio method for the evaluation of poultry feed supplements. Modifications associated with choice of dietary protein level for assay. J. Nutr. 105., 6, 688-700.

Buttery, P.J. and J.B. Soar 1975. A spectrofluorimetric assay of the tryptophan content of feedstuffs. J. Sci. Food. Agric. 26., 1273-1277.

Calloway, D.H. 1975. Nigrogen balance of men with marginal intakes of protein and energy. J. Nutr. 105., 7. 914-923.

Carpenter, K.J. and A.M. Ellinger 1955. The estimation of "available lysine" in protein concentrates. Biochem. J. 61., (a). XI.

Carpenter, K.J. and J. Opstvedt 1976. Application of chemical and biological assay procedures for lysine to fish meals. J. Agric. Food. Chem. 24., 389-392.

Carpenter, K.J. and A.A. Woodham 1974. Protein quality of feedingstuffs 6. Comparisons of the results of collaborative biological assays for amino acids with those of other methods. Brit. J. Nutr. 32., 647-659.

Columbus, A. 1951. Die Variabilität der biologischen Eiweisswertigkeit unter verschiedenen Bedingungen nach Stoffwechselversuchen an wachsenden Schweinen. Arch. Tierernähr. 1., 84-128.

Columbus, A. 1954 a. Stickstoff-Grundumsatz und Methodik der Bestimmung der biologischen Eiweisswertigkeit nach dem N-Bilanz-Verfahren bei wachsenden Ratten. Arch. Tierernähr. 4., 51-82.

Columbus, A. 1954 b. Problematik der Methoden zur Bestimmung der biologischen Eiweisswertigkeit. Wiss. Abh. DAL V/2, 327-354.

Duckworth, J., A.A. Woodham and I. McDonald 1961. The assessment of nutritive value in protein concentrate by the gross protein value method. J. Sci. Food Agric. 12., 407-417.

Eggum, B.O. 1970. Blood urea measurement as a technique for assessing protein quality. Brit. J. Nutr. 24., 983-998.

Eggum, B.O. 1973. A study of certain factors influencing protein utilization in rats and pigs. Kobenhavn.

Erbersdobler, H. 1962. Die Bestimmung von verfügbarem Lysin in Eiweissfuttermitteln mit Hilfe von Dinitrofluorbenzol. Diss. Tierärztl. Fak. Univ. München.

Evans, E., S.C. Carruther and R. Witty 1977. Comparison of Tetrahymena pyriformis and PER responses to meat and meat products. Nutr. Rep. Intern. 16., 4., 455-462.

Featherstone, W.R. 1972. Effect of diet on levels of amino acids in plasma and tissues. Poult. Sci. LI, 1. 17-27.

Fernell, W.R. and G.D. Rosen 1956. Microbiological evaluation of protein quality with Tetrahymena pyriformis W. 1. Characteristics of growth of the organismen and determination of relative nutritive values of intact protein. Brit. J. Nutr. 10., 2. 143-156.

Friedman, M. and J.W. Finley 1971. Methods of tryptophan analysis. J. Agr. Food Chem. 19., 4. 626-631.

Garlick, P.J. and D.J. Millward 1972. An appraisal of techniques for the determination of protein turnover in vivo. Proceedings Biochem. Soc., Biochem. J. 129., 2. 1-2.

Gebhardt, G. 1964. Zur Bewertung der Eiweissqualität von Nahrungs und Futtermitteln mit Hilfe des Tierversuches. In: Probleme der Eiweissanalytik. Tag-ber. DAL 64., 47-61.

Gebhardt, G. 1973. Parameter des N-Stoffwechsels und Wachstumsgesetzmässigkeiten. Wiss. Z., Marx Univ. Leipzig, Math. Natwiss. Reihe 22., 3. 201-213.

Gruhn, K. and B. Raue 1974. Ausscheidungen der Aminosäuren mit dem Harn und Kot von kolostomierten und nicht operierten Hennen-Beitrag zur Methode der Aminosäurenresorbierbarkeit. 1. Mitt. Abhängigkeit der Exkretion der Harnaminosäuren von Aminosäurenverzehr. Arch. Tierernähr. 24., 67-73.

Gundel, J. and E. Votisky 1974. Hydrolyse von Futterproteinen mit p-Toluolsulfonsäure und Tryptophanbestimmung in Fischmehl. Tagber. DAL 124., 59-63.

Hartfiel, W. 1961. Zur Bewertung von Futtermitteln im Tierversuch mit Hühnern. I. Über den Aufbau einer Stoffwechselbatterie sowie die Konservierung und Untersuchung der Exkremente. Arch. Tierernahr. 11., 225-232.

Hegedüs, M., U.P. Kralovánszky and T. Mátrai 1981. A takarmány-fehérjék minősítése. Mezőgazdasági Kiadó, Budapest.

Hegsted, D.M. 1975. Balance studies. J. Nutr. 106., 3. 307-311.

Hegsted, D.M. and Y. Chang 1965. a. Protein utilization in growing rats. I. Relative growth index as a bioassay procedure. J. Nutr. 85., 159-168.

Hegsted, D.M. and Y. Chang 1965.b. Protein utilization in growing rats at different levels of intake. J. Nutr. 87., 19-25.

Hegsted, D.M. and J. Worchester 1947.A study of the relation between protein efficiency and gain in weight on diets of constant protein content. J. Nutr. 33., 685-702.

Heiman, V.J., S. Carver and J.W. Cook 1939, 1955. b. A method for determining the gross value of protein concentrates. cit.: Carpenter, K.J. and G.M. Ellinger: Protein quality and "available lysine" in animal products. Poult. Sci. 34., 1451.

Hennig, A. 1958. Beiträge zur Ermittlung des Darmverluststickstoffes bei Schweinen. Z. Tierphysiol., Tierern. 13., 316-317.

Henning, A., K. Gruhn and G. Jahreis 1977. Incorporation of nitrogen 15 from lysine and wheat in the eggs and bodies of laying hens. In: Stable isotopes in the life sciences. Intern. Atomic Energy Agency. Vienna, 371-375.

Hohls, H.W. 1955. Die Berechnung des maximalen täglichen Eiweissansatzvermögens von Schweinen aus in der Literatur veröffentlichten Daten und dessen Bedeutung bei der Durchführung von Fütterungsversuchen. Z. Tierern. u. Futterm. 10., 1, 44-55.

Hohls, H.W. 1962. Zur Frage des Stickstoffverlustes bei Küken und Ratten. Arch. Tierernähr. 12., 179-187.

Hohls, H.W. 1967. Die Altersabhängigkeit verschiedener Stoffwechselgrössen bei wachsenden Hühnern. Arch. Geflügelk. 31., 184-205.

Holm, H. 1971. Micro-method for determination of non-N-terminal lysine in milk and similar products. J. Sci. Food Agric. 22., 378-381.

Horszcaruk, F. and H.-D. Bock 1963. Eine Modifikation des von K. Schiller vorgeschlagenen Stoffwechselkäfigs für Ratten. Z. Versuchstierkd. 2., 126-131.

Hurrell, R.F. and K.J. Carpenter 1976. An approach to the rapid measurement of "reactive lysine" in foods by dye binding. Proc. Nutr. Soc. 35., 23A.

Hurt, D., R.H. Forsythe and C.H. Krieger 1975. Factors which influence the biological evaluation of protein quality by the protein efficiency ratio method. In: Friedman, M. Protein nutritional quality of foods and feeds. Part 1. Marcel Dekker, Inc. New York, 87-112.

Kedenburg, C.-P. 1970. Beitrag zur Bestimmung des verfügbaren Lysins nach Carpenter. Landwirtschaftliche Forschung 23/II, Stand und Leistung agrikulturchemischer und agrarbiologischer Forschung XVII. 59-62.

Kihlberg, R. 1970. Changes in plasma-free amino acids in short growth studies with rats. In: Evaluation of novel protein products. eds. A.E. Bender, R. Kihlberg, B. Löfquist and L. Munck, Pergamon Press, Oxford and New York, 149-157.

Kment, A. and J. Leibetseder 1973. Zur Problematik der Proteinbewertung in der Tierernährung. Wien. Tierärztl. Mschr. 60., 2/3. 83-91.

Kofrányi, E. 1973. Evaluation of traditional hypothesis on the biological value of proteins. Nutr. Rep. Intern. 7., 1. 45.50.

Kofrányi, E., F.-K. Jekat and H. Müller-Wecker 1970. The determination of the biological value of dietary proteins, XVI. The minimum protein requirement of humans, tested with mixtures of whole egg plus potato and maize plus beans. Hoppe-Seyler. Z.f. Phys. Chem. 351., 1485-1493.

Kovács, J. and J. Ridly 1975, cit. in Hegedüs, M., U.P. Kralovánszky and T. Mátrai 1981. A takarmányfehérjék minősítése. Mezőgazdasági Kiadó, Budapest.

Kralovánszky U.P. and Mátrai T. 1980. A hús- és tejtermelés biológiája. Mezőgazdasági Kiadó, Budapest.

Kunze, B. 1968. Untersuchungen zum jahreszeitlichen Rhythmus des Stickstoff-Stoffwechsels wachsender Hähne. Diss. Martin-Luther-Universität Halle, GDR.

Leibetseder, J. and M.Y. Hamed 1968. Biologische Proteinbewertung an Küken. Z. Tierphysiol. Tierern. 23., 4. 239-242.

Lewis, A.J., P.J. Holden, R.C. Ewan and D.R. Zimmerman 1976. An automated fluorometric method for the measurement of tryptophan in plasma. J. Agric. Food Chem., 24., 5. 1081-1083.

Liappis, N., P. Anda and P. Bantzer 1975. Vergleich der freien Aminosäuren im Blutserum von Menschen und Tieren. 1. Mitt.: Mensch, Ratte, Maus, Huhn. Z. Tierphysiol. Tierern. 36., 1. 56-61. 2. Mitt.: Mensch, Kaninchen, Meerschweinchen, Schwein. Z. Tierphysiol. Tierern. 36., 2. 87-91.

Lintzel, W. and E. Mangold 1935. Die biologische Wertigkeit der Süsslupinensamen bei der Verfütterung an Schweine. Landw. Verss. 123., 133-146.

Lintzel, W. and J. Rechenberger 1940. Experimentelle Studien zur Theorie des Eiweisstoffwechsels. Biochem. Z. 304., 214. ff.

Lipton, S.H. and C.E. Bodwell 1977. A rapid method for detecting chemical alteration of Methionine. Agric. Food Chem. 25., 5. 1214-1216.

Maciejewicz-Rys, J. and A.M. Antoniewicz 1978. 2-Aminoethylphosphoric acid as an indicator of Tetrahymena pyriformis W. growth in protein-quality evaluation assay. Brit. J. Nutr. 40., 83-90.

Mangold, E. and A. Columbus 1937. Verdaulichkeit und biologische Wertigkeit von Kartoffeleiweiss beim Schwein. Landw. Verss. 129., 12-21.

Mangold, E. and A. Columbus 1938. Verdaulichkeit und biologische Eiweisswertigkeit der Samenkörner einer neuen gelben Süsslupine (Weiko) beim Schwein. Landw. Verss. 129., 110-123.

Mangold, E. and G. Behm 1955. Beziehungen zwischen Darmverlust-Stickstoff und Rohfasergehalt des Futters. Arch. Tierernähr. 5., 159-175.

Matheson, N.A. 1968. Available lysine. II. Determination of available lysine in feedingstuffs by dinitrophenylation. J. Sci. Food. Agric., 19., 496-502.

Matheson, N.A. 1973. The estimation of trypthophan. Proc. Nutr. Soc. 32., 3., 99A-100A.

Matheson, N.A. 1974. The determination of tryptophan in purified proteins and in feeding-stuffs. Brit. J. Nutr. 31., 3. 393-400.

McLaughlan, J.M. and M.O. Keith 1975. Bioassays for protein quality. In: Friedman, M., Protein nutritional quality of foods and feeds.Part 1. Marcel Dekker, Inc., New York, 79-85.

McLaughlan, J.M., G.O. Korsrud and J.E. Knipfel 1973. Plasma lysine as an indicator for lysine supplementation of wheat flour in rats. Nutr. Rep. Intern. 8., 1. 1-8.

Meier, H. and S. Poppe 1976. Zur Bestimmung der Stickstoffbilanz und der wahren Verdaulichkeit von Aminosäuren bei monogastrischen Tieren. Tag-ber. DAL 142., 33-51.

Menke, K.H. 1980. Proteinverwertung und Blutharnstoffkonzentration. Arch. Tierernähr. 30., 1/2. 51-54.

Mercer, L.P., P.H. Morgan, N.W. Flodin and A. Domm 1979. Prediction of food intakes and growth rates in weanling rats by the Four-Parameter model equation. Nutr. Rep. Intern. 19., 1. 1-8.

Millward, D.G. and P.J. Garlick 1972. The pattern of protein turnover in the whole animal and the effect of dietary variations. Proc. Nutr. Soc. 31., 257-263.

Millward, D.J., D.O. Nnanyelugo, W.P.T. James and P.J. Garlick 1974. Protein metabolism in skeletal muscle: the effect of feeding and fasting on muscle RNA, free amino acids and plasma insulin concentrations. Brit. J. Nutr. 32., 127-142.

Mitchell, H.H. 1924. a. A method of determining the biological value of protein. J. biol. Chem. 58., 873-903.

Mitchell, H.H. 1924. b. The biological value of protein at different level of intake. J. biol. Chem. 58., 905-922.

Mokady, S., S. Viola and G. Zimmermann 1969. A new biological method for estimating feed protein value. Brit. J. Nutr. 23., 491-495.

Munck, L. 1972. Improvement of nutritional value in cereals. Hereditas 72. 1-2.

Muramatsu, K., H. Takeuchi and K. Sakurai 1973. The relationship between weight gain and free amino acid concentration of plasma and liver in rats fed a diet supplemented with various amounts of lysine. J. Nutr. Sci. Vitaminol., 19., 277-285.

Müller, R. and D. Hötzel 1957. Zur Frage des Vergleichs von Ratte und Schwein bei der Proteinbewertung. Arch. Tierernähr. 7., 233-243.

Münchow, H. 1967. Untersuchungen über Beziehungen zwischen der biologischen Wertigkeit von Eiweissfuttermitteln und einigen biochemischen und biologischen Kenndaten bei Ratte und Schwein. Dissertationsschr. Humboldt-Universität Berlin.

Münchow, H. and H. Bergner 1967. Untersuchungen zur Proteinbewertung von Futtermitteln 2. Mitt.: Die Harnstoffkonzentration im Blut von Ratte und Schwein in Abhängigkeit vom biologischen Wert des gefütterten Nahrungsproteins. Arch. Tierernähr. 17., 3. 141-150.

Münchow, H. and H. Bergner 1968. Empfehlungen zur Proteinbewertung von Eiweissfuttermitteln anhand der Bestimmung der Harnstoffkonzentration im Blut von Ratte oder Schwein. Arch. Tierernähr. 18., 3. 222-228.

Münchow, H. and H. Bergner 1970. Vergleichende Untersuchungen zur Bestimmung der Thyreoideasekretionsrate (TRS) beim Schwein mittels Replacement- und Degradations - Verfahren. Arch. Tierernähr. 20., 3. 201-209.

Neale, R.J. and J.C. Waterlow 1974. a. The metabolism of ^{14}C-labelled essential amino acids given by intragastric or intravenous infusion to rats on normal and protein-free diets. Brit. J. Nutr. 32., 11-25.

Neale, R.J. and J.C. Waterlow 1974. b. Critical evaluation of a method for estimating amino acid requirements for maintenance in the rat by measurement of the rate of ^{14}C-labelled amino acid oxidation in vivo. Brit. J. Nutr. 32., 257-272.

Nehring, K. 1953. Die Bestimmung der biologischen Wertigkeit des Eiweisses. Landw. Forsch. Sonderheft. 4., 123.

Nehring, K. 1954. Untersuchungen über die biologische Wertigkeit von Eiweissfutterstoffen. 1. Mitt. Die Bestimmung der biologischen Wertigkeit und der Ergänzungswirkung von Eiweissfutterstoffen durch Versuche an wachsenden Ratten. Beih. Arch. Tierernähr. 4., 110-126.

Nehring, K. 1962. Methodik der N-Bilanzversuche zur Ermittlung der biologischen Wertigkeit des Eiweisses von Futtermitteln. Sitzungsberichte DAL XI., 1. 103-111.

Nehring, K. and H.-D. Bock 1961. Untersuchungen über die biologische Wertigkeit von Eiweissfutterstoffen an Ratten. Arch. Tierernähr., 11., 370-392.

Nehring, K., B. Knabe and H.-D. Bock 1964. Untersuchungen über den Stickstoffumsatz im tierischen Organismus. III. N-Bilanzversuche an Küken. Arch. Tierernähr. 14., 31-37.

Nehring, K. and W. Laube 1961. Untersuchungen über die biologische Wertigkeit des Eiweisses verschiedener Futterstoffe beim Schwein I. Eiweissfutterstoffe und Getreide. Z. Tierphysiol. Tierern. 16., 119-132.

Niess, E. and R. Müller 1972. Die Frage der Reproduzierbarkeit von Versuchen zur biologischen Proteinbewertung. Z. Tierphysiol. Tiererähr. 30., 177-192.

Njaa, L.R. 1959. a. A shortened version of the Mitchell method for determination of the biological value of protein. Growth rate as a source of error. Brit. J. Nutr. 13., 137-142.

Njaa, L.R. 1959. b. Biological value of herring-meal protein. Urinary nitrogen excretion in relation to protein content of diet and food intake. Brit. J. Nutr. 13., 142-150.

Njaa, L.R. 1966. Nitrogen balance experiments: some theoretical considerations. Nature, 211., 5056., 1413-1414.

Oddove, E.A. and S. Margen 1979, Nitrogen balance studies in humans: Long-term effect of high nitrogen intake on nitrogen accretion. J. Nutr. 109., 3., 363-377.

Ohno, T. and I. Tasaki 1976. Liver free amino acids in adult cockerels fed diets containing graded levels of protein. Nutr. Rep. Intern. 13., 3., 247-252.

Osborne, T.B., L.B. Mendel and E.L. Ferry 1919. A method of expressing numerically the growth-promoting value of proteins. J. biol. Chem. 37., 223-229.

Ostrowsky, H. 1969. A comparison of the Carpenter and Silcock methods for available lysine determination in protein concentrations and diets. Proc. Nutr. Soc. 28., 1. 3A-4A.

Poppe, S. 1976. Zur Bestimmung der wahren Aminosäurenverdaulichkeit. Tag-ber. DAL 142., 77-83.

Pruss, H.D . and K.H. Ney. 1972. Bestimmung des "verfügbaren" Lysins in Molkenpulver, Molkeneiweiss und labgefällten Casein mit dem Reaktivfarbstoff Remazolbrillantblau R.Z. Lebensm.Unters. Forsch. 148., 347-351.

Puchal, F., V.W. Hays, V.C. Speer, J.D. Jones and D.V. Catron 1962. The free blood plasma amino acids of swine as related to the source of dietary proteins. J. Nutr. 76., 11-17.

Robertson, E.I., J.S. Carver and J.W. Cook 1938., cit.: Butterworth, Poult. Sci. 17., (1962) 433.

Rolle, G. and B.O. Eggum 1971. A comparative protein evaluation with Tetrahymena pyriformis W. and rats. Acta Agric. Scand. 21., 69-72.

Rosen, G.D. and W.R. Fernell 1956. Microbiological evaluation of of protein quality with Tetrahymena pyriformis W. 2. Relative nutritive values of proteins in foodstuffs. Brit. J. Nutr. 10., 2., 156-168.

Rudérus, H. and Kihlberg, R. 1970. Determination of available lysine by column chromatography. In: Evaluation of novel protein products; ed. A.E. Bender, R. Kihlberg, B. Löfquist, L. Munck, Pergamon Press - Oxford and New York, 195-201.

Rufeger, H. 1972. Proteinbewertung und Berechnung exogener und endogener Grössen des N-Stoffwechsels monogastrischer Organismen mit Hilfe einer N-Bilanzfunktion. Zbl. Vet. Med. A., 19., 713-725.

Santarius, K. and H.-D.Belitz 1973. Eine einfache Methode zur Tryptophan-Bestimmung in Proteinen. Z. Lebensm. Unters. Forsch. 150., 279-282.

Sarwar, G. and J.M. McLaughlan 1981. Relative protein ratio method for evaluating protein quality. Nutr. Rep. Intern. 23., 6., 1157-1166.

Schadereit, R., H.-D. Bock, J. Wünsche and F. Kreienbring 1976. Untersuchungen über die wahre Aminosäurenverdaulichkeit bei Broilerküken. Tag-ber. DAL 142., 93-98.

Schiftan, H. 1932. Über die biologische Wertigkeit des Futtereiweisses bei wachsenden Schweinen. Wiss. Arch. Landw. B. 8., 212.

Schröder, I. and H.-D. Bock 1962. Bericht über die von der Forschungsgemeinschaft "Eiweiss in der Tierernährung" durchgeführten Enqueten über die Methoden zur Bestimmung der Aminosäuren-Zusammensetzung und der biologischen Wertigkeit von Futterproteinen. Arch. Tierernähr. 13., 241-246.

Shannon, b.M.,J.M. Howe and H.E. Clark 1972. Interrelationships between dietary methionine and cystine as reflected by growth, certain hepatic enzymes and liver composition of weanling rats. J. Nutr. 102., 4, 557-562.

Steinhart, H. 1979. Zur Abhängigkeit der mit verschiedenen Analysenmethoden ermittelten Tryptophangehalte von der Hydrolysenzeit bei alkalischen Hydrolysen. Arch Tierernähr. 29., 4., 211-220.

Steinhart, H. and J. Sandmann 1977. Determination of tryptophane in plasma with a spectrofluorometer system. Analyt. Chem. 49., 7., 950-953.

Stewart, A.M. 1974. Muscle cell size as an index of potential for growth in rats. Proc. Nutr. Soc. 33., 18A.

Stillway, L.W., A.C. Wiese and C.F. Petersen 1972. Selection of chicks to minimize variation in growth studies. J. Nutr. 102., 2., 205-208.

Stott, J.A. and H. Smith 1963. Microbiological evaluation of protein quality with Tetrahymena pyriformis W. 3. A simplified assay procedure. Brit. J. Nutr. 17., 2., 227-233.

Tayler, Y.S.M., N.S. Scrimshaw and V.R. Young 1974. The relationship between serum urea levels and dietary nitrogen utilization in young men. Brit. J. Nutt. 32., 107-411.

Thomas, K. 1909. Über di biologische Wertigkeit der N-Substanzen in verschiedenen Nahrungsmitteln. Arch. Anat. Physiol. 25., 219-305.

Walger, J. and B. Walger 1972. Metodikai kisérletek takarmány-fehérjék biológiai értékének mikroorganizmusokkal történő meghatározására. Kutatási jelentés (manuscript),OMFB Library, Budapest.

Walger-Kunze, B. 1972. Beeinflussung des Stickstoffstoffwechselswachsen der Hähne durch die Jahreszeit. 1. Mitt.: Beziehungen zwischen N-Erhaltungsbedarf und Jahreszeit. Arch. Tierernähr. 22., 6, 407-414. 2. Mitt.: Abhängigkeit des N-Stoffwechsels und der Wachstumsintensität von Jahreszeit und Klimaverlauf. Arch. Tierernähr. 22., 6., 415-422. 3. Mitt.: Die N-Ausscheidung als Kriterium für die Intensität des Stoffwechsels. Arch. Tierernähr. 22., 7., 475-478. 4. Mitt.: Orientierende Sticksstoffbilanzversuche mit Vollei - und Sojabohnenprotein. Arch. Tierernähr. 22., 7., 479-484.

Walz, O.P. and J.E. Ford 1972. The measurement of "Available Lysin" in protein foods. Z. Tierphysiol. Tierern. 30., 304-322.

Wetterau, H. 1953. Stickstoffgrundumsatz und biologische Eiweisswertigkeit bei wachsendem Geflügel. Diss. Martin-Luther-Universität Halle, GDR.

Wetterau, H. 1960. N-Bilanzversuche an wachsendem Geflügel. Arch. Geflügelz. Kleintierk. 9., 411-424.

Wirthgen, B. and H. Bergner 1970. Der Einfluss der Körpermasse der Versuchsratten auf die Enzymaktivität von GOT, GPT, LAP, OCT und Arginase in der Rattenleber bei quantitativ unterschiedlicher Eiweissernährung. Nahrung, 14., 3., 183-191.

Womack, M., D.A. Vaughan and C.E. Bodwell 1975. A modified PER method for estimating changes in the bioavailability of individual essential amino acids. In: Friedman, M., Protein nutritional quality of foods and feeds. Part 1. Marcel Dekker, Inc., New York, 113-123.

Wünsche, J. 1967. Bericht über die 3. Aminosäuren-Enquete des Themenkreises 9.1. Sitzungsberichte DAL XVI., 9., 17-24

Wünsche, J. 1969. Zur Tryptophanbestimmung in Hahrungs- und Futtermitteln nach der mirobiologischen Methode. Wiss. Univ. Rostock. Math.-Naturwiss. Reihe 18., 1/2. 177-181.

Wünsche, J., M. Meinl, T. Völker and H.-D. Bock 1978. Wahre Verdaulichkeit des Proteins und der essentiellen Aminosäuren von Kasein und Weizengluten bei Ferkeln in Abhängigkeit von verschiedenen Einflussfaktoren. Tag-ber., DAL 159., 49-60.

Yanez, E. and J.M. McLaughlan 1970. The effect of level of protein on protein quality of lysine-deficient foods. Can. J. Physiol. Pharm., 48., 3., 188-192.

Young, V.R., G. Vilaire, P.M. Newberne and R.B. Wilson 1973. Plasma insulin and amino acid concentrations in rats given an adequate or low protein diet. J. Nutr. 103., 5., 720-729.

Zausch, M. 1967. Verdaulichkeit und biologische Eiweisswertigkeit verschiedener Sorten von Luzerne, Rotklee und Grünerbsen bei Schweinen. Arch. Tierernähr. 17., 555-576.

Zausch, M. and B. Kunze 1968. Eiweissertrag und Eiweissverwertbarkeit einheimischer Kürnerleguminosen in Abhängigkeit von Einflussnahmefaktoren. Wiss. Z. Univ. Rostock, Math.-Naturwiss. Reihe 18., 1/2., 171-175.

Proc. Int. Assoc. Cereal Chem. Symp. Amino Acid Compn and Biol. Value of Cereal Proteins
Budapest, Hungary 1983, R. Lásztity, M. Hidvégi, eds

SPECIFICITY OF AMINO ACIDS FOR NUTRITIONAL EVALUATION OF PROTEINS

AKIRA YOSHIDA

Department of Agricultural Chemistry, Nagoya University, Nagoya 464, Japan

Abstract : From the idea of "Chemical Score" by Mitchell and Block, it is unexpectable that the supplementation of only one or two essential amino acid(s) to a nonprotein diet improves the nitrogen balance of animals. We observed the decrease in body weight of rats due to feeding of a nonprotein diet was significantly improved when the nonprotein diet was supplemented with a small amount of methionine and threonine. Nitrogen balance of rats was also significantly improved by the supplementation of these two essential amino acids. Single supplementation of methionine to the nonprotein diet also showed the improved nitrogen balance, but the nitrogen sparing effect of supplementation with both methionine and threonine was much greater than that due to single supplementation of methionine. The improved nitrogen balance was mainly due to the decreased urinary excretion of urea. Urinary excretion of allantoin and creatinine was not decreased by the dietary supplementation of methionine and threonine. The activities of liver enzymes relating to the degradation of amino acids and urea cycle were not decreased by such an amino acid supplementation. However, plasma concentration of amino acids was generally decreased and the expired $14CO_2$ from 14C-lysine was decreased in rats fed the amino acids supplemented diet. The polysome profile in the livers of rats fed the amino acids supplemented diet showed more aggregated pattern indicating the stimulation of protein syntheses.

Further supplementation of other essential amino acids to the nonprotein diet in addition to methionine and threonine didn't improve the nitrogen balance of rats. However, the additional supplementation with small amounts of isoleucine, valine and tryptophan to the nonprotein diet previously supplemented with 2.7% of nonessential amino acid mixture together with methionine and threonine further significantly improved the body weight change and nitrogen balance.

These results suggest that in rats fed the nonprotein diet, each essential amino acid is not equally deficient, but there may be a sequence of limitation in endogenously produced amino acids. Probably, methionine and threonine are the most limiting amino acids in rats fed the nonprotein diet followed by the group of amino acids such as isoleucine, valine and tryptophan. It may be important to consider these nutritional specificity of each amino acid for the nutritional evaluation of protein based on the amino acid composition, especially in low protein condition.

Relationships between the amino acid composition of proteins and biological values were well documented by Mitchell and Block in 1946(Block and Mitchell, 1946), and the idea is widely accepted and used as "Chemical Score" or "Amino Acid Score".

In this idea, all essential amino acids must present at the same time for protein synthesis and the nutritional specificity of each essential amino acid is not taken into account. However, in certain conditions, especially when dietary level of protein is low, some essential amino acids show specific nutritional effects which are not explainable on the basis of the theory of "Chemical Score".

During the course of our study on an amino acid imbalance and fatty liver we observed the decrease in body weight of rats due to feeding of a nonprotein diet was significantly improved when the nonprotein diet was supplemented with a small amount of methionine and threonine. Single supplementation of methionine showed only little improving effect. This improving effect of methionine and threonine is unexpectable and can not be explained by the present nutritional theory. Therefore, the mechanism of the effect of methionine and threonine was studied.

1. Nitrogen sparing effect of methionine and threonine in rats receiving a nonprotein diet.

When a nonprotein diet is supplemented with a small amount of methionine, rats produce fatty livers(Williams, Jr. and Jasik, 1963). We investigated the effect of threonine for this type of fatty liver. During the course of this study, it was realized that the supplementation of methionine and threonine to a nonprotein diet markedly reduced the body weight loss and urinary nitrogen excretion, and also liver lipid accumulation was partially prevented(Yoshida et al., 1966 ; Yoshida and Moritoki, 1974). Young adult female rats of the

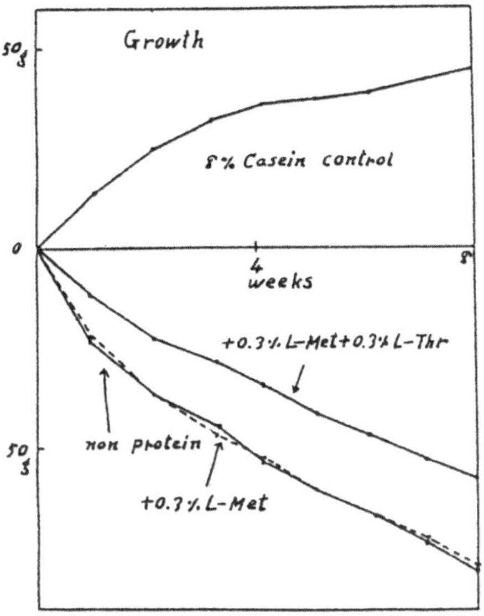

Fig. 1. Effect of supplementation of methionine and threonine to a nonprotein diet on body weight change of rats.

Wistar strain were fed a nonprotein-sucrose diet. These animals naturally lost their body weight(Fig. 1). However, the supplementation of 0.3% of L-methionine and 0.3% of L-threonine to this nonprotein diet, significantly reduced their body weight loss whereas single supplementation of methionine had almost no effect. Thus both methionine and threonine together were necessary for improvement of body weight loss of rats fed the nonprotein diet, although in later experiments single methionine supplementation showed some improving effect.

In the next experiments, effect of methionine and threonine on urinary nitrogen containing coumpounds were investigated.

As shown in Table 1, urinary excretion of urea of the nonprotein diet control group was 82mg for three days. But the rats on methionine and threonine supplemented group excreted only 23mg of urea for three days. Single supplementation of methionine also reduced the urinary excretion of urea, the amount was 56mg, not so significant as the case in methionine-threonine supplemented group. Urinary excretion of allantoin and creatinine

Table 1

Canges in urea, allantoin and creatinine contents in urine of rats fed Non-protein, Met and/or Thr supplemented diets

	urea mg/3days/100g BW	Avg mg/3days
(1) NP	114.9 ± 20.8	82.3
(2) NP+Met+Thr	31.4 ± 8.5	23.1
(3) NP+Met	78.6 ± 40.1	56.1
	allantoin mg/3 days	creatinine mg/3 days
(1) NP	1.23 ± 0.61	2.70 ± 0.52
(2) NP+Met+Thr	1.29 ± 0.72	3.54 ± 1.68
(3) NP+Met	1.28 ± 0.39	2.84 ± 1.02

Group 1 : Nonprotein diet. Group 2 : Nonprotein diet supplemented with methionine and threonine. Group 3 : Nonprotein diet supplemented with methionine.

was not affected by the supplementation of methionine or methionine plus threonine. The data show the nitrogen sparing effect of methionine and threonine in rats when they are supplemented to the nonprotein diet and the nitrogen sparing effect is mainly due to the reduced excretion of urea.

Because of a nonprotein diet was used as a basal diet, implication of the changes in digestibility of dietary protein is unlikely.

Willman et al.(Willman et al., 1945) indicated that the rats on 3.5% whole egg protein diet excreted less nitrogen than rats on protein poor diet. Brush, Willman and Swanson(Brush et al.,1947)further demonstrated that the nitrogen sparing effect of whole egg protein was mainly due to its methionine content. Allison et al.,(Allison et al., 1947) reported a similar observation with dogs. However, the mechanism of the nitrogen sparing effect of methionine has not been cleared yet. Furthermore, the nitrogen sparing effect of the combination of methionine and threonine in our observation is more significant than methionine alone.

We examined the effect of combination of methionine and one other amino acid on urinary nitrogen excretion. Glutamic acid was used to adjust the nitrogen content of the diet to be constant. Single addition of methionine to the nonprotein diet reduced the urinary nitrogen excretion and the more significant reduction in urinary nitrogen was observed by the addition of methionine and threonine;other combinations showed no more than the effect of methionine alone(Fig. 2A).

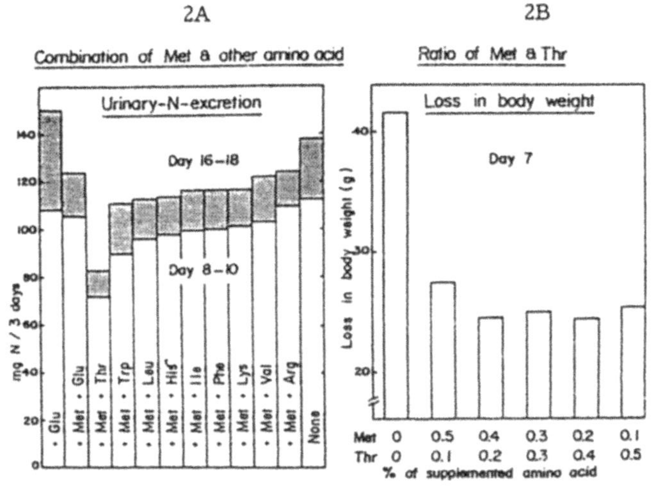

Fig. 2. Effect of amino acid supplementation to a non-protein diet on urinary nitrogen excretion (Fig. 2A) and on loss in body weight (Fig. 2B) of rats.

The ratio of supplemented methionine to threonine was variously changed keeping the total supplemental amount at 0.6%. Effect of the change in the ratio didn't affect on the loss in body weight significantly(Fig.2B) The amount of added methionine and threonine was gradually decreased and the nitrogen sparing effect was observed even as little as 0.02% of methionine and threonine(Yokogoshi and Yoshida 1976).

2. Effect of methionine and threonine on liver protein turnover.

At first, we supposed the effect of methionine and threonine would be some pharmacological ones through hormonal systems. But the adrenalectomy, diabetes or injection of growth hormone didn't affect the N-sparing effect of methionine and threonine.

There may be several mechanisms for the explanation of N-sparing effect of these amino acids.

Decreased degradation rate of body proteins, decrease in the rate of amino acid catabolism and urea formation, or increase in the reutilization of endogenously produced amino acids or combination of these factors are considered as possible mechanisms for N-sparing effect of methionine and threonine(Fig.3).

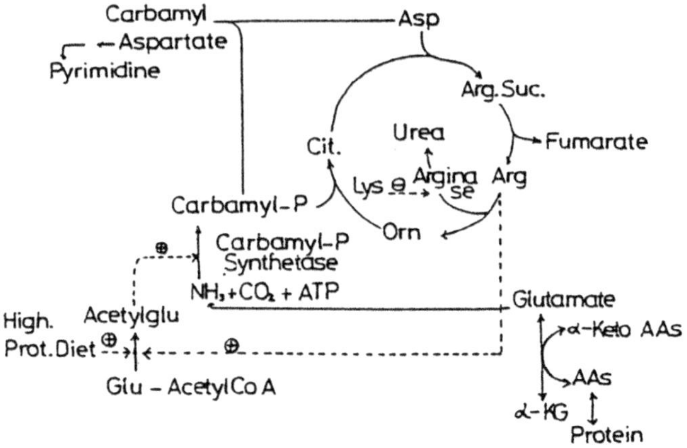

Fig. 3. General scheme of protein and amino acid metabolism, and urea cycle.

Effect of methionine and threonine on liver protein turnover was investigated. Some of the labeled amino acids released by protein breakdown is likely to be reincorporated into new protein molecules without leaving the tissues. It was proposed that 14C-arginine might be a useful tracer amino acid for the estimation of the rate of renewal of hepatic proteins. The high activity of liver arginase was thought to preclude a significant probability of reincorporation of labeled arginine arising from protein breakdown. Swick and Margot, however, surmised that there might be significant probability of reincorporation into hepatic proteins of labeled arginine derived from the breakdown of extrahepatic proteins, and suggested the use of 14C-sodium carbonate as a tracer. Therefore, 14C-sodium carbonate was used in the following experiments. Young female rats were fed a 25% casein-sucrose diet for 5 days. They were then injected 14C-sodium carbonate, and a group of rats was killed after 2 days. Others were fed the nonprotein diet or the methionine-threonine supplemented diet for another 9 and 20 days, respectively. Animals were killed and the radioactivities of liver proteins were determined by liquid scintillation spectrometer.

The decrease in total radioactivity of rats fed the nonprotein diet was greater than that of rats fed the methionine-threonine supplemented diet

(Fig. 4). In rats fed the amino acid supplemented diet, catabolism of liver proteins was slightly reduced together with the improved reutilization of other endogenously formed amino acids as compared with that of rats fed the nonprotein diet. Mortimore and Ward(Mortimore, G.E. and Ward, G.F. 1975) indicated that the addition of amino acids during pertusion strongly suppressed the intracellular protein degradation in livers and the most potent amino acid was methionine. These effects might contribute in part to the reduced excretion of urinary nitrogen.

3. Effect of methionine and threonine on the activities of enzymes relating to the amino acid metabolism.

Activities of some liver enzymes relating to the amino acid catabolism and urea cycle were determined. That were arginase, tyrosine-transaminase, alanine-transaminase, tryptophan-pyrolase, carbamoylphosphate synthetase, and others. But they were not decreased by supplement of methionine and threonine to the nonprotein diet(Table 2). Big effect was observed in tyrosine-transaminase. The activity of this enzyme was remarkably elevated by methionine supplement to the nonprotein diet. The increase of tyrosine transaminase activity by some amino acids and by corticosteroid has been reported(Kenney, 1963). But it is interesting the increase of the enzyme activity by dietary methionine was significantly prevented by simultaneous supplementation of threonine together with methionine. The reason why threonine supplementation prevented the elevation of tyrosine transaminase activity by methionine is not known. There may be an interaction between methionine and threonine for regulating the corticosteroid secretion.

McGivan et al.,(McGivan et al., 1974) reported that the rate of urea synthesis was regulated at the level of carbamoylphosphate synthetase activity, and N-acetylglutamic acid plays its important role in the regulation of urea biosynthesis through its activating effect on carbamoylphosphate synthetase(Shigesada, K. and Tatibana, M. 1971). However, the activity of carbamoylphosphate synthetase was not decreased by methionine-threonine supplementation and the daily injection of N-acetylglutamate in rats didn't affect the urea excretion(Yokogoshi et al., 1978).

4. Effect of methionine and threonine on tissue free amino acids and protein synthesis.

In liver, the level of most free amino acids of rats fed the nonprotein diet supplemented with methionine and threonine tended to decrease as

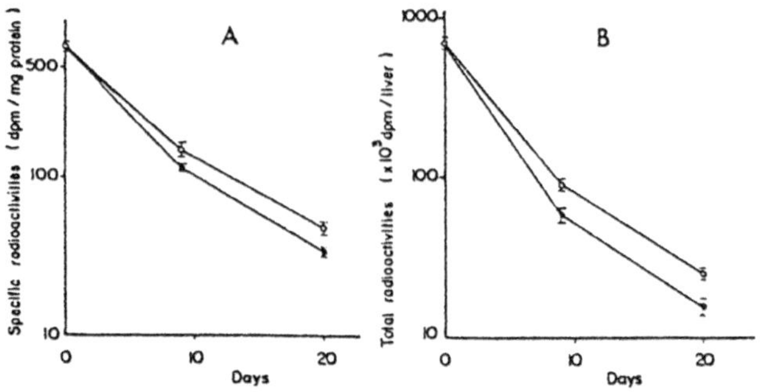

Fig. 4. Specific-(A, left) and total-(B, right) radioactivities of liver proteins of rats fed a protein free diet (●) or methionine and threonine supplemented diet (O). Body proteins of rats were previously labeled with 14C by injection of <u>14C-sodium carbonate</u> and then animals were fed the test diets. Radioactivity of liver proteins was determined 9 and 20 days on test diet. Vertical bars indicate standard deviations.

Table 2

T-134 ♀ 200g — Effect of Met-Thr Supplementation to a Protein-free Diet on Liver Enzyme Activities

	Non protein + Glu	Non protein + Met + Glu	Non protein + Met + Thr
Weight gain[1] 14 days	-44.4 ± 3.70	-28.4 ± 2.16[3]	-21.6 ± 2.77[3]
Liver Weight (g)	6.29 ± 0.382	8.02 ± 0.397[4]	8.72 ± 0.165[3]
Urinary N day 3-6	162 ± 14.2	123 ± 7.4[4]	100 ± 8.6[3]
Arginase mg Urea/100g B.W.	229 ± 20.8	209 ± 19.4	263 ± 14.7
Tyrosine transaminase[2] Total U/100g B.W.	521 ± 124.5	3176 ± 526.7[4]	1390 ± 299.8[4]
Alanine transaminase Total U/100g B.W.	649 ± 87.5	577 ± 98.1	569 ± 46.9

1) Initial body weight was about 200g.
2) mg P-hydroxyphenylpyruvic acid / 100g B.W.
3) Significantly different from group 1 ($P < 0.01$)
4) Significantly different from group 1 ($P < 0.06$)

compared with that of rats fed the control diet. Among the nonessential amino acids in rats fed the nonprotein diet supplemented with methionine and threonine, the concentration of aspartic acid, glutamic acid, serine and alanine were significantly reduced as compared with those of rats fed the nonprotein diet. Free lysine and histidine concentrations were also decreased. The contents of methionine and threonine in liver of rats fed the amino acid supplemented diet, however, tended to increase.

In plasma, as in liver, the concentration of lysine, histidine, serine, valine, leucine, and phenylalanine of rats fed the nonprotein diet supplemented with methionine and threonine were significantly reduced and the other amino acids also tended to decrease(Fig. 5)(Yokogoshi, H. et al., 1977). The results indicate that the changes in the level of some free amino acids might play an important role in the reduction in the amount of urea excreted in urine.

In the next experiments, the degradation of 14C-labelled amino acids to $14CO_2$ was investigated. Rats were fed the experimental diets, a nonprotein diet or methionine, threonine supplemented diet for 1 hour after overnight fasting. At the end of feeding, 14C-lysine, 14C-histidine or 14C-containing chlorella protein hydrolyzate was injected intraperitoneally, and the expired $14CO_2$ was collected. Radioactivity of the expired $14CO_2$ was determined by a liquid scintillation spectrometer.

When 14C-Lys or 14C-His was injected to rats fed the methionine and threonine supplemented diet, the expirations of $14CO_2$ were significantly decreased(Fig. 6). These phenomona also indicate the improved reutilization of tissue free amino acids by the supplementation of methionine and threonine.

Tissue polyribosomal profiles are considered to reflect the rate of protein synthesis. Rats were fed either a nonprotein diet or methionine-threonine supplemented diet for 5 days and the liver polyribosomal profiles were neasured. The postmitochondrial supernatant was applied to linear 0.5 to 1.5 M sucrose gradients, and were centrifuged 158,000 x g for 110 min. The ultraviolet absorption of the gradients at 254 nm was recorded. A population of monosome-disome area and polysome area was calculated. The ratio of monosome and disome to total ribosomes was significantly reduced suggesting the stimulated liver proteinsynthesis by methionine-threonine supplementation(Yokogoshi and Yoshida, 1979).

5. Sequence of limiting amino acids for the utilization of endogenous amino acids.

Animals on a diet devoid of one essential amino acid naturally show a

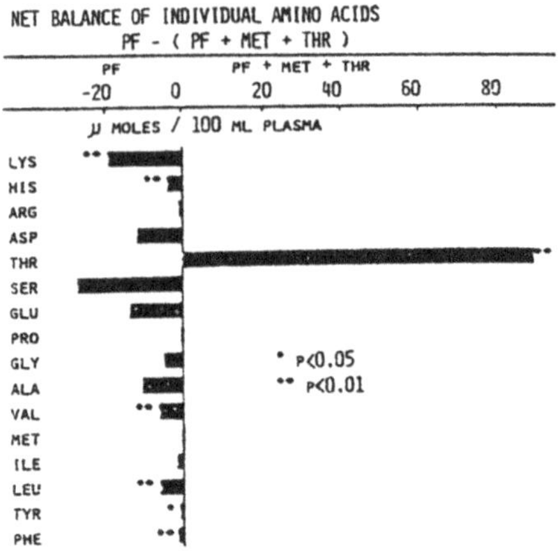

Fig. 5 Net balance of free amino acid contents in plasma of rats fed a nonprotein diet or methionine and threonine supplemented diet for 10 days. Net balance means the plasma concentration of nonprotein diet group minus that of methionine and threonine supplemented group.

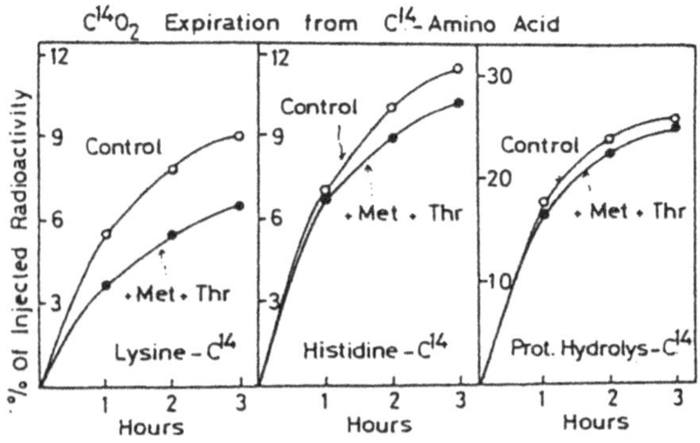

Fig. 6. Effect of supplementation of methionine and threonine to a nonprotein diet on $14CO_2$ expiration from 14C-lysine, 14C-histidine or 14C-protein hydrolyzates. Rats were fed the experimental diets, a nonprotein diet or methionine and threonine supplemented diet for 1 hour after overnight fasting. At the end of feeding, 14C-amino acid was injected intraperitoneally, and expired CO_2 was collected.

negative nitrogen balance. However, the effects of each essential amino acid deficiency on nitrogen balance are quite different from one essential amino acid to another even when the percentage deficiencies of these amino acids for the maintenance requirements were the same(Ashida and Yoshida, 1975, Yoshida and Ashida, 1972). Deficiency of either methionine and threonine caused the most severe negative nitrogen balance, whereas the deficiency of lysine or histidine showed little effect on nitrogen balance. These different effects might be the reflection of the limiting order of endogenous amino acids due to the differences in reutilization in the body of rats. Generally the first limiting amino acid or the sequence of limiting amino acid in dietary protein and foods is calculated from the amino acid composition of foods and the amino acid requirement without consideration of characteristic effect of each essential amino acid for nitrogen balance or nitrogen excretion. The limiting order of endogenous amino acids in animals has not been appraised. Nitrogen sparing effect of methionine and threonine might relate to this limiting order of

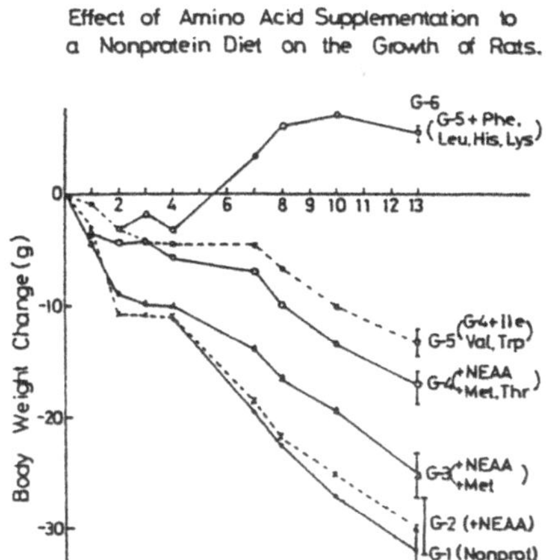

Fig. 7. Effect of supplementation of amino acids in addition to methionine and threonine to a nonprotein diet on body weight loss. Supplemented amounts of amino acids are as follows : nonessential amino acid mixture, 2.7% ; methionine, 0.14% ; threonine, 0.10% ; isoleucine, 0.16% ; valine, 0.16% ; tryptophan, 0.03% ; phenylalanine, 0.08% ; leucine, 0.18% ; histidine-HCl, 0.04% ; lysine-HCl, 0.05%

endogenous amino acids. Therefore, the effects of stepwise addition of essential amino acids to a nonprotein diet on body weight loss and nitrogen balance were investigated. We previously observed that further addition of a small amount of essential amino acids in addition to methionine and threonine didn't improve the body weight loss and nitrogen balance in rats on the nonprotein diet, and supposed that the nonspecific nitrogen source is the limiting factor. Thus 2.7% of nonessential amino acid mixture corresponding to 2.5% of egg protein was first supplemented to the nonprotein diet and then the supplemental effects of essential amino acids were observed.

The loss of body weight of rats fed the nonprotein diet was not reduced by the supplementation of nonessential amino acids alone, but was significantly reduced by the further supplementation of 0.14% of methionine(Fig. 7). Supplementation of 0.14% of methionine and 0.10% of threonine was more effective. When 0.16% of isoleucine, 0.16% of valine and 0.03% of tryptophan were added together with methionine and threonine further improved the body weight loss and nitrogen balance(Fig. 8)

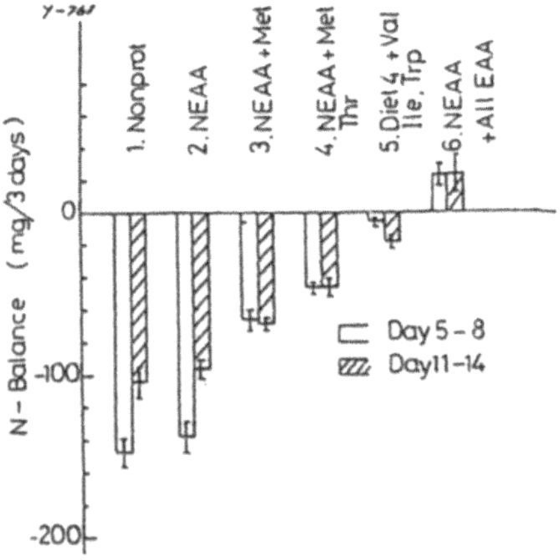

Fig. 8. Effect of supplementation of amino acids in addition to methionine and threonine to a nonprotein diet on nitrogen balance of rats. The amounts of supplemented amino acids were indicated in Fig. 7.

The further supplementation of the remaining essential amino acids(0.08% of phenylalanine, 0.18% of leucine, 0.04% of histidine and 0.05% of lysine) maintained the body weight and the nitrogen equlibrium.

From the results, it may be postulated that when rats were fed the non-protein diet that was deficient in all the amino acids, methionine was the first and threonine was the second limiting amino acid, and nonspecific nitrogen source would be the third and probably a group of isoleucine, valine and tryptophan was the fourth group. If it is the case, nitrogen sparing effect of methionine and threonine may be explained on this basis, and the utilization of endogenous amino acids would be very important for the nutritional evaluation of dietary proteins and for the supplementation of amino acids to the dietary proteins especially in low protein conditions.

6. Effect of supplementation of methionine and threonine to a rice or wheat diet in low protein condition.

From these experiments, we could expect that in low protein diet condition, methionine and threonine would be most limiting even when rice or wheat is used as a sole source of dietary protein in which lysine and threonine are generally considered to be most limiting.

In the next experiment, adult rats were fed a 20% rice diet in which rice was a sole source of protein, and dietary level of protein was 1.2%.

Animals fed this 20% rice diet showed negative N-balance. But when the diet was supplemented with small amounts of methionine and threonine or an amino acid mixture containing methionine and threonine rats showed positive N-balance(Fig. 9).

The limiting amino acids of rice protein for the growth of rats are usually lysine and threonine. However, methionine and threonine are most limiting amino acids if the diet contained very low level of rice protein.

Supplement of neither methionine nor threonine alone to the 20% rice diet, could improve the nitrogen balance so significantly as the combination of methionine and threonine.

In the next experiment, wheat was used as a sole source of dietary protein, and adult rats were fed a 12% of wheat diet. Animals showed the negative N-balance on this basal diet. By supplement with an amino acid mixture including 0.098% of isoleucine, 0.086% of methionine, 0.058% of threonine, 0.016% of lysine, and 0.087% of valine to the 12% wheat diet, rats showed almost N-equilibrium(control group). On deletion of either methionine or threonine from the supplemented amino acid mixture, animals showed the

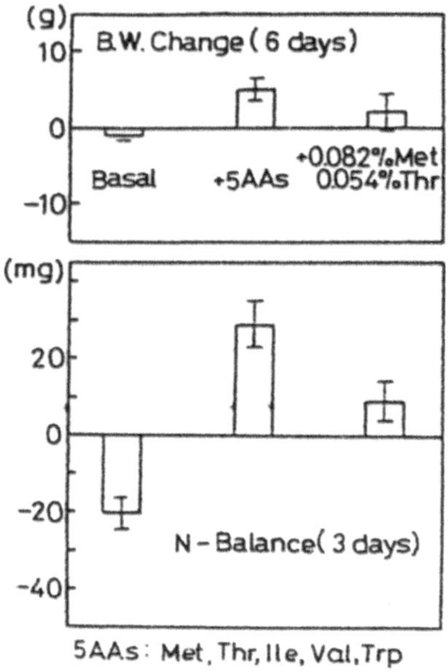

Fig. 9. Effect of supplementation of methionine and threonine to a 20% rice diet on body weight and nitrogen balance of adult rats. Rice is the only source of protein.

negative N-balance. But the deletion of lysine didn't induce negative N-balance,indicating again that methionine and threonine were most limiting in very low wheat protein diet, and lysine is not limiting in this condition.

7. Effect of one essential amino acid deficiency on nitrogen balance.

When rats were fed a diet deficient in one essential amino acid, N-balance is negative. However, the extent of negativity of N-balance is quite different depending on the kinds of deficient essential amino acids(Fig. 12).

When the deficient amino acid is methionine or threonine, rats showed severe negative N-balance. But if lysine or histidine is deficient in the diet, rats showed only slightly negative N-balance.

We can use this data for estimation of the limiting amino acid in a diet in lo protein condition considering the nutritional specificity of amino acids.

In Fig. 13 this is explained more clearly.

In this figure, the negativity of N-balance of rats is shown when

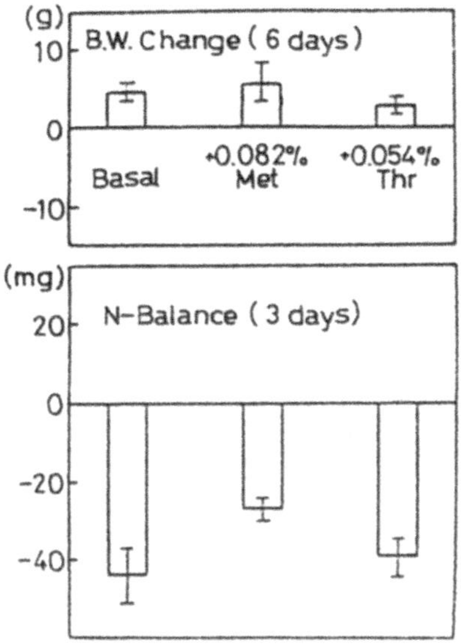

Fig. 10. Effect of supplementation of either methionine or threonine to a 20% rice protein diet on body weight and nitrogen balance of adult rats. Rice is the only source of protein.

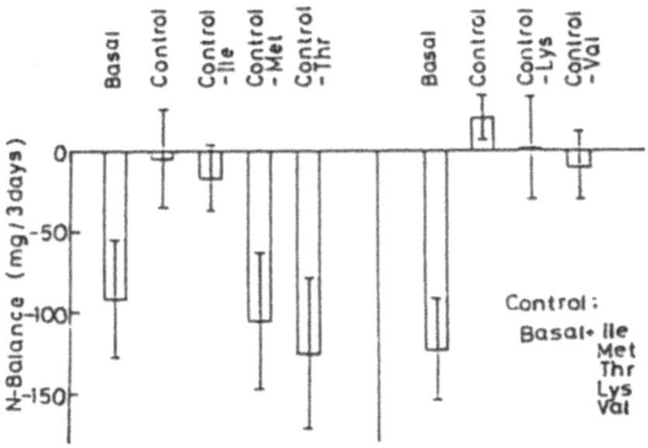

Fig. 11. Effect of supplementation of amino acids to a 12% wheat diet on nitrogen balance of adult rats. Basal diet contained 12% wheat flour as a sole source of protein. Control diet is the basal diet supplemented with 0.086% of methionine, 0.098% of isoleucine, 0.058% of threonine, 0.087% of valine and 0.016% of lysine.

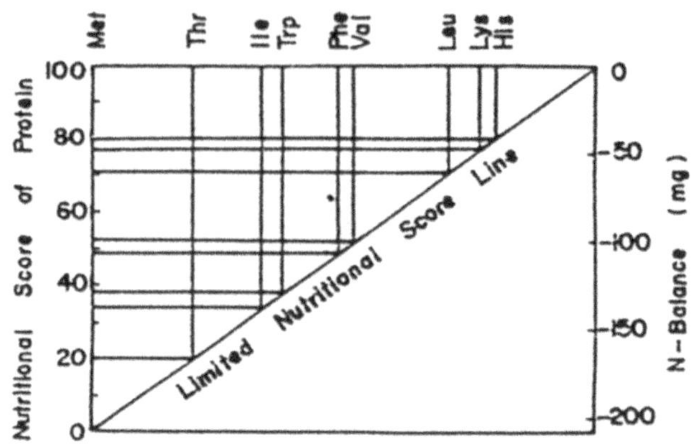

Fig. 12. Different effects of each essential amino acid deficiency on nitrogen balance of adult rats. Methionine deficiency cause severe negative nitrogen balance whereas lysine or histidine deficiency shows relatively slight negative nitrogen balance.

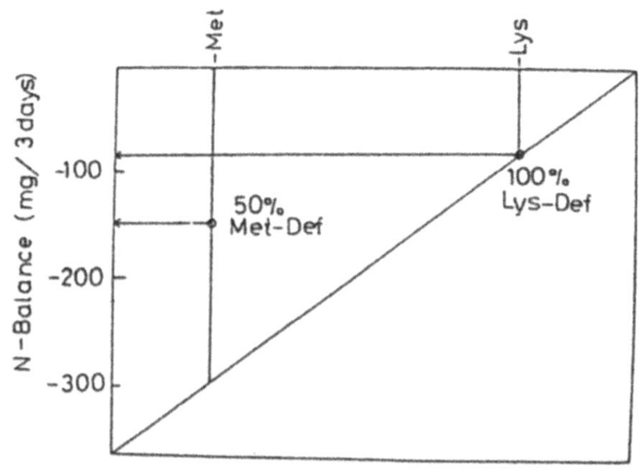

Fig. 13. Comparison of the effect of 50% deficiency of methionine and complete deficiency of lysine on nitrogen balance of adult rats. A 50% methionine deficient diet contains methionine of 50% maintenance requirement. From this figure it can be expected that rats on a 50% methionine deficient diet cause more severe negative nitrogen balance than on complete lysine deficient diet.

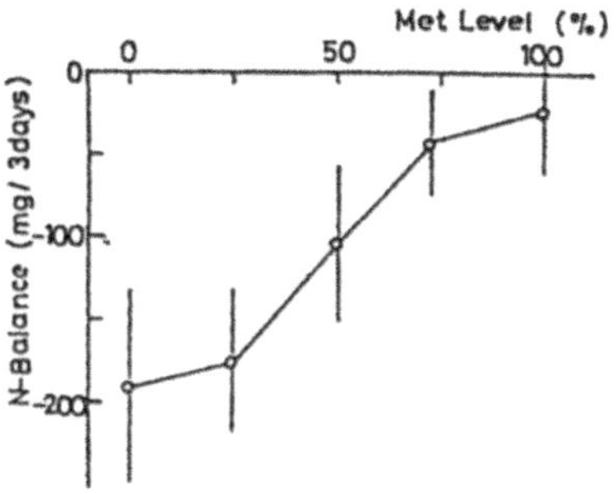

Fig. 14. Effect of dietary level of methionine on nitrogen balance of adult rats fed a nonlysine diet. Dietary level of methionine is expressed as percent of maintenance requirement. Nitrogen balance of rats is gradually improved even on the nonlysine diet.

methionine or lysine is omitted from the amino acid. The negativity of N-balance of rats fed a complete lysine deficient diet would be less than that of rats fed a diet containing 50% of maintenance requirement of methionine. This figure suggests simple percentage of deficiency for the requirement doesn't necessarily reflect the actual biological effect of deficiency of an amino acid.

In Fig. 14, the effect of methionine supplement to a lysine deficient diet on the N-balance of adult rats is indicated. Dietary level of methionine is expressed as percent of requirement for N-equlibrium.

Usually, people would not expect the improvement of N-balance of rats by methionine supplement to a complete lysine deficient diet.

However, as indicated in Fig. 14, along with the increase in the supplemental amount of methionine, the N-balance of rats was clearly improved even when lysine was completely omitted from the diet. This will be understandable if you remember the effect of methionine deficiency on N-balance is more severe than that of lysine deficiency as indicated in Fig. 13.

Thus specificity of amino acids would be important in a low protein diet condition for nutritional evaluation of proteins.

Sometimes people observe the biological value of egg protein is over 100 and this is generally considered as experimental error.

Egg proteins are abundant in both methionine and threonine. Feeding of a small amount of egg protein would increase the reutilization of endogenous amino acids together with the good utilization of egg proteins themselves. Accordingly, if the "Biological Value" is calculated assuming the endogenous urinary nitrogen is equal to that of the nonprotein diet condition, the "Apparent Biological Value" could be over 100.

The endogenous nitrogen excretion in urine is not constant, but is affected by dietary amino acids. This fact should be considered for the nutritional evaluation of proteins, especially in low protein conditions.

REFERENCES

Allison, J.B., Anderson, J.A. and Seeley, R.D. (1947). Some effects of methionine on the utilization of nitrogen in the adult dog. J. Nutrition 33, 361-370.

Ashida, K. and Yoshida, A. (1975). Nutritional specificities of essential amino acids and their relationships to evaluation of the nutritional quality of dietary proteins. Proceedings of Ninth Inter. Congr. Nutr., Mexico, 1972. 3, 321-331. (Karger, Basel)

Block and Mitchell (1946-47). The correlation of the amino acid composition of proteins with their nutritive value. Nutr. Abst. Rev., 16, 249-278.

Brusl, M., Willman, W. and Swanson, P.P. (1947). Amino acids in nitrogen metabolism with particular reference to the role of methionine. J. Nutrition 33, 389-410.

Kenney, F.T. (1963). Mechanism of hormonal control of rat liver tyrosine transaminase. Adv. Enz. Regulation(Weber, G., editor), Pergmon Press, Oxford. 1, 137-150.

McFarlane, A.S. (1963). Measurement of synthesis rats of liver produced plasma proteins. Biochem. J. 89, 277-290.

McGivan, J.D., Bradford, N.M. and Chappell, J.B. (1974). Adaptive changes in the capacity of systems used for the synthesis of citrulline in rat liver mitochondria in response to high and low protein diets. Biochem. J. 142, 359-364.

Mortimore, G.E. and Ward, W.F. (1975). Role of amino acids in the regulation of hepatic protein turnover. Proc. 10th Int. Congr. Nutrition. Kyoto. Abstract p.5.

Shigesada, K. and Tatibana, M. (1971). Role of acetyl glutamate in ureotelism. J. Biol. Chem., 246, 5588-5595.

Swick, R.W. (1958). Measurement of protein turnover in rat liver. J. Biol. Chem. 231, 751-764.

Swick, R.W. and Margot, M. (1974). Measurement of protein turnover in rat liver with 14C-carbonate. J. Biol. Chem. 249, 6836-6841.

Williams, J.N.Jr. and Jasik, A.D. (1963). A markedly antilipotropic action of methionine. Nature 200, 472.

Willman, W.P., Swanson, P.P., Stewart, G.F., Stevenson, G.T. and Bursh, M. (1945). Biological efficiency of egg proteins. Proc. Fed. Am. Soc. Exp. Biol. 4, 164.

Yokogoshi, H. and Yoshida, A. (1976). Some factors affecting the nitrogen sparing action of methionine and threonine in rats receiving a protein free diet. J. Nutrition 106, 48-57.

Yokogoshi, H., Hayase, K. and Yoshida, A. (1977). Effect of supplementation of methionine and threonine to a protein free diet on urinary excretion of nitrogen and tissue free amino acids in rats. J. Nutrition 107, 783-791.

Yokogoshi, H., Hayase, K. and Yoshida, A. (1978). Studies on carbamoylphosphate synthetase in livers of rats fed a protein free diet supplemented with methionine and threonine and injected with N-acetylglutamic acid. J. Nutrition 108, 1215-1221.

Yokogoshi, H. and Yoshida, A. (1979). Effect of supplementation of methionine and threonine on hepatic polyribosome profile in rats meal-fed a protein-free diet. J. Nutrition 109, 148-154.

Yokogoshi, H. and Yoshida, A. (1981). Sequence of limiting amino acids for the utilization of endogenous amino acids in rats fed a protein-free diet. Nutr. Rep. Inter., 23, 517-523.

Yoshida, A., Moritoki, K. and Noda, K. (1966). Plasma lipids of rat with fatty liver owing to amino acid imbalance. Japan. J. Food and Nutrition. 19, 291-296.

Yoshida, A. and Ashida, K. (1972). Nutritional specificity of amino acids and its application to the nutritional evaluation of food proteins. Riports of the research Committee of Essential Amino Acid(Japan). No. 56, 6.

Yoshida, A. and Moritoki, K. (1974). Nitrogen sparing action of methionine and threonine in rats receiving a protein free diet. Nutr. Rep. Inter. 9, 159-168.

Proc. Int. Assoc. Cereal Chem. Symp. Amino Acid Compn and Biol. Value of Cereal Proteins Budapest, Hungary 1983, R. Lásztity, M. Hidvégi, eds

AMINO ACID SCORING SYSTEMS AND THEIR ROLE IN THE ESTIMATION OF THE PROTEIN QUALITY OF CEREALS

PETER L. PELLETT

Department of Food Science and Nutrition, University of Massachusetts Amherst, Massachusetts 01003, USA

ABSTRACT

Cereals provide much of the protein in the diets of many areas of the world thus their protein quality is an important issue. It is however now more widely recognised that the protein value of the diet as a whole is of greater consequence than that of the individual proteins. While the concept of protein quality appears at first sight to be self-evident, it is difficult to define precisely since many factors beyond amino acid composition affect the capacity of a protein to meet the amino acid and nitrogen needs of the consumer. Nevertheless amino acid composition of proteins and/or dietaries in relation to human amino acid requirements, often termed protein scoring, has become the basis of chemical procedures used to measure protein quality. Several factors however limit the usefulness of protein scoring for the evaluation of protein quality. These include the facts that amino acid and protein requirements vary with age and physiological status of the consumer, digestibility and amino acid availability affect utilization, controversy still exists on the reliability and reproductibility of amino acid analysis in foodstuffs and finally that there is still no universal agreement on the standards with which amino acid composition should be compared. Several scoring systems have been devised and the derivation of the major scoring systems developed over the last four decades is described. The latest from FAO/WHO/UNU now advocates four different patterns depending on the age of the consumer. It is concluded that provided limitations are recognized and care is taken in interpretation, amino acid composition, especially with digestibility, may be used to predict the protein value of foods and dietaries with sufficient accuracy to meet all practical needs.

INTRODUCTION

Cereals are the major staples in almost all regions of the world. Total production is enormous being in excess of 1,600 million metric tons per annum in 1978 (FAO 1980). Wheat is now the major cereal produced comprising 28% of the total followed by rice (24%) maize (23%) and barley (12%). Cereals are also the major source of protein for many regions of the world (Table 1). It should be noted that the values shown are averages for large population groups, but poorer individuals within the poorer countries would certainly consume larger proportions than these.

Table 1: Proportion of protein consumed from the major food groups in various regions of the world.

	Population Millions	Protein per caput per day g.	Percentage of protein from major food groups				
			cereals	Roots + tubers	pulses + nuts	vegetables + fruits	meat, eggs fish, milk
North America	240	106	18	3	4	5	69
Western Europe	367	95	29	4	3	5	57
Eastern Europe+ USSR	369	103	37	5	3	4	50
Africa	344	55	51	8	16	4	20
Latin America	336	66	38	3	12	4	41
Middle East	196	74	62	1	8	6	21
Far East	1159	49	63	1	14	4	15

Calculated from Food Balance Sheets FAO 1980.

Nevertheless, even using these average values, over half of the protein consumed in Africa, the Middle East and the Far East comes from cereals. The protein quality of cereals thus becomes an important issue since cereals are generally poorer in quality (amino acid composition and digestibility) than animal foods. Cereals however are usually consumed along with other protein foods thus the protein quality of cereals by themselves is of less importance than the protein value of the dietary as a whole. Nevertheless for comparative purposes, consideration of cereal protein quality in isolation can be instructive. Amino acid composition data are of value both for the evaluation of individual protein values and for the estimation of complementary roles.

DETERMINATION OF PROTEIN QUALITY

The knowledge that proteins differed in their ability to support growth goes back to some of the earliest studies in nutrition but the concept of protein quality was not fully established until it was demonstrated by Wilcock and Hopkins in 1906 that the nutritive value of zein could be improved by addition of tryptophan (Lusk, 1933; McCollum, 1957; Munro, 1964). Nevertheless, several studies between 1840 and 1860 had demonstrated differences in the value of different dietary proteins. These studies surprisingly were not followed through for another 50 years (Munro, 1964). Techniques for the biological evaluation of proteins were quickly developed in the early years of the century, based both on nitrogen balance (Thomas, 1909) and on rat growth (Osborne et al., 1919). It took until the 1940's, however, before analytical techniques were sufficiently advanced for amino acid data to be used in the prediction of protein quality (Block and Mitchell, 1946).

Osborne however in studies extending from the 1890's to the late 1920's certainly recognized that proteins differed in amino acid composition and that this possibly related to nutritive value. This is illustrated in the following quotation (Osborne 1907):

> "The proportion of lysine in wheat gluten is likewise small especially compared with that obtained from the leguminous seeds. The amount of histidine, however, does not differ very greatly from that of the other seed proteins. What significance these differences have in respect to the nutritive value of these different proteins must be determined by future investigation, for it has only very recently been discovered that such differences exist. It is possible that feeding experiments with proteins of known character in respect to the relative proportions of their decomposition products will throw light on these important questions."

Osborne was also aware of the concept of protein complementation (Osborne 1919):

> "Experiments have demonstrated that combinations of cereal proteins with those of milk, meat or eggs are much more efficient for promoting the growth of young animals, and for renewing the tissues of adults than are the cereal proteins alone: and these are the very combinations which mankind eats whenever opportunity makes it possible."

Incidentally, Osborne (1908) also realized that growing animals have different amino acid requirement patterns from adults — a fact that has only now become explicitly recognized in the current FAO/WHO/UNU (1984) scoring patterns which show different requirement patterns at different ages.

The concept of protein quality seems at first sight to be self-evident; nevertheless, the more closely the concept is examined the more difficult it becomes to define precisely. The capacity of a protein, to meet the amino acid and nitrogen requirements of an organism is dependent not only on the amino acid composition and digestibility of the protein itself, but also upon the composition and adequacy of the diet as a whole and on the physiological, nutritional and health status of the animal or human consuming it. These factors further interact in a complex manner to modify overall utilization. In practice for assay purposes, many of these variable factors are either ignored, held constant or defined as being constant. Protein "quality" may thus only include consideration of amino acid composition and digestibility.

Proteins serve in the diets of the affluent as major sources of food energy and it is possible for a protein of poor amino acid composition to have poor bioavailability as a protein but to be fully available for energy purposes. In contrast proteins of low digestibility will be poorly bioavailable both as protein sources and as energy sources.

Further biochemical facts make the situation more complicated since all animals, including man, have the ability in some degree to reuse amino acids for the synthesis of protein, the rate of disposal of essential amino acids being dependent on the supply of the amino acid with conservation, taking place when intake is in deficit. Extensive reutilization must occur since 5-6 g of protein are synthesized for each gram protein allowance (Young and Scrimshaw, 1978). Anomalies related to this have been known for many years (Bender, 1961) since it has been demonstrated in the rat, that the net protein utilization (NPU) of a protein absolutely deficient in lysine (amino acid score = 0) is about 40. Hegsted (1971) has concluded that if anomalies such as this can occur the complete protein scoring system is valueless. This is an extreme viewpoint. A further conclusion from the data of Bender (1961) was that amino acids do not all behave in the same way when they are limiting or deficient. This followed from the observation that diets absolutely deficient in methionine or valine (scores = 0) had the expected zero response for NPU but that other essential amino acids behaved in an intermediate manner. Human plasma amino acid data also demonstrate that different responses occur with different deficiencies (Young, et al., 1977). Phenylalanine-tyrosine deficiency is not reflected in the short term by changes in plasma amino acid levels while valine and tryptophan deficiencies cause falls to about 50% of the normal value. Thus the experimental conditions suitable for studying a protein limiting in one amino acid are not necessarily the same if limitation is in another. This differs from simple protein quality and scoring theory where quality is defined solely in relation to the limiting (i.e., least proportion of "standard" or "requirement") amino acid.

Amino acid scoring has been discussed in several recent reviews and texts (Hackler 1977, Pellett 1978, Pellett and Young, 1980, Bodwell et al. 1981) as well as in a series of international reports (FAO 1957, FAO

1965, FAO/WHO 1973 and FAO/WHO/UNU 1984). The rationale behind amino acid scoring systems is both simple and logical since the role of dietary protein is to provide amino acids and nitrogen for the synthesis of body protein and other metabolically important nitrogenous metabolites. These nitrogen and amino acid requirements are, therefore, the logical yardstick by which to measure protein quality, and precise knowledge about these requirements is the basis for evaluation of the nutritional significance of dietary protein quality.

Several major factors, however, make application of scoring more difficult than the apparently simple and logical rationale behind it. These are 1) requirements vary with age and physiological state 2) there is no universal agreement on the "requirement" or standard to be used and 3) mere consideration of the amino acid composition of a protein following hydrolysis does not necessarily mean that the amino acids are all equally available to the consumer for protein synthesis.

DERIVATION OF SCORING SYSTEMS

Before consideration of the more general advantages and drawbacks of scoring procedures, the various scoring systems that have been derived will be discussed briefly. Several international recommendations have been made (FAO 1957, FAO/WHO 1965, FAO/WHO 1973, FAO/WHO/UNU 1984) but it was not until the 1974 edition of the US RDAs (NAS-NRC, 1974) that a U.S. pattern was presented for scoring protein. These various scoring patterns are shown in Table 2.

In 1946, Block and Mitchell introduced the concept of assessing the nutritional quality of a protein on the basis of its constituent amino acids and the value obtained was termed the "chemical score". Their method consisted of calculating, by the use of food tables or from direct analysis, the quantity of each essential amino acid contained in a protein or a mixture of proteins. The values were expressed individually as proportions in relation to the content of the corresponding amino acid in a suitable reference amino acid pattern. The amino acid that showed the lowest proportion was called the limiting amino acid and the value obtained was the score. Since egg was known to be a protein of high nutritional value from feeding experiments, Block and Mitchell used chemical score in relation to egg protein as a standard. In the years between the introduction of the concept of protein scoring by Block and Mitchell in 1946, and the 1955 FAO Committee, some data had accumulated on the amino acid requirements of adults and children and it became recognized that the Block and Mitchell scoring procedure did not always predict protein utilization with accuracy. While knowledge of human requirements for amino acids was still fragmentary, the 1955 Committee (FAO, 1957) believed information was sufficiently available to be used as a basis of developing a scoring system from human requirements rather than from comparison to a natural protein such as egg.

This hypothetical reference protein pattern replaced egg protein as a standard in 1957. The pattern was derived from human requirements and since the level of sulfur amino acids was considerably lower than that present in egg protein, improved agreement was found between scores and biological determinations of protein quality. The pattern was used with moderate success for several years, but discrepancies began to accumulate

Table 2: Some Reference Scoring Patterns

Essential Amino Acid	Whole Egg	FAO (1957)	FAO/WHO (1973)	NAS/NRC (1980)	FAO/WHO/UNU 1984 Infant (milk)	Preschool (2-5yrs)	School Age (10-12 yrs)	Adult
				mg/gm Nitrogen				
Histidine	-	-	-	106	162	125	113	100
Isoleucine	340	270	250	263	288	188	181	81
Leucine	540	306	440	440	580	438	288	119
Lysine	440	270	340	320	413	388	288	100
Total Sulfur Amino Acids	355	270	220	163	263	165	144	106
Total Aromatic Amino Acids	580	360	380	455	450	413	144	119
Threonine	294	180	250	220	269	225	181	56
Tryptophan	106	90	60	70	106	75	56	31
Valine	410	270	310	300	344	231	163	81
Total Essential Amino Acids								
+ Histidine				2340	2875	2244	1525	794
- Histidine	3060	2015	2215	2231	2713	2119	1413	694
Essential Amino Acids as Percentage of Protein	49.0	32.2	35.4	37.4	46.0	35.9	24.4	12.7

and the FAO/WHO 1965 report included recommendations for a new pattern based on a new procedure. Results from a series of investigations had tended to show that the tryptophan content of the FAO pattern was too high. Ironically, it was the tryptophan level of whole milk (90 mg/g nitrogen) that had been used in 1957 to allow for the conversion of a pattern based on tryptophan into a hypothetical reference protein. It was also found that the level of sulfur amino acids in the FAO(1957) pattern was too high (FAO/WHO 1965).

During this period it was demonstrated that proteins of generally high quality could be diluted with non-specific nitrogen to a greater extent than proteins of low quality without reducing their biological value. Thus the 1965 report emphasized, quite correctly, that the reqirements for amino acids or for nitrogen involved two components: 1) the essential amino acids that must be obtained from the diet because they could not be synthesized in the body and 2) the nitrogen from essential and non-essential amino acids that was also necessary for the synthesis of protein and other nitrogen containing compounds. In addition the 1957 pattern had originally been derived in relation to tryptophan taken as unity. The use of any single amino acid as a reference had two disadvantages: 1) the difficulty of finding an amino acid that was suitable as a reference standard, and 2) the fact that two proteins of very different nutritional value, could show very similar ratios of their essential amino acids to the amino acid chosen as a reference.

The new pattern recommended by the 1965 expert group used as its basis, the proportion of any amino acid present in relation to the total of the essential amino acids rather than in relation to the total nitrogen present. The standard used for the comparison was the proportion of the individual amino acid in the total essential amino acids in egg protein. The new procedure was cumbersome, and there were a number of theoretical objections raised to the scoring system. That pattern was not widely adopted and many researchers continued to use the 1957 pattern despite its shortcomings.

The approach to protein or amino acid scoring developed by the 1973 FAO/WHO expert group was essentially similar to the approach used in 1957 in that the pattern developed was based on human amino acid requirements. A moderate amount of new data on amino acid requirements in various age groups had accumulated, but, on examining these data, it became obvious that the proportion of essential amino acids to total nitrogen appeared to change with age. The infant needed some 35% to 40% of its amino acids in the form of essential amino acids, while the adult needed only 15%. Clearly, if, for scoring purposes, the low percentage of essential amino acids to total N required by adults were adopted, it would over-estimate the value of a protein for meeting the needs of children. In contrast, adoption of the child pattern would underestimate the value of a protein for the adult. The approach followed was that the best available data for the amino acid requirements of infants, children and adults were tabulated separately as milligrams of individual essential amino acids per kilogram body weight per day. Patterns were derived for each age group by dividing the amino acid requirements by the daily protein requirements of the same groups thus giving amino acid requirements in the form of patterns for each age in milligrams per gram protein (or nitrogen). The provisional pattern was developed by interpolation from these values and was close to that of the young child.

It was the opinion of the Committee that since protein quality was most critical for the younger age groups, scoring patterns appropriate to these age groups should be employed for all age groups. This in practice gave an extra margin of safety to adult needs. It should be noted that the pattern was not intended to cover the needs of very young infants, histidine would have to be included and adjustments of other values would also have been required, but was designed to meet the needs of children in the pre-school age group. It can be seen with hindsight that the committee did not have the courage of its convictions, since a single scoring system was eventually adopted despite the recognition of wide differences in amino acid requirements between adults and children. Significant changes in the pattern included lowering tryptophan and methionine and raising the levels of threonine and lysine (Table 2).

In both the 1974 and 1980 editions of the U.S. recommended dietary allowances, NAS-NRC 1980, a scoring pattern was presented which differed significantly from the FAO/WHO (1973) pattern. An especially important difference was in the level of the total sulphur amino acids, where the NAS/NRC pattern was nearly 30% below that of FAO/WHO (1973). Although it was claimed to be based on child requirements, from close reading of the text it can be seen to be based on amino acid compositional data. Agreed, there is an indirect relationship because it is known that a young child grows well on egg or milk protein. It is thus of interest that the low value for total SAA as recommended by NAS-NRC (1980) is similar to the FAO/WHO/UNU (1984) young child recommendations but for different reasons.

Returning to international recommendations, the next group report, which incidentally is far less well-known than the original 1973 document, was the recommendation by a joint FAO/WHO informal gathering of experts on energy and protein requirements (FAO/WHO 1975). The major concern of this group was on protein-energy relationships, but one important oversight of the 1973 report was corrected by this gathering of experts. It is widely misunderstood that the 1973 report, in using the term NPU, was specifically recommending a particular rat assay procedure. In fact, the term was intended to be used in a generic sense to indicate a measure of protein value that included both digestibility and the efficiency of utilization of absorbed nitrogen. The 1973 Committee, however, neglected to offer guidance on correction of the amino acid score for digestibility of dietary protein. When digestibility is high, NPU and amino acid score estimate similar values, however, since digestibility is a component of NPU, but is not a component of score, when digestibility is low, the two are no longer identical. The oversight of the 1973 Committee was corrected by the 1975 informal gathering of experts and it was recommended that the amino acid score be adjusted to 85% digestibility if the diet was based on coarse, whole grain cereals and vegetables and to 90% digestibility in the case of more refined diets. Some selected values for nitrogen digestibility in the human are shown in Table 3. If digestibility is known with accuracy for the diet being evaluated, the determined value should be used , rather than the 85% or 90% estimate values. Rapid in vitro procedures for digestibility (Satterlee et al 1979) are now available and may also be used to correct amino acid score.

The most recent recommendations for protein scoring are from the FAO/WHO/UNU Committee which met in Rome in 1982 and whose report is due to be published in 1984. This Group, like its predecessors, accepted the

Table 3: Values for the Digestibility of Protein in Humans

	True Digestibility % (mean ± SD)	Relative Digestibility
Egg	97±3	
Milk, cheese	95±3	100
Meat, fish	94±3	
Maize	85±6	89
Rice polished	88±4	93
Wheat whole	86±5	90
Wheat refined	96±4	100
Oatmeal	86±7	90
Millet	79	83
Soy Flour	86±7	90
Beans	78	82

Source: Selected from table in FAO/WHO/UNU 1984.

evidence of a relationship between the amino acid composition of proteins and their protein nutritional value and thus also proposed an amino acid scoring procedure. Amino acid requirements for various ages were derived from the best available data and were then divided by total protein requirements at the same ages to give a pattern of amino acid requirements. These, in mg amino acid per gram total nitrogen, are shown in Table 2. The values are different from those tabulated in the 1973 report, even though the estimates of amino acid requirements used, (in mg/kg body weight) were essentially unchanged. This was because the new total protein levels for adults and school children were higher than the 1973 figures and therefore the essential amino acids required per gram of protein were correspondingly reduced. The most innovative aspect is that they are now reported for four different age groups making it explicit that protein quality is not an unchanging attribute of a protein but can vary with the age of the consumer. For infants it was concluded that the amino acid pattern of human milk should be accepted as the requirement pattern. Proteins and diets with an essential amino acid content and pattern that effectively meet the needs of infants and young children will also be adequate for older children and adults, whereas the reverse may not be true. It will be noted that the level of requirements for all essential amino acids falls dramatically as age increases so that for adults few diets would fail to meet amino acid needs and indeed, as will be considered later, most cereals appear adequate in quality by themselves. The new view, to paraphrase a biblical expression, would thus indicate that man perhaps can live by bread alone but his wife and especially his children cannot. This statement is, of course, a gross oversimplification, but in practice it is no longer believed necessary that protein allowances be adjusted to take account of the amino acid composition of dietaries for adults. This, however, still remains necessary for children and perhaps also during pregnancy and lactation. A contrasting view may however emerge from the current work of Young and his associates at M.I.T. (see Young and Pellett 1983). In these studies, involving whole body leucine and lysine oxidation rates, it is concluded that the essential amino acid requirements of adults may be considerably underestimated by the currently used nitrogen balance techniques and may in fact not differ greatly from younger age groups when expressed as a proportion of the total protein needs.

In the FAO/WHO (1973) report the amino acid score was calculated without taking account of digestibility and as a result the capacity of a protein to meet physiological requirements was somewhat overestimated. In accordance with the suggestion of the Ad Hoc Consultative Group (FAO/WHO 1975), and in view of the importance of the digestibility of proteins in mixed diets, calculation of the capacity of a diet to meet the protein requirement should now incorporate an estimate both of the digestibility of the protein and of the amino acid score.

ADVANTAGES OF USING AMINO ACID "SCORING" PROCEDURES

Biological assays of protein quality such as PER (protein efficiency ratio) and NPR (net protein ratio) are functions of both digestibility and the limiting amino acid in the test protein source. Moreover, these tests *per se* neither provide any information about the identity of the limiting amino acid nor do they take into account information about any of the other amino acids in the test protein. Furthermore, the results of a rat bioassay procedure are, fundamentally, determined by the nutritional characteristics of the test species and these may not necessarily reflect those of the human consumer. Finally, because protein quality measurements using animal assays are made under conditions in which the protein is the limiting component of the diet, data from these assays are not necessarily indicative of the nutritional value of the protein for meeting human needs. With these and other limitations of rat assay values in mind, the advantages of using amino acid data emerge. Thus, knowledge of the amino acid content of proteins supplies information not only on the "limiting" amino acid but also on the other amino acids. The latter information may be more, or at least equally as important as that concerning the limiting amino acid. For example an understanding of the problem of amino acid complementation of food proteins, such as wheat and soy requires knowledge of both the lysine and sulphur amino acid composition of these two protein sources. Thus a potentially more complete description of the nutritional value of a protein can be obtained from a knowledge of its amino acid composition. To quote directly from the 1957 FAO Committee:

> "The concept of a desirable pattern of essential amino acids has one great advantage. By comparison with such a pattern, data on the amino acid content of food combinations can be appraised in a wide range of situations, in terms of possible defects of the diet and of methods of improving it. Comparisons, no doubt rough and approximate, can be made directly by the use of tables showing the content of foods in essential amino acids, regardless of the proportions in which individual foods are included in the diet. On the other hand, even when the biological value of each dietary component is known, a deduction cannot be made about the biological value of the diet as a whole."

Other advantages of scoring procedures are the obvious ones of cost, simplicity and the much shorter time needed when compared to the rat assay techniques. Against these strengths a series of weaknesses must also be considered. These are tabulated in Table 4. The importance of digestibility has already been discussed and it is necessary that it always be considered in conjunction with scores. The individual weaknesses listed in Table 4 have been elaborated upon by Pellett (1978) and by Pellett and Young (1980) and only problems of accuracy in amino acid analysis will be further discussed here.

Table 4: Weaknesses of amino acid scoring for assessing protein quality

1. Amino acid composition does not reveal protein digestibility or amino acid availability.

2. Protein utilization is not only affected by the level of the limiting amino acid but also by the levels of essential amino acids present in high amounts and by the amount of non-specific nitrogen.

3. While not strictly a protein quality consideration, the presence of toxic materials is not revealed by amino acid analysis. Such toxic materials however can affect biological response.

4. Because of amino acid recycling, especially when limited by lysine, there may be big discrepancies between score and biological response for low quality proteins.

5. Amino acid composition data is not always accurate and sufficiently reproducible.

6. Disagreements exist on the appropriate reference pattern to use and this may vary at different ages.

AMINO ACID ANALYSIS

The fundamental shortcomings of amino acid analysis in foodstuffs are the destruction of amino acids during acid hydrolysis and the discrepancy which can occur between amino acid content and nutritional availability. Unfortunately, the problems can be greatest with the essential amino acids likely to be limiting in practical diets - threonine, lysine, tryptophan, and total sulfur amino acids. Analytical problems have been extensively reviewed by Smyth and Elliot (1964), Kohler and Palter (1967), Tkachuk and Irvine (1969), Mondino and Bongiovanni (1970), Cavins et al. (1972), Davies and Thomas (1973), Spitz (1973), Robel (1973), Savoy et al. (1975), Concon (1975), Blackburn (1978) and Pellett and Young (1980). Ion-exchange chromatography remains the most utilized method of amino acid analysis, and most commercial analyzers available are based on the procedure of Spackman et al. (1958). Current equipment can be automated to include sequential sample loading and regeneration of the columns, together with peak area integration and direct calculation of results by use of an attached computer.

Other procedures exist but are far less widely used and have their own limitations. Analysis of amino acids using gas-liquid chromatography requires the quantitative conversion of the amino acids to volatile derivatives such as hydroxyacid methyl esters, trimethylsilyl esters, and n-butyl-N-trifluoracetyl esters.

Claims have been made that near-infrared reflectance spectroscopy (NIRS) may be satisfactory for the routine analysis of some amino acids in cereals in plant breeding programs (Williams, 1984). Microbiological assays for amino acids can be extremely useful when other equipment is not available or when only one amino acid, for which there is no convenient, specific color reaction, has to be determined in large numbers in grain and legume breeding programs.

Most amino acids in proteins can be satisfactorily determined with an automatic amino acid analyzer after properly controlled acid hydrolysis (Blackburn, 1978; Moore and Stein, 1963). Hydrolysis with 6N HCl at 110°C for 18 to 24 hr is commonly used for the determination of all amino acids except tryptophan. The hydrolysis time, which is often selected arbitrarily, has been repeatedly found to influence release of amino acids from proteins (Moore and Stein, 1963; Sarwar et al 1983; Cherry, 1981). Although cystine and methionine are determined in 6N HCl hydrolysates by some analysts, separate hydrolyses are preferred for analysis of sulphur amino acids since they are destroyed to varying degrees during acid hydrolysis. Cyst(e)ine and methionine are more accurately determined after oxidation by performic acid to their stable forms i.e. cysteic acid and methionine sulfone, respectively by the method of Moore (1963). Tryptophan is severely affected by acid hydrolysis and methods of tryptophan analysis have been critically reviewed by Friedman and Finley (1971). Alkaline hydrolysis is the most feasible way of quantitative determination of tryptophan in proteins when using an automatic analyser (Blackburn, 1978). Hugli and Moore (1972) have developed a simple procedure in which proteins are hydrolyzed with NaOH containing starch as an antioxidant, permitting accurate determination of tryptophan.

Several interlaboratory comparisons of amino acid analysis of proteins have been made (Knipfel et al 1971, Williams et al 1979, Happich et al 1981 and Sarwar et al 1983.) In the latter study the interlaboratory variation of tryptophan (coefficient of variation CV up to 24%), cystine and methionine (CV up to 17%) were greater than for all the other amino acids where the CV was generally less than 10%. The data for whole wheat flour in this study are shown in Table 5 together with the between and within laboratory variations. The CV for the limiting amino acid - lysine, is 7.3%; this would affect the score by about 4 units which is below the variation generally obtained in biological assays of protein quality. The high coefficients of variation for tryptophan and sulfur amino acids would, however, suggest there is need for improved standardization in the analytical techniques for these amino acids (Sarwar et al. 1983). The values for the essential amino acid content of the major cereals are shown in Table 6. These data originate from FAO (1970) but comparison with collaborative assay data for wheat (see Table 5) show almost identical results: the values differing by an average of less than 4%.

Table 5: Means and Coefficient of Variations of Whole Wheat Flour as Analyzed in a Collaborative Assay.

	Mean mg/g N	Coefficient of Variation % Between Laboratories	Within Laboratories
Arginine	269	13.0	2.8
Histidine	137	9.3	1.7
Isoleucine	209	7.2	2.2
Leucine	428	4.6	1.7
Lysine	166	7.3	2.7
Methionine	103	12.2	4.0
Cystine	139	14.1	2.0
Phenylalanine	304	8.6	1.0
Tyrosine	182	14.5	4.5
Threonine	183	9.7	1.5
Tryptophan	70	22.4	2.7
Valine	267	8.2	1.7
Alanine	218	4.8	1.5
Aspartic Acid	315	5.0	3.3
Glutamic Acid	1934	12.8	1.7
Glycine	247	4.8	1.5
Proline	653	7.5	1.7
Serine	274	9.0	3.0
Ammonia	208	17.7	3.3

Adapted from Sarwar et al. (1983).

In Table 7 the amino acid scores are shown in relation to the FAO/WHO 1973 and 1984 scores. It will be seen that, except for the comparison to adult requirements, lysine is the apparent limiting amino acid in almost all instances and scores increase as age increases. Second and third limiting amino acids vary from cereal to cereal but tryptophan and threonine would most frequently be the next limiting to lysine. What, however, is more important is the generally moderate - high levels of the total sulphur amino acids in cereals, thus demonstrating their ability to complement and be complemented by the high lysine, low sulfur amino acid legume proteins. The protein value of cereals is also dependent on their total protein content, rice only partly compensates for its low protein content by a slightly higher lysine value but oats are higher than other cereals in both quality and quantity. Both total protein and amino acid composition have been important considerations in plant breeding programmes but it is now generally agreed that yield is the most important attribute provided that current levels of protein quality and quantity can be maintained (Nygaad and Pellett, 1984).

It must be recognised that the protein quality of a cereal determined from its amino acid composition is only an estimate of a value under standardized conditions and the overall utilization of a protein is dependent on a variety of factors external to attributes of the protein

Table 6: Essential Amino Acid Composition of some Selected Cereals.

	Protein g/100g	Amino Acids mg/gN isoleucine	leucine	lysine	Total SAA	Total Aromatic	Threonine	Tryptophan	Valine	Histidine
Barley:dehulled (Hordeum vulgare)	11.0	224	417	216	246	515	207	96	315	132
Maize: grain (Zea mays)	9.5	230	783	167	217	544	225	44	303	170
Millet: grain (Pennisetum sp.)	9.7	256	598	214	302	504	241	122	345	153
Oats: meal (Avena sativa)	13.0	236	454	232	272	519	207	79	319	131
Rice: husked (Oryza sp.)	7.5	238	514	237	212	540	244	78	344	156
Rye: whole meal (Secale cereale)	11.0	219	385	212	210	396	209	46	297	138
Wheat: whole grain (Triticum sp.)	12.2	204	417	179	253	469	183	68	276	143

Source: Amino acid content of Foods FAO Nutrition Studies No. 24 FAO Rome 1970.

Table 7: Protein quality scores and limiting Amino Acids of cereals using FAO/WHO 1973 and the FAO/WHO/UNU 1984 Scoring Systems[1]

	FAO/WHO 1973	FAO/WHO/UNU 1984 Infant[2] (<1yr)	Preschool Child (2-5yr)	Child (10-12yr)	Adult
Barley	64(L)[3]	52(L)	56(L)	75(L)	100+
Maize	49(L)	41(L,T)	43(L)	58(L)	100+
Millet	63(L)	52(L)	55(L)	74(L)	100+
Oats	68(L)	56(L)	60(L)	80(L)	100+
Rice	70(L)	57(L)	61(L)	82(L)	100+
Rye	62(L)	43(T)	55(L)	74(L)	100+
Wheat	53(L)	43(L)	46(L)	62(L)	100+

1 for scoring patterns see Table 2.
2 pattern based on amino acid composition of human milk
3 limiting amino acid
L = Lysine, T = Tryptophan

food itself. Ultimate experimental confirmation should be made using humans of appropriate age and sex and of appropriate physiological and health status. Since this is generally impossible in practice, comparison is often made between predictions from amino acid composition and from animal assays. Some of these data are shown in Table 8 where several protein sources of known amino acid composition, analysed in a previous collaborative study (Sarwar et al. 1983), were determined for protein efficiency ratio (PER), net protein ratio (NPR) and relative NPR (RNPR) also by a collaborative assay (Sarwar et al. 1984). In Table 8 however, while the mean values used for the amino acid data originate from the collaborative assay, the biological determinations shown are the means (8 rats per group) from only one collaborating laboratory (University of Massachusetts) and must not be taken as representing the collaborative study. In addition to the original protein sources (casein, beef, soy, pea, wheat, rapeseed and egg white), casein, soy and pea were supplemented with methionine (0.1%), wheat was supplemented with lysine (0.2%), and wheat was also mixed (50% of the protein from each) with the other six protein sources. Digestibility was estimated from FAO/WHO/UNU (1984) values and the scores have been multiplied by digestibility to give estimated NPU's.

It will be seen that all the proteins and/or mixtures are all more than adequate (Score>100) for the adult and therefore no correlations with

Table 8: Comparison between the protein value determined biologically and from amino acid composition for some protein sources and mixtures.

A. Biological Determination

	Biological Determination[1]			Estimated Digestibility[2]
	PER	NPR	RNPR[3]	%
Casein	3.36	4.78	85	95
Minced beef	3.50	4.78	85	94
Soy assay protein	1.66	2.83	50	96
Pea flour	1.64	2.84	50	88
Whole wheat	1.23	2.44	43	86
Rapeseed protein concentrate	3.42	4.61	81	85
Egg White	3.85	5.28	94	97
Casein + methionine[4]	4.32	5.64	100	95
Soy assay protein + methionine[4]	2.72	3.89	67	86
Pea flour + methionine[4]	3.05	4.38	78	88
Whole wheat + lysine[5]	1.95	3.15	56	86
Whole wheat + casein[6]	3.21	4.32	76	90
Whole wheat + minced beef	3.08	4.23	75	90
Whole wheat + soy assay protein	2.41	3.58	64	86
Whole wheat + pea	2.29	3.49	62	87
Whole wheat + rape protein concentrate	2.35	3.58	64	86
Whole wheat + egg white	3.21	4.23	75	90

B. Amino Acid Composition

	Amino Acid Composition[7] mg/gm N			
	Lysine	Total S.A.A.	Threonine	Tryptophan
Casein	527	218	290	82
Minced beef	496	204	263	62
Soy assay protein	396	152	240	71
Pea flour	480	164	261	54
Whole wheat	166	242	183	70
Rapeseed protein concentrate	356	277	262	94
Egg White	436	451	293	91
Casein + methionine	527	296	290	82
Soy assay protein + methionine	396	230	240	71
Pea flour + methionine	480	242	261	54
Whole wheat + lysine	322	242	183	70
Whole wheat + casein	347	230	237	76
Whole wheat + minced beef	331	223	223	66
Whole wheat + soy assay protein	281	197	212	70
Whole wheat + pea	323	203	222	62
Whole wheat + rape protein concentrate	261	260	223	82
Whole wheat + egg white	301	329	238	81

C. Protein Quality from Amino Acid Data

	Estimated NPU (Amino Acid Score[8] X Digestibility) and Limiting Amino Acid [9]				
	FAO/WHO (1973)	FAO/WHO/UNO 1984			
		Infant	Young Child	School Age Child	Adult
Casein	94(S)	73(T)	100 -	100 -	100 -
Minced beef	87(S)	55(T)	77(T)	100 -	100 -
Soy assay protein	59(S)	50(S)	80(S)	89 -	100 -
Pea flour	66(S)	45(T)	63(T)	81(T)	100 -
Whole wheat	42(L)	34(L)	37(L)	47(L)	100 -
Rapeseed protein Concentrate	89(L)	73(L)	78(L)	100 -	100 -
Egg White	100 -	83(T)	100 -	100 -	100 -
Casein + methionine	100 -	73(T)	100 -	100 -	100 -
Soy assay protein + methionine	83(Th)	75(S)	82(T)	100 -	100 -
Pea flour + methionine	79(T)	45(T)	63(T)	81(T)	100 -
Whole wheat + lysine	63(Th)	58(Th)	70(Th)	82(Th)	100 -
Whole wheat + casein	85(Th)	65(T)	80(L)	100(L)	100 -
Whole wheat + minced beef	80(Th)	56(T)	76(L)	95(L)	100 -
Whole wheat + soy assay protein	70(L)	57(T)	62(L)	81(L)	100 -
Whole wheat + pea	77(Th)	50(T)	72(L)	92(T)	100 -
Whole wheat + rape protein concentrate	66(L)	54(L)	58(L)	77(L)	100 -
Whole wheat + egg white	79(L)	66(L)	70(L)	85(L)	100 -
Correlation Coefficient (R) between RNPR and score	0.95 (P<0.001)	0.75 (P<0.001)	0.75 (P<0.001)	0.71 (P<0.01)	NS

1. Determined at University of Massachusetts by standard procedures (Pellett and Young 1980) using eight rats per group.
2. Values from FAO/WHO/UNU 1984
3. NPR of casein + methionine taken as 100.
4. L(-)methionine 0.1%.
5. L(-)lysine 0.2%.
6. Mixtures of protein, 50% from each source.
7. From Collaborative Assay: Sarwar et al, 1983.
8. Using four amino acids only: pattern as in Table 2.
9. L=Lysine, T=Tryptophan, Th=Threonine and S= Sulphur amino acids.

the biological values can be performed. Protein quality is thus only relevant to younger age groups, this is not surprising since the biological determinations are made using growing rats. It will be seen that amino acid estimates of quality parallel biological estimates with correlation coefficients between estimated NPU's and RNPR values being significant with probabilities of $P<0.001$ for FAO/WHO 1973 and the FAO/WHO 1984 infant and young child patterns and $P<0.01$ for the school age child. The FAO/WHO 1973 pattern was, of course, also based on young child requirements and the high significance of its correlation is thus expected. Other correlations between scores and biological determinations have frequently demonstrated high significance. Seventy-one pairs of values extracted from the FAO/WHO (1970) book on amino acid data and biological values of proteins were correlated by Pellett (1978) and showed a correlation coefficient of $R=0.84$ ($P<0.001$) using the FAO/WHO 1973 scoring system. The new scoring systems involving several age groupings make comparison more difficult .

It is essential, as FAO/WHO/UNU (1984) so rightly emphasize, that the question be asked: protein quality for what? Protein quality is not a static value associated with a protein but is dependent on other dietary interactions and the age and physiological state of the consumer. The new scoring systems involving age, together with incorporation of digestibility make the relationships more rational if not more immediately predictable. For all practical purposes amino acid composition can be used to predict the protein value of foods and dietaries provided that its limitations and indeed the overall limitations of protein quality as a concept are borne in mind. The statement made some five years ago (Pellett 1978) remains true.

> "Since every other dietary component consumed with a protein source and the individual circumstances of the consumer affect the quality as measured, an absolute value for protein quality, true under all circumstances is an unattainable goal and searching for such a technique is regressive rather than progressive."

The steps taken by the new FAO/WHO/UNU(1984) Committee recognise these limitations and provided that care is taken in interpretation, amino acid composition and digestibility can be used to predict the protein value of foods and dietaries with sufficient accuracy to meet all practical needs.

REFERENCES

Bender, A.E. (1961). Determination of nutritive value of proteins by chemical analysis: In "Progress in meeting protein needs of infants and preschool children,: ed. L. Voris, Publ. 843, p. 407. Natl. Acad. of Sciences-Natl. Res. Council, Washington, D.C.

Blackburn, S. 1978. Sample preparation and hydrolytic methods. In "Amino Acid Determination, Methods and Techniques," 2nd ed., (Ed.) S. Blackburn. Marcel Dekker Inc., New York.

Block, R.J. and Mitchell, H.H. 1946. The correlation of the amino-acid composition of proteins with their nutritive value. Nutr. Abst. and Revs. 16:249.

Bodwell, C.E., Adkins, J.S. and Hopkins, D.T. (1981). Protein quality in humans: assessment and in vitro estimation. AVI Publishing Company, Westport, Connecticut.

Cavins, J.F., Kwolek, W.F., Inglett, G.E., and Cowan, J.C. 1972. Amino acid analysis of soybean meal: Interlaboratory study. J. Assn. Offic. Anal. Chem. 55:686.
Cherry, J.P. 1981. Progress report on topic: Amino acids. Presented at the Sixth Annual Spring Workshop of AOAC, Ottawa, Canada. May 12-14.
Concon, J.M. 1975. Chemical determination of critical amino acids in cereal grains and other foodstuffs. Chapt 18 in Friedman (1975), Part 1.
Davies, M.G. and Thomas, A.J. 1973. An investigation of hydrolytic techniques for the amino acid analysis of foodstuffs. J. Sci. Fd. Agric. 24:1525.
FAO. 1957. Protein requirements. FAO Nutr. Stud. No. 16. Food and Agric. Org., Rome.
FAO. 1970. Amino acid content of foods and biological data on proteins. FAO Nutr. Stud. No. 24. Food and Agric. Org., Rome.
FAO. 1980. Food Balance Sheets 1975-1977, Average and percaput food supplies FAO, Rome.
FAO/WHO. 1965. Protein requirements. FAO nutr. meetings, Rep. Ser. No.37 Food and Agric. Org. Rome.
FAO/WHO. 1973. Energy and protein requirements. Report of a joint FAO/WHO ad hoc expert committee on energy and protein requirements. World Health Org. Tech. Rep. Ser. No. 522, Geneva, Food and Agric. Org. Nutr. Rep. Ser. No. 52, Rome.
FAO/WHO. 1975. Energy and protein requirements. PAG. Bulletin 5.30-35. Protein Advisory Group, New York.
FAO/WHO/UNU. 1984. Protein and Energy requirements. FAO, Rome. In press.
Friedman, M. and Finley, J.W. 1971. Methods of tryptophan and analysis. J. Agr. Food Chem. 19:626.
Hackler, L.R. 1977. In vitro indices: Relationships to estimating protein value for the human. pages 55-67 in Evaluation of proteins for humans. C.E. Bodwell, Ed. AVI Publishing Co., Westport, Connecticut.
Happich, M.L., Bodwell, C.E., and Phillips, J.G. 1981. Collaborative studies of amino acid analyses: A review and preliminary observations from a nine-laboratory study. In "Protein Quality in Humans: Assessment and In Vitro Estimation," (ED.) C.E. Bodwell, J.S. Adkins, and D.T. Hopkins, p. 197. AVI Publishing Company Inc., Westport, Ct.
Hegsted, D.M. (1971). Nutritional research in the value of amino acid fortification: experimental studies in animals. In amino acid fortification of protein foods. N.S. Scrimshaw and A.M. Altschul Eds. M.I.T. Press Cambridge, Mass. pp 157-178.
Hugli, T.E. and Moore, S. 1972. Determination of the tryptophan content of proteins by ion-exchange chromatography of alkaline hydrolysates. J. Biol. Chem. 247(9):2828.
Knipfel, J.E., Aitken, J R., Hill, D.C., McDonald, B.E., and Owens, B.D. 1971. Amino acid composition of food proteins: Inter- and Intra-laboratory variation. JAOAC 54(4):777.
Kohler, G.O. and Palter, R. 1967. Studies on methods for amino acid analysis of wheat products. Cereal Chem. 44:512.
Lusk, G. 1933. "Nutrition." Hafner Pub. Co., New York. (Reprinted 1964.)
McCollum, E.V. 1957. "A History of Nutrition." Houghton Mifflin Co., Boston.
Mondino, A. and Bongiovanni, G. 1970. An experimental study of amino acid degration under open flask hydrolytic conditions. J. Chromat. 52:405.
Moore, S. 1963. On the determination of cystine as cysteic acid. J. Biol. Chem. 238 (1) 235

Moore, S. and Stein, W.H. 1963. Chromatographic determination of amino acids by the use of automatic recording equipment. In "Methods in Enzymology," Vol. 6, (Ed.) S.P. Colowick and N.O. Kaplan. Academic Press, New York.
Munro, H.N. 1964. Historical introduction. In "Mammalian Protein Metabolism," Vol. 1, Chapt. 1, ed. H.N. Munro. Academic Press, New York and London.
NAS-NRC. 1974. Recommended Dietary Allowances 8th Edition. National Academy of Sciences, Washington, D.C.
NAS-NRC. 1980. Recommended Dietary Allowances 9th Edition. National Academy of Sciences, Washington, D.C.
Nygaad, D. and P.L. Pellett, Eds. The interactions between agriculture, food science and nutrition in the Middle East. United Nations University, Tokyo in Press.
Osborne, T.B. 1907. The proteins of the wheat kernel. Carnegie Inst., Washington, Pub. No. 84.
Osborne, T.B. 1908. Our present knowledge of plant proteins. Science 28 417 -427.
Osborne, T . 1919. What and how much should we eat. Atlantic Monthly 122:332-341.
Osborne, T.B., Mendel, L.B. and Ferry, E.L. (1919). A method of expressing numerically the growth promoting property of proteins. J. Biol. Chem 37:223.
Pellett, P.L. 1978. Protein quality evaluation revisited. Food Tech. 32(5) 60-79.
Pellett, P.L. and V.R. Young, Eds. 1980. Nutritional evaluation of protein foods. United Nations University WHTR/UNUP 129. Tokyo.
Robel, E.J. 1973. Effect of the volume of HCl in minimizing amino acid losses when carbohydrate containing samples are hydrolyzed. Poultry Science 52:604.
Sarwar, G., D.A. Christensen, A.J. Finlayson, M. Friedman, L.R. Hackler, S.L. MacKenzie, P.L. Pellett and R. Trachuk 1983. Inter- and Intra-laboratory variation in amino acid analysis of food proteins. J. Food Sci. 48(2) 526-531.
Sarwar, G., R. Blair, M. Friedman, M. Gumbmann, L.R. Hackler, P.L. Pellett and T.K. Smith. 1984. Inter- and Intra-laboratory variability in rat growth assays for estimating protein quality of foods. In preparation.
Satterlee, L.D., H.F. Marshall and J.M. Tennyson. 1979. Measuring protein quality. J. Amer. Oil Chem. Soc. 56:103-109.
Savoy, C.f., Heinis, J.L., and Seals, R.G. 1975. Improved methodology for rapid and reproducible acid hydrolysis of food and purified proteins. Anal. Biochem. 68:562.
Smyth, D.G. and Elliott, D.F. 1964. Some analytical problems involved in determining the structure of proteins and peptides-A review. The Analyst 89:81.
Spackman, D.M., Stein, W.H., and Moore, S. 1958. Automatic recording apparatus for use in the chromatography of amino acids. Anal. Chem. 30:1190.
Spitz, H.D. 1973. A new approach for sample preparation of protein hydrolysates for amino acid analysis. Anal. Biochem. 56:66.
Tkachuk, R. and Irvine, G.N. 1969. Amino acid compositions of cereals and oilseed meals. Cereal Chem. 46:206.
Williams, A.P., Hewitt, D., and Cockburn, J.E. 1979. A collaborative study on the determination of cyst(e)ine in feeding stuffs. J. Sci. Food Agric. 30:469.

Williams, P.C. Regional research on processing and nutritional quality of cereals and legumes at ICARDIA. The interactions between agriculture, food science and nutrition in the Middle East. D. Nygaad and P.L. Pellett Eds. United Nations University, Tokyo in press.
Young, V.R. and Pellett, P.L. (1983). Some general considerations of amino acid and protein metabolism and nutrition. In Surgical Physiology J.F. Burke, Editor, W. B. Saunders Company, Philadelphia pp 51-74.
Young, V.R. and Scrimshaw, N.S. 1977. Human protein and amino acid metabolism and requirements in relation to protein quality. In "Evaluation of Proteins for Humans," ed. C.E. Bodwell. AVI Pub. Co., Westport, Conn.
Young, V.R., Rand, W.M., and Scrimshaw, N.S. 1977. Measuring protein quality in humans-A review and proposed method. Cereal Chem. 54:929.

Proc. Int. Assoc. Cereal Chem. Symp. Amino Acid Compn and Biol. Value of Cereal Proteins Budapest, Hungary 1983, R. Lásztity, M. Hidvégi, eds

MATHEMATICAL MODELING OF PROTEIN NUTRITIONAL QUALITY FROM AMINO ACID COMPOSITION

M. HIDVÉGI, F. BÉKÉS

Department of Biochemistry and Food Technology, Technical University of Budapest, H-1111 Budapest, Müegyetem rkp. 3, Hungary

ABSTRACT

Amino acid composition has long been known to determine the nutritive value of food- and feed proteins and several mathematical formulae have been constructed to describe this relationship. In the paper an attempt is made for a generalized treatment of the various models in order to develop a general concept to construct new types of models and to define fields of applications. Another aim of this article is that through collecting the various equations together a guide should be given for supporting their easy use in everyday practice. The detailed algorithms of the models will be demonstrated in the APPENDICES of this paper.

INTRODUCTION

In contradistinction to the aversion for use of *in vitro* methods evaluating nutritional quality of food and feed proteins, it is beyond all question that they have their own and unreplaceable role in areas of the widely defined food production and consumption. There are at least two kinds of situations where the application of *in vitro* techniques are inevitable:

- situations requiring an immediate or fast treatment or observation (i.e., process control), where the time limit rejects the investigation of the *existing* sample by *in vivo* methods;
- cases where the sample does *not exist* at all, and the composition of a food- or feed blend is looked for just by the computation of the predicted nutritional values in an optimization process.

Besides, *in vitro* methods have a true advantage from financial point of view, as well.

The whole idea prerequires the existence of reliable, accurate reproducible, relatively simple *in vitro* methods having good correlation with the corresponding *in vivo* method.

Under the term "corresponding *in vivo* method" we mean such an assay which is able to distinguish the various nutritional values according to the species-, age-, sex-, physiological conditions, etc. differences of the consumer. It would lead the present treatment too far to discuss that a corresponding *in vitro* method can be better than an uncorresponding *in vivo* one.

Perhaps the most powerful possibility to investigate the nutritional value by *in vitro* methods is the use of amino acid composition data of the sample applying a mathematical model describing the relationship between this data set and protein nutritional value. These mathematical models are called chemical indices. Since the year 1946 when the first chemical index was introduced, numerous calculating procedures have been developed. Certain of them are able to rank proteins according to their qualities only, while the others can even measure protein quality on a given scale. The background of the difference between the information contents of these two groups is that the latter models were fitted to *in vivo* data by statistical methods.

When dealing with chemical indices there are many open questions. The judgement of "goodness" of a chemical index comparing it to *in vivo* or to other *in vitro* methods and the decision to choose the appropriate index is actually the most important factor. Excellent reviews concerning this topic can be found in the literature. However, because of the contradictory statements of these works, to make a sound decision in a given situation is quite hard.

Another branch of the problems is the appearance of the widespread variety of methodical realizations. These difficulties are underlined by the different reproducibility, accuracy, etc. of the techniques used.

As in every interdisciplinary area of science, there is a problem of the uniform use and interpretation of different notions, technical terms which sometimes results in confusion.

The aim of this work is to give an overview on the families of chemical indices going back to the origins, citing the original definitions of terms and grouping the indices in a chronological order and in such a way which points to the underlying unities of the mathematical formulations.

Generally speaking, the nutritive value of a protein is characterized by a biological response, R, which is considered to be a function of the amino acid composition of the food or feed.

$$R = f\ (a_1, a_2, a_3, \ldots , a_n) \tag{1}$$

R, the biological response, can be BV (biological value), TD (true digestibility), NPU (net protein utilization), PER (protein efficiency ratio), or any type of growth response. On the other hand, the a_i values represent the crude amino acid data of the input as determined by chemical methods and usually, no correction is made for availability or any type of variance in utilization. In the case of a single a_i variable Eq. (1) will be called the amino acid increment model, which reflects the response of an organism to increasing one amino acid in the diet. The amino acid increment model can be described by either linear or non-linear (saturation-, sigmoidal- or maximum-type) functions. The effects of more amino acids in the diet can be described as either as the sum or as the product of the individual response curves. Thus, f, the function in Eq. (1) is, as a rule, a complex one, because it is constructed of transformed amino acid data. These transformations also reflect the logical background behind the models.

POSSIBLE WAYS FOR GROUPING THE MODELS

There are numerous possibilities of grouping the different models. The most convenient one is based on the chronological order, following the appearances of the subsequent contributions to the field. Though this system is the simplest, it may be considered too positivistic, for neglecting our attitude to the development and present state of art. Another way of grouping is to treat the models according to the nature of the mathematical approach used. It is a more abstract methodology and can elegantly demonstrate the rationale behind the models. From the point of view of better understanding, a suitable grouping is possible through the principles - resulting from the accumulated knowledge in the science of nutrition - governing the constructions of the formulae. These are the principle of limiting amino acids, the principle of the harmonic amino acid patterns and Kofrányi's principle. A more practical grouping is available according to the implicit biological information contained in the different indices: whether the given formula carries specific reference (requirement) data, or the equation is the result of a regression on an experimental data base (feeding trials vs. amino acid compositions), or coming from purely theoretical considerations.

In case of regression, which kind of biological response should be used? For which kind of consumer has been the index constructed, in view of the reference data and/or the test organism?

Anyhow, it can be concluded that a precise grouping of chemical indices is problematical; however, some elegant reviews have been published (Sheffner 1967; Hackler, 1977; Pellett and Young, 1980; Bodwell, 1981).

CHEMICAL INDICES - HISTORICAL OVERVIEW

Let stand here a quotation from a classical paper (Block and Mitchell, 1946):

> "McCollum, as quoted by Mendel (1923) too, remarked that the investigations carried out during the period between 1910 and 1920 on protein foods of plant origin 'leave no room for doubt that all the amino acids necessary for the nutrition of an animal are contained in the proteins found in each of these foods. Certain of these are, however, present in such limited amounts as to restrict the extent to which the remaining ones, which are more abundant, can be utilised...' "

Perhaps, McCollum's words give the first explicit definition of a paradigm, as nowadays we call it, the principle of limiting amino acids, that is - in the words of Mitchell and Block (1946):

"... the nutritive value of a protein or mixture of proteins for any biological function or combination of functions is limited by the relative proportions of the essential amino acids contained in it..."

This principle can be considered as an analogy to the minimum law of Liebig, that is in plant nutrition the assimilation of soil minerals is limited by the inorganic component being present in minimal relative concentration.

Historically, the first model expressing protein nutritional quality by amino acid composition is based on the principle mentioned above, and is called Chemical Score, developed in 1946 by two pioneer scientists, Harold H. Mitchell, a pioneer in nitrogen balance experiments and Richard J. Block, a path-breaker in amino acid analysis.

The original computing procedure of Mitchell and Block was as follows: first, the ratios of the quantity of each essential amino acid of the test protein - standardized to a nitrogen content of 16 per cent - compared to the quantity of the given amino acid in a reference protein were calculated, and referred to as percentage values. (See, Mitchell and Block, 1946, Block and Mitchell, 1946, and also APPENDIX 1). For the reference amino acid composition Mitchell and Block proposed the amino acid requirements of the rat for growth. Because of those data were unknown at that time, they used the proteins of the dried whole egg, as an "amino acid mixture that is very highly digestible and almost perfectly utilizable in rodent metabolism".

Originally, Mitchell and Block introduced the term, percentage deviation which was equal to the difference between the percentage value and 100. In the case of negative percentage deviation, the latter was referred as percentage deficit. The percentage deficit with the greatest absolute value was called the greatest percentage deficit. The amino acid with the greatest percentage deficit was called the limiting amino acid. Chemical Score was defined by the following procedure: the greatest percentage deficit (the percentage deficit in the limiting essential amino acid) substracted from 100. The greater the percentage deficit in the limiting essential amino acid, the poorer the protein "as a source of amino acids for the growing rat", as well as, the larger the Chemical Score, the better the protein.

The names of Mitchell and Block - concerning the field of chemical scoring - were associated to the Chemical Score only, however, their research activities covered a methodologically wider spectrum of chemical indexing. In the two classical papers, cited above, Mitchell and Block gave equations of the type Eq. (1). These were linear ones and have one independent variable, the percentage deficit in the limiting essential amino acid. The dependent variables were PER and BV. (Also, NPU data were given, but the equation for predicting NPU from percentage deficit was missing; however, it could be calculated by the reader, as all the sufficient information was presented.) The equations resulting in the linear regressions had fairly good coefficients of correlation, -0.86 for BV and -0.89 for PER, which latter was statistically indistinguishable from that of BV. However, the equations themselves have no practical use today because of the relatively small size of the data base determined by the simple methods (there were no automatic amino acid analysers at that time, etc.) Yet, the methodology itself, i.e. the comparative view of chemical and biological techniques, must be considered a very modern one, as it was emphasized by Bender (1973).

The next contribution to the art is associated with the name of J. Kühnau, whose index is historically the first integrated amino acid index (Kühnau, 1946, 1949). The paradigm behind the integrated amino acid models is that - in contrast with the theory of limiting essential amino acids - by the words of Oser (1951):

> "It is characteristic of proteins that their food value must be considered in the light of their amino acid picture as a whole.
> ... It seems more reasonable, however, that a protein quality rating should be based on the contribution a protein makes in respect to all of the essential amino acids rather than simply the one in greatest deficit, because each essential amino acid is specific in its own right and all are equally essential."

These expressive words define the paradigm, as now we call it, the principle of harmonic amino acid pattern, the declaration of which has greatly been influenced by the pioneering works of Rose (1936), the expander of the concept of nutritive essentiality of amino acids.

The method proposed by Kühnau (see, APPENDIX 2) for evaluating protein nutritional quality solely from amino acid analysis data uses the amino acid composition of human milk, as reference pattern, (grams per 16 grams of nitrogen), Kühnau divides the sum of the concentrations of each essential amino acid (histidine, lysine, methionine, cystine, phenylalanine, tyrosine, leucine, isoleucine, valine, threonine, tryptophan and arginine) of the sample protein with that of the proteins of human milk, and, this ratio, multiplied by 100, is referred to as the Total Value. (Histidine should be omitted when formula for the evaluation of protein value for man is used.) However, this calculation overestimates the nutritive value, because the amino acids in excess of those occurring in the standard protein increase the numerical value of the index. It also follows from the mathematical nature of summation, because the addends contribute to the sum independently. In order to avoid this problem, Kühnau introduces the so-called Pure Value, which can be computed in a similar way to that of the Total Value, but with the restraint that if the concentration of any of the amino acids in the protein tested is greater than that of the reference pattern, then it is equal, not superior, to the standard value. The difference between the Total and the Pure Values is called Supplementary Value, which, in turn, reflects the possibility of using the sample protein for supplementing other proteins being deficient in those amino acids which occur in excess in the test protein.

Enriched by both the egg ratio concept of the Chemical Score and the "integrated" attitude of Kühnau, it was Bernard L. Oser, who proposed an integrated model, the so-called Essential Amino Acid Index (Oser, 1951). The principal novelty of Oser's method lies upon its mathematics, namely, that the

Essential Amino Acid Index is the geometric mean of the nutritional egg ratios. (See also APPENDIX 3.) This approach reflects the complexity of the interactions among nutritionally important amino acids, as well as the mutual dependence of amino acids upon each other. The same consequences can be arrived at when we consider the connections between the mathematical description of probability of events occurring simultaneously: the expression of the protein value by Oser's index, i.e. the probability of the event that all the essential amino acids will be available at the polyribosomes within a tissue, being a function of the product of their concentrations, as it has also been noticed by Sheffner (1967). In his empirical formula Oser has originally taken into consideration the following essential amino acids: lysine, tryptophan, isoleucine, valine, arginine, threonine, leucine, phenylalanine, histidine and the sum of methionine and cystine. It can be seen that Oser did not consider tyrosine in the formula at first, but later - as it will be discussed - influenced by Mithell's ideas, he did include tyrosine in the index, too. It follows from the mathematical character of the Essential Amino Acid Index that the value of a protein, being completely lacking in one or more essential amino acids, becomes zero. In order to avoid the discrepancy between this nature of the formula and the fact that the *in vivo* biological values of proteins, known to have complete deficiency in one indispensable amino acid, is low but finite which, in turn, is due to re-use of the products of tissue catabolism (endogen losses) and coprophagy by the target animal applied in the test, Oser makes the assumption: the minimum egg ratio be one per cent. And, no credit is given for any excess amino acid input, that is, similarly to Kühnau's solution of this problem, if the concentration of an amino acid is higher than that of the reference, it should be equal to, not greater, than the standard.

Oser has also investigated the correlation between his index and the *in vivo* biological value. He found not only a rather good correlation ($r = 0.85$), but also a numerically similar run of *in vivo* and *in vitro* data. Another important perception of Oser is that the basis for computing the Essential Amino Acid Index can be modified or extended concerning the reference protein, as well as the target species for which the index is intended to be used. For instance, he said that glycine might be included in the evaluation of protein for avian nutrition. On the other hand, Oser emphasizes that his formula cannot be applied to insoluble, incompletely digested proteins. This note has prompted some nutritionists to improve Oser's method from the point of view of amino acid availability.

Prior to dealing with these and other modifications of the Essential Amino Acid Index, the chronologically next model will be discussed here. This is called Bigwood's Index as it was constructed by E.J. Bigwood in 1953. The method of Bigwood is simple, as his formula is based merely on the ratio of the sum of certain essential amino acids to that of the total amino acid (see APPENDIX 4). Thus Bigwood's Index describes the proportion of total protein derived from threonine, methionine, valine, isoleucine, leucine, phenylalanine, lysine and tryptophan, the amino acids considered to be essential in Rose's pioneering studies. Generally, Bigwood's Index gives a low estimate of protein nutritional value.

Now, let us return to the Essential Amino Acid Index, more precisely to its modified version which was suggested by the classic of the art, Mitchell, in 1954. One of Mitchell's proposals was to eliminate arginine from the calculation, which idea did not meet that of Oser's, however, Oser accepted Mitchell's other proposal to include the semi-essential amino acids, tyrosine and cystine, in the index. Yet, if the essential amino acid of the pair is present in excess to that in the reference, this excess can be used to supplement the deficiency of the semi-essential amino acids however, the reverse does not hold true. Therefore the potential excesses in cystine and tyrosine cannot be taken into account in the egg ratios of sulphur-containing and aromatic amino acids, respectively. Thus, the relevant amino acids at the calculation of the Modified Essential Amino Acid Index are: histidine, lysine, methionine, cystine, methionine + cystine, phenylalanine, tyrosine, phenylalanine + tyrosine, leucine, isoleucine, valine, threonine and tryptophan (see APPENDIX 5).

As it was mentioned above, intensive efforts have been made to include availability data into the Essential Amino Acid Index.

The first model of this type, published by Sheffner et al. (1956), accepted the proposal of Melnick and co-workers (1946) that "in addition to the total amino acid composition, the rate of release of amino acids from protein by pancreatic digestion was also an important factor in the nutritional quality of a protein." So, the aim of Sheffner et al. was "to develop an *in vitro* procedure which could accurately estimate the nutritional value of proteins by the patterns of amino acids released by digestive enzymes". The digestive process was simulated by a 24 hours pepsin digestion with an enzyme/substrate ratio of 0.025. The qualitative description of the Sheffner -Eckfeldt--Spector's Pepsin Digest Residue Index is the following (for details see APPENDIX 6.): the essential amino acids, lysine, methionine, cystine, phenylalanine, tyrosine, leucine, isoleucine, valine, threonine and tryptophan are used when the index is calculated for humans and histidine is also included when the screening procedure is made for the growing rat. Sheffner and co-workers introduce the term 'residue fraction' which is the difference between the concentrations of a given amino acid in the completely hydrolyzed protein and in the pepsin digest, respectively. The concentrations are expressed as the percentages of the sum of the total amino acid. The so-called egg ratios are then calculated by dividing the respective ratio of the test protein by that of the reference, the whole egg protein. Egg ratios should not be larger than 1 or less than 0.01 for any of the amino acids taken into consideration, similarly with that at the Essential Amino Acid Index. Furthermore, methionine and cystine, as well as phenylalanine and tyrosine are considered as a unit. Excess inputs at these amino acid pairs are described similarly to that at the Modified Essential Amino Acid Index. The mathematical novelty of the Pepsin Digest Residue Index lies upon the correcting and weighting of the geometric means of the computed egg ratios. Terms, "corrected geometric means" are used for the geometric means of the pepsin digest and the residue fractions, respectively, multiplied by their proteolysis factors which, in turn, can be obtained by summing the concentrations of the amino acids in the test fractions and dividing the totals by the sum of the respective amino acids in the reference protein, the whole egg. Moreover, the weighting exponents for the digest and the residue fractions are the proportions of amino acids the fractions represent in the total reference protein (APPENDIX 6). The Pepsin Digest Residue Index for the test protein can be obtained by multiplying the corrected and weighted geometric means of the digest and residue fractions, respectively.

For the sake of chronological accuracy two simple scoring procedures proposed by FAO (1957) will be mentioned now.

The so-called E/N ratio is the ratio of essential amino acids to non-essential amino acids in a food protein (APPENDIX 7). This ratio is generally used in the investigations of the effects dietary proteins cause in the amino acid concentration of body fluids.

The so-called E/T ratio is the proportion of the total nitrogen derived from essential amino acids. (See APPENDIX 8). The importance of the E/T index manifests itself when it is the non-essential nitrogen which is limiting factor in the diet.

A great problem or question associated with the reliable application of the Chemical Score is the nutritional character of the reference amino acid composition, that is the definition and the determination of that. Really, the reference pattern deeply influences the results as it is evident from the computing procedure. Therefore, during the fifties, intensive efforts have been devoted improving the reliability of the Mitchell and Block's method. The 1955 FAO Committe's (FAO, 1957) most important achievement was the suggestion of a theoretically conceived reference pattern derived from human amino acid requirements. For details, see APPENDIX 9 and Pellett (1984).

This concept of an "ideal protein" also was applied by A.E. Bender (1958) who calculated an "ideal" requirement pattern for rats on the basis of feeding trials. This standard amino acid mixture had an NPU of 92. (Bender's Chemical Score is shown in APPENDIX 10).

At the time when the determination of amino acids had been carried out by microbiological procedures it was an important proposal to reduce the number of amino acids taken into consideration in chemical scoring. This was done by McLaughlan et al. in 1959 introducing the so-called Simplified Chemical Score. The Score can be calculated from lysine and the sulphur-containing amino acids only, as for almost all practical diets these amino acids are the most important limiting ones. It was also shown that the Simplified Chemical Score had correlated well with results of PER determinations on the same foodstuffs: r = 0.96 was found for proteins deficient in lysine and r = 0.83 was obtained for protein foods deficient in sulphur-containing amino acids. Nowadays, when laboratories are well supplied with automatic amino acid analysers, the significance of the Simplified Chemical Score is rather historical than practical. (For details see APPENDIX 11.)

Historically, the next, rather little known result in the calculation of protein value from amino acid composition was developed by István Korpáczy, Károly Lindner and Károly Varga (1961). Their efforts were devoted to include the contributions of both essential and non-essential amino acids to the nutritive value of proteins into one formula. The index of Korpáczy and his co-workers can be considered an extended version of Oser's method. The modifications concern the following shortcomings of the Oser's index:

- the quantity of non-essential nitrogen was not included in the Essential Amino Acid Index;
- the negative nutritional effects associated with the excess amino acid intakes were not considered.

The first deficiency is corrected by taking into account the relative quantity of non-essential amino acids applying the observation of Rose et al. (1955) that the nitrogen balance of humans fed with only essential amino acids became negative, and after administrating 25 per cent of disposable nitrogen, originating from non-essential amino acids, the balance values returned to the normal level. Thus, Korpáczy et al. broke down the formula into two terms. The first one is, practically, the Essential Amino Acid Index multiplied by 0.75. The excess amino acid intake is taken into consideration by the constrain: if any of the egg ratios is greater than 1.0, its reciprocal must be used. The empirical background of this way of calculating excess intakes lies in the empirical findings where excess inputs of essential amino acids turned to degrade the biological value of proteins for the test animals (Korpáczy et al. 1961). The ratio of the difference between the sums of the concentrations of non-essential amino acids in the test protein and the reference, the egg, respectively, and the sum of non-essential amino acids in the egg only, multiplied by 25, gives the term. The index of Korpáczy, Lindner and Varga is the sum of the above mentioned two terms (APPENDIX 12).

Miller and Payne (1961) proposed an equation for the prediction of protein values from chemical data. Their index calculates net dietary calories per cent as a function of Chemical Score and protein calories (see APPENDIX 13). The method was well applicable to a wide range of protein mixtures and concentrations.

Although the chronologically next contribution, that is the Pepsin Pancreatin Digest Index of Akeson and Stahmann (1964), does not differ from the index of Sheffner et al. (1956) in its mathematics, the modification of the chemical procedure is considerable, since a combined digestion using pepsin and followed by pancreatin, as well as automatic amino acid analysis are applied (for details see APPENDIX 14).

A new method for scoring proteins on the basis of their limiting essential amino acids was proposed by the Joint FAO/WHO Expert Group on Protein Requirements at a Geneva meeting in 1963 and was published in a report in 1965 (FAO, 1965). As a matter of fact, this new method, the FAO-WHO Index, carries a theoretical setback because it goes back to the antiquated theory of limiting essential amino acids. The index measures "the extent to which a food or food combination supplies the limiting amino acid as compared with the provisional pattern" which reflects the amino acid requirements of humans. The FAO/WHO procedure introduces the so-called A/E ratio which describes the "relationship between the content of an individual essential amino acid in a food protein and the total essential amino acid content. It may be expressed either as milligrams of the individual amino acid per gram of total essential amino acids, or as grams of nitrogen from the individual amino acid per gram of nitrogen from all essential amino acids." The A/E ratios of each of the essential amino acids in the test protein divided by those in the reference pattern and multiplied by 100 can be called the FAO/WHO percentage values. Then, the FAO/WHO Index is defined as the smallest percentage value. (See APPENDIX 15). The greater the smallest percentage value the better the protein. The amino acid with the smallest percentage value is called the First Limiting Essential Amino Acid. Evidently, the amino acid with the second smallest percentage value is the Second Limiting Essential Amino Acid, etc. Very often, the words "FAO/WHO" are followed by a date of year and then the word "Index". The year refers to the date when the reference pattern was published.

(For the sake of chronological priority, we note that the pattern: ratio of each essential amino acid to the total content of essentials, was originally introduced by Sheffner et al. (1956)).

The first attempt "to ascertain whether a mathematical formula instead of the chemical score would not give a protein quality index more respondent to biological reality" is ascribed to the year 1969 when a group in Rome, after a large work of collecting data, published the results of a multiple correlation study of biological value or protein efficiency ratio with essential amino acids (Cresta et al. 1969).Equations resulting in the computer-aided investigations are shown in APPENDIX 16. The data set used in the study was also published in the form of a book (FAO, 1970) and comprised the amino acid composition of 274 different protein sources; the biological value of 87 of these and the protein efficiency ratio of the remaining 187 proteins were also presented. These data were the results of a great literary survey made by the FAO Nutrition Division. The coefficients of correlation in the equations of Cresta et al. are about 0.7. The chemical analyses and the feeding tests were not carried out on the same samples.

The work of Cresta, Périssé, Autret and Lombardo comprised a major advance in the exact description of protein value from amino acid composition. Their efforts inspired several investigators to continue the work following the words of Cresta and co-workers; "... any contribution towards the solution of this problem of assessing protein quality should originate in a series of biological experiments (BV, PER, NPU) carried out on a sufficiently extensive number of foods and diets; it is also essential that the amino acid composition of these foods and diets should be ascertained by column chromatography. Results could then be subjected to the same kind of mathematical processing as we have used."

The next contribution to the art of protein quality evaluation is again an integrated index using *in vitro* digestion. This was first published in 1970 by an expert from Nestlé's Research Laboratory (Mauron, 1970a, b). The method, the Pepsin Pancreatin Digest Dialysate Index (PPDD) takes the advantages of both the *in vitro* digestion procedure with simultaneous dialysis for the determination of amino acid availability and the computing procedure developed by Sheffner et al. (1956). The method proposed by Mauron (for further information see APPENDIX 17) is an ingenious simulation of proteins' 'fate' *in vivo* and, therefore "will not only yield a PPDD index as an estimate of the nutritive value, but also supply data on amino acid availability ... In many cases the latter information is more useful than the former. Indeed, the nutritive value of a protein food as sole protein source does not give much information on the supplementary value of such a protein in a mixed diet. The basis for such an evaluation is given by the data on amino acid availability."

In 1972 a new amino acid scoring pattern was proposed by Pellett and Kaba (1972). This was based on rat carcass amino acid data (APPENDIX 18). Scoring on this new pattern had a rather good correlation with NPU data, i.e., may be useful in predicting true limiting amino acids (Kaba and Pellett, 1975).

Starting from the pioneering idea of Cresta et al. (1969) that a protein measure system could be constructed from corresponding *in vivo* and *in vitro* data, it was Niels Glem Hansen and Bjørn O. Eggum who carried out a great correlation study between biological value and amino acid composition of proteins (Glem Hansen and Eggum, 1973). Their calculations comprised 221 samples and, contrary to the calculations of the working in Rome group, the *in vivo* and *in vitro* measurements had been performed on identical material. The data set was statistically worked up by the method of least squares comprising multiple regression analyses, correlation studies and analyses of variance. Their first index, called Total Amino Acid Value (TAAV) provides expressions of biological value as a function of the gross amino acid composition, i.e. on the basis of the threonine-, valine-, isoleucine-, leucine-, tyrosine-, phenylalanine-, lysine-, histidine-, methionine-, cystine-, tryptophan-, aspartic acid-, serine-, glutamic acid-, glycine-, alanine- and arginine content. We mentioned 'expressions' because Hansen and Eqqum carried out the computer runs on the entire material and also on different groups separated according to origins (extracted oil cakes, grain products, fruits and vegetables, non-heat-treated animal samples, heat-treated animal samples, pig- and poultry mixtures and mixtures for mink, dogs and cats, respectively).

The coefficient of the multiple correlation, in case of the entire material, was found to be 0.74; however, it increased up to 0.85 when the regressions were run individually on the different groups. A further implicite, but important benefit of this grouping is that the effects of certain antinutritive factors associated with some of the groups of the samples are included into the numerical value of the coefficients of the equations. The other index, the Essential Amino Acid Value (EAAV), was gained by similar procedures, however, on the essential amino acids only. Thus the independent variables at the EAAV are threonine, valine, isoleucine, leucine, tyrosine, phenylalanine, lysine, histidine, methionine, cystine, and tryptophan. Elimination of non-essential amino acids resulted in a slight decrease in the value of the correlation coefficient from 0.85 to 0.82. According to the above-mentioned authors this fact may be due to the influence that the non-essential amino acids exert on the biological value. A practical demonstration of the use of TAAV and EAAV indices is presented in APPENDICES 19 and 20.

The 1973 FAO/WHO report proposed a new reference scoring pattern as the suggestion by the 1965 FAO/WHO Expert Group was not widely used and also some new data on human amino acid requirements has already been assembled. Although the pattern developed by the 1971 Joint FAO/WHO Ad Hoc Expert Committee (FAO, 1973) gave an extra margin of safety concerning the true amino acid requirements of adult humans (Hackler, 1977, Pellett, 1984), its success can be well documented by the fact that, even nowadays, it is the most widely adopted reference pattern in the field. Particulars regarding the use of the FAO/WHO 1973 Index are shown in APPENDIX 21.

In 1974 the US National Research Council - National Academy of Sciences reported a reference amino acid pattern based on human requirements (NAS/NRC, 1974). The main differences between this pattern and that of the FAO/WHO (1973) are:

- the NAS/NRC (1974) pattern takes the histidine into consideration, too;
- there are 26 per cent reduction and 22 per cent increase in the values of the sulphur-containing and the aromatic amino acids, respectively (APPENDIX 22).

An examplary, precise mathematical attempt to deduce formulae from amino acid compositions and corresponding *in vivo* (protein efficiency ratio) data was published in 1974 by an USDA team (Alsmeyer et al. 1974). These authors estimated multiple variabled linear equations from the data by three, correctly applied, mathematical statistical procedures. First, a multiple regression was performed, "setting leucine and proline as the independent variables with PER as the dependent variable. Leucine and proline were selected for this regression because they had a high positive correlation and a high negative correlation, respectively, with PER and also because they had a low simple correlation with each other." The equation gained by the multiple regression (APPENDIX 23) had a correlation coefficient of 0.99 and only one significant variable, the leucine. This equation seemed to be useful in estimating the PER values for meat and poultry products. The other approach was a stepwise regression with backward elimination, which recalculated the t test values of the variables, after each step of regression. Independent variables having smaller t values than the minimal one needed for signification were eliminated from the equation. Thus, the regression was terminated with two variables, leucine and tyrosine (APPENDIX 24) and had a multiple correlation coefficient of 0.95. The third procedure, applied, was a straightforward stepwise regression which calculated t values only at the start of the regression and proceeded to add all variables having t values greater than the required minimum. There remained four variables, methionine, leucine, histidine and tyrosine, in the formula which had a multiple correlation coefficient of 0.98 (APPENDIX 25). The equations developed by Alsmeyer and his co-workers had extremely high coefficients of correlation, however, it was important to test the equations, because the high correlations might be due to the relatively small size of data base used in the regressions. The data base comprised only eight observational units (eight samples), although homogeneous ones (all were beef tissues). For example, it could have been expected that equations resulting on "beef tissue data" could have been successfully applied in situations predicting PER of beef tissues only. Another reason why testing was necessary was described by the authors themselves (and actually it is a general reason):

> "Keep in mind that regression analysis is only a mathematical analysis that determines the mathematical relationship between a dependent variable (PER in this case) and one or more independent variables. There is no causal relationship determined or implied. The amino acids selected are not to be regarded as having more biological significance than other amino acids present, but only as having a more significant mathematical relationship to PER. In other words, the changes in amounts of these amino acids have value in predicting the changes in PER, but may not have a direct relation to PER..."

The next contribution to protein quality evaluation by chemical indices was the so-called Enzyme Score of Stahmann and Woldegiorgis (1975). Enzyme Score was calculated from the amount of threonine, valine, methionine, isoleucine, leucine, phenylalanine, aromatic amino acids, lysine, tryptophan, histidine, released by pepsin followed by pancreatin digestion, in the same way as the Chemical Score. For reference, amino acids released from whole egg solids by the combined *in vitro* digestion was used. Tested on nine samples, a correlation coefficient of 0.87 was found between Enzyme Score and PER. (For details see APPENDIX 26).

The perception of the fact, that a gap existed between chemical indices based on animal experiments and their use in testing proteins for humans prompted Erling S. Olesen and Inge-Lise K. Mørup to develop a new index on data from *in vivo* human experiments (Olesen and Mørup 1975, Mørup and Olesen 1976). These authors sensitively took notice of an oeuvre to re-evaluate the traditional hypotheses on the *in vivo* biological value of proteins. The data and conclusions considered by Olesen and Mørup were taken from the works of Ernst Kofrányi and his colleagues (Friedrichkarl Jekat and Hildegard Müller-Wecker) at the Max-Planck-Institut für Ernahrungsphysiologie, Dortmund. Kofrányi et al. performed long term dietary experiments with adult human males using both single protein source and different mixtures of two-two protein sources of different biological value. Ernst Kofrányi and his co-workers were interested in the biological value of food proteins for human nutrition because it had been suggested (e.q. Jekat and Pabst, 1969) that the biological values obtained with humans and rats were quite different and, in addition, no data existed regarding the extent of improvement of biological value obtained by combining food proteins. The exact execution of the experimental procedures enabled the authors to obtain exceptionally reproducible results (± 1.5 per cent for measurements on one subject) for the biological value of protein and protein mixtures (Kofrányi et al., 1970).

"Healthy adult males between 20-30 years of age were used as experimental subjects. They were accomodated in the Institute where they ate, slept and gave their excrements, but were allowed to carry out their normal daily occupations. Before accepting a subject, his general physiological condition was determined by medical examination and clinical tests upon blood and urine. If satisfactory, the individual was contracted to the Institute for the duration of a test series (6-12 months)... The bulk of the nitrogen in a diet was provided by the sources being tested... Supplementation with vitamines and minerals was necessary due to the length of tests (12-20 days). Agar-Agar and cellulose were included in some diets to ensure peristaltic movement and stool formation. From the basic diets, mixtures of constant nitrogen content were prepared... Caloric loss due to change in one major component was compensated by addition of fat, sugar or maize starch. When, during a test, the nitrogen content of a diet was adjusted to achieve equilibration of intake and output, the calorie content was also adjusted to ensure that the body-weight of the subject was constant or increased slightly... Before beginning a test and also between the different tests the nitrogen balance with normal mixed food was determined for about 10 days. The tests were divided into periods of 3 to 4 days. The nitrogen balance during the first part of the test period was measured and the input for subsequent periods adjusted accordingly until slight negative balances were achieved. The first part of the test period required 5 to 11 days. The test was then continued for 10-12 days with slight negative balances. Only values from this part of the test period were used in our calculations. During the normal food periods we ensured that the "labile protein pool" was replenished and positive balances were achieved (1.0 to 1.5 g N/day). When starting with a new subject his minimum requirement for whole egg nitrogen was determined. The value obtained was used for standardization of data... At the end of each test the serum levels of aspartate aminotransferase and alanine aminotransferase were measured to determine whether these had been altered by the diet... "

Nitrogen loss from skin peeling, perspiration, nail and hair were also estimated. The biological value of a diet was also defined:

"as the reciprocal of the minimum protein requirement (g protein per kg body weight and day) determined under condition of nitrogen balance. The value obtained with whole egg was set equal to 100%... The initial body weight of a subject was taken for calculation throughout the tests. The minimum requirement for any one protein, calculated as g per kg and day, varied between individuals. Therefore in order to compare the resutls obtained with different subjects we standardized our data. The standardization factor used by ourselves was based upon the minimum protein requirement of a subject for our whole egg diet. The average minimum requirement was 0.5 g protein per kg and day (determined in our laboratories with 28 subjects who showed a range of 0.37-0.64)."

The 0.5 value divided by the actual minimum requirement for egg gave the standardization factor for a particular subject. The standardized requirement values (requirement values multiplied by the factor) of different subjects could be compared. Kofrányi and his co-workers performed more than 200 long term balance experiments. They tested individual protein sources, egg, rice, wheat, maize, potato, bean, milk, veal, etc., and also two-component mixtures of these raw materials (usually at four different mixing ratios) for biological value (Kofrányi and Jekat 1964a, b, 1967, Kofrányi et al. 1970, Kofrányi 1972, 1973). The authors published also the amino acid compositions of the proteins tested (Kofrányi and Jekat 1964a). Some of their results were unexpected. They found that "certain mixtures of the two protein sources had a higher biological value than the single sources in isolation." The highest biological value was achieved with the 35 per cent whole egg-N plus 65

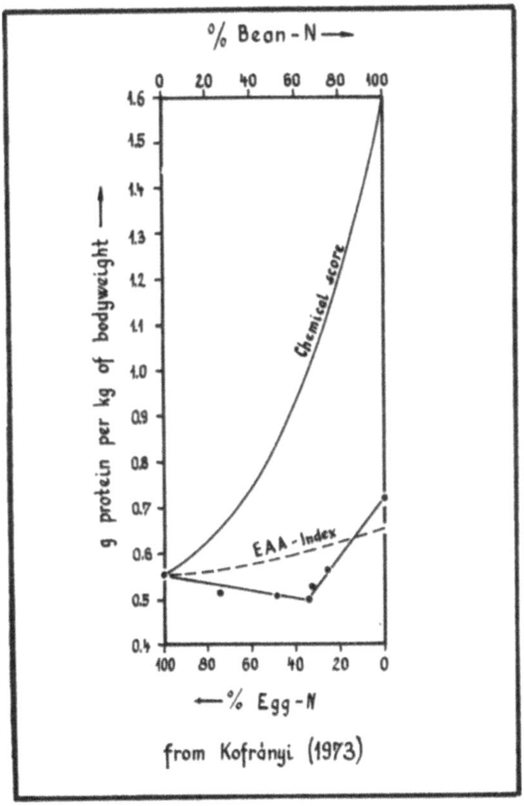

Fig. 1. Measured and calculated protein qualities of egg-bean 2-component mixtures

per cent potato-N. If the biological value of the 100 per cent egg-N sample was set as 100, this former mixture had a value of 136 (Kofrányi et al., 1970). By using both the Chemical Score and Essential Amino Acid Index it failed to predict these synergic phenomena (Kofrányi and Jekat, 1964a, Kofrányi, 1972, 1973) (Fig. 1).

Eventually, the following inferences were drawn by Kofrányi (1973):

> "An optimal proportion of amino acids exists in food mixtures. Each deviation from this proportion will produce a lower biological value. Employing mixtures of pure amino acids in balance tests, we sought to obtain the mathematical formula of the law which is the basis for biological value. Indeed, there are essential amino acids and surely they should not decrease below a certain critical level in nutrition. The hypothesis of the "limiting essential amino acids" could have an effect with extreme diets such as the mixture of egg with more than 50 per cent gelatine. This always occurred at the time in our balance tests when the straight lines of the minimum requirement became hyperbolas. But, for a somewhat normal nutrition, the hypothesis of the "limiting essential amino acids" is not, in our opinion, valid. Hence, the minimum requirement of each single essential amino acid depends on the proportion of all the other amino acids and therefore data can be given only for special cases."

The words cited above represent an idea that is known now as Kofrányi's principle. Kofrányi's thoughts were left unregarded, although they would have been worthy of attention. The theory of limiting amino acids was dogmatized, most of the experts have not even heard about Kofrányi's experiments. Among the inevitable reasons why these ideas could not come into prominence a primary one was that Kofrányi's works did not arouse the interest of important professional forums.

In Kofrányi's experiments, curves representing the minimum protein requirements from a two-component mixture of proteins supplied in different proportions may be of different values, however, their slope has the same tendency and all have a breaking point at a given nitrogen ratio (Kofrányi, 1971). It also means that the minimum quantity of protein requirement, the value of the curve on the ordinate, depends on the individual, while the value of the break point on the abscissa is determined by the quality of the proteins (Kerese, 1976). Figure 1 shows minimum protein requirements from mixtures of whole egg and bean protein of various ratios for humans and essential amino acid indices and chemical scores corresponding to these compositions. Although, with the reduction of egg protein the minimum requirement also decreases to a 32 per cent share of the former, the Essential Amino Acid Index increases in proportion to the reduction of egg protein, while Chemical Score gives a steeply ascending hyperbolic curve (Kerese, 1976). Figure 2 demonstrates the calculated amino acid quantities corresponding to 0.5 g whole egg protein, 0.51 g potato protein and a 0.37 g mixture of whole egg protein (35%) and potato protein (65%).

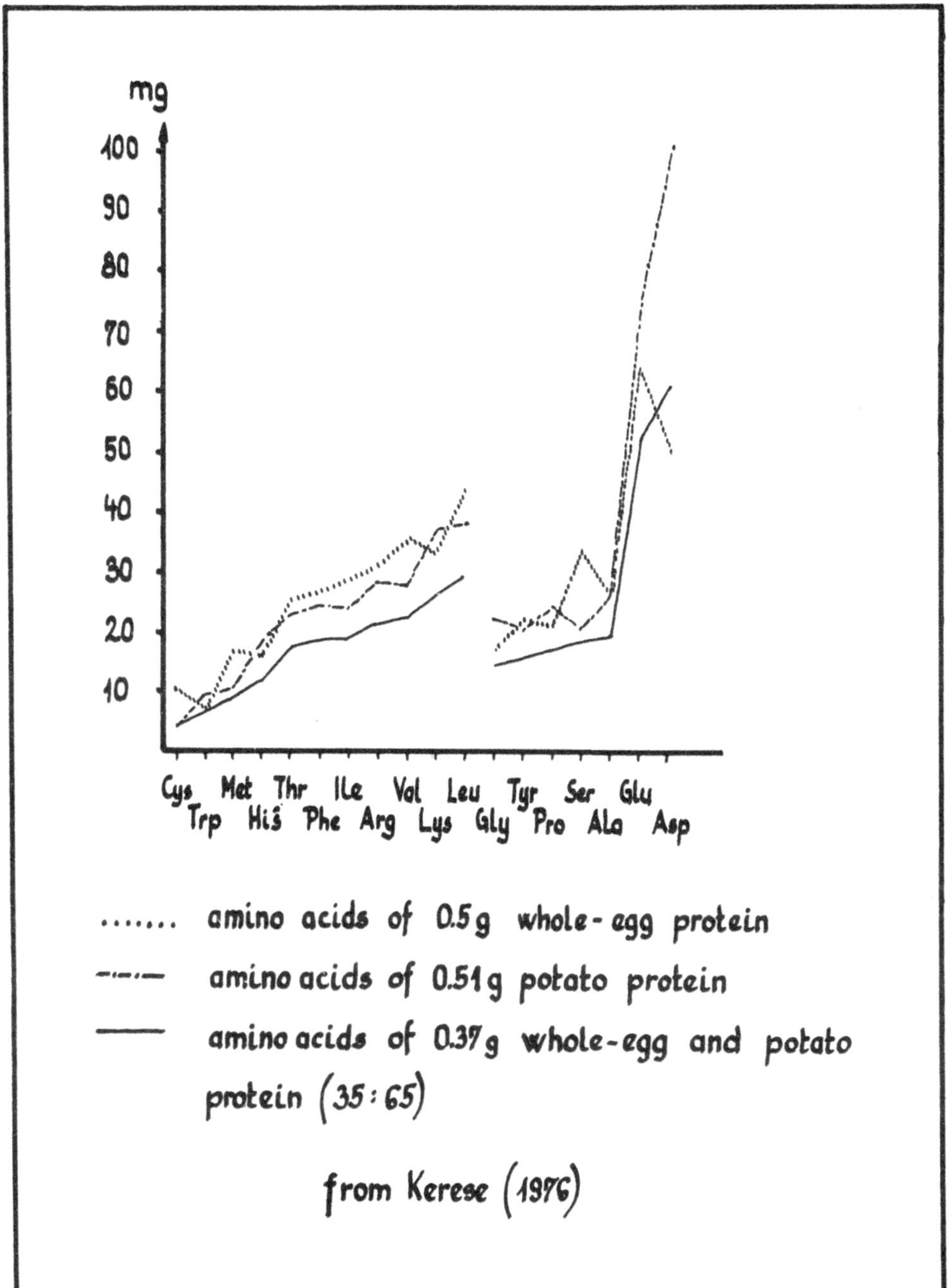

Fig. 2. Comparison of amino acid contents of egg, potato and of their mixture

A clear explanation of Kofrányi's principle was done in the same figure by Kerese (1976):

> "Whole egg protein given by itself, as well as potato protein and the quantities chosen here of their 35:65 ratio mixture are of equal biological value, since these weights satisfy minimum requirements. Since all amino acids of 0.5 g whole egg protein are required in larger quantities than those found in a 0.37 g mixture of whole egg and potato protein of 35:65 ratio (and in most cases in mixtures of other ratios, too), all essential amino acids of this last curve should be considered limiting. Further, on the basis of curves running side by side, we can conclude that the biological value of biologically equal proteins, or of protein mixtures of different composition, is not decided by the quantity of a certain amino acid (e.g. Lys) but by the proportions that the individual essential amino acids bear to each other. The possibility of different proportions of essential amino acids is clearly seen if we take as a basis for our calculations those quantities of the differently composed mixtures of whole egg and potato protein whose identical weights ensure the nitrogen balance of the organism..... These data prove the possibility of different proportions of the necessary amounts of essential amino acids being of equal biological value, notwithstanding the theory of the limiting character of essential amino acids. The cause of correlation between the essential amino acid ratios and their biological values will be revealed by physiological investigations..."

Returning to the method we have started to discuss, Olesen and Mørup tried to put the results of Kofrányi et al. into a mathematical model. The Mørup-Olesen Index was constructed on the assumption that the essential amino acid pattern in terms of the mutual amino acid ratios - not the absolute amounts - has major significance. Therefore the individual amino acid ratios were formed analogously to those of the FAO/WHO Index but using a different reference pattern. Thus, the variables of the Mørup-Olesen Index resulted from dividing the content of each of the essential amino acids - expressed in mg per g of total essential amino acids - by that of the reference pattern, which, in turn, was called provisional reference.

Provisional reference comprised the amino acid pattern of the 35:65 mixture of whole egg and potato protein from Kofrányi's experiments, but with two slight modifications due to the relatively low leucine and tryptophan contents of the optimum quality potato-egg mixture. Amino acid imbalances caused by excess intakes were taken into consideration - similarly to those at the index of Korpáczy et al. - by the following constrain: if any of the amino acid terms (q_i) is greater than 1.0, its reciprocal should be used.

The Mørup-Olesen Index, the so-called Predictive Value was constructed as follows:

$$PV = 10^{\alpha_o} \prod_{i=1}^{8} q_i^{\alpha_i} \qquad (2)$$

where q_i is the i-the amino acid ratio and α_0 and α_i are weighting factors determined by statistical procedures. The essential amino acids considered were isoleucine, leucine, lysine, phenylalanine + tyrosine, methionine + cystine, threonine, tryptophan and valine. The experimental data set used for these studies was taken from Kofrányi's works: 27 *in vivo* biological value data and corresponding essential amino acid patterns. On the basis of these biological *vs.* chemical data the alpha weighting factors were looked for where the sum of the squared differences of *in vivo* and predicted biological values was minimal. The problem as formulated above - in contrast to the text described by Mørup and Olesen (1976) - could not be considered as a regression on the logarithm of Eq (2), because it had to be fulfilled for every alpha weighting factors that those must be zero or positive as it was also put in the paper of Mørup and Olesen (1976). Thus, the exact mathematical method applied by the authors is unknown. (However, it has been shown (Békés et al. 1982) that following an appropriate transformation of the vector of alpha weighting factors, as

$$\alpha_i = a + b \sin^2 \gamma_i \, , \qquad (3)$$

the minimization of the squared differences mentioned above could be done using Eq. (3) type quadratic sinusoidals by a non-linear optimization applying the Hooke-Jeeves algorithm.) Mørup and Olesen eliminated alpha exponents not significantly related to biological value from the equation. From the eight factors three turned out to be zero. Thus, it means that isoleucine, leucine and valine have no individual q_i values in the final formula. However, their amount is taken into account in each q_i values (see APPENDIX 27). The Mørup-Olesen Index (APPENDIX 27) gave a very close correlation with the experimental values determined by Kofrányi (r=0.95) and truely reflected the synergism phenomena discovered by this author. Nutritional values of protein mixtures could be well predicted. Chronologically, it was the first *in vitro* method having this important characteristic. It is why the Mørup-Olesen Index and its modified versions (Gaussian-type indices, Tailing Index, see later) could be successfully used in different food industrial situations (Békés et al., 1979, 1981, 1982a, b, 1984, Békés and Zsigmond, 1980, Hidvégi, 1983a, b, Kemény et al., 1982, Wöller et al., 1977).

An enzymatic ultrafiltrate digest (EUD) assay was developed in Italy during the year 1975. The method can be regarded as a modification of Mauron's Pepsin Pancreatin Digest Dialysate Index because it involved digesting by pepsin, trypsin and pancreatin and then determining the liberated amino acids by analyzing the ultrafiltrate of the enzyme digest (Floridi and Fidanza, 1975). Testing the method against *in vivo* (rat) biological value data resulted in good correlation. (EUD assay is not included in the APPENDICES of the present paper due to the partial information available for us.)

The fact that the amino acid score, recommended by the 1973 FAO document, does not include corrections for digestibility has motivated this international organization to take also into consideration digestibility of dietary protein, because the 1973 score failed to predict protein quality of foods with low digestibilities. Thus, a joint FAO/WHO informal gathering of experts on energy and protein requirements decided to include digestibility into the FAO/WHO Index, i.e. the Index should be reduced being multiplied by a digestibility factor (FAO/WHO 1975). It was recommended that the FAO/WHO 1975 Index be adjusted to 85 per cent digestibility in case of coarse, whole grain cereals and vegetables and to 90 per cent digestibility in the case of more refined proteins (Pellett, 1984, APPENDIX 28)

However, the next contribution, the so-called Computed Protein Efficiency Ratio (C-PER) method of Lowell D. Satterlee and his co-workers needed " ...5 years of work to develop, modify and test" and, therefore, its final version was published in a very elegant article in 1982 (Satterlee et al. 1982). We insert the method in the chronology here, because its first version was published in 1977 (Satterlee et al., 1977), although the present treatment will follow the last version. (For the subsequent publications see Satterlee et al., 1977, 1979, 1981, 1982, Hsu et al., 1978, Jewell, 1979.) Actually, the first contribution made by the authors was an essential amino acid score we shall refer to as the Nebraska Score, which can provide for itself quite apart from the C-PER technique, too. The Nebraska Score is a further modification of the Essential Amino Acid Index although using the FAO/WHO 1973 reference. The Score is corrected also for digestibility. It comprised a four-enzyme procedure of the authors. Furthermore, authors introduced weighting factors to multiply the amino acid terms in the Score. The weighting factors were determined by least squares methods; they are common for all amino acids and depend only on the sample/reference amino acid ratios (APPENDIX 29). It was suggested that the Nebraska Score is a useful procedure in evaluating protein quality also for humans (Bodwell 1981).

C-PER assay includes all the advantages of "Nebraska scoring" because C-PER algorithm starts with the calculation of Nebraska Scores for the sample and for a standard protein (casein). In order to get better prediction and also to eliminate the necessity of any *a priori* knowledge on the "antecedents" of the proteins tested, C-PER assay comprises discriminant analysis. This latter is a pure mathematical-statistical technique for grouping of data. Thus, it can be said that there are four (discriminant analysis resulted in four groups) C-PER assays concerning the four different - by means of abstract characteristics - types of protein groups. Actual equations giving the C-PER values are quadratic ones and their independent variables express the ratio of the sample's Nebraska Score and that of the casein (APPENDIX 30). As the C-PER index was constructed from samples with known amino acid composition having corrected *in vivo* (rat) PER data ranging from 0.67 and 3.22, the model was not designed to operate outside this range. The standard error of estimate of the method was about $\pm$ 0.36 PER units, however, it may be smaller. The following real advantages of C-PER over the rat PER assay were summarized by the original researchers:

> " (a) can yield a predicted PER in 72 hr or less and at a much lower cost than can the rat PER assay; (b) is biologically explainable in that the factors used to predict the protein quality are its degree of protein digestibility as well as its essential amino acid profile; (c)

provides information as to why the PER is high or low by indicating the degree of protein digestibility and by quantitating the degree each essential amino acid is limiting in the protein; (d) and, is sensitive to trypsin inhibitors and changes in protein structure, which occur during processing and that affect in vitro protein digestibility and ultimately protein quality."

It was also recommended that all calculations used to determine a C-PER should be based on the nitrogen content of the sample, in order to eliminate the selection of an incorrect Kjeldahl factor.

The next publication on prediction of protein quality from amino acid analysis is dated from 1978 and was made by meat scientists for the purpose of predicting PER of meats (Lee et al., 1978). Although the main objective of their study was to determine the influence of a wide range of connective tissue contents on amino acid composition and protein efficiency ratio, the authors also developed two linear equations computing PER from amino acid composition. Amino acid contents and rat-PER data of 14 different beef mixtures were used in the investigations. Lee et al. simply correlated the E/T values with protein efficiency ratios. The independent variable of the first equation was the sum of ten essential amino acids: arginine, histidine, isoleucine, leucine, lysine, methionine, phenylalanine, threonine, tryptophan and valine, while that of the second equation was the sum of isoleucine, leucine, lysine, methionine, phenylalanine, threonine and valine expressed as grams of amino acid residue per 100 g of total amino acid residues. Correlation coefficients for both equations were as high as 0.98 (APPENDICES 31-32).

On the basis of the experimental data used in the development of the C-PER method and after drawing some conclusion from the use of the latter, a combined assay for predicting protein efficiency ratio solely from amino acid compositional data was worked out also by the team of Satterlee, at the University of Nebraska (Jewell 1979, Jewell et al. 1980). As it was mentioned, the method, the Discriminant Computed Protein Efficiency Ratio assay is a combined one, because it involves another procedure, the so-called Discriminant In Vitro Protein Digestibility assay. Therefore, first, this latter technique will be reviewed. Doing so, these procedures will be reviewed according to Satterlee et al. (1982), too.

Experiences, reported on the increase of accuracy of predictions of *in vitro* protein quality, when the methods were applied on distinct protein groups separated according to origins or by discriminant analysis, led to the research work in course of which multiple regressions on *in vivo* (rat) digestibility data as dependent variables and on the corresponding amino acid contents as independent variables were run, using samples grouped by discriminant analysis prior to regressions. As it was reported (Jewell et al., 1980), the resulting estimates of *in vivo* digestibility were more accurate than those obtained with multienzyme assays (APPENDIX 33).

The algorithm of the DC-PER method is similar to that of the C-PER, aside from the taking into consideration of digestibility, because the latter is done by the above-mentioned Discriminant In Vitro Protein Digestibility assay. Thus, DC-PER algorithm includes two discriminant analyses which makes the assay more abstract (APPENDIX 34) as it is based only on the amino acid profile; that is why the accuracy of the DC-PER method is in the range of accuracy of the amino acid analysis.

Besides some known procedures, two simple, however strikingly useful scores, based on the theory of limiting essential amino acids, were used by Bodwell in a great comparative study concerning the applicability of different chemical indices to predict protein nutritive values for adults (Bodwell, 1981). In one of these indices (Lysine-Tryptophan-Methionine+Cystine, LTMC, Score), the total amount of cystine was reckoned in the methionine + cystine value, although for the other (Lysine-Tryptophan-Methionine+Adjusted Cystine, LTMAC, Score), levels of cystine in excess of that of methionine were not included (APPENDICES 35 and 36). For the calculations - as reference values - the FAO/WHO 1973 and the NRC 1974 patterns were recommended.

A specific reference pattern for two years old children and a scoring procedure was proposed by Torún et al. in 1981. Benjamin Torún and his co-workers suggested the use of "an amino acid scoring pattern based exclusively on the amounts of essential amino acids that must be absorbed from the diet by a 2-year old child to satisfy his requirements for each amino acid." The authors introduced the so-called Amino Acid Quality Index (AAQI), which is a kind of chemical score based on the limiting amino acid concept. In the calculation of AAQI, first the concentrations of the essential amino acids (isoleucine, leucine, lysine, methionine + cystine, phenylalanine + tyrosine, threonine, tryptophan and valine) of the sample have to be divided by those of the scoring pattern. The lowest ratio thus obtained - indicating the first limiting amino acid - should be multiplied by the *in vivo* true digestibility (possibly from child studies) of the sample protein to obtain the AAQI (APPENDIX 37). Amino Acid Quality indices can be used for comparative purposes, too. The so-called Relative Nutritive Quality (RNQ) of a test protein to a given reference protein can be calculated by dividing the two AAQI values and multiplying this ratio by 100 (APPENDIX 38). The RNQ should be subscripted with the name of the reference protein. RNQ value can also be used in estimating the safe level of intake of the test protein if that of the reference protein is known. Thus, the safe level of intake of the test protein is the ratio of the safe level of intake of the reference protein to the AAQI of test protein: AAQI of reference protein) ratio.

Speculations on the mathematics of PDR-type computations developed by Sheffner et al. (1956) and the calculation of the Enzyme Score of Stahmann and Woldegiorgis (1975) led Nina Marable and George Sanzone to express protein nutritional quality in forms of rate functions. The authors developed two equations (Marable and Sanzone 1981). The independent variables were the so-called limiting relative rate and the limiting relative rate multiplied by the Essential Amino Acid Index, respectively, while, the dependent variable for both cases was the biological value (APPENDICES 39 and 40). Actually, the limiting relative rate was the Enzyme Score itself. The non-linear (saturation-type) models of Marable and Sanzone used data as obtained by the PPDD digestion procedure of Mauron (1970a).

It was mentioned that the Mørup-Olesen Index models excess amino acid intakes by a reciprocal-forming - in the same way as does the method of Korpáczy et al. This results in a mathematical discontinuity over the set of the independent variables. In order to overcome this problem, a continuous function for the individual amino acid terms was proposed by Békés and co-workers (1982a, b). Their so-called Gaussian Index can be described as follows: the overall form of the index is shown in Eq. (2), the q_i is, however, a Gaussian function of a_i, the concentration of the i-th essential amino acid, expressed as grams per 100 g of total essentials. Thus q_i is a Gaussian function of the respective a_i, so that if a_i is equal to $a_{i,ref}$, the i-th essential amino acid of the reference pattern, the value of q_i equals to 1 and, if the sample does not contain the given essential amino acid, the value of q_i equals to zero, because it was stated that the half-width of the Gaussian bell curve is equal to the reference value of the corresponding amino acid. The reference pattern for the Gaussian Index is the same as that of the Index of Mørup and Olesen. (For details see APPENDIX 41). The alpha weighting factors were determined by the non-linear optimization method, described previously. For the fitting of the model, the *in vivo* human biological values and the associated essential amino acid compositions, published by Kofrányi et al., were used. On the basis of these data and by the technique described, several Gaussian indices were elaborated (Békés et al., 1984). They differed from each other in the number of essential amino acids, considered. In some cases arginine was taken into account as an essential amino acid, furthermore, methionine and cystine, as well as phenylalanine and tyrosine were taken as units or individually. Originally, eight different Gaussian indices were presented, although, under the term "Gaussian Index" we mean only the one with the best coefficient of correlation (0.99) and this index is presented in APPENDIX 41.

Following from the non-linear nature of the Gaussian Index, if the Index is twice as great, it does not mean that the protein is twice as good. Thus sometimes, for comparative assays the so-called Transformed Gaussian Index is more useful. This latter was defined (Békés et al., 1982b) as the geometric mean of the individual amino acid terms, multiplied by 100 (APPENDIX 42). Transformed Gaussian Index changes proportionally to the protein quality on a zero-to-hundred scale.

It has also been proposed by the authors that digestibility could be taken into account by multiplying the Transformed Gaussian Index by a digestibility factor resulting in the so-called Transformed Gaussian Index Corrected for Digestibility (APPENDIX 43).

Sometimes, it is important to investigate both qualitative and quantitative aspects in a combined manner. For such, however, only comparative purposes, a so-called Protein Nutritional Value Index was suggested (Békés et al. 1982b), which was defined as the geometric mean of the Transformed Gaussian Index and the digestible protein content of the protein tested (APPENDIX 44).

The last derivative of the Gaussian Index was the so-called Extended Gaussian Index (Békés et al. 1982a, 1984, Hidvégi 1983a, b) which was defined in the following way: all the alpha weighting exponents in the Gaussian Index should be equal to 1 and, then, a Transformed Gaussian Index be formed. The reference amino acid pattern, used in the given Extended Gaussian Index, should be constructed from the amino acid requirement data of the given consumer (adult, child, infant, different kinds of domestic animals, etc...). So, the Extended Gaussian Index is a consumer-specific assay (APPENDIX 45).

A further modification of scoring patterns were proposed by the 1982 Rome FAO/WHO/UNU Committee (FAO/WHO/UNU, 1984, Pellett, 1984). The Committee suggested four different amino acid scoring patterns for humans considering four different age groups. The joint Committee also introduced more accurate digestibility factors into the scoring procedure (APPENDIX 46).

Similarly to the Gaussian Index, a new equation was developed on the data of Kofrányi's experiments, but using, a different mathematical model. Effects of individual amino acids were described - in contrast to the Gaussian Index - by a non-symmetrical "tailing" function (see next sub-chapter) which resulted in smaller decreases of predicted biological values in the case of excess amino acid intakes, than at deficits (Hidvégi, 1983a, Hidvégi et al., 1984, APPENDIX 47). The non-linear optimization technique mentioned at the Gaussian Index was modified as well, because at the same time, both weighting factors and the reference pattern were optimized.

"Last, but not least", however chronologically the last method for protein quality evaluation on the basis of amino acid contents is published in the present book (Sarwar, 1984). The method is called the Available Amino Acid Score and follows the theory of the limiting essential amino acids. Available amino acid ratios are defined as the ratios of mg of available amino acids (mg of total amino acid multiplied by *in vivo* (rat) true amino acid digestibility) in 1 g of test protein to the mg of amino acids in 1 g of reference protein (FAO/WHO 1973 pattern). The smallest ratio multiplied by 100 gives the AAA Score (APPENDIX 48).

MATHEMATICAL MODELING OF PROTEIN QUALITY FROM AMINO ACID DATA - GENERAL CONSIDERATIONS

In this section a formal mathematical description of different chemical indices will be outlined in order to develop a general concept to construct new types of models.

In a mathematical sense, nutritional quality of a protein is characterized by a function (f) constructed of amino acid compositional data. The function models protein nutritional quality (PNQ):

$$PNQ \longrightarrow f \quad , \qquad (4)$$

that is a set of certain attributes of PNQ is translated into an abstract formalism. Thus, there are three important terms:

"a set of certain attributes", "translated" and "abstract formalism". What do they really mean?

It is a platitude that nutritional value is a very complex characteristic of proteins. It is influenced by several chemical factors from the side of the protein (absolute and relative amounts of essential amino acids, even the sequence of the amino acids due to the specific substrate-binding character of the digestive enzymes, etc.), as well as by many biological factors from the side of the consumer (genetical and physiological factors concerning amino acid requirements, metabolic size and rates, etc., social and psychological factors, etc.).

We wish to emphasize that besides the above mentioned, nutritional value of protein sources depends on the other compounds of the food or feed, as fiber, vitamins, minerals, etc. Therefore, it does have a significance to choose an appropriate "set of certain attributes" of PNQ for modeling. This is, usually, a kind of biological response (change of body mass, nitrogen balance, etc.). However, the set of attributes can comprise any hypothetical yardstick of PNQ measurement. (It is the case when models are not fitted to experimental data.)

The "abstract formalism" is a mathematical function with amino acid data as independent variables, within or without a given algorithm. "Amino acid data" represent the crude amino acid input as determined by chemical methods, possibly even with correction made for availability or any type of variance in utilization.

The term "translated" means the very essence of modeling. It includes "logistic" assumptions made *a priori*, however, guided by principles and intuition, and the structure of mathematical formulation. It is important - if possible - to fit the model to the experimental data.

The term "amino acid increment models" will be introduced here which describes the biological (real or hypothetical) response of an organism to increasing one amino acid concentration in the diet. Thus, R, the biological response is a function (g) of individual increments (q_i):

$$R = g\ (q_i) \qquad (5)$$

The i-th increment term is a function (h) of the concentration of the i-th amino acid (a_i):

$$q_i = h\ (a_i) \qquad (6)$$

Therefore, the overall function in relation (4) is the following:

$$f = g(h) \qquad (7)$$

Obligate characteristics of q_i functions are:

(1) $a_i \geqq 0$; (8)

(2) $q_i \leqq 1$ (exclusive of the linear models); (9)

(3) $h(0) = 0$ (see note below); (10)

(4) $q_{i,max} = h(a_{i,ref}) = 1$ (exclusive of the linear and the asymptotic models) (11)

If there is a small, but positive response at a zero amino acid input - due to endogen losses, etc. - then

$$h(0) = q_{i,min} \tag{12}$$

The effect of more amino acids in a diet can be described as either as the sum or as the product of the individual response curves. That is, the function g in Eq. (5) can represent summation, product formation or minimum search.

The concept of individual terms covers the fact that specific interactions between amino acids, such as antagonism or synergism, are not included in the models; however, these effects can implicitly be involved by fitting to the experimental data. However, replacability of certain amino acids can be incorporated by using common terms as for the aromatic and for the sulphur-containing amino acids, respectively.

Models may comprise two types of constants: individual and common ones. The term "individual" refers to individual amino acids, while "common" is valid for the whole index. Constants can be given *a priori*, or can be determined by mathematical-statistical procedures. In the latter case, constants will be subscripted with "st".

In the following, chemical indices will be treated according to the nature of the mathematical approach used in forming amino acid increment models, i.e., according to the mathematical description of q_i functions.

Chemical indices with linear increment models

These models assume a simple linear dependence of q_i on the a_i values, as demonstrated in Fig. 3.

The linear models are: Mitchell and Block's Chemical Score, Kühnau's Total Value, Bigwood's Index, E/N, E/T, FAO 1955 Score, Bender's Chemical Score, Simplified Chemical Score, Miller and Payne's equation, the FAO/WHO 1965 Index, equations of Cresta et al., Pellett and Kaba's Index, the TAAV, EAAV, FAO/WHO 1973 Index, NRC/NAS Index, PER equations of Alsmeyer et al., the Enzyme Score, FAO/WHO 1975 Index, PER equations of Lee et al., Discriminant *In Vitro* Protein Digestibility Assay, the LTMC Score, LTMAC Score, AAQI, RNQ, FAO/WHO/UNU 1984 Index, AAA Score.

The type of calculation for the different chemical scores and FAO/WHO indices is the minimum search (function g in Eq. (5)). That for the others is summation. Individual constants for the different "scores" and FAO/WHO indices are the $a_{i,ref}$ values. The same holds for the Total Value, the AAQI and for the RNQ. Equations of Cresta et al. and Alsmeyer et al., as well as, the EAAV and TAAV indices and the Discriminant *In Vitro* Protein Digestibility Assay have both individual constants$_{st}$ and common constants$_{st}$. There are only common, but "st" type constants in the PER equations of Lee et al.

It is an over-simplification to model nutritional response in a linear way, however, it can be exact if "working ranges" for independent variables (amino acid concentrations) are given

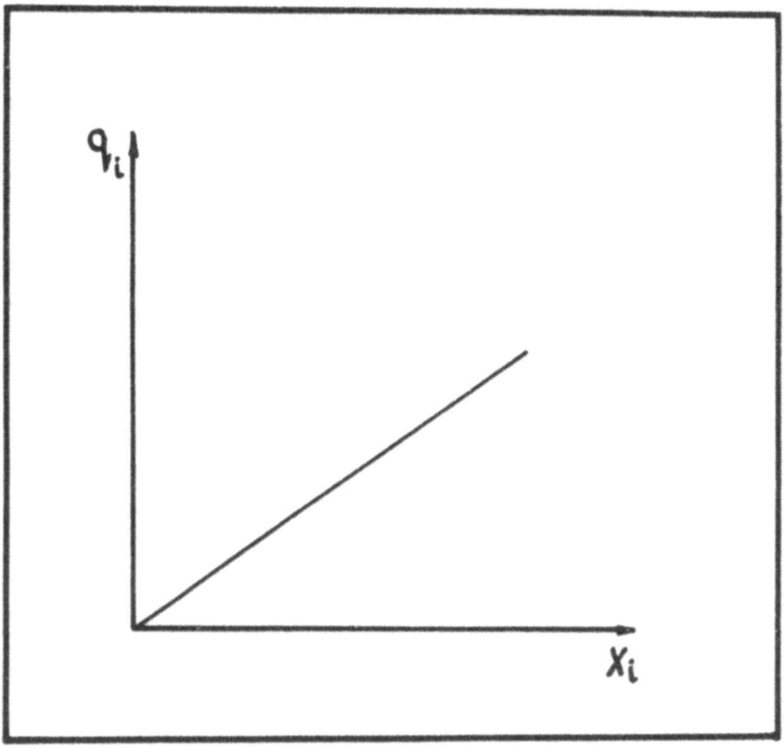

Fig. 3. Linear model

(see PER equations of Alsmeyer et al.). Actually, this note is valid only for models having "st" type constants.

Chemical indices with saturation increment models

The paradigm behind saturation-type increment models is that there is no difference between reference (requirement) and excess amino acid intakes. Negative nutritional effects are associated only with deficits.

There are two kinds of saturation-type increment models of chemical indices: smooth saturation and saturation with breakpoint. The latter is shown in Fig. 4.

The following chemical indices have "saturation with breakpoint"-type increment models: Kühnau's Pure Value, the Nebraska Score, C-PER, DC-PER. The type of calculation is summation in these methods. The common constants are: weighting factors_{st} in the Nebraska Score, C-PER and DC-PER; furthermore, C-PER and DC-PER indices have more common, but "st" constants. The individual constants are: $a_{i,ref}$ for each of the methods; in addition, special "st" constants at the C-PER and DC-PER indices.

A "smooth saturation"-type increment model can be seen in Fig. 5. Equations proposed by Marable and Sanzone can be

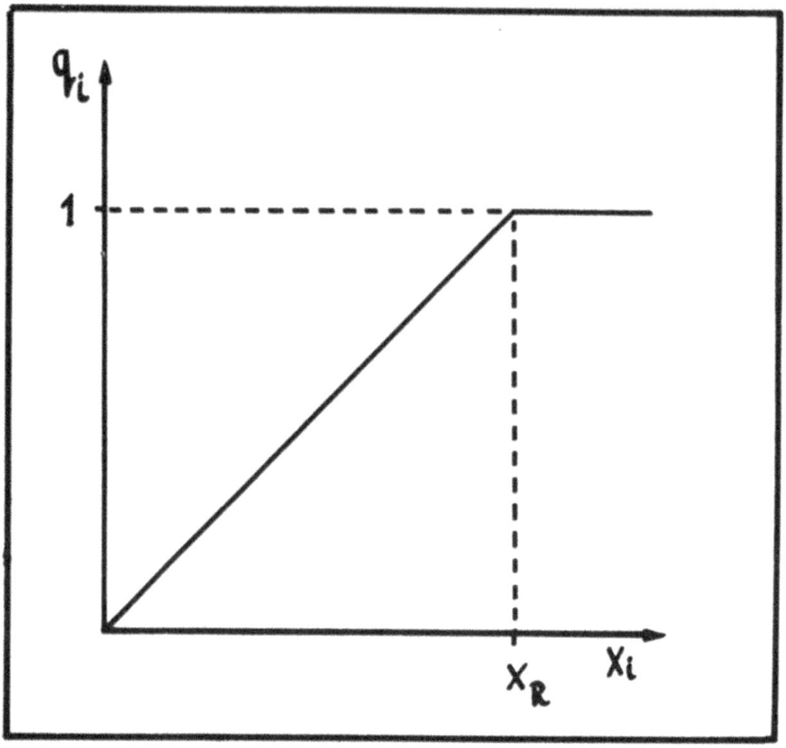

Fig. 4. Saturation model with breakpoint

assigned to this category. The type of calculation is minimum search for these indices. There are individual and common st constants in the equations of Marable and Sanzone.

Marable and Sanzone's equations are the only published chemical indices of the sort "smooth saturation". A model describing the effects of individual essential amino acids on protein nutritional quality by a Michaelis-Menten relation was proposed by one uf us (Hidvégi 1983a) giving a logical and generally accepted basis for these types of models. This amino acid increment model is the following (see also Fig. 5):

$$q_i = (q_{MAX} \times X_i) / (X_K + X_i) \tag{13}$$

where $q_{MAX} = 1$. If we assume that q_R (which is close to 1) is the dependent variable associated with a reference amino acid intake ($a_{i,ref}$), and the independent variables (X_i) are the individual ($a_i/a_{i,ref}$) ratios, where a_i is the concentration of the i-th essential amino acid in the test protein, and X_K is the independent variable concerning the half-maximal value of the dependent variable, we can write:

$$q_i = X_i / (((1-q_R) / q_R) + X_i) \tag{14}$$

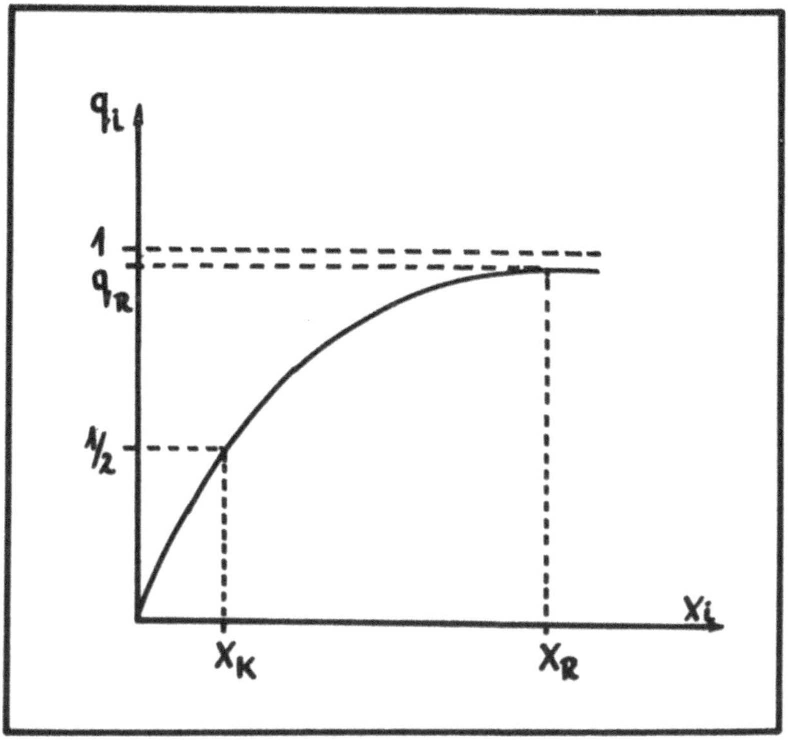

Fig. 5. Smooth-type saturation model

(Although Eq. (14) has not been fitted to experimental data, it might be a possible candidate for a new index to be developed.)

Chemical indices modeled with threshold response curves

Threshold response models assume that nutritive value (nutritive response) depends on whether the input amino acid concentration is above or below a critical level. Threshold response is essentially a sigmoidal response - sometimes called as logistic - and can be described either by a curve with two breakpoints or by a smooth function. A model with two breakpoints is shown in Fig. 6. This type of increment models can be found in case of the following indices: the EAA Index of Oser, Modified EAA Index, PDR Index, PPD Index, PPDD Index. These all are calculated through product formation and they have the $a_{i,ref}$ individual constants as well.

Smooth sigmoidals have not been used in chemical indexing yet, although these types of models could easily be constructed. The imporatance of using smooth sigmoidals to describe nutritional response when changing one amino acid concentration in the diet becomes more even accentuated in the light of some very recent *in vivo* experiments, where the measured response

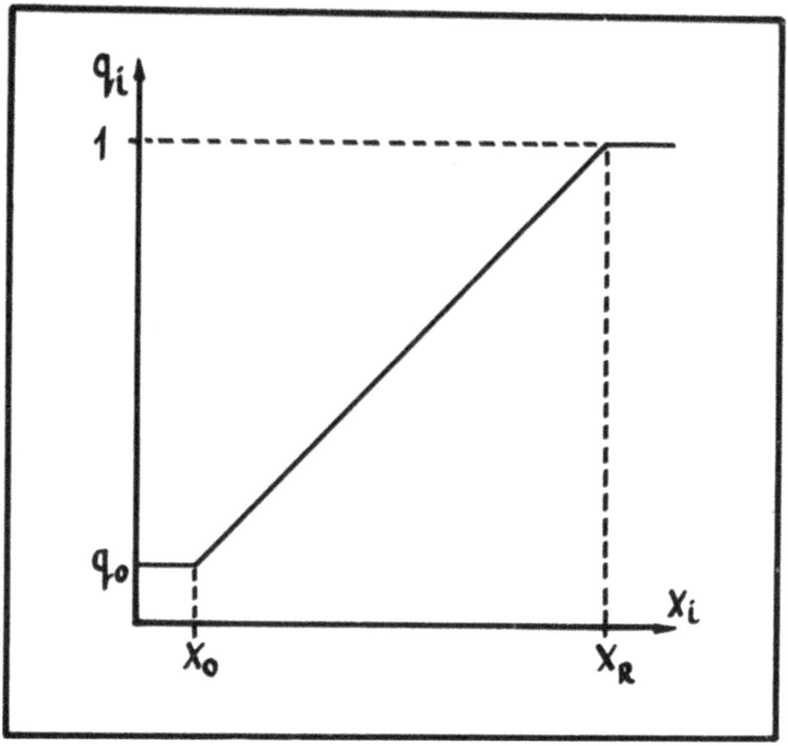

Fig. 6. Sigmoidal model with breakpoints

curves followed sigmoidal behaviour (Mercer, 1983). Thus, the so-called Four-Parameter Model of Mercer (see, e.g. Mercer, 1984) could be a good candidate for a smooth sigmoidal model (see Fig. 7):

$$q_i = ((q_o \times X_K^m) + X_i^m) / (X_K^m + X_i^m) \tag{15}$$

where X_i is the ratio of the actual and the reference concentrations of the i-th amino acid. Furthermore,

$$q_R = ((q_o \times X_K^m) + 1) / (X_K^m + 1) \tag{16}$$

thus,

$$q_i = (q_o \times ((1-q_R) / (q_R-q_o)) + X_i^m) / ((1-q_R) / (q_R-q_o) + X_i^m) \tag{17}$$

where m is an individual$_{st}$ constant of the model.

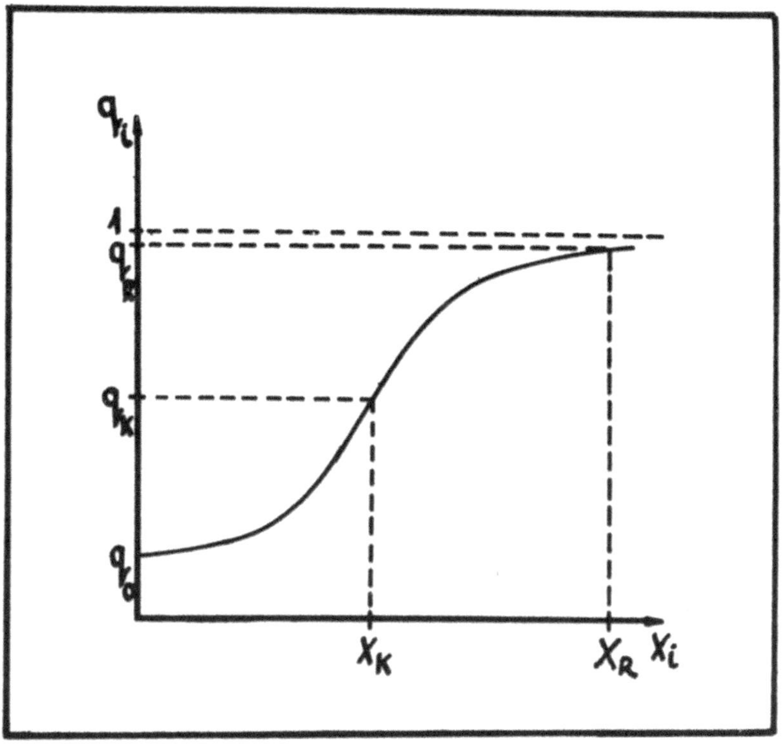

Fig. 7. Smooth sigmoidal model

Chemical indices with maximum-type increment models

These strategies say that there does exist an optimal (reference, requirement) intake of the given essential amino acid, or even there is an optimal distribution of them. Any deviation from this input (concentration) displays negative effects on the nutritive value.

A general graph for maximum-type increment models with breakpoint is shown in Fig. 8.

The index of Korpáczy et al. and the equation proposed by Mørup and Olesen apply this kind of model. Both indices are calculated by product formation. Individual constants are the $a_{i,ref}$ values for these indices and, moreover, there are $individual_{st}$ constants (exponents) and one $common_{st}$ constant in the Mørup-Olesen Index.

There are two sorts of smooth maximum-type models, i.e. symmetrical and asymmetrical. A symmetrical model is shown in Fig. 9. The Gaussian Index and its derivatives have increment models of this type. They are calculated by product formation. These indices have one $common_{st}$ constant and individual $a_{i,ref}$ constants, as well as $individual_{st}$ constants (exponents).

In contrast to the symmetrical models which states that excess amino acid inputs and deficits decrease nutritive value

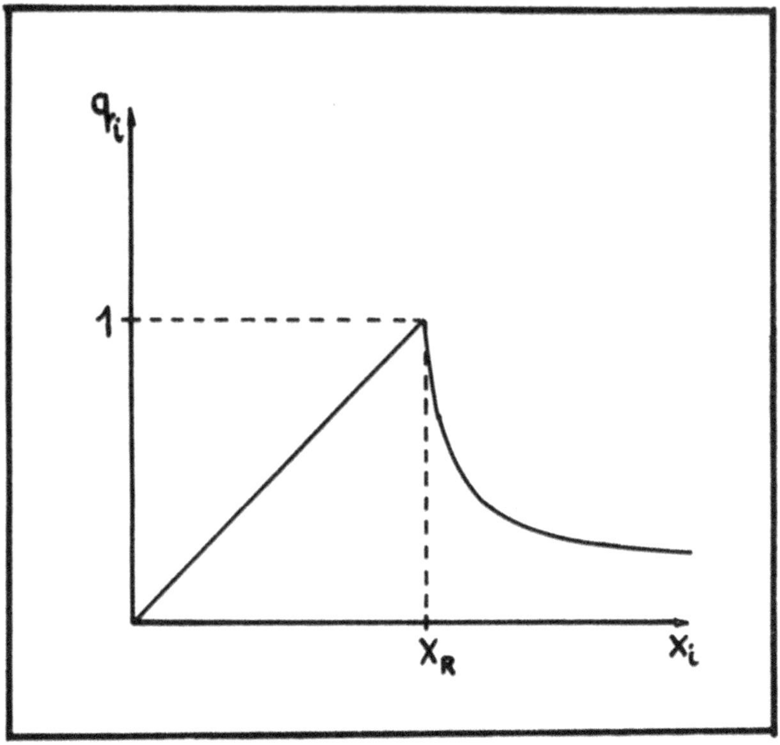

Fig. 8. Maximum-type increment model with breakpoint

in equal proportion, assymmetric models make distinction between the two negative effects, they judge excess intakes less severely (see Fig. 10). Our Tailing Index is a typical representative of this type. It is calculated in a similar way and has the same type constants as the Gaussian Index. (See APPENDIX 47.)

Closing remarks

It is readily seen that to search for a good amino acid increment model is essentially the search for a real growth model. Moreover, it is also conceivable that an amino acid increment model is basically a dose-response situation, too. Thus, when the task is to construct a model of protein nutritional quality with amino acid data, mathematical theories of growth and dose-response relationships should be connected and applied. It may open up new vistas in research.

Finally, it should be emphasized again that chemical indices are *in vitro* methods having their advantages and limitations, as well. It is always the facts and practice which prompts the researchers to improve these methods. However, the words of Poincaré should be kept in mind:

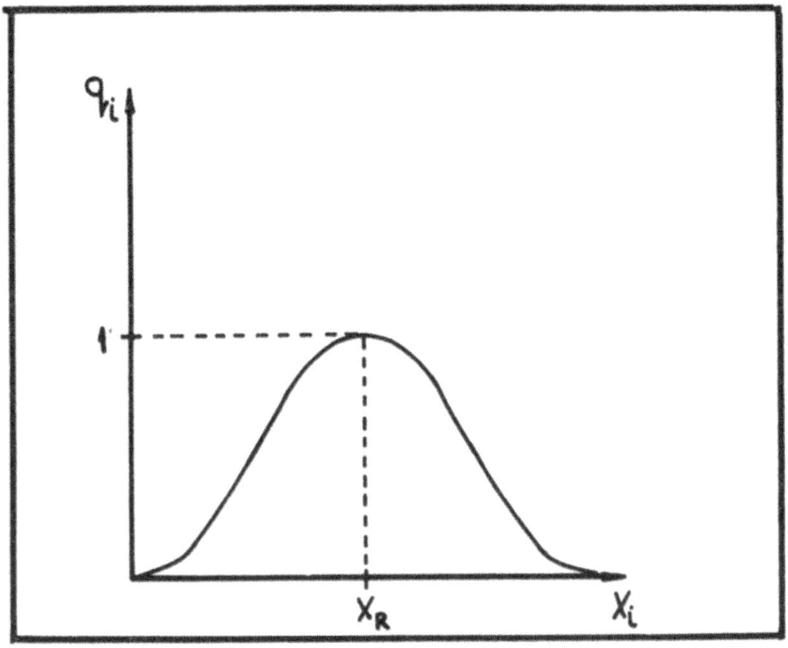

Fig. 9. Symmetrical smooth maximum-type model

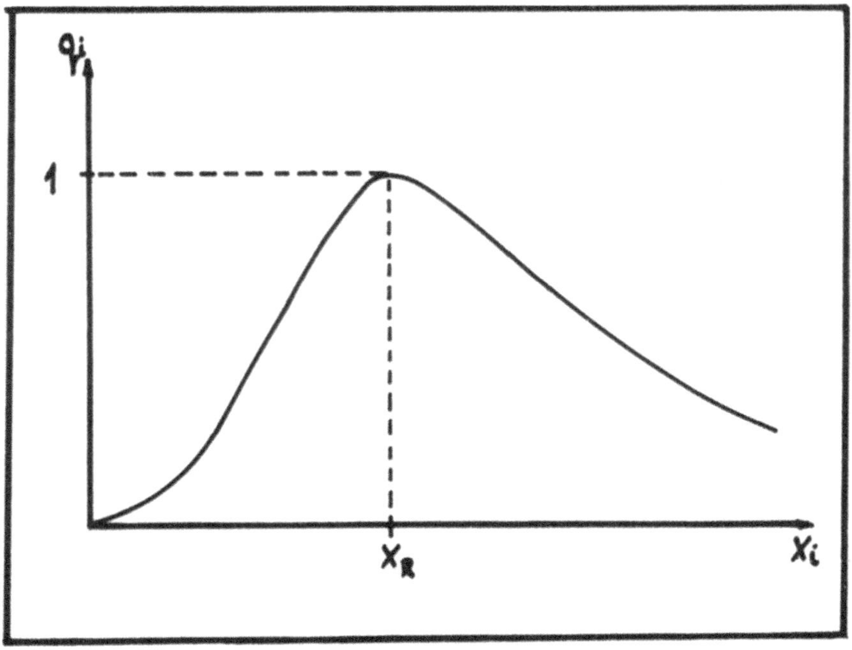

Fig. 10. Asymmetrical smooth maximum-type model

"The man of science must work with method. Science is built up of facts, as a house is built of stones; but an accumulation of facts is no more a science than a heap of stones is house. Most important of all, the man of science must exhibit foresight."

ACKNOWLEDGMENT

The authors will always remember those valuable discussions which they had the opportunity to lead with the late dr. István Kerese about the subject.

APPENDICES

COMPUTATION OF *IN VITRO* INDICES FOR EVALUATING PROTEIN NUTRITIONAL QUALITY: A BRIEF MANUAL

In the following, practical computation procedures for the different chemical indices and formulae, discussed in the text, are presented. The methods are listed chronologically. As a sample, the proteins of Selkirk wheat will be used. The mean amino acid composition of the whole Selkirk wheat is taken from a paper by Tkachuk and Irvine (1969) and listed in table O.

Table O. Amino acid composition (grams of amino acid per 16 grams of nitrogen) of Selkirk wheat (whole seed, Western Canada, 1966 composite, nitrogen content: 2.63%)

Amino acid	Selkirk wheat
Arginine	3.98
Histidine	2.21
Lysine	2.32
Tyrosine	2.67
Phenylalanine	4.75
Total aromatic	7.42
Tryptophan	1.53
Cystine	2.59
Methionine	1.68
Total sulphur-containing	4.27
Threonine	2.77
Leucine	6.72
Isoleucine	3.82
Valine	4.46
Ammonia	3.57
Aspartic acid	4.67
Serine	5.01
Glutamic acid	33.1
Proline	11.1
Glycine	3.76
Alanine	3.26

APPENDIX 1

Mitchell and Block's Chemical Score

The Chemical Score is defined by the equation:

$$CS = 100 \times MIN \left(\frac{a_i}{a_{i,ref}}\right) \qquad (1.1)$$

where

a_i: concentration of the i-the essential amino acid in the sample (g per 16 g N);

$a_{i,ref}$: concentration of the i-the essential amino acid in the reference (whole dried egg, see Table 1.1) protein (g per 16 g N).

The ratio in Eq. (1.1) is called egg ratio, and the smallest egg ratio multiplied by 100 gives the Chemical Score. If cystine is the most deficient amino acid, the sum of methionine and cystine should be used in calculating the Chemical Score. When methionine is the most deficient amino acid, only the methionine content should be used. The same relationship should not be considered for the aromatic amino acids. Results are demonstrated in Table 1.1.

APPENDIX 2

Kühnau's indices

The mathematical forms of Kühnau's indices are the following:

$$\text{Total Value} = 100 \times \frac{\sum_{i=1}^{11} a_i}{\sum_{i=1}^{11} a_{i,ref}}, \qquad (2.1)$$

where a_i and $a_{i,ref}$ stand for the concentration of the i-th essential amino acid in the sample and the reference protein, respectively. The amino acid concentration can be expressed in grams per 16 grams of nitrogen. The eleven amino acids accounted in Kühnau's formulae are: histidine, lysine, tyrosine, phenylalanine, tryptophan, cystine, methionine, threonine, leucine, isoleucine, valine. It is generally accepted now, that arginine should not be included in the calculation. As reference the amino acid composition of proteins in human milk is used (see Table 2.1).

Table 1.1. Calculation of Mitchell and Block's Chemical Score for Selkirk wheat. (Chemical Score is underlined.)

Essential amino acids (g per 16 g N)	Whole egg, the reference protein	Egg ratios
Arginine	6.4	62
Histidine	2.1	105
Lysine	7.2	<u>32</u>
Tyrosine	4.5	59
Phenylalanine	6.3	75
Tryptophan	1.5	102
Cystine	2.4	108
Methionine	4.1	41
Total sulphur-cont.	6.5	66
Threonine	4.9	57
Leucine	9.2	73
Isoleucine	8.0	48
Valine	7.3	61
Limiting amino acid	LYS	

$$\text{Pure Value} = 100 \times \frac{\sum_{i=1}^{11} a_i}{\sum_{i=1}^{11} a_{i,ref}}, \tag{2.2}$$

and, in addition to Eq. (2.2),

if $a_i > a_{i,ref}$, then be

$$a_i = a_{i,ref} \tag{2.3}$$

Table 2.1. Essential amino acid contents of human milk. (Grams of amino acid per 16 grams of nitrogen)

Essential amino acid	Orr and Watt (1957)	FAO (1970)	FAO (1973)
Histidine	2.2	2.5	2.2
Lysine	6.6	6.8	6.6
Tyrosine	5.2	3.3	-
Phenylalanine	4.3	3.5	-
Total aromatic	9.5	6.8	9.5
Tryptophan	1.6	1.7	1.6
Cystine	2.0	1.3	-
Methionine	2.0	1.6	-
Total sulphur-containing	4.0	2.9	4.1
Threonine	4.5	4.5	4.5
Leucine	9.1	8.8	9.1
Isoleucine	5.5	4.1	5.5
Valine	6.3	4.5	6.2
Sum of individual amino acids	49.3	42.6	49.3

The amino acids taken into consideration are the same as in Eq. (2-1).

$$\text{Supplementary Value} = \text{Total Value} - \text{Pure Value} \quad (2.4).$$

The results of calculations are shown in Table 2.2.

Table 2.2. Kühnau's indices for Selkirk wheat protein

Kühnau's indices	Orr and Watt (1957)	FAO (1970)	FAO (1973)
Total Value	69	80	69
Pure Value	69	77	69
Supplementary Value	0	3	0

APPENDIX 3

<u>Oser's Essential Amino Acid Index</u>

$$\text{EAA Index} = 100 \times \sqrt[10]{\prod_{i=1}^{10} \frac{a_i}{a_{i,ref}}}\,, \tag{3.1}$$

where a_i and $a_{i,ref}$ stand for the concentration of lysine, tryptophan, isoleucine, valine, arginine, threonine, leucine, phenylalanine, histidine and the sum of methionine and cystine in the sample and the reference, the egg protein, respectively (g/16 g N). There are two additional constraints to Oser's formula, that is,

$$\text{if } \frac{a_i}{a_{i,ref}} < 0.01, \text{ then } \frac{a_i}{a_{i,ref}} = 0.01, \tag{3.2}$$

and, similarly to Eq. (2.3),

$$\text{if } \frac{a_i}{a_{i,ref}} > 1.00, \text{ then } \frac{a_i}{a_{i,ref}} = 1.00 \tag{3.3}$$

For $a_{i,ref}$ the reference data, see Table 1.1. The results of computations are shown in Table 3.1.

Table 3.1 Computation of EAA Index for Selkirk wheat. The $a_i/a_{i,ref}$ values, using the Mitchell and Block (1946) reference pattern and, in the last line, the EAA Index are presented

Essential amino acid	$a_i/a_{i,ref}$	Corrected $(a_i/a_{i,ref})$
Arginine	0.62	0.62
Histidine	1.05	1.00
Lysine	0.32	0.32
Phenylalanine	0.75	0.75
Tryptophan	1.02	1.00
Methionine + cystine	0.66	0.66
Threonine	0.57	0.57
Leucine	0.73	0.73
Isoleucine	0.48	0.48
Valine	0.61	0.61
EAA Index	64	

APPENDIX 4

Bigwood's Index

$$BI = 100 \times \frac{\sum_{i=1}^{8} ea_i}{\sum_{i=1}^{18} a_i} \tag{4.1}$$

where the numerator involves the sum of the concentration of threonine, methionine, valine, isoleucine, leucine, phenylalanine, lysine and tryptophan and, the denominator does the same for every amino acid. Bigwood's Index of the Selkirk wheat protein is 28.

APPENDIX 5

Oser's Essential Amino Acid Index as modified by Mitchell

The formula of the MEAA Index coincides with that of the EAA Index, that is

$$\text{MEAA Index} = 100 \times \sqrt[9]{\prod_{i=1}^{9} \left(\frac{a_i}{a_{i,ref}}\right)} \quad , \qquad (5.1)$$

however, the amino acids taken into consideration are: histidine, lysine, methionine, cystine, methionine + cystine, phenylalanine, tyrosine, phenylalanine + tyrosine, leucine, isoleucine, valine, threonine and tryptophan for both the sample sample and the reference, the egg protein, respectively. Equations (3.2, 3.3) are valid for the MEAA Index, too, but it is important - as it was also emphasized in the text - that the excess in the sulphur-containing and in the aromatic amino acid pairs can be used to supplement the deficiency of the semi-essential amino acids only. The results of the calculation are shown in Table 5.1.

Table 5.1. Computation of the MEAA Index for Selkirk wheat. The $a_i/a_{i,ref}$ values, using the Mitchell and Block (1946) reference pattern and, in the last line, the MEAA Index are presented

Essential amino acid	$a_i/a_{i,ref}$	Corrected $a_i/a_{i,ref}$
Histidine	1.05	1.00
Lysine	0.32	0.32
Methionine	0.41	-
Cystine	1.08	-
Methionine + cystine	0.66	0.63*
Phenylalanine	0.75	-
Tyrosine	0.59	-
Phenylalanine + tyrosine	0.69	0.69
Leucine	0.73	0.73
Isoleucine	0.48	0.48
Valine	0.61	0.61
Threonine	0.57	0.57
Tryptophan	1.02	1.00
MEAA Index		64

*Because $(a_{CYS}/a_{CYS,ref})>1$, therefore be $a_{CYS} = a_{CYS,ref} = 2.4$ (instead of 2.59), thus, be $a_{MET+CYS} = 4.08$ (instead of 4.27) and $(a_{MET+CYS}/a_{MET+CYS,ref}) = 0.63$.

APPENDIX 6

Sheffner-Eckfeldt-Spector's Pepsin Digest Residue Index

The formula of Sheffner et al. is the following:

$$\text{PDR Index} = K \times G \ , \qquad (6.1)$$

where

$$K = \left[\frac{\sum_{i=1}^{n} a_i}{\sum_{i=1}^{n} a_{i,ref}} \sqrt[n]{\prod_{i=1}^{n} \frac{\dfrac{a_i}{\sum_{i=1}^{n} a_i}}{\dfrac{a_{i,ref}}{\sum_{i=1}^{n} a_{i,ref}}}} \right]^{\left[\frac{\sum_{i=1}^{n} a_{i,ref}}{\sum_{i=1}^{n} A_{i,ref}}\right]} \quad (6.2)$$

and

$$G = \frac{\sum_{i=1}^{n} A_i - \sum_{i=1}^{n} a_i}{\sum_{i=1}^{n} A_{i,ref} - \sum_{i=1}^{n} a_{i,ref}} \sqrt[n]{\prod_{i=1}^{n} \frac{\dfrac{A_i - a_i}{\sum_{i=1}^{n} (A_i - a_i)}}{\dfrac{(A_{i,ref} - a_{i,ref})}{\sum_{i=1}^{n} (A_{i,ref} - a_{i,ref})}}}^{\left[\frac{\sum_{i=1}^{n} (A_{i,ref} - a_{i,ref})}{\sum_{i=1}^{n} A_{i,ref}}\right]} \quad (6.3)$$

where a_i: concentration of the i-th amino acid considered in the pepsin digest, for the test protein. By the original method, the pepsin digests were prepared by incubating 1 g of protein (N x 6.25) with 25 mg of pepsin (USP 1:10 000) in 30 ml of 0.1 N H_2SO_4 for 24 hours at 37°C. The samples were covered with toluene during incubation and stirred occasionally. At the end of the indicated incubation period the digests were heated in a boiling water bath for 10 minutes, cooled and adjusted to pH 2. One volume of 10 per cent sodium tungstate and one volume of 2/3 N H_2SO_4

were then added for each eight volumes of the digest. The mixtures were allowed to stand for ten minutes and filtered. The clear filtrates were adjusted to pH 6.8, as well as diluted to the appropriate amino acid concentration and stored frozen until analyzed. In the case of starchy samples, starch was removed by centrifugation before the digest was heated. Following hydrolyses, the amino acid analyses were originally performed by microbiological procedures.

$a_{i,ref}$: concentration of the i-th amino acid in the pepsin digest, for the reference, the whole egg.

A_i: concentration of the i-th amino acid in the "crude" sample, in the total hydrolysate.

$A_{i,ref}$: concentration of the i-th amino acid in the undigested reference protein, the "crude" egg.

n: number of the amino acids considered. When the protein is evaluated for humans, n = 8 because the amino acids taken into consideration are lysine, methionine + cystine, phenylalanine + tyrosine, leucine, isoleucine, valine, threonine and tryptophan, while when a protein is tested for the growing rat, n = 9, because then histidine is also taken into account.

The constraints imposed upon the egg ratios are:

$$\text{if} \quad \frac{\dfrac{a_i}{\sum_{i=1}^{n} a_i}}{\dfrac{a_{i,ref}}{\sum_{i=1}^{n} a_{i,ref}}} > 1.00, \text{ then it is to be taken equal to 1.00,} \tag{6.4}$$

and

$$\text{if} \quad \frac{\dfrac{a_i}{\sum_{i=1}^{n} a_i}}{\dfrac{a_{i,ref}}{\sum_{i=1}^{n} a_{i,ref}}} < 0.01, \text{ then it is to be taken equal to 0.01} \tag{6.5}$$

If the essential precursor amino acid of the methionine-cystine and phenylalanine-tyrosine pairs is present in excess of that in egg, the excess can be used to make up the deficiency of the non-essential amino acid, but the reverse does not apply.

Results of computations are shown in Tables 6.1.-6.5. However, because of no experimental data concerning the pepsin digest of Selkirk wheat are available, data originally used by Sheffner et al. (1956) are presented. The test protein is therefore casein. (Histidine is also taken into consideration.)

Table 6.1. Calculation of the PDR Index for casein. Amino acid composition of fractions in the whole egg, the reference protein

Amino acid (mg/g)	Total hydrolysate	Pepsin digest*	Residue fraction
Histidine	26.8	0.45	26.4
Lysine	82.8	2.9	79.9
Methionine	31.6	7.2	24.4
Cystine	21.4	0.54	20.9
Phenylalanine	55.4	11.4	44.0
Tyrosine	36.3	5.9	30.4
Leucine	80.7	52.5	28.2
Isoleucine	55.4	38.2	17.2
Valine	66.3	11.7	54.6
Threonine	49.0	25.9	23.1
Tryptophan	13.5	6.8	6.7
Sum	519.2	163.5	355.8

*Corrected for enzyme blank.

Table 6.2. Calculation of the PDR Index for casein. Amino acid composition of fractions in casein

Amino acid (mg/g)	Total hydrolysate	Pepsin digest*	Residue fraction
Histidine	31.8	0.07	31.7
Lysine	80.8	0.34	80.5
Methionine	30.4	0.16	30.2
Cystine	3.4	0.07	3.3
Phenylalanine	55.4	4.8	50.6
Tyrosine	52.0	6.2	45.8
Leucine	98.4	38.2	60.2
Isoleucine	58.1	5.9	52.2
Valine	72.5	1.1	71.4
Threonine	41.2	12.5	28.7
Tryptophan	11.6	4.0	7.6
Sum	535.6	73.3	462.2

*Corrected for enzyme blank.

Table 6.3. Calculation of the PDR Index for casein. Amino acid composition - as the percentage of the sum of the 11 amino acids - and egg ratios of the pepsin digest

Amino acid (%)	Whole egg	Casein	Egg ratio
Histidine	0.28	0.10	35.7
Lysine	1.77	0.46	26.0
Methionine	4.40	0.22	
Cystine	0.33	0.10	
Sulphur-cont.	4.73	0.32	6.8
Phenylalanine	6.97	6.55	
Tyrosine	3.61	8.46	
Aromatic	10.58	10.16	96.0
Leucine	32.11	52.11	100.0
Isoleucine	23.36	8.05	34.5
Valine	7.16	1.50	20.9
Threonine	15.84	17.05	100.0
Tryptophan	4.16	5.46	100.0

Table 6.4. Calculation of the PDR Index for casein. Amino acid composition - as the percentage of the sum of the 11 amino acids - and egg ratios of the residue fraction

Amino acid (%)	Whole egg	Casein	Egg ratio
Histidine	7.42	6.86	92.5
Lysine	22.46	17.42	77.6
Methionine	6.86	6.53	
Cystine	5.87	0.71	
Sulphur-cont.	12.73	7.24	56.9
Phenylalanine	12.37	10.95	
Tyrosine	8.54	9.91	
Aromatic	20.91	19.49	93.2
Leucine	7.92	13.02	100.0
Isoleucine	4.83	11.29	100.0
Valine	15.34	15.45	100.0
Threonine	6.49	6.21	95.7
Tryptophan	1.88	1.64	87.2

Table 6.5. Calculation of the PDR Index for casein. Results of final computations

Parameters	Pepsin digest	Residue fraction
Geometric mean	42.3	88.0
Corrected geometric mean	(42.3 x 73.3/163.5) = 18.96	(88.0 x 462.2/355.8) = 114.32
PDR Index	65	

APPENDIX 7

E/N ratio

$$E/N = \frac{\sum_{i=1}^{n} ea_i}{\sum_{i=1}^{m} nea_i}, \quad (7.1)$$

where ea_i is the concentration of the i-the essential amino acid in the sample and nea_i is that of the i-th non-essential, while n and m stand for the number of essentials and non-essentials, respectively. Their actual values depend on the biochemical status of the consumer, which the protein is evaluated for. Assume that the Selkirk wheat is assayed for an adult. In this case the calculation results in an E/N ratio of 0.50.

APPENDIX 8

E/T ratio

$$E/T = \frac{\sum_{i=1}^{n} ea_i}{\sum_{i=1}^{m} a_i}, \qquad (8.1)$$

where ea_i is the content of the i-th essential amino acid in the sample and a_i is that of every amino acid; n and m denote the number of the essential and the total amino acids, respectively (m=18). For the value of n see APPENDIX 7. The E/T ratio of Selkirk wheat for an adult is 0.33.

APPENDIX 9

Chemical Score as modified by the 1955 FAO Committee

For calculation see APPENDIX 1, but use the following reference pattern (FAO provisional pattern, expressed as grams of amino acid per 100 g of protein): isoleucine=4.2, leucine= =4.8, lysine=4.2, phenylalanine=2.8, tyrosine=2.8, total aromatic=5.6, methionine=2.2, cystine=2.0, total sulphur-cont.= =4.2, threonine=2.8, tryptophan=1.4, valine=4.2.

A value of 55 (lysine) can be calculated for Selkirk wheat by the use of this method.

APPENDIX 10

Bender's Chemical Score

For calculation see APPENDIX 1, but use the following reference pattern (amino acid requirements of the laboratory rat in terms of percentage composition of the ideal protein): histidine=1.8, lysine=5.2, tryptophan=0.7, phenylalanine=3.8, cystine=2.0, methionine=2.7, threonine=4.1, leucine=7.5, isoleucine=4.3, valine=5.0.

Bender's Chemical Score of Selkirk wheat is 45 (lysine).

APPENDIX 11

McLaughlan-Rogers-Chapman-Campbell's Simplified Chemical Score

For the calculation of SCS see APPENDIX 1, use, however, lysine, methionine and cystine, only. The SCS value of Selkirk wheat is 32 (lysine).

APPENDIX 12

Korpáczy-Lindner-Varga's Modified Essential Amino Acid Index

The formula for calculating the KLV Index is the following:

$$KLVI = 100 \times (0.75\ K + 0.25\ G), \tag{12.1}$$

where

$$K = \sqrt[8]{\prod_{i=1}^{8} \frac{a_i}{a_{i,ref}}}\ , \tag{12.2}$$

where

a_i: concentration of the i-th essential amino acid in the sample (g per 100 g of protein);

$a_{i,ref}$: concentration of the i-th essential amino acid in the reference, the whole egg, protein (g per 100 g of protein).

Furthermore,

$$G = 1 - \frac{\Sigma C_i - \Sigma C_{i,egg}}{\Sigma C_{i,egg}} , \qquad (12.3.)$$

where

ΣC_i: sum of the non-essential amino acids of the sample;

$\Sigma C_{i,egg}$: sum of the non-essential amino acids in the egg.

In addition to Eqs (12.1.-3.), the constraint, i.e.

$$\text{if} \quad \frac{a_i}{a_{i,ref}} > 1,$$

then the reciprocal of that egg ratio should be used, must be satisfied.

An example for the computation is shown in Table 12.1.

Table 12.1. Calculation of Korpáczy-Lindner-Varga's Modified Essential Amino Acid Index for Selkirk wheat

Amino acids (g/100 g prot.)	Reference (whole egg) composition	Egg ratios
Isoleucine	7.7	0.50
Leucine	9.2	0.73
Lysine	7.0	0.33
Methionine	4.0	0.42
Phenylalanine	6.3	0.75
Threonine	4.3	0.64
Tryptophan	1.5	0.98
Valine	7.2	0.62
Sum of alanine, arginine histidine, aspartic acid, cystine, glutamic acid, glycine, proline, serine and tyrosine	51.2	"G"-value 1 - 0.41
"G" value	0.59	
"K" value	0.59	
KLVI	59	

APPENDIX 13

Miller and Payne's NDpCals Index

The equation proposed by Miller and Payne is the following:

$$\text{NDpCals per cent} = \text{"score"} \times P\,(54-P)/(54-P_m), \qquad (13.1)$$

where

NDpCals per cent: net dietary protein calories %, the utilizable protein content of a diet in terms of calories expressed as a percentage of the total metabolizable calories, *in vivo* data;

"score": modified Chemical Score by the 1955 FAO Committee, (see APPENDIX 9);

P: protein calories per cent, the protein content of a diet in terms of calories expressed as a percentage of the total metabolizable calories:

$$100 \times \text{(protein calories)}/\text{(total metabolizable calories)} \tag{13.2}$$

where term, protein calories is the metabolizable energy of dietary proteins obtained by multiplying the crude protein content by 4:

$$N \times 6.25 \times 4 = N \times 25, \tag{13.3}$$

where

N: nitrogen content of the sample (%);

P_m: 400/"score", protein calories per cent, required for maintenance.

As the metabolizable energy content of Selkirk wheat is not available for us, no demonstration for calculation of NDpCals % for Selkirk wheat will be given here. We note that protein calories per cent values are, usually, between 20 and 40, while, NDpCals % values are, generally, between 3 and 12. These are, however, only rough estimates.

APPENDIX 14

Akeson and Stahmann's Pepsin Pancreatin Digest Index

Method for measuring and calculating the PPD Index is the following:

100 mg protein were incubated with 1-5 mg pepsin in 15 ml of 0.1N HCl at 37°C for 3 h. After neutralization with 7.5 ml of 0.2N sodium hydroxide and addition of 4 mg pancreatin in 7.5 ml of pH 8.0 phosphate buffer, the digestion mixtures were incubated for an additional 24 h at 37°C. Enzyme blanks were prepared by incubation under the described conditions with the protein sample omitted. Merthiolate was added to prevent growth of microorganisms. Ten milliliters of digestion mixture were added to 50 ml of 1 per cent picric acid solution and centrifuged for 30 min at 1000xg to remove undigested protein and larger peptides. Fifty milliliters of supernatant were passed

through a column containing anion exchange resin in chloride form into a 250 ml lyophilizing bottle. The effluent was dried by lyophilization. The dried samples were dissolved in pH 2.2 buffer and analyzed for their amino acid content by the ion exchange method of Moore et al. Analyses of pepsin hydrolyzates were unsatisfactory since large concentrations of peptides obscured peaks of some amino acids, many of which were present in small concentrations. Chromatograms of the pepsin followed by pancreatin hydrolyzates gave excellent resolution of the amino acid, but in some areas small amounts of peptides influenced the base line of the chromatograms.

Another sample of the protein was acid hydrolyzed. The amino acids were also determined by ion exchange chromatography and provided a measure of total amino acid content. Tryptophan was determined in a separate alkine hydrolyzate.

PPD Index was calculated in essentially the same manner as the PDR Index (APPENDIX 6) with slight modifications.

The amino acid concentrations were expressed as grams per 100 g total amino acid rather than as milligrams per gram of protein. The amino acids used for calculation were the same as those used by Sheffner with the exception of cystine and tryptophan. Tryptophan was destroyed during the picric acid procedure and could not be determined in the enzyme hydrolyzates. A correction for tryptophan was therefore included in the geometric mean of each fraction for some calculations. This correction was the ratio of total tryptophan in the sample to total tryptophan in the whole egg protein. It was found that this correction had very little influence on the Index unless the protein had a very low tryptophan content. The final values obtained were called the Pepsin Pancreatin Digest Index (PPD).

For computation see APPENDIX 6.

APPENDIX 15

FAO/WHO 1965 Index

We note that the way of computation is common to all of the FAO/WHO indices, they differ in only the reference patterns To calculate the FAO/WHO Index:

(1) Add up the contributions of all the essential amino acids, together with those of cystine and tyrosine;

(2) Calculate the ratios, the so-called A/E ratios, of the individual essential amino acids to the total:

$$\frac{a_i}{\sum_{i=1}^{n} a_i}, \tag{15.1}$$

where

a_i: concentration of the i-th essential amino acid in the sample, expressed as grams per 100 g of protein;

n: 8, number of the essential amino acids, which, in turn, are: isoleucine, leucine, lysine, phenylalanine+ +tyrosine, methionine+cystine, threonine, tryptophan and valine;

(3) Calculate the A/E ratios for the reference values. The reference values, $a_{i,ref}$, for the FAO/WHO *1965* Index are those of APPENDIX 9;

(4) Calculate the eight ratios of the A/E values;

(5) The smallest ratio multiplied by 100 results in the Index:

$$\text{FAO/WHO Index} = 100 \times \text{MIN} \frac{(a_i / \sum_{i=1}^{n} a_i)}{(a_{i,ref} / \sum_{i=1}^{n} a_{i,ref})} \tag{15.2}$$

The FAO/WHO 1965 Index of Selkirk wheat is 54. The limiting essential amino acid is lysine.

APPENDIX 16

Cresta-Périssé-Autret-Lombardo's Equations

This group of Rome proposed multivariate linear regression formulae for calculating biological values and protein efficiency ratios. The first two equations contain all the variables, while the second two formulae comprise the amino acids with ($t > 1.5$) significant coefficients only. Concentrations are expressed in mg of amino acid per g of nitrogen.

$$\begin{aligned} BV = {} & 32.831 - 0.07897\ \mathrm{ILE} + 0.03628\ \mathrm{LEU} + \\ & + 0.06267\ \mathrm{LYS} + 0.02171\ (\mathrm{MET+CYS}) - \\ & - 0.01694\ (\mathrm{PHE+TYR}) + 0.02649\ \mathrm{THR} + \\ & + 0.20899\ \mathrm{TRP} + 0.01048\ \mathrm{VAL} - \\ & - 0.00079\ \mathrm{NON\text{-}ESS\ AA} \end{aligned} \tag{16.1}$$

$$\begin{aligned} PER = {} & - 1.2689 + 0.00237\ \mathrm{ILE} - 0.00046\ \mathrm{LEU} + \\ & + 0.00214\ \mathrm{LYS} + 0.00249\ (\mathrm{MET+CYS}) + \\ & + 0.00018\ (\mathrm{PHE+TYR}) + 0.00033\ \mathrm{THR} + \\ & + 0.00587\ \mathrm{TRP} + 0.00462\ \mathrm{VAL} \end{aligned} \tag{16.2}$$

$$\begin{aligned} BV = {} & 30.556 - 0.06543\ \mathrm{ILE} + 0.03381\ \mathrm{LEU} + \\ & + 0.06814\ \mathrm{LYS} + 0.21581\ \mathrm{TRP} \end{aligned} \tag{16.3}$$

$$\begin{aligned} PER = {} & - 1.25482 + 0.00210\ \mathrm{ILE} + 0.00229\ \mathrm{LYS} + \\ & + 0.00256\ (\mathrm{MET+CYS}) + 0.00706\ \mathrm{TRP} + \\ & + 0.00412\ \mathrm{VAL} \end{aligned} \tag{16.4}$$

Multiple correlation coefficients are 0.707, 0.724, 0.688 and 0.722, respectively.

Calculated protein qualities for Selkirk wheat are 60.4, 2.07, 59.6 and 2.09, consecutively.

APPENDIX 17

Mauron's Pepsin Pancreatin Digest Dialysate Index

Chemical details for the method were described as follows: An amount of sample corresponding to 4 gm protein was first dialysed against tap water and subsequently against 0.1N HCl. This step is not essential and can be omitted in foods containing no low molecular weight sugars. The sample was then incubated under stirring with 50 mg pepsin at a pH of about 2 and at 30°C for 16 h. After neutralization to pH 7.4 with sodium hydroxide 100 mg pancreatin were added and the sample was transferred into a dialysis bag. Toluene and iodine were added to prevent growth of microorganisms. The digestion mixture was incubated for 24 h at 50°C in an apparatus which enables the automatic adjustment of the pH, stirring, heating and the taking of dialysate fractions at regular intervals; 27 fractions are taken in 24 h. Aliquots of each dialysate fraction were pooled,acidified to pH 4.5. The volume of the final pool was reduced to one-sixth by concentration in a rotary evaporator at 40°C. An aliquot of this concentrated pool was taken for the determination of the amino acids by automatic chromatography.

The PPDD Index was calculated in the same way as the PDR Index (APPENDIX 6).

APPENDIX 18

FAO/WHO Index as modified by Pellett and Kaba

For calculation, see APPENDIX 15, but, use the following reference pattern: isoleucine=3.6, leucine=7.6, lysine=7.2, sulphur-cont.=3.9, aromatic=7.5, threonine=4.6, tryptophan=1.2 and valine=4.5. Values are expressed in g per 100 g protein. By this method a value of 39 can be calculated for Selkirk wheat. Lysine is the limiting amino acid.

APPENDIX 19

Glem Hansen and Eggum's Total Amino Acid Value Index

$$\begin{aligned} \text{TAAV Index} = c_j &+ 7.285\ \text{THR} + 2.122\ \text{VAL} - 4.090\ \text{ILE} - \\ &- 0.018\ \text{LEU} - 0.059\ \text{TYR} - 1.055\ \text{PHE} + \\ &+ 0.954\ \text{LYS} - 1.019\ \text{HIS} + 9.745\ \text{MET} + \\ &+ 1.977\ \text{CYS} + 3.889\ \text{TRP} + 1.202\ \text{ASP} + \\ &+ 1.397\ \text{SER} - 0.192\ \text{GLU} - 0.622\ \text{GLY} - \\ &- 2.839\ \text{ALA} + 0.207\ \text{ARG}, \end{aligned} \tag{19.1}$$

where c_j is the constant calculated for the j-th feedstuff group.

The constans are:
extracted oil cakes: 23.09,
grain products: 31.52,
fruits and vegetables: 4.60,
non-heat-treated animal samples: 24.99,
heat-treated animal samples: 21.03,
pig- and poultry mixtures: 38.26,
mixtures for mink, dogs and cats: 28.71,
if no distinction is made: 24.81.

Concentrations of amino acids should be expressed in g per 16 g N.

TAAV Index of Selkirk wheat is 63.2.

APPENDIX 20

Glem Hansen and Eggum's Essential Amino Acid Value Index

$$\begin{aligned} \text{EAVV Index} = d_j &+ 3.751\ \text{THR} + 4.211\ \text{VAL} + 0.163\ \text{ILE} - \\ &- 2.274\ \text{LEU} + 2.553\ \text{TYR} - 1.129\ \text{PHE} + \\ &+ 1.990\ \text{LYS} + 0.065\ \text{HIS} + 9.820\ \text{MET} + \\ &+ 3.407\ \text{CYS} + 0.365\ \text{TRP}, \end{aligned} \tag{20.1}$$

where d_j is the constant for the j-th sample group:
extracted oil cakes: 11.97,
grain products: 15.16,

fruits and vegetables: -5.14,
non-heat-treated animal samples: 5.48,
heat-treated animal samples: 3.05
pig- and poultry mixtures: 22.67,
mixtures for mink, dogs and cats: 12.73,
if no distinction is made: 9.60.

Amino acid contents should be expressed as g per 16 g N. EAAV Index of Selkirk wheat is 61.8.

APPENDIX 21

FAO/WHO 1973 Index

For steps of computation see APPENDIX 15, but, use the following reference pattern (g per 100 g protein): isoleucine==4.0, leucine=7.0, lysine=5.5, sulphur-cont.=3.5, aromatic=6.0, threonine=4.0, tryptophan=1.0 and valine=5.0.

FAO/WHO 1973 Index of Selkirk wheat is 46, lysine being the limiting amino acid.

APPENDIX 22

FAO/WHO Index as modified by NRC/NAS/1974

For steps see APPENDIX 15, but, with the following reference pattern (g per 100 g protein): isoleucine=4.2, leucine=7.0, lysine=5.1, sulphur-cont.=2.6, aromatic=7.3, threonine=3.5, tryptophan=1.1 and valine=4.8. When the sample is tested for infants, the value of n in Eqs (15.1-2) is 9 and also histidine is taken into consideration with a reference concentration of 1.7. By this method a value of 49 (with lysine) can be calculated for Selkirk wheat.

APPENDIX 23

Alsmeyer-Cunningham-Happich's PER Equation (A)

$$PER = -0.684 + 0.456\ LEU - 0.047\ PRO, \qquad (23.1)$$

where the amino acid values are grams of amino acid residue per 100 grams of total amino acid residues. Eq (23.1) can only be assumed to be linear over the ranges:

LEU: 3.8 - 9.3 (23.2)

PRO: 3.6 - 13.8 . (23.3)

The PER value of Selkirk wheat as calculated by Eq (23.1) is 1.85.

APPENDIX 24

Alsmeyer-Cunningham-Happich's PER Equation (B)

$$PER = -0.468 + 0.454\ LEU - 0.105\ TYR, \qquad (24.1)$$

where concentrations are the same as in Eq (23.1). The ranges are:

LEU: Eq. (23.2)

TYR: 0.9 - 4.8 (24.2)

By the use of Eq. (24.1) a PER value of 2.29 can be calculated for Selkirk wheat.

APPENDIX 25

Alsmeyer-Cunningham-Happich's PER Equation (C)

$$PER = -1.816 + 0.435\ MET + 0.780\ LEU + 0.211\ HIS - 0.944\ TYR, \qquad (25.1)$$

where for concentrations and ranges see Eqs (23.1-2, 24.2), consecutively. Additional ranges are:

$$\text{MET: } 0.7 - 2.7 \tag{25.2}$$

$$\text{HIS: } 0.8 - 3.8 \tag{25.3}$$

Prediction of PER for Selkirk wheat by this equation is 2.12.

APPENDIX 26

Enzyme Score of Stahmann and Woldegiorgis

For experimental details, see APPENDIX 14.

$$\text{Enzyme Score} = 100 \times \text{MIN} \left(\frac{a_i}{e_i} \right), \tag{26.1}$$

where

a_i: concentration of the sample's i-th amino acid in the digest (expressed as gram per cent released based on acid hydrolysis and corrected for release from enzyme alone);

e_i: the same for the whole egg standard.

Amino acids considered are: threonine, valine, methionine, isoleucine, leucine, phenylalanine, aromatic amino acids, lysine, tryptophan, histidine.

Since as no digestion data for Selkirk wheat are available, for the way of calculation see APPENDIX 1.

APPENDIX 27

Mørup and Olesen's Index

$$\text{MOI} = 10^{2.15} \times q_{LYS}^{0.41} \times q_{AROM}^{0.60} \times q_{SULPH}^{0.77} \times q_{THR}^{2.4} \times q_{TRP}^{0.21}, \tag{27.1}$$

where

$$q_i = \frac{a_i / \sum_{i=1}^{n} a_i}{a_{i,ref} / \sum_{i=1}^{n} a_{i,ref}} . \qquad (27.2)$$

If

$g_i > 1$,

then, its reciprocal is to be used. (27.3)

In Eq. (27.2) n=8, and the a_i and $a_{i,ref}$ values stand for the concentrations of the respective essential amino acids in the sample and the reference protein, respectively. Reference ratios for the eight essential amino acids considered are given in Table 27.1.

Table 27.1. Calculation of the Mørup-Olesen Index for Selkirk wheat

Amino acids mg per g total essentials	Sample	Reference	q_i
Isoleucine	115	110	-
Leucine	202	179	-
Lysine	70	141	0.496
Aromatic	223	212	0.951
Sulphur-cont.	128	89	0.695
Threonine	83	99	0.838
Tryptophan	46	30	0.652
Valine	133	140	-
MOI	46.5		

APPENDIX 28

FAO/WHO 1973 Index Corrected for Digestibility = FAO/WHO 1975 Index

$$\text{FAO/WHO 1975 Index} = \text{FAO/WHO 1973 Index} \times \text{digestibility}, \qquad (28.1)$$

where

$$0 < \text{digestibility} < 1 \qquad (28.2)$$

Recommended values for digestibility are: 0.85 for coarse, whole grain cereals and vegetables, and 0.90 for more refined diets. FAO/WHO 1975 Index of Selkirk Wheat = 46 x 0.85 = 39 (lysine).

APPENDIX 29

Satterlee-Kendrick-Banjo-Hsu-Marshall-Miller-Sutton-Tennyson's Nebraska Score

Steps for computing Nebraska Score are as follows:

(1) Express each essential amino acid as percentage of the unrounded FAO/WHO 1973 standard and correct for digestibility:

$$\%\ \text{FAO}_i = (a_i / a_{i,ref}) \times \%\ \text{digestibility}, \qquad (29.1)$$

where

a_i:
concentration of the i-th essential amino acid in the sample, expressed as g amino acid per 16 g N. When combining MET+CYS and PHE+TYR, the CYS and TYR can be not> 50% of MET+CYS and PHE+TYR, respectively. (If MET=2 and CYS=3, use 4 for MET+CYS total, because max. CYS can only be 50% of MET+CYS total.);

$a_{i,ref}$:
reference values, are: lysine=5.44, methionine+cystine= =3.52, threonine=4.00, isoleucine=4.00, leucine=7.04,

valine=4.96, phenylalanine+tyrosine=6.08 and tryptophan= =0.96;

% digestibility:

can be calculated as

$$\% \text{ digestibility} = 234.84 - 22.56 \times H \,, \qquad (29.2)$$

where H is an *in vitro* measure determined in the following way: use sample in a quantity containing 10 mg N. Place it in labeled vial containing magnetic stirring bar. Add 10 cm^3 H_2O and let soak 1 h. Using pH meter, 37°C bath, and stirrer, equilibrate sample to pH 8 $\pm$ 0.03 at 37°C by the use of diluted HCl and NaOH. At this time also equilibrate enzyme solutions to pH 8 $\pm$ 0.03 at 37°C. Replace enzymes on ice. Hold sample at 37°C. To equilibrated vial add 1 cm^3 enzyme solution A, while stirring.

Enzyme solution A:

dissolve 227 040 BAEE units of trypsin (porcine pancreatic trypsin, type IX, Sigma) plus 1860 BAEE units of α-chymotrypsin (bovine pancreatic α-chymotrypsin, type II, Sigma) plus 0.520 L-leucine β-naphthylamide units of peptidase (porcine intestinal peptidase, grade I, Sigma) in 10 cm^3 H_2O. Exactly 10 min after addition of solution A, add 1 cm^3 enzyme solution B, and then transfer vial to 55°C H_2O bath.

Enzyme solution B:

dissolve 65 casein units of bacterial protease (Pronase P or E, Sigma) in 10 cm^3 H_2O. Exactly 19 min after adding solution A, transfer vial back to 37°C bath, insert pH electrode, and read pH at 20 min. This pH value is signed as H in Eq. (29.2).

(2) Examine each % FAO_i and adjust as follows: if all percentages are $\geq$90% (before rounding to nearest integer) of the FAO/WHO standard, and LEU is <135% (before rounding to nearest integer) proceed to Step (3), otherwise, if any percentage is >100, reduce to 100.

(3) Compute the following:

$$K = \sum_{i=1}^{n} ((1/\%\ FAO_i) \times wt_i) \qquad (29.3)$$

$$G = \sum_{i=1}^{n} wt_i \ , \qquad (29.4)$$

where wt_i values are shown in Table 29.1, n=8.

Table 29.1. wt_i weighting factors for the Nebraska Score

% FAO_i (round to nearest integer)	wt_i
100	1
91-99	2
81-90	2.83
71-80	4
61-70	5.66
51-60	8
41-50	11.31
31-40	16
21-30	22.63
11-20	32
0-10	45.25

(4) Nebraska Score = G/K (29.5)

Choosing a 85 per cent digestibility for Selkirk wheat (no real date is available) the calculation of the Nebraska Score for this sample is shown in Table 29.2.

Table 29.2. Calculation of Nebraska Score for Selkirk wheat

Amino acids	% FAO_i		wt_i
Lysine	36.25		16
Sulphur-cont.	81.14		2.83
Threonine	58.86		8
Isoleucine	81.18		2.83
Leucine	81.14		2.83
Valine	76.43		4
Aromatic	100.00		1
Tryptophan	100.00		1
K value		0.719	
G value		38.49	
Nebraska Score		53.5	

APPENDIX 30

Satterlee-Kendrick-Banjo-Hsu-Marshall-Miller-Sutton-Tennyson's C-PER Index

Steps computing C-PER Index are:

(1) Calculate Nebraska Score for a standard protein, for ANRC reference casein, and for the sample.

(2) Divide Nebraska Score of sample by that of reference casein. If this ratio is between 0.99 and 1.01, then PER of sample is 2.5, i.e., the sample is casein or its equivalent. Proceed to Step (3), otherwise:

(3) Calculate: Z = ratio of scores x 2.5 (30.1)

(4) Compute 4 discriminant values to determine group into which sample is to be classified. Discriminant equations are:

$$\begin{aligned}\text{Group 1} = &- 671.8418 - 6.57689\ \text{LYS} + 3.56696\ (\text{MET+CYS}) + \\ &+ 13.10145\ \text{THR} + 2.54503\ \text{ILE} + 16.99881\ \text{LEU} - \\ &- 0.43395\ \text{VAL} - 11.5244\ (\text{PHE+TYR}) + 31.55321\ \text{TRP} + \\ &+ 14.59278\ \%\ \text{digestibility} \qquad (30.2)\end{aligned}$$

$$\text{Group 2} = -666.4492 - 2.78584\,\text{LYS} + 5.17441\,(\text{MET+CYS}) + 13.08564\,\text{THR} + 4.61808\,\text{ILE} + 16.22603\,\text{LEU} - 1.63223\,\text{VAL} - 10.13673\,(\text{PHE+TYR}) + 32.60196\,\text{TRP} + 14.11668\,\%\,\text{digestibility} \quad (30.3)$$

$$\text{Group 3} = -619.0813 - 3.13909\,\text{LYS} + 4.26918\,(\text{MET+CYS}) + 10.00988\,\text{THR} - 1.42144\,\text{ILE} + 15.7547\,\text{LEU} + 5.6604\,\text{VAL} - 11.28705\,(\text{PHE+TYR}) + 30.49168\,\text{TRP} + 13.79953\,\%\,\text{digestibility} \quad (30.4)$$

$$\text{Group 4} = -744.7122 - 0.37674\,\text{LYS} + 6.03697\,(\text{MET+CYS}) + 11.51527\,\text{THR} + 1.63251\,\text{ILE} + 17.29687\,\text{LEU} + 3.0294\,\text{VAL} - 11.5033\,(\text{PHE+TYR}) + 37.88725\,\text{TRP} + 14.68169\,\%\,\text{digestibility} \quad (30.5)$$

(5) That of Eqs (30.2-5) with the largest discriminant value will indicate the group into which the sample is classified. PER is to be calculated by the one of the following equations:

$$\text{C-PER (Group 1)} = 1.12683 - 1.61426\,Z + 0.99306\,Z^2 \quad (30.6)$$

$$\text{C-PER (Group 2)} = -7.25391 + 8.14063\,Z - 1.79517\,Z^2 \quad (30.7)$$

$$\text{C-PER (Group 3)} = 4.30469 - 1.99609\,Z + 0.45996\,Z^2 \quad (30.8)$$

$$\text{C-PER (Group 4)} = 12.75 - 8.21484\,Z + 1.66016\,Z^2 \quad (30.9)$$

(As no real data are available, computation of C-PER for the Selkirk wheat will not be presented.)

APPENDIX 31

Lee-Elliott-Rickansrud-Hagberg's PER Equation (A)

$$PER = - 0.1539 + 0.06320 \times \sum_{i=1}^{n} a_i , \qquad (31.1)$$

where a_i: concentration of the i-th essential amino acid, expressed as grams of amino acid residue per 100 g of total amino acid residues;

n: 10, the amino acids being: arginine, histidine, isoleucine, leucine, lysine, methionine, phenylalanine, threonine, tryptophan, valine.

Equation (31.1) can only be used for meats.

APPENDIX 32

Lee-Elliott-Rickansrud-Hagberg's PER Equation (B)

$$Per = - 0.1094 + 0.08084 \times \sum_{i=1}^{n} a_i , \qquad (32.1)$$

where a_i: see APPENDIX 31;

n: 7, the amino acids being those in APPENDIX 31, except tryptophan, arginine and histidine.

Equation (32.1) can only be used for meats.

APPENDIX 33

Satterlee-Jewell-Kendrick's AD Index

By the use of this method apparent protein digestibility can be calculated from amino acid compositions. The procedure comprises discriminant analysis, too. The first step is to compute discriminant values for the sample:

$$Group\ 1 = -203.7537 - 2.59402\ LYS + 9.27153\ LEU + 19.36964\ ASP + 4.19676\ PRO + 12.46035\ CYS + 34.3075\ AMMONIA \quad (33.1)$$

$$Group\ 2 = -150.3707 - 0.78115\ LYS + 7.6239\ LEU + 15.46558\ ASP + 3.8947\ PRO + 12.79949\ CYS + 29.74493\ AMMONIA \quad (33.2)$$

$$Group\ 3 = -155.9532 + 4.61135\ LYS + 7.85429\ LEU + 13.25949\ ASP + 4.68431\ PRO + 13.2907\ CYS + 19.89403\ AMMONIA \quad (33.3)$$

Equation with the highest discriminant value gives the group number for the relevant digestibility equation. Apparent digestibility equations are:

$$AD\ (Group\ 1) = 67.8263 + 0.60144\ LYS - 1.73309\ LEU + 2.48377\ ASP + 2.03523\ PRO - 0.97312\ CYS - 6.44299\ AMMONIA \quad (33.4)$$

$$AD\ (Group\ 2) = 160.5607 + 5.7998\ LYS - 2.20744\ LEU - 7.35627\ ASP - 0.85275\ PRO + 6.11058\ CYS - 14.54944\ AMMONIA \quad (33.5)$$

$$AD\ (Group\ 3)) = 116.5451 + 0.99537\ LYS - 4.37473\ LEU - 0.10243\ ASP - 0.06304\ PRO - 0.14005\ CYS + 3.48679\ AMMONIA \quad (33.6)$$

Independent variables in Eqs. (33.1-6) are expressed as g per 16 g N. Calculated apparent digestibility of Selkirk wheat is 79.25 (Group 2).

APPENDIX 34

Satterlee-Jewell-Kendrick's DC-PER Index

(1) Compute AD Indices for the sample and for the ANRC casein, the reference protein.

(2) Compute Nebraska Scores for sample and reference, but use AD Index instead of % digestibility in Eq. (29.1).

(3) Calculate Z value acoording to Eq. (30.1).

(4) Substitute following discriminant group equations for sample:

$$\text{Group 1} = -350.9675 + 2.34642\ \text{LYS} - 8.60862\ (\text{MET+CYS}) - 13.80721\ \text{THR} + 11.71013\ \text{ILE} + 11.7984\ \text{LEU} - 12.10787\ \text{VAL} + 9.68089\ (\text{PHE+TYR}) + 46.88927\ \text{TRP} + 7.291\ \text{AD Index} \quad (34.1)$$

$$\text{Group 2} = -454.6516 + 7.83575\ \text{LYS} - 14.3054\ (\text{MET+CYS}) - 15.64592\ \text{THR} + 13.32306\ \text{ILE} + 14.1817\ \text{LEU} - 17.40405\ \text{VAL} + 12.36894\ (\text{PHE+TYR}) + 64.39914\ \text{TRP} + 8.00712\ \text{AD Index} \quad (34.2)$$

$$\text{Group 3} = -405.9275 + 5.01252\ \text{LYS} - 8.46439\ (\text{MET+CYS}) - 15.014\ \text{THR} + 10.1986\ \text{ILE} + 11.91023\ \text{LEU} - 9.50181\ \text{VAL} + 9.46879\ (\text{PHE+TYR}) + 49.43095\ \text{TRP} + 7.78124\ \text{AD Index} \quad (34.3)$$

$$\text{Group 4} = -488.5569 + 9.3207\ \text{LYS} - 11.36379\ (\text{MET+CYS}) - 15.24675\ \text{THR} + 10.60119\ \text{ILE} + 13.93578\ \text{LEU} - 12.14625\ \text{VAL} + 10.15707\ (\text{PHE+TYR}) + 63.1489\ \text{TRP} + 8.22588\ \text{AD Index} \quad (34.4)$$

(5) The one of Eqs (34.1-4) with the highest value indicates the group into which the sample is classified. Respective equations computing PER values are:

$$\text{DC-PER (Group 1)} = 1.254 - 2.04932\ Z + 1.30629\ Z^2 \quad (34.5)$$

$$\text{DC-PER (Group 2)} = -4.08594 + 5.125\ Z - 1.08398\ Z^2 \tag{34.6}$$

$$\text{DC-PER (Group 3)} = 4.66406 - 2.29297\ Z + 0.50586\ Z^2 \tag{34.7}$$

$$\text{DC-PER (Group 4)} = 10.44141 - 5.93359\ Z + 1.13281\ Z^2 \tag{34.8}$$

(As no real data for casein are available, DC-PER Index for Selkirk wheat is not presented here.)

APPENDIX 35

Bodwell's Lysine-Tryptophan-Methionine+Cystine Score

For calculating the LTMC Score, see APPENDIX 1, use, however, lysine, tryptophan and methionine+cystine, only. As reference pattern either the FAO/WHO 1973 or the NRC/NAS 1974 can be used. (See APPENDICES 21-22.) LTMC Scores of the Selkirk wheat by the use of these reference patterns are 42 and 45, respectively.

APPENDIX 36

Bodwell's Lysine-Tryptophan-Methionine+Adjusted Cystine Score

For calculating the LTMAC Score, see APPENDIX 35, however, levels of cystine in excess of that of methionine shall not be taken into account. LTMAC Scores of Selkirk wheat are 42 and 45, respectively.

APPENDIX 37

Torún-Pineda-Viteri-Arroyave's Amino Acid Quality Index

$$\text{AAQI} = \text{TD} \times \text{MIN} \left(\frac{a_i}{a_{i,ref}} \right) \tag{37.1}$$

where TD: % true digestibility of the sample protein;

a_i: composition of the i-th essential amino acid of the sample, expressed as mg amino acid per g protein;

$a_{i,ref}$: reference value, expressed in the same manner; the values are: isoleucine=31, leucine=73, lysine=64, sulphur-cont.=27, aromatic=69, threonine=37, tryptophan=12.5, valine=38.

The AAQ Index should be used for predicting protein quality for 2-year old children.

APPENDIX 38

Torún-Pineda-Viteri-Arroyave's Relative Nutritive Quality Index

The RNQ Index of a test protein compared to a standard protein is calculated as:

$$RNQ = 100 \times (\text{AAQI of test protein/AAQI of standard protein}) \quad (38.1)$$

Usually the name of the standard is written as a subscript of RNQ.

APPENDIX 39

Marable and Sanzone's Saturation index (A)

A predicting equation for the biological value is:

$$BV = 100 \times (1 - \exp(-2.9 \times ES)), \quad (39.1)$$

where ES is the Enzyme Score (see APPENDIX 26).

APPENDIX 40

Marable and Sanzone's Saturation Index (B)

$$BV = 100 \times (1 - \exp(-0.038 \times ES \times EAAI)), \qquad (40.1)$$

where ES is the Enzyme Score (see APPENDIX 26) and EAAI is the Essential Amino Acid Index (see APPENDIX 3).

APPENDIX 41

Békés-Hidvégi-Zsigmond-Lásztity's Gaussian Index

$$GI = 10^{2.16} \times q_{LYS}^{0.28} \times q_{TRP}^{0.19} \times q_{THR}^{3.32} \times q_{MET+CYS}^{0.67} \times q_{PHE+TYR}^{0.72} \qquad (41.1)$$

where

$$q_i = \exp\left((-4.5) \times \left(\frac{a_i - a_{i,ref}}{a_{i,ref}}\right)^2\right), \qquad (41.2)$$

where a_i and $a_{i,ref}$ stand for the concentrations of the essential amino acids in the sample and the reference pattern, respectively, expressed as mg per g total essentials.

Calculations and data are given in Table 41.1.

Table 41.1. Calculation of Gaussian Index for Selkirk wheat

Amino acids mg per g total essentials	Selkirk wheat	Reference	q_i
Isoleucine	115	110	-
Leucine	202	179	-
Lysine	70	141	0.319
Aromatic	223	212	0.988
Sulphur-cont.	128	89	0.421
Threonine	83	99	0.889
Tryptophan	46	30	0.278
Valine	133	140	-
GI	30.9		

APPENDIX 42

Békés-Hidvégi-Zsigmond-Lásztity's Transformed Gaussian Index

$$TGI = 100 \times \left[\frac{GI}{10^{2.16}}\right]^{0.2} , \qquad (42.1)$$

where for GI see APPENDIX 41.

The TGI of Selkirk wheat is 73.4

APPENDIX 43

Békés-Hidvégi-Zsigmond-Lásztity's Transformed Gaussian Index Corrected for Digestibility

$$TGICD = \%\ \text{digestibility} \times \frac{GI}{10^{2.16}}^{0.2} , \qquad (43.1)$$

where for GI see APPENDIX 41.

The TGICD of Selkirk wheat is 62.4, if a digestibility of 85 per cent is taken into account for the sample.

APPENDIX 44

Békés-Hidvégi-Zsigmond-Lásztity's Protein Nutritional Value Index

$$PNVI = \left[\frac{GI}{10^{2.16}}\right]^{0.2} \times \%CP \times \%D , \qquad (44.1)$$

where GI is the Gaussian Index (APPENDIX 41), % CP is the crude protein content as g per 100 g sample, and % D is the digesti-bility of the protein.

The PNVI of Selkirk wheat, with a Kjeldahl factor of 5.7 and a digestibility of 85%, is 30.6.

APPENDIX 45

Békés-Hidvégi-Zsigmond-Lásztity's Extended Gaussian Index

$$EGI = \%D \times \sqrt[n]{\prod_{i=1}^{n} q_i}, \qquad (45.1)$$

where %D: digestibility of the sample (in lack of such data, it may be 100);

q_i: see Eq. (41.2), but for $a_{i,ref}$ use the amino acid requirements of that consumer whom the index is calculated for;

n: number of the amino acids which are essential for the given consumer.

EGI is also useful in evaluating protein quality of feeds for different livestock if the specific amino acid requirements are known.

APPENDIX 46

FAO/WHO Index as modified by the 1982 Rome FAO/WHO/UNU Committee

For steps see APPENDIX 28, but use the following reference patterns and digestibility factors (Tables 46.1,2).

Table 46.1. Reference patterns proposed by the 1982 Rome FAO/WHO/UNU Committee (FAO/WHO/UNU 1984)

Essential amino acid, g per 16 g N	Infant	Child 2-5 yrs	Child 10-12 yrs	Adult
Histidine	2.59	2.00	1.81	1.60
Isoleucine	4.61	3.01	2.90	1.30
Leucine	9.28	7.01	4.61	1.90
Lysine	6.61	6.21	4.61	1.60
Sulphur-cont.	4.21	2.64	2.30	1.70
Aromatic	7.20	6.61	2.30	1.90
Threonine	4.30	3.60	2.90	0.90
Tryptophan	1.70	1.20	0.90	0.50
Valine	5.50	3.70	2.61	1.30

Calculated protein qualities of Selkirk wheat for the 4 different age groups are 39, 33, 30 and 45, respectively; lysine is the limiting factor. For digestibility see Table 46.2.

Table 46.2. Digestibility values suggested by the 1982 Rome FAO/WHO/UNU Committee (FAO/WHO/UNU 1984)

Protein	% Digestibility
Egg	97
Milk, cheese	95
Meat, fish	94
Maize	85
Polished rice	88
Whole wheat	86
Refined wheat	96
Oatmeal	86
Millet	79
Soy flour	86
Beans	78

APPENDIX 47

Hidvégi-Örsi-Békés-Lásztity's Tailing Index

$$TI = (TI_c)^{1.12} , \tag{47.1}$$

where

$$TI_c = 10^{2.4301} \times q_{ILE}^{3.34} \times q_{LYS}^{1.74} \times q_{PHE+TYR}^{1.46} \times \times q_{MET+CYS}^{2.86} \times q_{THR}^{8.87} \times q_{TRP}^{0.51} , \tag{47.2}$$

where

$$q_i = \frac{a_i}{a_{i,ref}} \times \exp \left(1 - \frac{a_i}{a_{i,ref}}\right) , \tag{47.3}$$

where a_i and $a_{i,ref}$ represent the concentrations of the essential amino acids in the sample and the reference pattern, respectively, expressed as mg per g total essentials. Calculations are shown in Table 47.1. It must be noted here, that the index is not valid over BV = 140.

Table 47.1. Calculation of Tailing Index for Selkirk wheat

Amino acids mg per g total essentials	Selkirk wheat	Reference	q_i
Isoleucine	115	89.2	0.965
Leucine	202	279.0	-
Lysine	70	111.4	0.911
Aromatic	223	130.8	0.842
Sulphur-cont.	128	80.8	0.883
Threonine	83	139.4	0.892
Tryptophan	46	52.3	0.992
Valine	133	117.1	-
TI	62.3		

(We note that modified versions of the Tailing Index, according to APPENDICES 42-45, may also be used.)

APPENDIX 48

Sarwar's Available Amino Acid Score

$$\text{AAA Score} = 100 \times \text{MIN} \left(\frac{aa_i}{a_{i,ref}}\right) \quad (48.1)$$

If AAA Score > 100, then it is to be taken equal to 100. (48.2)

Symbols in Eq. (48.1):

aai: available concentration of the i-th essential amino acid in the sample, calculated as total amino acid x true amino acid digestibility and expressed as mg per g protein;

$a_{i,ref}$: concentration of the i-th essential amino acid in the reference protein, the FAO/WHO 1973 pattern, expressed as mg per g protein.

AAA Score of Selkirk wheat, with a 79 per cent of true lysine digestibility, is 36.

REFERENCES

Akeson W.R. and Stahmann M.A. (1964): A pepsin pancreatin digest index of protein quality evaluation. J. Nutr. 83, 257-261.

Alsmeyer R.H., Cunningham A.E. and Happich M.L. (1974): Equations predict PER from amino acid analysis. Fd. Techn. 34-40.

Bender A.E. (1958): The amino-acid standards for calculating chemical score. Proc. Nutr. Soc. 17, XXXIX.

Bender A.E. (1973): Chemical scores and availability of amino acids. In: Proteins in human nutrition, Porter J.W.G. and Rolls B.A. (eds.), Academic Press, New York, pp. 167-178.

Békés F. and Zsigmond A. (1980): In vitro determination of the biological value of food and feed proteins. In: Abstracts of COMECON conference on nutritive value of food proteins.

Békés F., Zsigmond A. and Juhász Á. (1979): Investigation of the nutritive value of Hungarian dry sausages. In: Proc. 25-th Meat Res. Congr., pp. 339-343.

Békés F., Hidvégi M., Kemény G., Pokorny T., Lásztity R., Kós I. and Fórizs, K. (1981): Process and equipment for development of optimal mixing ratios of components of foods and feeds based on the biological value and/or the price. Hung. Pat. 3872/81.

Békés F., Lásztity R. and Hidvégi M. (1982a): Evaluation of food proteins on the basis of chemical indices, II. Off-line amino acid analyzer-computer system and its applications in the food industry. Élelm. Ip. 36, 402-410.

Békés F., Hidvégi M., Zsigmond A. and Lásztity R. (1982b): A novel mathematical method for determining in vitro biological value of proteins and its application for non-linear optimization of the nutritional quality of food and feed formulas. Paper presented at the 7-th World Cereal and Bread Congress held at Prague 28 June - 4 July 1982. (In: Progress in cereal chemistry and technology, (Vol.5B), Holas J. and Kratochvil J. (eds.), Elsevier, Amsterdam, 1983, pp. 1213-1218.

Békés F., Hidvégi M., Zsigmond A. and Lásztity R. (1984): Studies on the evaluation of the in vitro biological valu of food proteins. Acta Alim. 13, 135-158.

Bigwood E.J. (1953): Gegenwartsprobleme der Ernahrungsforschu Symposium Basel. Experimentia Supplementum I, Birkhäuser, Basel and Stuttgart, pp. 88.

Block R.J. and Mitchell H.H. (1946): The correlation of the amino-acid composition of proteins with their nutritive value. Nutr. Abst. Rev. 16, 249-278.

Bodwell C.E. (1981): Use of amino acid data to predict protei nutritive value for adults. In: Protein quality in humans assessment and in vitro estimation, Bodwell C.E., Adkins J.S. and Hopkins D.T. (eds.), Avi, Westport, Conn., pp. 340-373.

Cresta M., Périssé J., Autret M. and Lombardo E. (1969): Stud of the correlations between biological and chemical measu ments of food protein quality. Nutr. Newslett. FAO 7, 1-'

FAO (1957): Protein requirements. FAO Nutr. Stud. No. 16, Rom

FAO (1965): Protein requirements. FAO Nutr. Meet. Rep. Ser. No. 37, Rome.

FAO (1970): Amino acid content of foods and biological data c proteins. FAO Nutr. Stud. No. 24, Rome.

FAO (1973): Energy and protein requirements. FAO Nutr. Meet. Rep. Ser. No. 52, Rome.

FAO/WHO (1975): Energy and protein requirements. PAG Bull. 5, 30-35, PAG, New York.

FAO/WHO/UNU (1984): Protein and energy requirements. Rome (in press).

Floridi A. and Fidanza F. (1975): The enzyme-ultrafiltrate-digest (EUD) assay for measuring protein. Riv. Sci. Tech. Alim. Nutr. Um. 5, 13-18.

Hansen Glem, N. and Eggum B.O. (1973): The biological value c proteins estimated from amino acid analyses. Acta Agr. Sca 23, 247-251.

Hackler L.R. (1977): In vitro indices: relationships to estin ing protein value for the human. In: Evaluation of prote: for humans, Bodwell C.E. (ed.), Avi, Westport, Conn., pp. 55-67.

Hidvégi M. (1983a): Modeling of protein nutritional quality from amino acid data. Ph.D. Thesis, Technical University, Budapest.

Hidvégi M. (1983b): New methods of protein evaluation for gra and feed products. Gabonaip. 30, 46-49.

Hidvégi M., Örsi F. and Békés F. (1984): Equations predict BV TD and NPU from amino acid analyses. In: Cereals - health food for all, Steller W. (ed.) C. Kersting, St. Augustin, pp. 106.

Hsu H.W., Vavak D.L., Satterlee L.D. and Miller G.A. (1977): A multienzyme technique for estimating protein digestibility J. Fd. Sc. 42, 1269-1273.

Jekat F. and Pabst V. (1969): Vergleich zwischen der Stickstoffbilanzierung beim Menschen und bei der Laboratoriumsratte. Z. ges. exp. Med. 150, 70.

Jewell D.K. (1979): An economic evaluation of a rapid protein quality programmed model. M.S. Thesis, University of Nebraska, Lincoln.

Jewell D.K., Kendrick J.G. and Satterlee L.D. (1980): The DC-PER assay: a method for predicting protein quality solely from amino acid compositional data. Nutr. Rep. Int. 21, 25-38.

Kaba H. and Pellett P.L. (1975): Prediction of true limiting amino acids using available protein scoring systems. Ecol. Fd. Nutr. 4, 109-116.

Kemény G., Pokorny T., Fórizs K., Kós I., Békés F., Hidvégi M. and Lásztity R. (1982): Feed advisory system based on NIR ingredient data. Paper presented at the 7-th World Cereal and Bread Congress held at Prague 28 June - 4 July 1982. In: Progress in cereal chemistry and technology, (Vol. 5A.), Holas J. and Kratochvil J. (eds), Elsevier, Amsterdam,1983, pp. 601-606.

Kerese I. (1976): Differences and correlations between the biological value and in vitro examination results of proteins. Acta Agron. 25, 473-484.

Kofrányi E. (1971): Nitrogen balance in adults. In: Protein and amino acid functions, Bigwood E.J. (ed.), Pergamon Press, Oxford, pp. 40-45.

Kofrányi E. (1972): Die biologische Wertigkeit von Eiweiss- und Aminosäure-Gemischen. Med. Mitt. (Melsungen), 46, 15-23.

Kofrányi E. (1973): Evaluation of traditional hypotheses on the biological value of proteins. Nutr. Rep. Int. 7, 45-50.

Kofrányi E. and Jekat F. (1964a): Zur Bestimmung der biologischen Wertigkeit von Nahrungsproteinen, VIII. Die Wertigkeit gemischter Proteine. Z. physiol. Chem. 335, 174-179.

Kofrányi E. and Jekat F. (1964b): Zur Bestimmung der biologischen Wertigkeit von Nahrungsproteinen, X. Vergleich der Bausteinanalysen mit dem Minimalbedarf gemischter Proteine für den Menschen. Z. physiol. Chem. 338, 159-167.

Kofrányi E. and Jekat F. (1967): Zur Bestimmung der biologischen Wertigkeit von Nahrungsproteinen, XII. Die Mischung von Ei mit Reis, Mais, Soja, Algen. Z. physiol. Chem. 348, 84-88.

Kofrányi E., Jekat F. and Müller-Wecker H. (1970): The determination of the biological value of dietary proteins, XVI. The minimum protein requirement of humans tested with mixtures of whole egg plus potato and maize plus beans. Z. physiol. Chem. 351, 1485-1493.

Korpáczy I., Lindner K. and Varga K. (1961): Recent contributions to the composition of foods, VII. Improved method for the calculation of the biological value of food proteins. Élelmiszervizsgálati Közl. 7, 11-17.

Kühnau J. (1946): Artzl. Wochenschr. 1, 161.

Kühnau J. (1949): Biochemie des Nahrungs Eiweisses. Angew. Chem. 61, 357-365.

Lee Y.B., Elliott J.G., Rickansrud D.A. and Hagberg E.C. (1978): Predicting protein efficiency ratio by the chemical determination of connective tissue content in meat. J. Fd. Sc. 43, 1359-1362.

Marable N.L. and Sanzone G. (1981): In vitro assays of protein quality utilizing enzymatic hydrolyses. In: Protein quality in humans: assessment and in vitro estimation, Bodwell C.E., Adkins J.S. and Hopkins D.T. (eds.), Avi, Westport, Conn., pp. 261-277.

Mauron J. (1970a): Nutritional evaluation of proteins by enzymatic methods. In: Improving plant protein by nuclear techniques. IAEA, Vienna, pp. 303-318.

Mauron J. (1970b): Nutritional evaluation of proteins by enzymatic methods. In: Evaluation of novel protein products, Bender A.E., Löfqvist B., Kihlberg R. and Munck L. (eds.), Pergamon Press, Oxford, pp. 211-234.

McLaughlan J.M., Rogers C.G., Chapman D.G. and Campbell J.A. (1959): Evaluation of protein in foods, IV. A simplified chemical score. Can. J. Biochem. Physiol. 37, 1293-1299.

Melnick D., Oser B.L. and Weiss S. (1946): Rate of enzymic digestion of proteins as a factor in nutrition. Science 103, 326.

Mendel L.B. (1923): Nutrition: the chemistry of life. Yale Univ. Press, New Haven, Conn.

Mercer L.P. (1983): Personal communication.

Mercer L.P. (1984): Protein nutritional quality: a modeling approach. (In this book.)

Miller D.S. and Payne P.R. (1961): Problems in the prediction of protein values of diets: the use of food composition tables. J. Nutr. 74, 413-419.

Mitchell H.H. (1954): In: Symposium on methods for the evaluation of nutritional adequacy and status, Spector H., Peterson M.S. and Friedemann T.E. (eds.), NRC, Washington D.C., pp. 13.

Mitchell H.H. and Block R.J. (1946): Some relationships between the amino acid contents of proteins and their nutritive values for the rat. J. Biol. Chem. 163, 599-620.

Mørup I.K. and Olesen E.S. (1976): New method for prediction of protein value from essential amino acid pattern. Nutr. Rep. Int. 13, 355-365.

NAS/NRC (1974): Recommended dietary allowances. NAS, Washington D.C.

Olesen E.S. and Mørup I.K. (1975): Prdiction of protein value in human nutrition. New index based on revised evaluation of amino acid pattern. In: Abstracts of the X-th Int. Congr. Nutr., Kyoto, Japan.

Orr M.L. and Watt B.R. (1957): Amino acid content of foods. Home Economics Res. Rep. No. 4., USDA, Washington D.C.

Oser B.L. (1951): Method for integrating essential amino acid content in the nutritional evaluation of protein. J. Amer. Diet. Assoc. 27, 396-402.

Pellett P.L. (1984): Amino acid scoring systems and their role in the estimation of the protein quality of cereals. (In this book.)

Pellett P.L. and Kaba H. (1972): Carcass amino acids of the rat under conditions of determination of net protein utilization. J. Nutr. 102, 61-68.

Pellett P.L. and Young V.R. (eds.) (1980): Nutritional evaluation of protein foods. UNU, Tokyo.

Rose W.C. (1936): The nutritive significance of the amino acids. Physiol. Rev. 18, 109.

Rose W.C., Wixon R.L., Lockhart H.B. and Lambert G.F. (1955): The amino acid requirements of man, XVI. The role of nitrogen intake. J. Biol. Chem. 217, 997.

Sarwar G. (1984): Available amino acid score: method for protein quality evaluation. (In this book.)

Satterlee L.D., Kendrick J.G. and Miller G.A. (1977): Rapid in vitro assays for estimating protein quality. Fd. Technol. 31 (6), 78-81.

Satterlee L.D., Marshall H.F. and Tennyson J.M. (1979): Measuring protein quality. J. Am. Oil Chem. Soc. 56, 103-109.

Satterlee L.D., Kendrick J.G., Jewell D.K. and Brown W.D. (1981): Estimating apparent protein digestibility from in vitro assays. In: Protein quality in humans: assessment and in vitro estimation, Bodwell C.E., Adkins J.S. and Hopkins D.T. (eds.), Avi, Westport, Conn., pp. 316-339.

Satterlee L.D., Kendrick J.G., Marshall H.F., Jewell D.K., Ali R.A., Heckman M.M., Steinke H.F., Larson P., Phillips R.D., Sarwar G. and Slump P. (1982): In vitro assay for predicting protein efficiency ratio as measured by rat bioassay: collaborative study. J. Assoc. Off. Anal. Chem. 65, 798-809.

Sheffner A.L. (1967): In vitro protein evaluation. In: Newer methods of nutritional biochemistry, Vol. III, Albanese A.A. (ed.), Academic Press, New York, pp. 125.

Sheffner A.L., Eckfeldt G.A. and Spector H. (1956): The pepsin-digest-residue (PDR) amino acid index of net protein utilization. J. Nutr. 60, 105-120.

Stahmann M.A. and Woldegiorgis G. (1975): Enzymatic methods for protein quality determination. In: Protein nutritional quality of foods and feeds. Part 1. Assay methods - biological, biochemical and chemical, Friedman M. (ed.), Marcel Dekker, Inc., New York, pp. 211-234.

Tkachuk R. and Irvine G.N. (1969): Amino acid composition of cereals and oilseed meals. Cereal Chem. 46, 206-218.

Torún B., Pineda O., Viteri F.E. and Arroyave G. (1981): Use of amino acid composition data to predict protein nutritive value for children with specific reference to new estimates of their essential amino acid requirements. In: Protein quality in humans: assessment and in vitro estimation, Bodwell C.E., Adkins J.S. and Hopkins D.T. (eds.), Avi, Westport, Conn., pp. 374-393.

Wöller L., Békés F. and Lásztity R. (1977): Evaluation of food proteins on the basis of chemical indices, I. Computing of data of amino acid analysators. Élelm. Ip. 31, 15-21.

Proc. Int. Assoc. Cereal Chem. Symp. Amino Acid Compn and Biol. Value of Cereal Proteins
Budapest, Hungary 1983, R. Lásztity, M. Hidvégi, eds

PREDICTION OF PROTEIN NUTRITIVE VALUE OF CEREAL-LEGUME BLENDS USING RAT BIOASSAYS AND AMINO ACID SCORES

F. W. SOSULSKI, G. SARWAR*

Department of Crop Science and Plant Ecology, University of Saskatchewan, Saskatoon, Sask. S7N OWO, Canada
*Bureau of Nutritional Sciences, Food Directorate, Health Protection Branch, National Health and Welfare, Tunney's Pasture, Ottawa, Ontario, K1A OL2, Canada

ABSTRACT

Cereal grains and root crops provide the major portion of the world food supply, resulting in widespread deficiencies in dietary protein and essential amino acids. The utilization of legumes and oilseed meals to overcome the lack of lysine, tryptophan and threonine requires high levels of protein supplementation and introduces the problem of methionine deficiency. These dicotyledonous protein sources contain flatulence and antinutritive factors which limit protein utilization and raise protein requirements even further. Amino acid scores (chemical scores) based on the amino acid requirements of the rat gave excellent prediction of feed intake, weight gain, protein efficiency ratio and true biological value in rat bioassays of cereal-legume blends. It is suggested that AA scores based on the amino acid requirements of the human would represent the protein nutritive value more accurately than the rat bioassay. Variations in the digestibilities of the cereal-legume blends examined in this study indicate the need for a specific measure of digestibility as a correction factor for AA score.

INTRODUCTION

Protein efficiency ratio (PER) has been the most widely used procedure for the evaluation of nutritive value in proteins. The official PER method employs a 4-week test using male weanling rats and a control diet containing a casein standard, and all PER values are corrected to obtain a constant value of 2.50 for the casein (Association of Official Agricultural Chemists, 1975). The PER test makes no allowance for body maintenance, assuming that all the protein is utilized for growth. It is also criticized for being expensive to conduct, the duration of the feeding trial being too long for routine use during food processing. Also the general public has not understood the scale values relative to casein = 2.50.

Another basic weakness of the rat assay is the high requirement by the rat for the sulfur-containing amino acids (5.0 g/16 g N) and lysine (7.5 g/16 g N) (National Academy of Sciences, 1972). The requirements for methionine and cystine (met + cys) and lysine (lys) for the growing child have been established at 3.5 and 5.5 g/16 g N, resp., by the FAO/WHO

(1973). A scoring pattern for an ideal protein, based on safe levels of intake for a 2-yr old child, were recently reported to be 2.7 and 6.4 g/16 g N for met + cys and lys, resp., by Torun et al. (1981). The NRC (1980) use values of 2.6 and 5.1, resp., for these amino acids in their amino acid requirements for man.

Amino acid requirements for the adult are substantially less than the growing child, and neither rat assay nor amino acid scores appears to provide accurate prediction of protein nutritive value for the mature adult (Bodwell, 1979).

Amino acid score

With the development of automation and short columns for amino acid analysis, a large body of data is now available on the variations in composition of the common protein sources in human and animal diets. Also, techniques for plasma amino acid analysis has led to the elaboration of amino acid requirements for man and animal species with a reasonable degree of accuracy. Therefore, many investigators have examined the possibility of utilizing the essential amino acid (EAA) data for the diet to predict their sufficiency for meeting the human or animal requirements. The essential amino acid index (EAAI), which is the geometric mean of the ratios of ten EAA in the test protein to the proportions in a reference protein or an EAA requirement pattern, has not been particularly useful for the prediction of protein nutritive value. However, the amino acid score (AA score), formerly chemical score, has shown high correlations with the results of rat bioassays. This has led to the suggestion that the protein nutritive value of foods and feeds might be more accurately predicted from AA score than from the PER value which requires the use of another animal species as test organism. The purpose of this review is to examine this proposal on data collected in our laboratory on nutritive value of cereal-legume blends.

The AA score is calculated directly from the EAA composition of the protein source and the corresponding values in a reference protein or in the EAA requirement pattern for an animal species or man. For each EAA, the calculation is:

$$\frac{\text{mg of amino acid in 1 g of test protein}}{\text{mg of amino acid in 1 g of reference protein}} \times 100$$

The lowest percentage value is the AA score for the dietary protein source. This calculation also identifies the first limiting amino acid. Because the percentage values for AA score encompass the scale of 0-100%, the significance of any specific value is readily apparent to the consumer or public.

Protein digestibility

The validity of AA scores has been questioned because of variations among plant sources in the digestibility of proteins. An additional problem is associated with the low availability of the most limiting amino acids in certain proteins. In wheat, the availability values for lys (80-85%) and tyrosine (tyr) (82-87%) were lower than the values for other amino acids (90-97%) and for nitrogen (92-95%) (Sarwar and Bowland, 1975). Among three legume species (soybean, field pea and fababean), met and cys were least available (70-85%), threonine (thr) and tyr were intermediate (80-86%) and lys was highly available (85-91%) relative to N digestibility (80-87%) (Sarwar et al., 1975a). The equal blends of legume + wheat proteins showed met and cys availabilities of 81-90%, and that of lys and tyr was 82-86%. There appears to be merit in correcting the amino acid score for low digestibility. At the present time Recommended Dietary Allowances (NRC, 1980) are adjusted for poor utilization of protein in mixed diets as compared with the reference protein. The correction applied assumes 75% efficiency of utilization of the poorer protein, and further adjustment may not be necessary unless specific protein factors are to be applied.

Cereal-legume blends

The calculation of AA score is simplified because mixed diets usually contain satisfactory proportions of most EAA, and only two or three have the potential of becoming limiting amino acids if protein intake is controlled. Cereal-legume diets may be deficient in one or more of lys, met, thr and tyr for growth purposes. Therefore, attention is directed to these critical amino acids in the following discussion.

Milled rice and corn products are dietary staples which typically contain less than 10% protein on a dry basis (Table 1). Rice proteins have a favorable amino acid balance as compared to the several deficiencies in corn proteins. Lysine is the first limiting amino acid in rice proteins but the AA score of 71 indicated that low protein content would be the major nutritional problem in rice-based diets (Sarwar et al. 1975b).

Table 1. Protein (%), EAA (g amino acid/100 g protein) and AA scores (FAO/WHO, 1973) for cereals, grain legumes and oilseed flour

Protein source	Protein N x 6.25	Arg	His	Ile	Leu	Lys	Met+ Cys	Phe+ Tyr	Thr	Try	Val	AA score
Casein	96.0	3.4	2.6	4.9	8.7	7.8	3.2	10.2	3.8	2.9	6.2	91
Cereals												
Milled rice	9.1	9.1	2.4	4.5	8.9	3.9	4.8	10.8	3.8	0.9	6.4	71
Wheat flour	15.6	3.5	2.1	3.3	6.2	2.0	4.9	7.6	2.4	1.5	3.6	36
Grain legumes												
Field pea	21.1	8.8	2.5	4.4	7.4	7.7	2.4	8.3	3.8	1.3	4.9	69
Field bean	24.5	5.8	2.7	4.9	8.7	7.0	2.2	9.6	4.4	1.0	5.7	63
Lentil	21.3	7.1	2.5	4.5	7.4	8.1	2.1	8.0	3.8	0.8	5.0	60
Broad bean	26.9	8.7	2.4	4.0	7.0	6.3	2.0	6.9	3.4	0.7	4.6	57
Fababean	27.8	8.4	2.3	3.9	6.9	6.1	2.0	6.9	3.3	1.0	4.3	57
Oilseed flour												
Soybean	52.3	7.3	2.5	4.4	7.6	6.4	2.6	8.5	3.8	1.8	4.9	74
AA requirements												
Human	-	-	-	4.0	7.0	5.5	3.5	6.0	4.0	1.0	5.0	-
Rat	-	5.0	2.5	4.6	6.2	7.5	5.0	6.7	4.2	1.3	5.0	-

[1]FAO/WHO (1973). [2]NAS (1972).

On the other hand, cereals like wheat and oat groats contain 10-18% protein (Table 1). Wheat proteins are seriously deficient in lys, as well as thr, and the AA score was only 36%. The correlation coefficients between lys and protein contents in hard red spring wheats are in the range of -0.75**, and low protein samples have up to 3.0% lys (Sosulski et al., 1966). Otherwise nutritional problems with wheat-based diets would be quite severe.

While grain legumes are excellent sources of lys to complement the deficiencies in cereals, their met + cys values are low (Table 1). Also several species have comparatively low protein contents, averaging 19-22%, including field pea, lentil, chickpea, cowpea and lima bean. Oilseed meals and flours, after oil extraction, are concentrated sources of protein, and lys in the case of soybean. However, oilseed species such as sunflower and peanut have little complementary effect on the lys deficiency in cereals except through excess consumption.

The protein nutritive values of five grain legumes, soybean flour and casein were evaluated in equal blends with wheat flour or milled rice in feeding trials with weanling male rats (Sarwar et al., 1975b). Relative to rat requirements (NAS, 1972), the wheat-based blends were seriously deficient in lys, the AA scores ranged from 54 to 65 (Table 2). The AA scores and essential amino acid indexes (EAAI) were higher in legume blends with milled rice than with wheat flour. Lys, met + cys or try were first limiting in the rice-legume blends.

Feed intakes of the legume-rice blends averaged 40 g higher than the legume-wheat diets but weight gains were more than proportionately greater than in the latter diet (Table 2). Therefore, the PER values for rice blends were higher than for wheat blends even though the true protein digestibilities (TPD) were greater in the wheat blends.

AA score and EAAI gave good prediction of feed intake, weight gain, PER and true biological value (TBV) but not TPD (Table 3). The range in TPD was 84-94% in the legume-wheat diets and 81-92% in the legume-rice diets, which suggested that AA score should be supplemented with data on protein digestibility.

Amino acid supplementation

In a subsequent feeding trial, the nutritive values of soybean, field pea and fababean proteins were evaluated alone and in equal protein blends with wheat flour (Sarwar et al., 1975a). The nature of the deficiencies exhibited by these diets were explored by supplementation with 0.2% L-met or 0.2% L-met, 0.4% lys and 0.1% Thr (Table 4). The legumes alone were very deficient in met + cys (AA scores = 40-52) and weight gains were very low relative to casein, especially for the fababean diet. Supplementation with met increased the AA scores to 77-88%, and the feed intakes, weight gains and PER for soybean and field pea diets were comparable to the casein diet, but not the casein plus met diet.

Table 2. Relationship between amino acid composition and the feed intake, weight gain and protein utilization of cereal-legume diets by rats (Sarwar et al. 1975b)

Protein source in diet	Amino acid composition of diet: Lys	Met+Cys	Thr	Try	AA score %	EAAI %	Feed intake g	Weight gain g	TPD %	PER adj.	TBV %
	% of rat requirements										
Legume-Wheat blends											
Casein	65[1]	81	74	170	65	71	410	133.8	96	2.50	60
Soybean	56	75	74	127	56	70	338	83.5	92	2.04	46
Field pea	65	73	74	108	65	70	318	85.5	94	2.13	52
Field bean	60	71	81	96	60	70	360	95.9	88	1.96	51
Lentil	67	70	74	88	67	67	298	74.7	84	1.88	57
Broad bean	55	69	69	85	55	65	294	68.5	90	1.82	49
Fababean	54	69	69	96	54	65	293	63.4	87	1.72	44
Legume-rice blends											
Casein	78	80	90	146	78	82	420	151.8	97	2.62	63
Soybean	69	74	90	104	69	78	424	136.8	91	2.29	63
Field pea	77	72	90	85	72	77	376	119.9	92	2.31	61
Field bean	73	70	98	73	70	78	321	88.1	84	1.99	58
Lentil	80	69	90	65	65	76	351	94.0	81	1.94	54
Broad bean	68	68	86	62	62	73	340	92.3	88	1.96	55
Fababean	67	68	85	73	67	72	350	90.2	84	1.86	56

[1] First limiting amino acid(s) is underlined.

Table 3. Correlation coefficients between amino acid indices and rat performance data for cereal-legume blends (Sarwar et al. 1975b)

	AA score	EAAI	Feed intake	Weight gain	TPD	PER
EAAI	0.85**					
Feed intake	0.62**	0.72**				
Weight gain	0.73**	0.77**	0.97**			
TPD	0.53*	0.47	0.47	0.49		
PER	0.81**	0.79**	0.88**	0.96**	0.55*	
TBV	0.84**	0.74**	0.69**	0.80**	0.67**	0.87**

*Significant at P = 0.05. **Significant at P = 0.01.

Table 4. Effects of protein sources and amino acid supplementation on feed consumption, weight gain and protein utilization by rats (Sarwar et al. 1975a)

Protein and amino acids in diet	Amino acid composition of diet: Lysine (% of rat requirements)	Met+Cys	AA score	EAAI	Feed intake	Weight gain	TPD %	PER adjusted
Legumes alone								
Casein	104	64[1]	64	80	344	118.7	99	2.50
Soybean	85	52	52	78	274	68.2	87	1.81
Field pea	103	48	48	76	181	36.5	85	1.47
Fababean	81	40	40	67	140	10.0	80	0.52
Legumes plus met								
Casein	104	104	68	83	357	152.7	100	3.10
Soybean	85	92	85	78	378	127.0	90	2.43
Field pea	103	88	88	79	407	141.7	88	2.53
Fababean	81	80	77	70	343	100.0	83	2.11
Legume-wheat blends								
Casein	65	81	65	71	405	141.2	99	2.54
Soybean	56	75	56	70	291	74.2	92	1.85
Field pea	65	73	65	70	303	84.2	94	2.02
Fababean	54	69	54	65	323	80.0	90	1.80
Legume-wheat plus lys, met and thr								
Casein	119	121	69	80	388	168.2	98	3.15
Soybean	109	115	84	79	392	150.5	92	2.78
Field pea	118	113	84	78	365	144.7	91	2.88
Fababean	107	109	78	73	372	135.7	91	2.66

[1]First limiting amino acid is underlined.

The legume-wheat blends had AA scores of 54-65% due to lys deficiencies (Table 4). For these diets the feed intakes, weight gains and PER were intermediate between those of legumes alone and legumes plus met diets. Supplementation of these diets with lys, met and thr resulted in uniformly high values for all rat growth parameters. The PER values for these amino acid-supplemented legume-wheat blends were 2.7-2.9. Note that the chemical scores for these blends were 78-84%, based on isoleucine (ile) and valine (val) being the first limiting amino acids in each legume blend. It did not appear that low concentrations of ile or val had adverse effects on rat growth and development.

For the amino acid supplemented diets, the AA score gave excellent prediction of feed intake, weight gain and PER, the coefficients varied from +0.83** to +0.90** (Table 5). On the other hand, EAAI showed only a low significant correlation with PER. The results of both rat trials indicate clearly that only AA score gives consistent prediction of rat growth performance.

Table 5. Correlation coefficients between amino acid indices and rat performance data for amino acid supplemented legume-wheat blends (Sarwar et al. 1977a)

	AA score	EAA1	Feed intake	Weight gain	TPD
EAA1	0.52*				
Feed intake	0.83**	0.32			
Weight gain	0.90**	0.49	0.94**		
TPD	0.43	0.39	0.62**	0.69**	
PER	0.88**	0.55*	0.89**	0.97**	0.73**

*Significant at P = 0.05.
**Significant at P = 0.01.

On the other hand, TPD values were not predicted by either AA score or EAAI (Table 5). Obviously the factors which had adverse effects on protein digestibility were not associated with the composition of EAA or the first limiting amino acid. The legumes exhibited a range in TPD, the values being 87, 85 and 80%. However, the blends with wheat were higher in digestibility, the range being 90-94%. Unlike legumes alone, supplementation with amino acids did not affect the TPD for the legume-wheat blend.

CONCLUSION

The present data demonstrate that, when AA scores are based on rat requirements for EAA, this index gives excellent predictions of rat growth performance and utilization of dietary protein. It is suggested that AA scores based on human requirements for EAA would also give good prediction of protein value for the human. On the other hand, the high requirements for lys and met by the rat indicate that this species would respond differently than man to the same dietary protein source. There is need for an accurate bioassay for protein digestibility since AA score and digestibility were not correlated in the present study of cereal-legume blends.

REFERENCES

Association of Official Agricultural Chemists (AOAC). 1975. Official methods of analysis. 12th ed. AOAC, Washington, D.C.

Bodwell, C.E. 1979. The nutritive value of the same protein preparations as estimated by human, rat and chemical assays. J. Amer. Oil Chem. Soc. 56: 156-159.

FAO/WHO. 1973. Energy and protein requirements. Technical report series No. 522. World Health Organization, Rome.

National Academy of Sciences. 1972. Nutrient Requirements of domestic animals. No. 10. Nutrient requirements of laboratory animals. 2nd Ed. Printing and Publishing Office, N.A.S., Washington, D.C.

NRC. 1980. Recommended dietary allowances. 9th ed. National Research Council, Nat. Acad. Sci., Washington, D.C.

Sarwar, G. and Bowland, J.P. 1975. Availability of amino acids in wheat cultivars used in diets for weanling rats. Can. J. Animal Sci. 55: 579-586.

Sarwar, G., Sosulski, F.W. and Bell, J.M. 1975a. Nutritive value of field pea and fababean proteins in rat diets. Can. Inst. Food Sci. Technol. J. 8: 109- 112.

Sarwar, G., Sosulski, F.W. and Holt, N.W. 1975b. Protein nutritive value of legume-cereal blends. Can. Inst. Food Sci. Technol. J. 8: 170-174.

Sarwar, G., Sosulski, F.W. and Bell, J.M. 1977. Availability of amino acids in legumes and legume-wheat blends. Can. Inst. Food Sci. Technol. J. 10: 31-35.

Sosulski, F.W., Lin, D.M. and Paul, E.A. 1966. Effects of moisture, temperature, and nitrogen on the yield and protein content of Thatcher wheat. Can. J. Plant Sci. 46: 583-588.

Torun, B., Viteri, F.E. and Young, V.R. 1981. Nutritional role of soya protein for humans. J. Amer. Oil Chem. Soc. 58: 400-405.

Proc. Int. Assoc. Cereal Chem. Symp. Amino Acid Compn and Biol. Value of Cereal Proteins Budapest, Hungary 1983, R. Lásztity, M. Hidvégi, eds

DIFFERENCES BETWEEN DIGESTIBILITIES OF PROTEIN AND FIRST LIMITING AMINO ACID IN SOME PLANT PRODUCTS

G. SARWAR

Bureau of Nutritional Sciences, Food Directorate, Health Protection Branch, National Health and Welfare, Tunney's Pasture, Ottawa, Ontario K1A OL2, Canada

ABSTRACT

Values /percent/ for true digestibility /TD/ of protein and essential amino acids /EAA/ in some cereals, legumes and oilseeds and their mixtures have been determined by the rat or pig fecal /balance/ method. In milling and utility wheats, the TD /bioavailability/ values of lysine /80-85/ were up to 12 percent lower than those of protein /92-95/ and other EAA /90-96/. As in wheat, lysine /the first limiting amino acid in cereals/ had the lowest bioavailability in barley /72/, oat /73/, rye /72/ and sorghum /71/. The TD values of protein and bioavailability of other EAA in barley, oat, rye and sorghum were, 82, 79-89; 79, 77-87; 81, 74-89 and 85, 83-87, respectively. The bioavailability values of methionine /the first limiting amino acid in legumes/ in field pea /75/, fababean /70/, lentil /60/ and navy bean /61/ were markedly lower than the TD values of protein /80-85/ and bioavailability of other EAA /80-96 in field pea, 78-90 in fababean, 67-90 in lentil/. Limiting amino acids were also less digestible than protein in soybean, rapeseed, sunflower and groundnut and blends of wheat with legumes and oilseeds. These data suggest that protein digestibility may not be a good preditor of bioavailability of the first limiting amino acid. Therefore, the rapid in vitro methods based on the amount of first limiting amino acid /amino acid score/ plus enzymatic digestibility may not accurately predict protein quality of foods. A preferable approach would be to obtain information on bioavailability of individual amino acids and then correct amino acid score for bioavailability of individual amino acids. Amino acid score corrected for true digestibility /bioavailability/ of individual amino acids has been termed as "available amino acid score". The positive correlation /r = 0.92/ between available amino acid score and relative net protein ratio /RNPR, the most suitable rat growth method for evaluating protein quality/ was highly significant. Protein digestibility and amino acid bioavailability has been a problem in preventing widespread acceptance of amino acid score. Available amino acid score provides a solution to this problem.

INTRODUCTION

Theoretically, the most logical method of estimating protein quality is by consideration of essential amino acid content of a food with human amino acid requirements /Harper, 1979; Pellett, 1978/. In this approach, the level of each dietary essential amino acid is expressed as a % of the amount of that specific amino acid in the reference protein such as human milk, egg or calculated reference mixture of essential amino acids based on human requirements. That amino acid which gives the lowest percentage value is the most /or first/ limiting amino acid and would presumably determine the nutritive value. The term "amino acid score" /mg of amino acid in 1 g of test protein/mg of amino acid in 1 g of reference protein x 100/ was used in the FAO/WHO/1973/ report which suggested a new scoring pattern based on the more recent assessment of human amino acid requirements. The procedure of scoring proteins from amino acid composition is simple and provides information about the supplementary or complementary value of proteins. Nevertheless, a serious weakness of the scoring procedure is that /unlike bioassay methods/ amino acid scores do not take into account digestibility of protein and bioavailability of amino acids.

In diets based on a sole source of protein, first limiting amino acid can usually be easily predicted from amino acid compositions. However, in the case of protein mixtures in which the protein sources may differ in digestibility and availability of amino acids, it is often difficult to predict the true first limiting amino acid /Sarwar et al. 1983/. Similarly, the amino acid score technique does not accurately predict the protein nutritional value of foods where processing has affected protein digestibility and amino acid bioavailability /Satterlee et al. 1981/. Rapid in vitro tests for estimating protein digestibility have been developed /Satterlee et al. 1982/. Digestibility of protein is a useful parameter for protein nutrition but it may not provide an appropriate correction factor for amino acid score. There is evidence that digestibility of individual amino acids may differ considerably from digestibility of total nitrogen in a protein source /Eggum, 1968; Sarwar and Bowland, 1975; Sarwar et al. 1977/. The objectives of this paper were twofold: /a/ to review data on true digestibility of protein and amino acids in some cereals, legumes, oilseeds and their blends; /b/ to report new values for digestibility of protein and amino acids in some plant products obtained in the Health Protection Branch laboratories, Ottawa, Canada.

METHODS FOR DETERMINING BIOAVAILABILITY OF AMINO ACIDS

The fecal /also called balance method/ method as proposed by Kuiken and Lyman /1948/ is the most widely used animal assay for the estimation of bioavailability of individual amino acids. In this method, true digestibility /bioavailability/ of amino acid is calculated using the following equation:

$$\text{True digestibility } /\%/ = \frac{AAI - (FAA - MFAA)}{AAI} \times 100$$

Where, AAI = total intake of amino acid, FAA = fecal excretion of amino acid, MFAA = metabolic fecal amino acid /determined by analyzing the feces of animal fed nitrogen-free diet/.

The determination of bioavailability of amino acid by balance trials is criticized on the grounds that the intestinal microflare may modify dietary amino acids especially the non-essential amino acids /Elwell and Soares, 1975/. This modification may overestimate bioavailability of amino acids, particularly in foods damaged by processing. Measurement of the disappearance of amino acids from the small intestine /ileal recovery/ has been proposed as an accurate measure of their bioavailability /Payne et al. 1968/. Cho and Bayley /1972/ compared the amino acid profiles of ileal and rectal digests of pigs fed soybean or rapeseed meal diets and found no significant difference in the proportions of most amino acids. The ileal recovery method neglects the absorption in the large intestine. Therefore, this method may underestimate bioavailability of amino acids because 30-40% of the amino acids present in rat's ileum were reported to be absorbed in the large intestine

/Slump and Beek, 1975/. Growth assays have been frequently used to estimate amino acid bioavailability /Gupta et al. 1958; Carpenter et al. 1963; Netke and Scott, 1970/. However, this method is limited to the determination of bioavailability of single amino acid and tends to overestimate or underestimate its availability due to growth response to unknown dietary factors /Elwell and Soares, 1975; Sarwar et al. 1975/. Although the plasma amino acid ratios have been found useful in assessing the effect of processing on availability of amino acids, the development of a method for estimating amino acid bioavailability by the plasma analyses had only limited success /Elwell and Soares, 1975; Vaughan et al. 1977/. In the light of the above discussion, the fecal /balance/ method appears to be the most suitable technique at present for estimating bioavailability of amino acids. The accuracy of bioavailability results obtained by the balance method is determined by the nature of the endogenous protein /Slump and Beek, 1975/. Whether the endogenous amino acids represent real body loss /unabsorbed residues of gastro-intestinal secretions and cells of mucosa of the intestinal lining/ or microbial proteins, true digestibility coefficients are useful as a measure of amino acid bioavailability with respect to amino acid balance for an animal.

The data reported in this paper have been taken from those studies in which protein and amino acid digestibilities were determined by the rat or pig balance method.

DIGESTIBILITY OF PROTEIN AND AMINO ACIDS IN SOME CEREALS, LEGUMES AND OILSEEDS AND THEIR BLENDS /LITERATURE REPORTS/

Cereals

True digestibility values /%/ of total nitrogen and essential amino acids /EAA/in No. 1 Canada Western Red Spring milling wheat, Neepawa; and No. 1 Utility wheats, Glenlea and Norquay are shown in Table 1. The digestibility values /as determined by rat balance method/ of nitrogen and EAA in the two types of wheats were similar. Except for lysine, the digestibility values for other EAA /90-96%/and protein /92-95%/ in wheats were high. The digestibility values of lysine /the first limiting amino acid/ were 10-12 percentage units lower than those of protein.

As in wheat, lysine /the first limiting amino acid in cereals/ has the lowest digestibility in barley /72%/, oat /73%/, rye /72%/ and sorghum /72%, Table 2/. The digestibility values /as determined with pigs/ of lysine were 6 to 14 percentage units lower than those of protein in these four cereals. The digestibility of other EAA varied from 78-89% in barley; 77-87% in oat; 74-89% in rye; and 83-87% in sorghum. In corn, isoleucine /88%/ and lysine /89%/ appeared lower in digestibility than nitrogen and other EAA /90-95%, Table 2/.

Grain Legumes

Values for true digestibility of protein and EAA in field pea and fababean /as determined by rat balance method/ are shown in Table 3. The digestibility of methionine /the first limiting amino acid in legumes/ was 10 percentage units lower than the digestibility of protein in these two grain legumes. The digestibility of other EAA varied from 80-96% in field pea and 78-90% in fababean.

Oilseeds

Values for true digestibility of protein and EAA in soybean, rapeseed, sunflower and groundnut meals are reviewed in Table 4. In soybean meal, methionine /the first

Table 1. Values /%/ for true digestibility of nitrogen and essential amino acids in wheats[1].

Wheat	Neepawa /Milling/	Glenlea /Utility/	Norquay /Utility/
Nitrogen	93	95	92
Arginine	94	95	93
Histidine	92	93	92
Isoleucine	93	93	90
Leucine	94	94	93
Lysine	83[2]	85	80
Methionine	94	94	93
Phenylalanine	95	95	94
Threonine	91	92	90
Tryptophan	96	96	95
Valine	94	95	93

1 Sarwar and Bowland /1975, 1976/.
2 The lowest digestibility value is underlined.

Table 2. Values /%/ for true digestibility of nitrogen and essential amino acid in five cereals[1].

Cereal	Barley	Oat	Rye	Sorghum	Corn
Nitrogen	82	79	81	85	90
Arginine	89	87	88	87	95
Histidine	88	85	89	85	93
Isoleucine	79	78	74	83	88[2]
Leucine	84	82	81	87	93
Lysine	72	73	72	71	89
Methionine	77	77	74	85	94
Phenylalanine	81	79	80	85	92
Threonine	78	77	74	83	90
Tryptophan	ND[3]	ND	ND	ND	ND
Valine	82	79	90	85	90

1 Eggum /1968/.
2 The lowest digestibility value is underlined.
3 ND = not determined.

Table 3. Values /%/ for true digestibility of nitrogen and essential amino acids in two grain legumes[1].

	Field pea /*Pisum sativum arvense*/	Fababean /*Vicia faba* minor/
Nitrogen	85	80
Arginine	95	90
Histidine	96	90
Isoleucine	82	78
Leucine	86	82
Lysine	91	85
Methionine	75[2]	70
Phenylalanine	89	82
Threonine	80	78
Tryptophan	ND[3]	ND
Valine	84	80

[1] Sarwar et al. /1977/.
[2] The lowest digestibility value is underlined.
[3] ND = not determined.

Table 4. Values /%/ for true digestibility of nitrogen and essential amino acids in some oilseeds.

Oilseed meal Experimental animal	Soybean[1] rat	Soybean[2] pig	Rapeseed[3] rat	Sunflower[2] pig	Groundnut[2] pig
Nitrogen	87	90	85	90	91
Arginine	94	96	90	96	95
Histidine	95	94	88	95	92
Isoleucine	85	90	85	91	90
Leucine	87	91	88	92	91
Lysine	88	92	83[4]	87	88
Methionine	84	87	91	92	89
Phenylalanine	90	91	85	91	92
Threonine	85	90	84	90	87
Tryptophan	94	ND[5]	90	ND	ND
Valine	86	89	83	91	90

[1] Sarwar et al. /1977/.
[2] Eggum /1968/.
[3] Sarwar et al. /1975/.
[4] The lowest digestibility value is underlined.
[5] ND = Not determined.

limiting amino acid/ had the lowest digestibility /84% with rats and 87% with pigs/. The digestibility values for other EAA and protein in soybean meal as determined with rats and pigs were 85-95% and 89-96%, respectively.

Methionine, tryptophan, arginine and histidine /88-91%/ appeared more digestible than other EAA and protein /83-85%/ in rapeseed meal /Table 4/. In sunflower meal, lysine /the first limiting amino acid, Sarwar et al. 1973/ had the lowest digestibility /87%/ whereas the values for protein and other EAA varied from 90-96%, Table 4. In the case of groundnut meal, threonine, lysine and methionine /limiting amino acids; Mir and Hill, 1979/ appeared less digestible /87-89%/ than protein and other EAA /90-95%, Table 4/.

Plant Protein Mixtures

Values for true digestibility /as determined by rat balance method/ of protein and EAA in blends of wheat with soybean, fababean and field pea are reported in Table 5. The limiting amino acids in these blends such as lysine, methionine and threonine were less digestible than protein. The digestibility of lysine, the first limiting amino acid in blends of wheat with soybean and fababean, was 8 percentage units lower than the digestibility of proteins in these two blends. In wheat-pea blend, threonine /the first limiting amino acid, Sarwar et al. 1983/ was 6 percentage units less digestible than protein.

NEW CONFIRMATORY DATA

The literature reports /Tables 1-5/ about the differences between the digestibilities of protein and first limiting amino acid in plant products were confirmed by the new data which are given in Table 6.

The author of this paper has recently completed a series of rat balance studies for the determination of true digestibility of protein and amino acids in a number of protein sources and their complementary and supplementary mixtures. The results for whole wheat flour, peas, lentil and navy bean have been calculated and are reported in Table 6.

As reported in the literature /Tables 1 and 2/, lysine /the first limiting amino acid in cereals/ was less digestible than protein and other EAA in wheat flour /Table 6/. Similarly, the digestibility of methionine /which is the first limiting amino acid in legumes/ was markedly lower than the digestibility of protein in peas, lentil and navy bean /Table 6/. The difference between the digestibilities of protein and methionine was as high as 25 percentage units in the case of lentil, 23 units in the case of navy bean and 22 units in the case of pea. Tryptophan and threonine /other limiting amino acids/ were also considerably less digestible than protein in lentil, navy bean and pea.

CONCLUSIONS

The data presented in this paper suggest that true digestibility or bioavailability of the limiting amino acids /especially the first limiting amino acid/ may be considerably lower than digestibility of protein in a plant product. In other words, digestibility of protein may not be a good predictor of bioavailability of the first limiting amino acid. Therefore, the rapid in vitro methods based on the amount of first limiting amino acid /amino acid score/ plus enzymatic digestibility may not

Table 5. Values /%/ for true digestibility of nitrogen and essential amino acids in some blends[1].

Blend	Wheat-Soybean	Wheat-Fababean	Wheat-Field pea
Nitrogen	92	90	94
Arginine	94	94	94
Histidine	93	91	94
Isoleucine	88	85	87
Leucine	90	88	90
Lysine	<u>84</u>[2]	<u>82</u>	<u>86</u>
Methionine	90	<u>81</u>	<u>85</u>
Phenylalanine	93	90	91
Threonine	86	84	<u>85</u>
Tryptophan	ND[3]	ND	ND
Valine	90	86	88

1 Sarwar et al. /1977/.
2 The lowest digestibility value is underlined.
3 ND = Not determined.

Table 6. New confirmatory values /%/ for true digestibility of nitrogen and essential amino acids in wheat and grain legumes[1].

	Wheat flour /whole/	Field pea /Pisum satiuum/	Lentil /Lens culinaris/	Navy bean /Phaseolus vulgaris/
Nitrogen	87	85	85	84
Arginine	91	90	90	89
Histidine	93	88	82	87
Isoleucine	84	79	80	81
Leucine	91	82	84	83
Lysine	<u>79</u>[2]	85	86	82
Methionine	87	<u>63</u>	<u>60</u>	<u>61</u>
Phenylalanine	94	84	85	85
Threonine	87	75	77	77
Tryptophan	ND[3]	75	67	73
Valine	90	79	81	77

1 Results of the rat balance studies conducted in the Health Protection Branch Laboratories, Ottawa, Canada.
2 The lowest digestibility value is underlined.
3 ND = Not determined.

accurately predict protein quality of foods. A preferable approach would be to obtain information on availability of individual amino acids and then calculate amino acid score corrected for availability of amino acids.

Amino acid score corrected for true digestibility of individual amino acids, as determined by rat balance method, has been termed as "available amino acid score" /Sarwar, 1984/. Sarwar /1984/ calculated available amino acid scores for 17 foods /mainly mixtures/ and reported a highly significant correlation /r = 0.92/between available amino acid score and relative net protein ratio /RNPR, the most suitable rat growth method for evaluating protein quality/. Sarwar /1984/ suggested that regulating agencies should take the lead in generating data on true digestibility of essential amino acids in common foods. The available amino acid scoring method is simple and would be accurate and applicable to a wide variety of foods. In the interium, the available amino acid score would probably be as expensive as rat growth methods for evaluating protein quality such as PER, NPR, RNPR, etc., but much cheaper when the amino acid digestibility /bioavailability/ tables come into use.

ACKNOWLEDGMENTS

The author is grateful to Mrs. Agnes Kemeny for reading this paper at the ICC Symposium on 'Amino Acid Composition And Biological Value of Cereal Proteins', May 31 - June 1, 1983, Budapest, Hungary.

REFERENCES

Carpenter, K.J., Milner, C.K. and Campbell, R.C. /1963/. A growth assay with chicks for the lysine content of protein concentrates. Brit. J. Nutr. 17, 309-323.

Cho, C.Y. and Bayley, H.S. /1972/. Amino acid composition of digesta taken from swine receiving diets containing soybean or rapeseed meals as sole source of protein. Can. J. Physiol. Pharmacol. 50, 513-522.

Eggum, B.O. /1968/. Nutritional evaluation of proteins by laboratory animals. In: Evaluation of Novel Protein Products. Proc. of International Biological Program (IBP) and Wenner-Gren Centre Symposium, Stockholm, Swededn, Bender, A.E. Kihlberg, R., Lofquist, B. and Munck, L. /ed./, Pergamon Press, New York, pp. 117-125.

Elwell, D. and Soares, J.H. Jr. /1975/. Amino acid bioavailability: a comparative evaluation of several assay techniques. Poult. Sci. 54, 78-85.

FAO/WHO. /1973/. Energy and protein requirements. Food and Agriculture Org. Nutr. Rep. Ser. No. 52, Rome; World Health Org. Techn. Rep. Ser. No. 522, Geneva.

Gupta, J.D., Dakroury, A.M., Harper, A.E. and Elvehjem, C.A. /1958/. Biological availability of lysine. J. Nutr. 64, 259-270.

Harper, A.E. /1979/. Human requirements for lysine and sulphur-containing amino acids. In: Soy Proteins and Human Nutrition, Wilcke, H.L., Hopkins, D.T. and Waggle, D.H. /ed./, Academic Press, New York, pp. 171-186.

Kuiken, K.A. and Lyman, C. /1948/. Availability of amino acids in some foods. J. Nutr. 36, 359-368.

Mir, Z. and Hill, D.C. /1979/. Nutritional value of peanut meals from Ontario grown peanuts. Can. Inst. Food Sci. Technol. J. 12, 56-60.

Netke, S.P. and Scott, H.M. /1970/. Estimates of the availability of amino acids in soybean oil meal as determined by chick growth assay: methodology as applied to lysine. J. Nutr. 100, 281-288.

Payne, W.L., Combs, G.F. and Kifer, R.R. /1968/. Investigation of protein quality-ileal recovery of amino acids. Federation Proc. 27, 1199-1203.

Pellett, P.L. /1978/. Protein quality evaluation revisited. Food Technol. 32, 61-79.

Sarwar, G. /1984/. The available amino acid score for evaluating protein quality of foods. J. Assoc. Off. Anal. Chem. /In Press/.

Sarwar, G. and Bowland, J.P. /1975/. Availability of amino acids in wheat cultivars used in diets for weanling rats. Can. J. Anim. Sci. 55, 579-586.

Sarwar, G. and Bowland, J.P. /1976/. Availability of tryptophan in wheat and oilseed proteins for weanling rats. Can. J. Anim. Sci. 56, 433-437.

Sarwar, G., Peace, R.W. and Botting, H.G. /1983/. Validity of rat plasma amino acids in predicting first limiting amino acid in protein mixtures. Nutr. Rep. Int. 28, 613-620.

Sarwar, G., Shannon, D.W.F. and Bowland, J.P. /1975/. Effects of processing conditions on the availability of amino acids in soybean and rapeseed proteins when fed to rats. Can. Inst. Food Sci. Technol. J. 8, 137-141.

Sarwar, G., Sosulski, F.W. and Bell, J.M. /1973/. Nutritional evaluation of oilseed meals and protein isolates by mice. Can. Inst. Food Sci. Technol. J. 6, 17-21.

Sarwar, G., Sosulski, F.W. and Bell, J.M. /1977/. Availability of amino acids in legumes and legume-wheat blends. Can. Inst. Food Sci. Technol. J. 10, 31-35.

Satterlee, L.D., Kendrick, J.G., Jewell, D.K. and Brown, W.D. /1981/. Estimating apparent protein digestibility from in vitro assays. In: Protein Quality in Humans: Assessment and In Vitro Estimation, Bodwell, C.E., Adkins, J.S. and Hopkins, D.T. /eds./. AVI Publishing Company Inc., Westport, C.T., pp. 316-339.

Satterlee, L.D., Kendrick, J.G., Marshall, H.F., Jewell, D.K., Ali, R.A., Heckman, M.M., Steinke, H.F., Larson, P., Phillips, R.D., Sarwar, G. and Slump, P. /1982/. In Vitro assay for predicting protein efficiency ratio as measured by rat bioassay: Collaborative Study. J. Assoc. Off. Anal. Chem. 65, 798-809.

Slump, P. and Beek, V. /1975/. Amino acids in feces related to digestibility of food proteins. In: Protein Nutritional Quality of Foods and Feeds. Part I. Assay Methods - Biological, Biochemical and Chemical, Friedman, M. /ed./, Marcel Dekker, Inc. New York, pp. 67-78.

Vaughan, D.A., Womack, M. and McClain, P.E. /1977/. Plasma free amino acid levels in human subjects after meals containing lactalbumin, heated lactalbumin or no protein. Am. J. Clin. Nutr. 30, 1709-1712.

Proc. Int. Assoc. Cereal Chem. Symp. Amino Acid Compn and Biol. Value of Cereal Proteins
Budapest, Hungary 1983, R. Lásztity, M. Hidvégi, eds

AVAILABLE AMINO ACID SCORE: METHOD FOR PROTEIN QUALITY EVALUATION

G. SARWAR

Bureau of Nutritional Sciences, Food Directorate, Health Protection Branch, National Health and Welfare, Tunney's Pasture, Ottawa, Ontario K1A OL2, Canada

ABSTRACT

Amino acid score corrected for true digestibility of individual amino acids /as determined by the rat balance method/ has been described as "available amino acid score". Available amino acid scores have been calculated for 7 protein sources /casein, egg white, beef, soy assay protein, pea flour, rapeseed protein concentrate and whole wheat flour/ and their 10 mixtures. Available amino acid scores for the 17 foods were similar to their relative net protein ratio /RNPR/ values and the positive correlation between available amino acid score and RNPR was highly significant /r=0.92/. Available amino acid score is a simple and quantitative measure of protein quality.

INTRODUCTION

Amino acid score /FAO/WHO, 1973/, a rapid and common method of estimating protein quality, does not include corrections for digestibility of protein and amino acids. In calculating amino acid scores, the use of determined or literature values for protein digestibility has been suggested /UNU, 1980/. However, the correction for protein digestibility would be of limited applicability because true digestibility of individual amino acids may differ considerably from the digestibility of total nitrogen in the same protein source /Sarwar, 1984/. Moreover, in a processed food product, digestibility of protein may not be a good predictor of bioavailability of those individual amino acids which are more susceptible to processing loss, such as lysine in early Maillard reactions /Hurrell and Carpenter, 1981/. Therefore, it is necessary to correct amino acid scores for bioavailability /true digestibility/ of individual amino acids. Amino acid score corrected for true digestibility of individual amino acids /as determined by the rat balance method/ has been termed "available amino acid score" /Sarwar, 1984a/.

CALCULATION OF AVAILABLE AMINO ACID SCORE

Sarwar /1984a/ calculated available amino acid scores according to the following formulae:

Available amino acid score

$$= \frac{\text{mg of available amino acid in 1 g of test protein}}{\text{mg of amino acid in 1 g of reference protein}} \times 100$$

where, Available amino acid = Total amino acid x true amino acid digestibility,

$$\text{True amino acid digestibility} = \frac{\text{AAI-/FAA-MFAA/}}{\text{AAI}} \times 100,$$

where AAI = amino acid intake, FAA = fecal amino acid, MFAA = metabolic fecal amino acid; estimates of metabolic amino acids were made by analyzing the feces of rats fed the nitrogen-free diet, Reference protein = provisional amino acid scoring pattern as recommended by FAO/WHO /1973/.

RELATIONSHIP BETWEEN AVAILABLE AMINO ACID SCORES AND RELATIVE NET PROTEIN RATIO (RNPR) VALUES

Sarwar /1984a/ calculated available amino acid scores for 7 protein sources /casein, egg white, beef, soya assay protein, pea flour, rapeseed protein concentrate and whole wheat flour/ and their ten mixtures /casein + methionine, soya protein + methionine, pea flour + methionine, wheat flour + lysine, wheat flour + casein, wheat flour + egg white, wheat flour + beef, wheat flour + soya protein, wheat flour + pea flour and wheat flour + rapeseed concentrate, Table 1/.

The available amino acid scores and RNPR values of the 17 diets, which were recently tested in a collaborative rat growth study, are given in Table 2. Available amino acid scores were similar to the RNPR values, the differences being less than 10 units in most cases. In general, RNPR values were slightly lower than available amino acid scores which reflected the higher essential amino acid requirements of the growing rat than humans. The positive correlation between available amino acid scores and RNPR values of the 17 diets was highly significant /r=0.92/.

The calculation of available amino acid score is simple and this method is applicable to a wide variety of protein products including processed foods. When data for digestibility of amino acids in typical foods become available, the determination of available amino acid score would be no more expensive than analysis of amino acids. In the Canadian Health Protection Branch Laboratories, values for the true digestibility /bioavailability/ of amino acids are being tabulated for a range of protein sources.

Additional information on the differences between digestibilities of protein and of individual amino acids in the same protein sources, as well as standardization of procedures for amino acid analysis and digestibility determinations are required before the available amino acid score can be recommended for routine application. Moreover, consideration would have to be given to the selection of the most appropriate human amino acid requirement pattern. Although the FAO/WHO /1973/ pattern was used in the calculation of available amino acid scores, it now appears that the NRC /1980/ pattern would be more appropriate for humans, especially in terms of sulphur amino acids.

Table 1. Available essential amino acids /EAA/ provided by protein sources expressed as a % of human requirements /calculation of available amino acid scores/[1,2,3]

EAA	Ile	Leu	Lys	Met + Cys	Phe + Tyr	Thr	Trp	Val
Protein Sources								
Casein	129	139	151	93	190	114	130	134
Casein + Met	129	143	151	130	190	114	130	134
Egg White	129	122	123	183	171	112	142	133
Beef	101	107	140	90	113	102	95	89
SAP[4]	109	114	108	62	153	88	107	92
SAP + Met	108	112	107	98	151	88	105	91
Pea flour	91	98	129	61	129	90	71	90
Pea flour + Met	89	98	129	98	127	90	72	88
RPC[5]	97	103	97	117	108	94	139	98
WW[6]	70	89	38	99	120	63	101	76
WW + Lys	74	92	77	104	123	67	104	79
WW + casein	94	112	92	95	151	84	109	101
WW + egg white	96	103	79	141	142	85	117	102
WW + beef	82	95	84	91	113	77	88	77
WW + SAP	86	99	70	78	129	72	102	83
WW + pea flour	82	95	84	86	125	75	87	82
WW + RPC	78	94	65	108	112	77	116	85

[1] Sarwar /1984a/.

[2] Available essential amino acid = Total amino acid x true amino acid digestibility.

[3] The lowest ratio is the available amino acid score. The scores of above 100 were considered as 100.

[4] Soya assay protein.

[5] Rapeseed protein concentrate.

[6] Whole wheat flour.

Table 2. Available amino acid scores and relative NPR values

Diets	Available amino acid score, %[1]	RNPR, %[2]
Casein	93	86
Casein + Met	100	100
Egg white	100	95
Beef	89	91
SAP	62	51
SAP + Met	88	70
Pea flour	61	54
Pea flour + Met	72	81
RPC	94	87
WW	38	44
WW + Lys	67	55
WW + casein	84	79
WW + egg white	79	77
WW + beef	77	79
WW + SAP	70	64
WW + pea flour	75	66
WW + RPC	65	63

[1] Sarwar /1984a/.

[2] Sarwar et al. /1984/, $\text{RNPR} = \frac{\text{NPR of test protein}}{\text{NPR of reference protein}} \times 100$, where

$$\text{NPR} = \frac{\text{weight gain of rats fed test diet + weight loss of rats fed non-protein diet}}{\text{protein consumed by rats fed test diet}}$$

REFERENCES

FAO/WHO /1973/. Energy and protein requirements. Food and Agriculture Org. Nutr. Rep. Ser. No. 52, Rome; World Health Org. Techn. Rep. Ser. No. 522, Geneva.

Hurrell, R.F. and Carpenter, K.J. /1981/. The estimation of available lysine in foodstuffs after Maillard reactions. Prog. Food Nutr. Sci. 5: 159-176.

NRC /1980/. Recommended Dietary Allowances, National Research Council. Natl. Acad. Sciences, Washington, D.C.

Sarwar, G. /1984/. Differences Between Digestibilities of Protein and First Limiting Amino Acid in Some Plant Products. In: Amino Acid Composition and Biological Value of Cereal Proteins, R. Lasztity and M. Hidvegi /Eds./. D. Reidel Publishing Company, Boston, U.S.A. /in press/.

Sarwar, G. /1984a/. The available amino acid score for evaluating protein quality of foods. J. Assoc. Off. Anal. Chem. /in press/.

Sarwar, G., Blair, R., Friedman, M., Gumbmann, M.R., Hackler, L.R., Pellett, P.L. and Smith, T.K. /1984/. Inter- and intralaboratory variability in rat growth assays for estimating protein quality of foods. J. Assoc. Off. Anal. Chem. /in press/.

UNU /1980/. Nutritional Evaluation of Protein Foods. P.L. Pellett and V.R. Young /Eds./. The United Nations University, Tokyo, Japan, pp. 103-117.

Proc. Int. Assoc. Cereal Chem. Symp. Amino Acid Compn and Biol. Value of Cereal Proteins Budapest, Hungary 1983, R. Lásztity, M. Hidvégi, eds

SIMPLE ENZYMIC METHODS FOR PREDICTION OF PLANT PROTEIN DIGESTIBILITY

ANDRÁS SALGÓ, KATALIN GANZLER, JOLÁN JÉCSAI*

Department of Biochemistry and Food Technology, Technical University of Budapest, H-1111 Budapest, Müegyetem rkp. 3, Hungary
*Department of Physiology, Institute for Animal Nutrition, Research-Center for Animal Production, H-2053 Herceghalom, Hungary

For the investigation of the digestibility of plant proteins a two-digestive-enzyme /trypsin, pancreatin/ in vitro measuring technique was used in the pH-decrease and pH-stat methods respectively. Parallel to the in vitro measurement, true and apparent digestibility were investigated in in vivo experiments on rats. It was established from data obtained for 45 test proteins that results obtained with the pH-stat method in a digestive period of 10' are closely correlated /r=0.91/ with in vivo data, digestibility can be well predicted from the in vitro data.

The two-enzyme method, using pH-stat technique, gives a similar correlation to that of multi-enzyme techniques. The costs of the method are less than a third of that of multi-enzyme tests.

In processes accompanied by change in protein quality, the method is suitable for the rapid screening of digestibility.

INTRODUCTION

Surveys /Pellett 1978, Bodwell 1981/ on the methods of determination of the nutritive properties of proteins of different origin, of the quality of proteins, indicate the main trends of the various biological, microbiological and chemical /enzymic/ methods of testing.

However, many questions arise during the use of the qualifying methods:

- What parameters are characteristic, among others, for protein quality? Biological value, PER, digestibility, etc.
- What is the relationship between the characteristic measured and the effective biological "response"? /Is the model correct?/
- What is the reliability of the method used?
- How much does the method used cost?

Investigating these important aspects, the general tendency will be noted that instead of slow, costly in vivo methods with large standard deviation, in vitro methods which model the biological process steadily gain ground, and after appropriate correction are suitable for the replacement of in vivo qualifying processes.

This offers a possibility to predict the nutritive properties of proteins, properties of which digestibility is one of the best usable parameters according to Pedersen and Eggum /1983/.

The single-enzyme methods used for the measurement of protein digestibility by Buchanan /1969/, Maga et al. /1973/, the two-enzyme methods of Akeson et al. /1964/, Saunders et al. /1973/, and the multi-enzyme techniques of Ford et al. /1966/ substantially differ with respect to the enzymes used, the methods of product separation and the detection of the products.

The three-digestive-enzyme process /trypsin, chymotrypsin, peptidase/, described by Hsu et al. /1977, 1978/, introduced a new mode of detection, the measurement of the departing COO^- end-groups on the basis of the decrease in pH.

Using a digestion period of 10 minutes, in vitro results are in good correlation with in vivo data in rats. A similarly good correlation was obtained by Pedersen and Eggum /1981/ for proteins of plant and combined /plant-animal/ proteins. Satterlee et al. /1979/ introduce even a four-enzyme digestion technique, in which protease from Streptomyces griseus is the fourth digestive enzyme, and the basis of detection is here too, the decrease in pH. The four-enzyme in vitro methods and parallel in vivo results are evaluated somewhat contradictorily by Rich et al. /1980/ and by Bodwell et al. /1980/.

Authors found that on grouping the proteins according to origin /plant, plant-animal, animal/, the correlation of in vivo and in vitro data is reliable only within the single groups e.g. Marshall et al. /1979/.

However, the use of the pH-decrease method alone raises several problems:

- The buffer capacity of the substance must be measured and taken into consideration in correction.
- It must be taken into consideration that digestive enzymes exert their action at changing pH values because of the decrease in pH.
- Processes of protein digestion proceed in vivo in the small intestines at a constant pH value of about 8, and this fact is not taken into account in the model measuring on the basis of pH-decrease.

The possibilities of substances of high buffer capacity and of antinutritive properties in digestibility tests were thoroughly elucidated by Pedersen and Eggum /1981/.

The error of the pH-decrease method was similarly eliminated by Pedersen and Eggum /1983/ by the introduction of the pH-stat technique /pH=8.0/. Using three- and four-enzyme digestion, they show by both pH-decrease and pH-stat method that the pH-stat method subsequently gives in the case of various protein sources better correlation with in vivo data /r=0.95; 0.97; 0.98 plant - combination - animal/, than the pH-decrease method /r=0.90; 0.93/.

Their method models also more truly in vivo pH conditions, and is suitable for the determination of the digestibility of substances with high buffer capacity.

Multienzymic pH-stat technique, supplemented by pre-digestion with pepsin, further improves in vivo - in vitro relationships, diminishing the effects of antinutritive substances /protease inhibitors, lectins, tannin, etc./. The multienzymic process with pepsin pre-digestion simulates more closely in vivo digestion conditions.

In our present work, a simplified two-enzyme modification of multienzyme techniques was developed for the testing of cereals and feed components of plant origin, by both pH-decrease and pH-stat methods. The correlation of in vivo and in vitro data was investigated. Our aim was to develop a rapid, simple and relatively cheap method, suitable for the rapid screening of protein digestibility.

Materials and methods

Test materials and enzymes

Investigations concerned the digestibility of cereals /n=18/ and other vegetal feed components /legumes n=27/, involving in most of the cases samples of defined varieties distinguishing between years of cultivation and storage conditions. Our samples were ground before the test, sifted on a sieve to mesh 80, and stored at room temperature. Raw protein content was calculated from Kjeldahl N data /AOAC 1975/.
Digestive enzymes used for the test:

Trypsin /Merck 24579, crystalline, lyophilized, 2.0 U/mg/.
Pancreatin /Sigma P-1750, crystalline Grade VI, Grade 4xNF/.

In vitro protein digestibility methods

For each test protein two parallel in vitro methods were used /pH-decrease and pH-stat/ with digestion periods of 10 and 15 minutes, respectively. According to the three-enzyme method of Hsu et al. /1977/ we used two digestive enzymes. The test substance containing 200 mg of protein was suspended in 25 ml of bidistilled water, and the pH of the suspension was adjusted at 37 °C ± 0.1 °C to pH=8.00, while mixing continuously. Simultaneously 0.5 ml of trypsin solution of 8 mg/cm^3 concentration and 0.5 cm^3 of pancreatin solution of 20 mg/cm^3 concentration /freshly prepared and put in ice/, exactly adjusted to pH=8.00, were injected into the test solution. The change in pH was measured for exactly 10 and 15 minutes, respectively. /Digital pH-meter, RADELKIS/. In giving the in vitro digestibility, pH values measured at the end of 10 and 15 minutes were used.

In the pH-stat method the test protein and enzyme quantities given above were used. The pH of the suspension is kept by the automatic titrator /Radiometer, Copenhagen/ at a value of pH=8.00, using 0.05 N NaOH as titrant. The quantity /µl/ of the alkali consumed is measured from the moment of injection for 10 and 15 minutes, respectively. From these data in vitro digestibility values are calculated. In both processes, mentioned above, 3 parallel tests were carried out.

In vivo apparent and true digestibility methods

In vivo experiments were carried out according to the method of Eggum /1973/. Every test substance was fed to each of a group of 6 young male Wistar rats. In the special metabolic room animals were kept under air conditioning /23 °C; 75 % rel. humidity/ in separate metabolic cages. The weight of the experimental animals varied between 90 and 130 g. The experiment consisted of 4-day prefeeding and 6-day experimental period. During the latter the quantity of feed ingested was measured and the urine and faeces of the animals were collected. The quantity of nitrogen, taken up with the feed and evacuated in the urine and faeces was determined by the Kjeldahl method /AOAC 1975/, apparent /AD/ and true /TD/ digestibilities were calculated, too. Composition of the diet fed: 9.5 % raw protein, starch, oil, sugar, fibre cellulose, vitamin mixture, mineral substances, as it has been given in the literature.

Mathematical methods

Statistical analyses were performed according to Czakó /1982/. Linear correlation method was used for the determination of the correlation of in vivo and in vitro data series.

Result and discussion

In the digestibility model system used by us, in vitro digestibility results obtained for 45 protein samples of vegetal origin give satisfactory correlation with in vivo data in rats /Table 1/.

Correlation data obtained by us approximate data yielded by three- and four-enzyme digestibility tests. Our simplified

Table 1.

Linear regression coefficients between in vivo and in vitro results in 45 plant protein samples as affected by procedure and incubation time

Procedure	pH drop		pH stat	
Incubation time /min/	10	15	10	15
TD	0.74	0.72	0.91	0.89
AD	0.78	0.74	0.87	0.86

TD: true digestibility /%/

AD: apparent digestibility /%/

model follows closely in a wide range in vivo results. Taking into consideration that pancreatin contains several proteolytic enzyme components, the technique used by us can be also considered as multienzymic. Detecting digestibility with the pH-decrease method, in the case of substances of low digestibility great deviations from in vivo data can be observed /Fig.1/. By the introduction of the pH-stat technique our simplified model follows well in vivo data /r=0.91/ /Fig.2 /. The accuracy of both procedures is better when a 10 minute digesting period is used. As concerns in vivo techniques, there is no substantial difference between the correlation of the TD and AD data series. In the pH-stat method the correlation of TD is somewhat better. Regression equations suitable for the prediction of in vivo digestibility are contained in Table 2.

On comparing our equations with the relationships given by Pedersen and Eggum /1981/ for plant proteins, in the range of high digestibility /TD 90 %/ identical results were obtained, while our method predicts considerably lower TD in the case of plant proteins of low digestibility.

This difference can be attributed to the fact that our test substances include a broader range with respect to digestibility.

In view of the results discussed above, pH-stat methods will be preferentially used because of the incertitudes of the pH-decrease techniques /Table 2/.

Data unequivocally indicate that with respect to both TD and AD the in vitro data of the pH-stat technique are more accurate. Results measured with pH-decrease method reveal a considerably higher discrepancy. Using our two-enzyme method, differences in the digestibility of legums can be readily detected. Within the single species different varieties substantially differ with respect to digestibility. Of the fodder peas, for example, the variety Dukát is of the poorest digestibility.

Characteristic of the sensitivity of our method is its suitability for the detection of differences in the digestibility of each of 4 maize samples true to variety, stored in wet and dry state, respectively /Table 3/. Proteins of maize stored in dry state are easier digested.

These two examples show that the simplified two-enzyme method, using the pH-stat technique, is suitable for the qualification of the effects of various technological processes /milling, hydrothermal, etc. operations/ on protein quality. Compared with multienzyme, three-, four-enzyme processes, the costs of our method are less than a third of that of the method of Hsu et al. /1977/ or Satterlee et al. /1979/. The sensitivity of two-enzyme technique can be further improved at a small increase in costs by the introduction of Pedersen and Eggum's /1983/ modification of the pre-digestive step with pepsin. This modification would simulate also in vivo conditions more correctly.

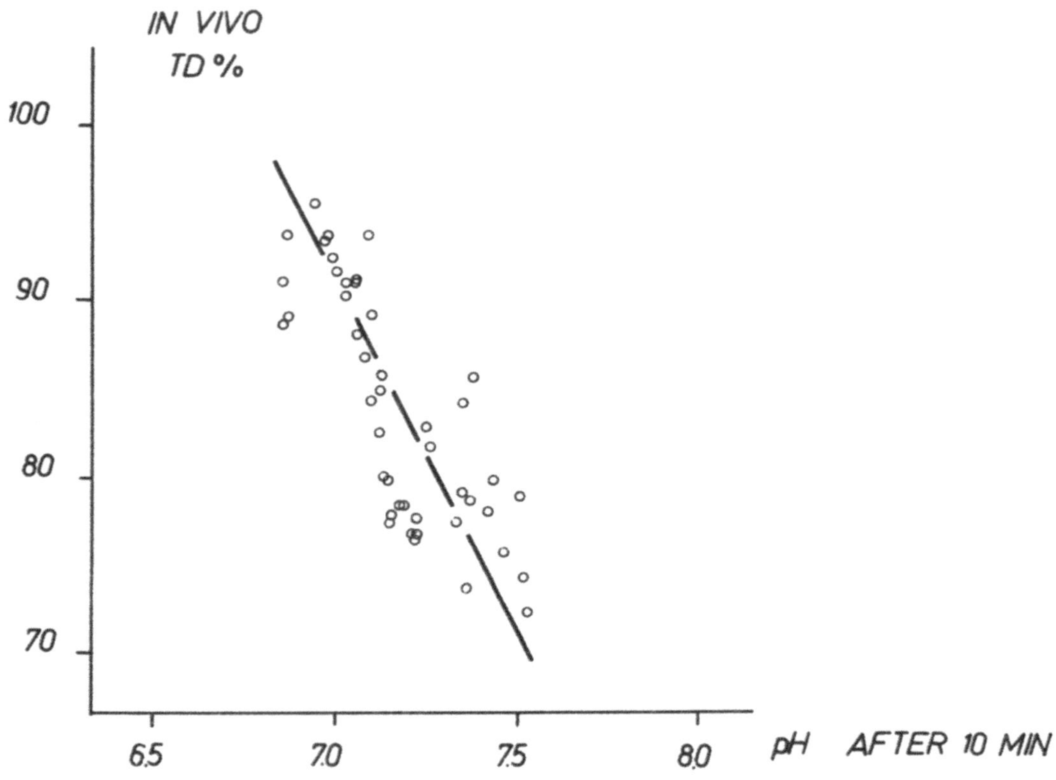

Figure 1. Relationship between in vivo digestibility and pH value after 10 minutes in vitro digestion

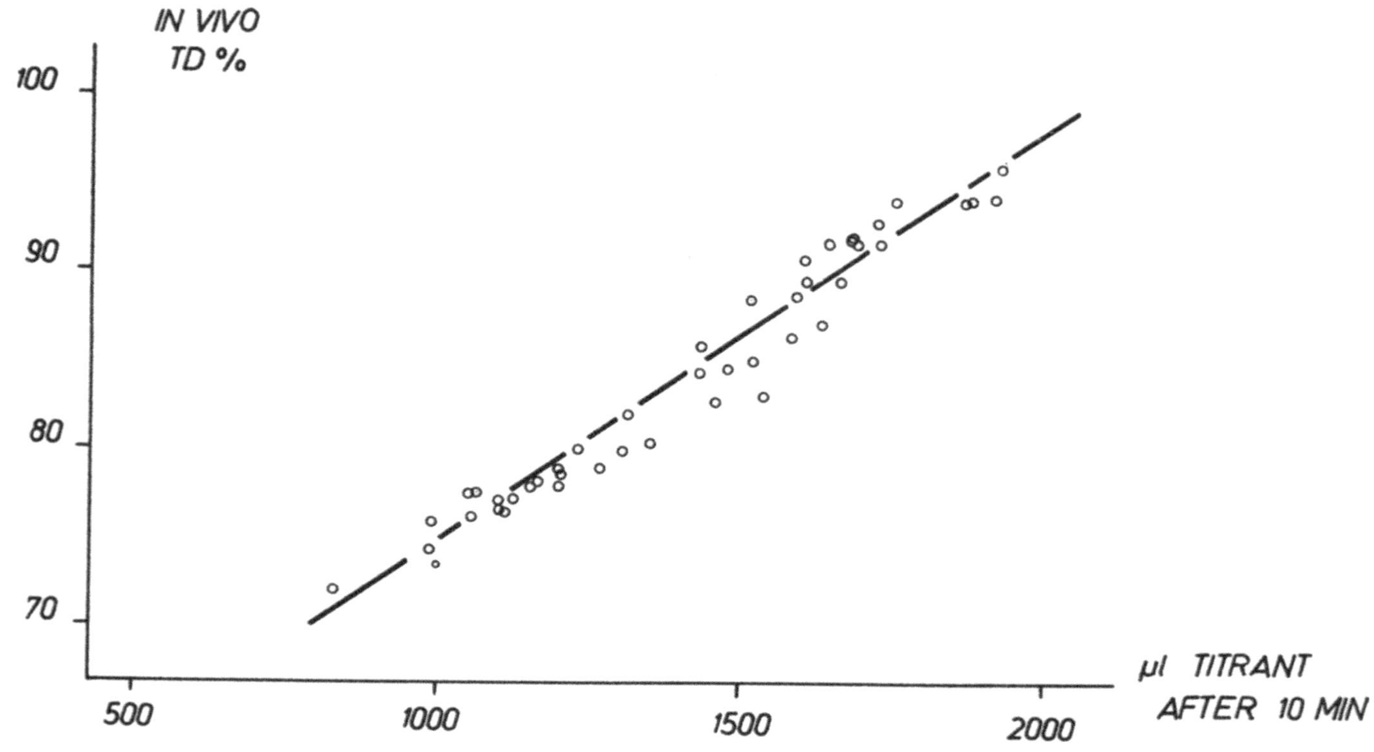

Figure 2. Relationship between in vivo digestibility and amount of titrant added during the in vitro pH-stat digestion procedure

Table 2.

Regression equations between in vivo and in vitro protein digestibility using pH-drop and pH-stat methods, respectively

$$TD\ \% = 425.78 - 47.64\ pH_{10}$$

$$AD\ \% = 392.51 - 44.84\ pH_{10}$$

pH_{10}: pH value of the digested mixture, recorded exactly 10 minutes after the enzyme injection

$$TD\ \% = 52.00 + 0.0223\ B_{10}$$

$$AD\ \% = 36.97 + 0.0236\ B_{10}$$

B_{10} µl: amount of titrant /0.05 N NaOH/, added during 10 min of digestion

Table 3.

A comparison of in vitro and in vivo protein digestibility in a variety of plant protein sources

Samples	In vitro pH-drop		In vitro pH-stat		In vivo	
	TD %	AD %	TD %	AD %	TD %	AD %
Feeding peas vs. Maxi /1981/	74.2	61.6	84.0	70.8	85.6	72.5
- " - vs. IP8 -"-	75.2	62.5	84.0	70.7	84.2	70.7
- " - vs. Dukát -"-	81.1	68.1	76.5	62.9	76.6	64.4
Horsebean vs. Erfordia /1981/	69.7	57.3	74.1	60.4	75.7	62.4
- " - vs. Lippai -"-	71.6	59.1	75.4	61.7	77.4	64.0
- " - vs. Fribo -"-	70.9	58.4	79.5	66.0	79.9	66.5
Lupine /yellow/ vs.Borluta /1981/	84.2	71.0	76.5	62.9	77.1	66.8
- " - vs.R 60-22 -"-	85.6	72.3	84.6	71.4	82.7	69.2
- " - vs.Refusa N -"-	80.6	67.6	78.8	65.3	78.5	66.6
Lupine/white/ vs.Watt /1981/	82.1	69.0	78.8	65.3	78.1	58.4
- " - vs.Horizont -"-	82.3	69.2	77.7	64.1	78.0	64.6
- " - vs.Nyirségi -"-	80.4	67.4	75.5	61.8	76.2	65.5
Feeding peas vs. Maxi /1982/	83.7	70.5	81.2	67.8	79.9	66.5
- " - vs. IP 8 -"-	84.4	71.2	82.1	68.8	80.2	66.8
- " - vs. Dukát -"-	83.5	70.3	75.8	62.1	77.5	64.1
Horsebean vs. Erforida /1982/	73.7	61.1	78.0	64.4	78.1	64.8
- " - vs. Lippai -"-	75.2	62.5	77.2	63.6	77.2	63.8
- " - vs. Fribo -"-	74.0	61.3	74.3	60.5	73.5	58.4

Lupine /yellow/ vs.Borhuta /1982/	87.3	73.9	84.8	71.6	84.4	70.8
- " - vs.Ventus -"-	85.9	72.6	85.9	72.8	84.9	71.4
- " - vs.Refusa -"-	81.8	68.7	76.9	63.3	76.4	62.7
Lupine /white/ vs.Watt /1982/	74.7	62.0	80.3	66.9	79.0	65.6
- " - vs.Horizont -"-	78.7	68.4	86.4	73.3	82.9	69.4
- " - vs.Nyirségi -"-	78.5	65.6	81.3	68.0	81.9	68.5
Soyabean vs. S 1346 /1982/	66.6	54.4	70.5	56.5	72.1	58.8
- " - vs. Ewans -"-	67.5	55.3	78.8	65.3	78.7	65.3
- " - vs. 1. s. 15. -"-	67.1	54.8	74.1	60.3	74.2	60.9
Wheat: 1	98.3	84.2	87.6	74.5	88.5	75.2
2	98.3	88.0	89.1	76.2	89.3	76.0
3	98.5	84.4	89.7	76.8	91.2	77.9
4	97.3	83.3	93.7	81.0	93.8	80.4
5	87.5	74.1	88.4	75.4	86.8	73.5
6	90.2	76.6	90.6	77.7	91.2	77.9
7	86.8	73.4	94.8	82.2	93.9	80.6
8	88.3	74.8	89.5	76.6	91.2	77.8
9	87.1	73.7	87.8	74.8	89.3	76.0
10	84.9	71.7	87.3	74.3	85.9	73.7
Maize: vs. Pioneer SC 3978	91.6	77.9	89.5	76.6	91.6	77.0
wet vs. - " - 3901	90.4	76.8	87.7	74.7	90.3	72.6
stored vs. SC 3390	88.0	74.6	85.8	72.7	88.2	74.9
vs. Iris G 303 DC	88.5	75.0	88.7	75.7	91.1	76.7
vs. Pioneer SC 3978	94.2	80.4	95.1	82.5	95.5	80.9
dry vs. - " - 3901	92.3	78.6	90.4	77.6	92.5	78.4
stored vs. SC 3390	93.3	79.5	91.1	78.2	93.4	79.0
vs. Iris G 303 DC	92.8	79.1	93.9	81.3	93.7	79.6

REFERENCES

Akeson, W.R., - Stahmann, M.A. /1964/: A pepsin-pancreatin digest index of protein quality. J. Nutr. 83. 257-261.

A.O.A.C. /1975/: "Official Methods of Analysis", 12th ed. Association of Official Analytical Chemists, Washington, D.C. p. 45.

Bodwell, C.E., - Satterlee, C.D., - Hackler, L.R. /1980/: Protein digestibility of the same protein preparations by human and rat assays and by in vitro enzymic digestion methods. Amer. J. Clin. Nutr. 33. 677-686.

Bodwell, C.E.,- Adkins, J.S., - Hopkins, D.T. /1981/: Protein Quality in Humans: Assessment and in Vitro Estimation, AVI Publishing Company; Inc. Westport, Connecticut.

Buchanan, R.A. /1969/: In vivo and in vitro methods of measuring nutritive value of leaf protein concentrates. Brit. J. Nutr. 23. 533-545.

Czakó, J. /1982/: Design and evaluation of livestock-breeding tests. Akadémiai Kiadó, Budapest.

Eggum, B.O. /1973/: 406. Beretn., National Institute of Animal Science, Copenhagen.

Ford, J.E., - Salter, D.N. /1966/: Analysis of enzymatically digested food proteins by Sephadex gel filtration. Brit. J. Nutr. 20. 843-860.

Hsu, H.W., - Vavak, D.L., - Satterlee, C.D., - Miller, G.A. /1977/: A multienzyme technique for estimating protein digestibility. J. Food Sci. 42. 1269-1273.

Hsu, H.W., - Sutton, N.E., - Banjo, M.O., - Satterlee L.D.,- Kendrick, J.G. /1978/: The C-PER and T-PER assays for protein quality. Food Technol. 32/12/. 69-73.

Maga, J.A., - Lorenz, K., - Onayemi, O. /1973/: Digestive acceptability of proteins as measured by the initial rate in in vitro proteolysis. J. Food Sci. 38. 173-174.

Marshall, H.F. - Wallace, G.W. - Satterlee, L.D. /1979/: Prediction of protein digestibility by an in vitro procedure using human, porcine and rat pancreatin preparations. Nutr. Rep. Int. 19. 901-913.

Pedersen, B. - Eggum, B.O. /1981/: Prediction of protein digestibility by in vitro procedures based on two multi-enzyme systems. J. Anim. Physiol. and Anim. Nutr. 45. 190-200.

Pedersen, B. - Eggum, B.O. /1983/: Prediction of protein digestibility by an in vitro enzymatic pH--stat procedure. J. Anim. Physiol. and Anim. Nutr. 49. 265-277.

Pellett, P.L. /1978/: Protein quality evaluation revisited. Food Technol. 32/5/, 60-79.

Rich, N. - Satterlee, L.D. - Smith, J.L. /1980/: A comparison of in vivo apparent protein digestibility in man or rat to in vitro protein digestibility as determined by using human and rat pancreatins and commercially available proteins. Nutr. Rep. Int. 21. 285-300.

Satterlee, L.D. - Marshall, H.F. - Tennyson, J.M. /1979/: Measuring protein quality. J. Am. Oil Chemist's Soc. 56. 103-109.

Saunders, R.M. - Connor, M.A. - Booth, A.N. - Bickoff, E.M. - Koehler, G.O. /1973/: Measurement of digestibility of alfalfa concentrates by in vivo and in vitro methods. J. Nutr. 103. 530-535.

Proc. Int. Assoc. Cereal Chem. Symp. Amino Acid Compn and Biol. Value of Cereal Proteins Budapest, Hungary 1983, R. Lásztity, M. Hidvégi, eds

OPTIMIZATION OF LYSINE COMPOSITION IN PLANT BREEDING PROGRAMMES AND IN FEED TECHNOLOGY BY THE DYE-BINDING ANALYSIS

LARS MUNCK

Carlsberg Research Laboratory, Department of Biotechnology, Gamle Carlsberg Vej 10, DK-2500 Copenhagen Valby, Denmark

The dye-binding capacity (DBC) method employs Acid Orange-G which binds to basic amino groups of proteins including lysine. This fast analytical method is used in plant breeding of high-lysine barley and to screen feed raw materials such as barley, fish meal, meat-bone meal, and soybean meal and practical feedlots of these raw materials. Interactions with calcium can be counteracted with addition of oxalic acid to the dye solution. The DBC-analyses may be used for

1. Controlling lysine level when used in combination with the Kjeldahl protein analysis
2. Controlling and minimizing the variation of protein within a specific feed mix or recipe
3. Controlling and minimizing variation of minor additives such as vitamins and minerals by controlling the variation of free calcium level of the mix.

The benefits of the DBC-analyses are discussed.

INTRODUCTION

The development of rapid and reliable methods for the measurement of the essential amino acids has been a rather slow process (Munck 1983). In spite of the tedious techniques developed from 1882-1900 by E. Fischer, T.B. Osborne and L.B. Mendel could in 1914 define the limiting amino acids - tryptophane and lysine - for growth in rats fed on the diet of the maize protein zein. In 1950 when Moore and Stein invented the chromatograpic methods, accurate amino acid analyses could be performed for the first time although the analysis took 24 hours for a complete aminogram.

As early as at the turn of the century 1800-1900, however, the dormant idea of a rapid analysis for one of the most important and essential amino acids - lysine - rested unnoticed. The potential know-how of such an analysis was embodied in the textile industry where diazo dyes at that time were introduced as a stain for proteinaceous textile fibre such as wool. It was already at that time clear that the diazo dyes had the capability to bind to the basic amino groups of a protein at a low pH (Fraenkel-Conrat and Cooper 1944, Rosenberg and Klötz 1960). The amino acids contributing to the free amino groups of protein are mainly lysine, arginine and histidine. In 1950 Udy (Udy 1954, 1971) introduced the diazo dye acid orange-12 or acilane-orange in a convenient method for estimating Kjeldahl protein (nitrogen x 6.25) in grains and feed. A fixed amount of the finely ground sample was reacted with the dye solution buffered at a pH of 2.0. The dye suspension was filtered and the decolorization of the filtered solution measured in a colorimeter with a short pathway cuvette was correlated to the protein content of the sample. As seen in Table 1, different commodities have different regression lines. In 1962-67 the dye-binding capacity (DBC) method according to Udy was tested on barley which was heat-treated at different

Table 1: Regression lines protein - dye-binding for various raw materials

Protein System $\% P = A(C_I - C)^*$	$\frac{1}{\text{Slope}}$ A	Intercept C_1	Sample Weight (mg)
Barley	26.7	1.064	800
Corn (Maize)	18.4	1.100	1000
Cotton seed meal	67.7	1.320	140
Fish meal	88.5	1.320	120
Soybean meal	61.5	1.320	160
Wheat	27.4	1.052	800

*) According to Udy: P = % protein, C = Dye concentration after the reaction

temperatures and water contents in closed bottles (Munck 1968, 1972). In an experiment demonstrated in Figure 1 it is seen that lysine is preferentially destroyed at a water content of around 15% when heating barley seeds. Treatment at 67°C for 168 hours did more effectively destroy lysine compared to 85°C in 24 hours. The ratio dye-binding to Kjeldahl protein (DBP:KP) varied in a similar way as the analyses for total lysine and available lysine. There was also a good correlation between gain in protein of laboratory mice and dye-binding (DBP:KP). Addition of lysine to the treated diets eliminated the growth differences (Munck 1968). The studies cited were made in cooperation with Mossberg who in 1969 proposed the DBC-method with acid orange-12 as a screening method for lysine and basic amino acids. The method was found to work with such different cereals as wheat, maize, barley, rye, and triticale. Fortunately, the intercorrelations between the basic amino acids are high in most protein materials which ensures that the DBC-method based on the sum of arginine, histidine, and lysine could give a representative estimate of lysine. Obviously the different slopes (A) obtained in the regression lines for DBC to Kjeldahl proteins demonstrated in Table 1 are proportional to the amount of basic amino acids and lysine in the various commodities listed, starting with fish meal and cotton seed meal at the upper end and finishing with maize which is especially low in lysine.

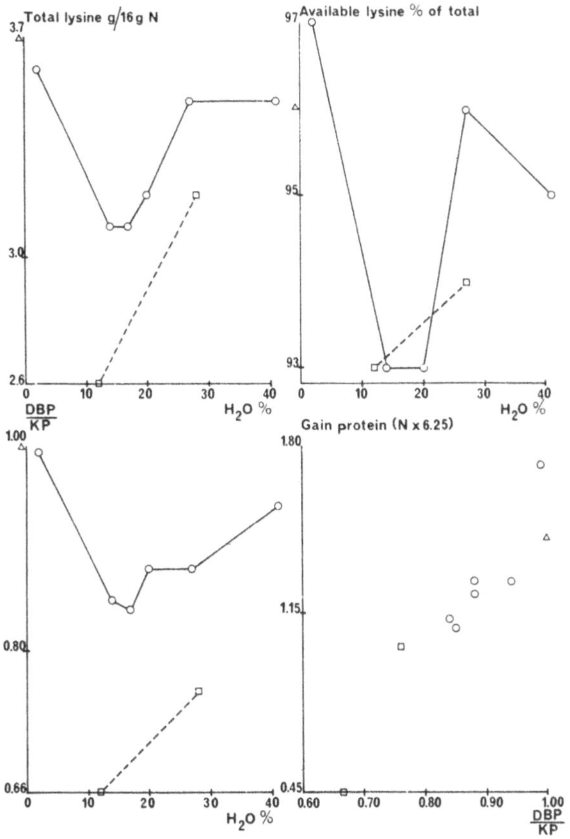

Fig. 1. The effect of heat-treatments of barley seeds on total lysine g/16 g N, available lysine % of total, and dye-bound protein: Kjeldahl protein ratio (DBP:KP) as related to water content during heat-treatment. Mouse gain in carcass protein is also correlated with dye-binding (DBP:KP). (Open circles: treatment 85°C for 24 hrs, open squares 67°C for 168 hrs, untreated control is marked with a triangle).

USE OF THE DBC-METHOD IN PLANT BREEDING PROGRAMMES

In 1966 the DBC-method combined with Kjeldahl protein analysis was used to select the first high-lysine barley line Hiproly from the world barley collection (Munck et al. 1970). The Hiproly gene lys was found to be inherited recessively. Figure 2 shows how high-lysine segregants (single plants in F_2) from a cross Hiproly x normal barley could be differentiated from the normal lysine types by plotting their DBC/kg against their protein content. In Figure 3 the lysine content of the two classes from Figure 2, high and low in DBC, are verified. The correlation between the sum of the basic amino acids lysine, arginine and histidine and the DBC-analysis is reasonable (Fig. 4) while the correlation between DBC and lysine is less optimal (Fig. 5), which again proves the limitation of

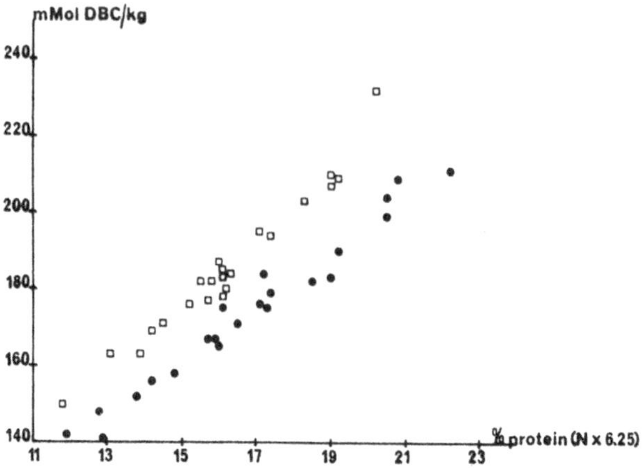

Fig. 2. Relation between dye-binding (mMol/kg) and crude-protein percentage in high-lysine (squares) and normal lysine (dots) barley segregants from a cross between Hiproly and normal barley.

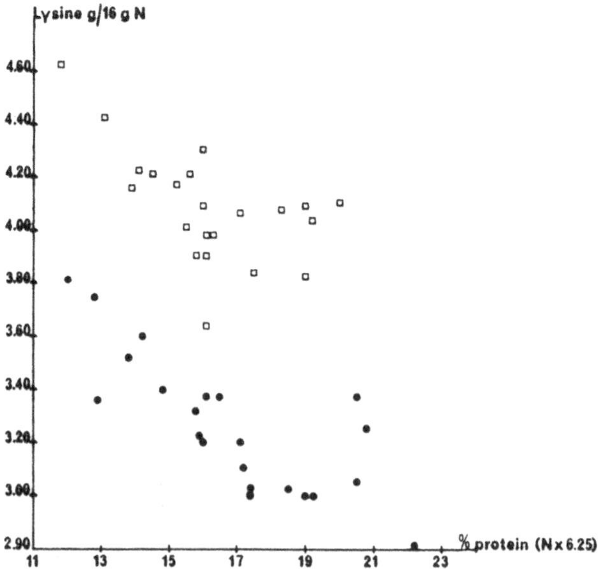

Fig. 3. Segregation for lysine (g/16 g N) at different crude-protein levels in F_2 from the material in Fig. 2.

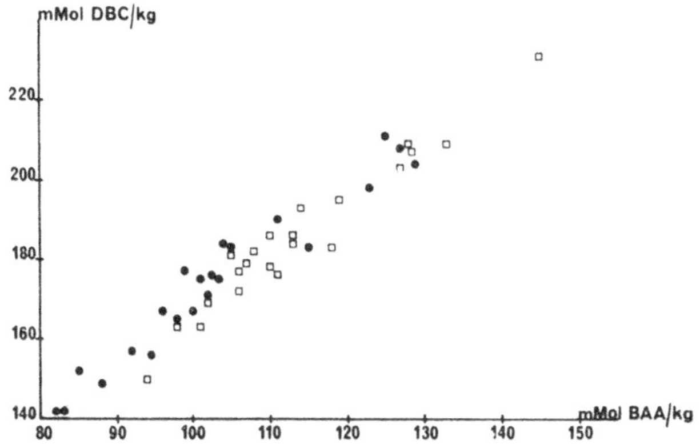

Fig. 4. Relation between dye-binding (mMol DBC/kg) and basic amino acids (mMol/kg; lysine, histidine and arginine). Material from Fig. 2.

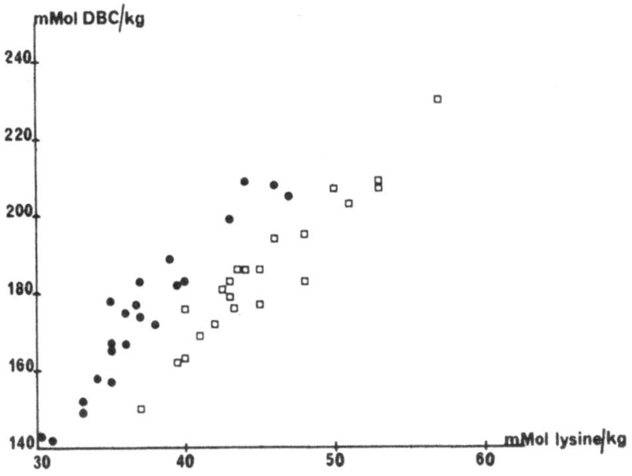

Fig. 5. Relation between dye-binding (mMol/kg) and lysine (mMol/kg) in high-lysine (squares) and normal lysine (dots) barley segregants from Fig. 2.

the DBC-method when used as an estimate for lysine. The intercorrelation between the basic amino acids is, however, good enough for the DBC-method to be used as a selection method for the high-lysine types (Munck 1976).

In fact, the DBC-method could be used for all cereals to estimate lysine also including the high-lysine types found in maize, sorghum, and barley (Munck 1980). In 1974 Doll et al. published a paper on an extreme lysine barley, mutant M-1508, using the DBC-Kjeldahl protein analysis as a selection criterium.

Table 2: Feeding trials with slaughter pigs with unsupplemented high-lysine and normal barley as compared to an optimal feed mixture

	Optimal Feed mixture	M 1508 type	Normal barley
Protein, g	189	143	99
Lysine, g	8.8	5.8	2.9
Methionine + cystine, g	6.5	4.9	3.4
Threonine, g	6.6	4.9	2.7
Feeding trials (20-90 kg)			
Feed mixture, kg	206	209	538
Number of feeding days, day	100	112	269
Daily growth, g	703	635	261
Relative performance (%)	100	98	34

A feeding trial with slaughter pigs, in Table 2, demonstrates the drastic nutritional effect of the improved lysine level of M-1508 barley. Normal barley has 2.9 g lysine/kg and M-1508 has 5.8 g lysine/kg compared to 8.8 g/kg in an optimal feed mixture. It is seen that the daily growth has increased from 261 g/day for normal barley to 635 g/day with M-1508, both fed without protein additives. In a complete barley-soybean meal diet, the daily growth was 703 g/day.

The main problem with high-lysine barley mutants, however, is that they are too low in yield and in starch and energy content. After 17 years of work, breeding for the high-lysine character in barley, I am, however, still optimistic. At the Carlsberg Research Laboratory we have now improved M-1508 types obtained by intense crossing and selection which are as high yielding as the controls displaying an improved starch content. Without the DBC-method this breeding work would have been impossible.

Due to the low price of soybean meal in comparison with the price of cereals (ratio 2:1 or less) in the western world, the economical benefit of breeding high-lysine cereals as demonstrated in Table 3 is low (Bach Knudsen and Munck 1981). In other countries, e.g. in Eastern Europe, however, there is a lack of protein additives and thus the advantage of the improvement of lysine in feed commodities is more appreciated in agricultural development programmes.

Table 3: Chemical composition (g/kg) and economical value of normal and high-lysine barley at two extreme protein levels

	Feed* barley	Normal lysine barley 8% protein	Normal lysine barley 16% protein	High lysine barley 8% protein	High lysine barley 16% protein
Protein, g	108	80	160	80	160
Lysine, g	3.9	3.2	4.8	4.2	8.3
Methionine + cystine, g	4.2	3.1	6.2	3.1	6.2
Threonine, g	3.6	2.6	5.3	3.2	5.3
Economical value (%)**	100	99.6	100.6	100.4	103.1

*) Table values for chemical composition
**) Based on soybean meal price to barley 2:1.

USE OF DBC-ANALYSES IN FEED TECHNOLOGY

Protein additives such as fish meal are expensive, and a quality control of these commodities with regard to lysine is thus important. Processing might introduce heat damage which is especially critical for the available lysine content. In Figure 6 and Table 4 the variation of available lysine and total lysine of fish meal, meat-bone meal, and soybean meal is demonstrated showing large variations particularly with regard to fish meal. As indicated before, DBC will reflect changes in lysine due to both heat-treatment as well as to the natural variation.

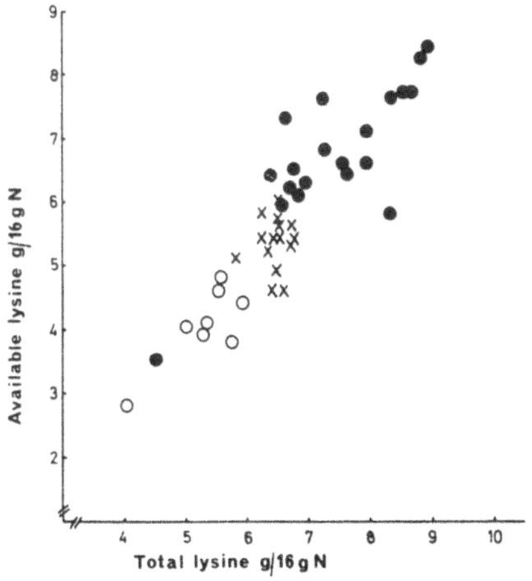

Fig. 6. Relation between available lysine (g/16 g N) and total lysine (g/16 g N) in feed supplements. (Full circles: fish meal, open circles: meat-bone meal, crosses: soybean meal).

Table 4: Chemical composition (g/kg) and economical value of extreme samples of fish meal, meat and bone meal, and soybean meal

	Fish meal			Meat + bone meal			Soybean meal		
	Min	Table Value	Max	Min	Table Value	Max	Min	Table Value	Max
Protein, g	500	702	760	372	512	605	435	450	510
Lysine, g	22.5	55.5	68.4	18.6	25.0	35.0	25.2	27.0	30.6
Methionine + cystine, g	23.0	26.7	28.9	6.8	9.3	11.0	13.8	14.3	16.2
Threonine, g	22.0	35.1	38.0	10.8	14.8	17.5	16.0	16.6	18.8
Economical value (%)	78.2	100	106.2	95.1	100	110.9	98.5	100	103.5

Table 5: The combined effect of extreme negative and positive compositions of feedstuffs on the chemical composition and performance value of a feed mixture for slaughter pigs (FU_p and g/kg). Material from Table 3 (normal barley) and from Table 4 and Figure 6. See also Munck 1972.

		Min	Max	Theory Δ	Found in practice Munck 1972 Δ
FU_p	0.98	0.96	0.99		
Crude protein, g	161	148	169	21	26
Lysine, g	7.7	5.9	8.7	2.8	1.9
Calcium, g	8	7.5	9.5	2.0	6.0
Phosphorus, g	6	5.4	7.5	2.1	3.5
Performance value (%)	100	92	101		

Recipe (%): Barley 74.2, wheat 11.0, soybean meal 3.6, fish meal 5.0, meat and bone meal 2.1, molasses 3.0, limestone flour 1.0, vitamin - micro-nutrients 0.2.

Cereal protein is an important contributor to lysine in feed mixtures for monogastric animals, and a check on the lysine and protein content of cereals could therefore spare protein additives. Normally, table values of e.g. barley (Table 3) and protein supplements (Table 4) are used for feed optimization. In order to obtain a guaranteed limit of lysine and protein in the diet, protein additives have to be given in excess as a precaution. This problem is demonstrated in Table 5 where the extreme diets as regards crude protein, lysine, calcium, and phosphorus are constructed from the raw materials in Tables 3 (normal barley only) and 4 (protein supplements) to show the maximal theoretical variation in performance value with the given variation in raw material composition. While an oversupplementation only increases the calculated animal performance with 1%, undersupplementation decreases performance with 8%. The actual variation found in a survey of the quality of commercial pig feeds (Munck 1972) was slightly less with regard to lysine but as great as the theoretical maximal variation with regard to crude protein and still higher for calcium and phosphorus, presumably depending on the difficulty of mixing small amounts of fine mineral powders evenly with large amounts of feed.

The question is now how the DBC-method could be used to control the feed quality and its variation.

Firstly, it is possible to use the DBC-method in combination with the Kjeldahl protein analysis to assess lysine (basic amino acids) in both feed raw materials and in feed mixtures. Materials containing free calcium give analytical problems with the original DBC-method because calcium precipitates the dye. This could be fully counteracted by the addition of oxalic acid to the dye buffer. Oxalic acid forms an insoluble complex with calcium and eliminates the interaction between calcium and acid-orange 12.

Secondly, the DBC-method can also be used in order to control the Kjeldahl protein content within a feed mix if a defined mixture of raw materials is selected and thus the content of basic amino acids on protein base is constant. The DBC-analysis can thus be used to check the mixing efficiency of cereals and protein additives in the feed plant and to secure a thorough economical dosage of the protein additives (Fig. 7). Such a check would provide security in obtaining the guaranteed standard of feed product delivered without oversupplementing expensive protein additives. Thus a minimization of variation in protein and lysine content in the feed mixture would secure increased profits to the feed plant operation by sparing expensive additives. Also the animal breeders would appreciate a more constant feed quality because in practice a too high level of protein may e.g. increase the incidence of swine dysentery and risk the health of the lactating sow.

The third way of using the DBC-method is to check the mixing-in of limestone meal as a representative of a minor finely milled additive. The full feed is analysed with dye solutions with and without oxalic acid. The difference (Δ-DBC) is proportional to the free calcium (e.g. from limestone) in the mix (Fig. 8). Minor components with a small particle size such as vitamins and minerals are often more difficult to mix accurately and evenly than the more coarse protein additives. The Δ-DBC tells the feed mill operator the accurate function of the mixing equipment with regard to the mixing-in of the minor components. The Δ-DBC cannot be used as a measurement of total calcium in the feed mix using protein with mineral components from animals because it does not measure bound calcium (e.g. calcium phosphate).

The feed industry in general is rather conservative and is slow in introducing and utilizing modern analytical methods such as the DBC-

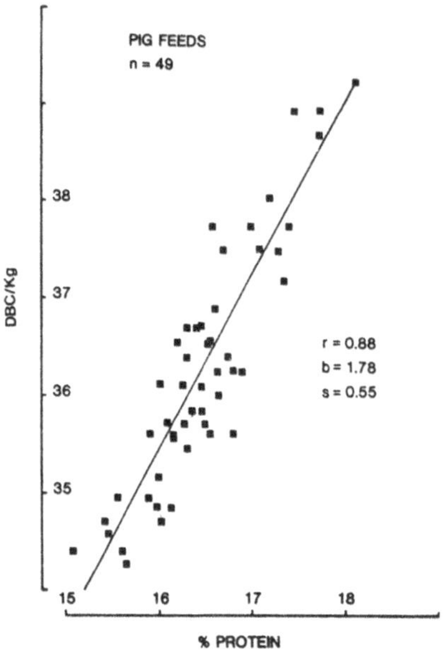

Fig. 7. Relation between DBC/kg and Kjeldahl protein % in pig feed samples.

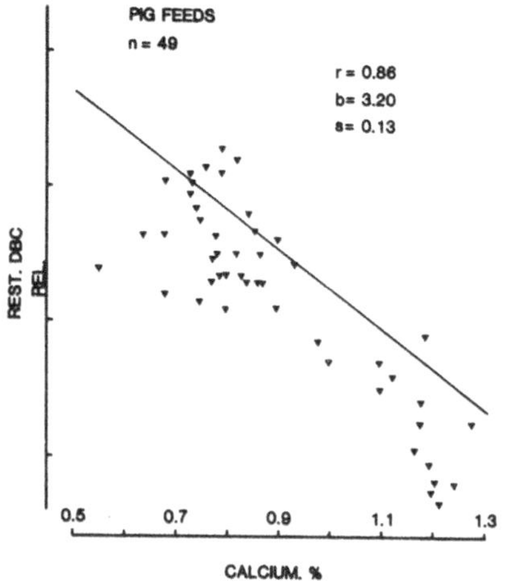

Fig. 8. Relation between calcium % and Δ-DBC (see text) in pig feeds with added limestone meal.

technique (Munck 1979). After having investigated the use of the DBC-technique in an operating feed mill, we have obtained positive evidence that the DBC-analysis is capable of

1) controlling lysine level on raw materials and feed mixtures if used in combination with the conventional Kjeldahl protein analysis

2) controlling and minimizing the variation of Kjeldahl protein within a specific feed mix (or recipe)
3) controlling and minimizing the variation of minor additives (vitamins and minerals) by controlling the variation of the free calcium level of the mix.

These new methods need basic understanding, preferably in combination with computer-based optimization of recipes, in order to be applied. If properly practiced, however, they will greatly contribute to the economical success of the feed mill involving merely the expenses of the wages of one skilled technician or engineer and of a small laboratory.

ACKNOWLEDGEMENT

The assistance of lic.agro. Knud Erik Bach Knudsen regarding the economical calculations and of Kirsten Kirkegaard for typing the manuscript is gratefully acknowledged.

REFERENCES

Doll, H., Køie, B. and Eggum, B.O. (1974). Induced high lysine mutants in barley. Rad. Bot. 14: 73-80.

Fraenkel-Conrat, H. and Cooper, M. (1944). The use of dyes for determination of acid and basic groups in proteins, J. Biol. Chem. 154: 239.

Knudsen, K.E. Bach and Munck, L. (1981). The feasibility of breeding barley for feed quality exemplified by the nutritional analysis of the botanical components of Bomi and the 1508 high lysine mutant. 4th Int. Barley Genetics Symp., Edinburgh, pp. 320-329.

Mossberg, R. (1969). Evaluation of protein quality and quantity bye dye-binding capacity: A tool in plant breeding. New Approaches to Breeding for Improved Plant Protein. Proc. Panel Röstånga. International Atomic Energy Agency, Vienna 151.

Munck, L. (1968). Cereals for feed - quality and utilization. J. Swed. Seed Ass. 78: 137-201.

Munck, L., Karlsson, K.E., Hagberg, A. and Eggum, B.O. (1970). Gene for improved nutritional value in barley seed protein. Science 168: 985-987.

Munck, L. (1972). Improvement of nutritional value in cereals. Hereditas 72: 1-128.

Munck, L. (1976). Aspects of the selection, design and use of high lysine cereals. Proc. Evaluation of Seed Protein Alterations by Mutation Breeding. International Atomic Energy Agency, Vienna.

Munck, L. (1979). Genetic potential for improved crop quality. Proc. Workshop on Agricultural Potentiality Directed by Nutritional Needs. Hungarian Academy of Sciences, Budapest. (Ed. S. Rajki, Akadémiai Kiadó, Budapest).

Munck, L. (1980). The genetical basis for protein improvement in cereals. Proc. XIV Congress of Genetics, Moscow, 1978). (Ed. M.E. Vartanian, MIR Publishers, Moscow), pp. 249-259.

Munck, L. (1981): Barley for food, feed and industry. Proc. Conference Cereals: A Renewable Resource, Theory and Practice, Copenhagen (Eds. Y. Pomeranz and L. Munck, The American Association of Cereal Chemists, St. Paul, Minn., U.S.A.), pp. 427-460.

Munck, L. (1983). Nutrition and health aspects on cereals in human diet. Conf. Food Production-Nutr.-Health, Royal Swedish Academy of Science, Uppsala, 1981 (Akadémiai Kiadó, Budapest).

Rosenberg, R.M. and Klötz, I.M. (1960). Dye-binding methods. A Laboratory Manual of Analytical Methods of Protein Chemistry (Eds. P. Alexander and R.J. Block). Pergamon Press, New York, pp. 133.

Udy, D.C. (1954). Dye-binding capacities of wheat flour protein fractions. Cereal Chem. 31: 389.

Udy, D.C. (1971). Improved method for estimating protein. J. Am. Oil Chem. Soc. 48: 29A.

Proc. Int. Assoc. Cereal Chem. Symp. Amino Acid Compn and Biol. Value of Cereal Proteins Budapest, Hungary 1983, R. Lásztity, M. Hidvégi, eds

DETERMINATION OF REACTIVE LYSINE BY DYE-BINDING

BARÁTH A., HALÁSZ A.

Central Food Research Institute, H-1525 Budapest, P.O.B.76, Hungary

The availability of essential amino acids highly influences the biological value of foods. Among essential amino acids, as a limiting amino acid, lysine has a distinguished importance and its availability can be measured chemically as well. The greatest part of in vitro methods known for the rapid and routine-like determination of available lysine content is based on the principle that the availability of lysine depends on the free state of the ε-amino group of the lysine molecule.

In recent years, the selective dye-binding method of HURREL and CARPENTER (1976) got widespread fot the determination of the available amount of lysine. WALKER (1979) applied the dye-binding method as well to follow up the availability of the lysine content in the production of plant protein concentrates.

In our laboratory this latter method has been adapted, being a modified alternative of the HURREL and CARPENTER procedure.

Principle of the procedure

The dye-binding method is based on the bond of the azodye Acid Orange 12 to the alkaline amino groups of the proteins. A free amino group of this kind is contained in lysine, in histidine, in arginine, thus these three amino acids are determined by the s.c. dye-binding capacity (DBC). In case the ε-amino group of the lysine is blocked with anhydrous propionic acid, the reactive (available) lysine content can be determined specifically by the difference between the two dye-binding capacities. As there is a selective bond of the anhydrous propionic acid to the ε-amino acid group of the lysine, it is not capable to bind this dye after blockage, thus by deducing the DBAP value (=ARG+HIS) of the propionated sample of the DBC value (=ARG+HIS+rLYS) of the unpropinated sample, we get as a result the reactive lysine content (DBL = dye-binding lysine).

The main steps of the determination can be seen on Fig.1.

The main steps of the determination

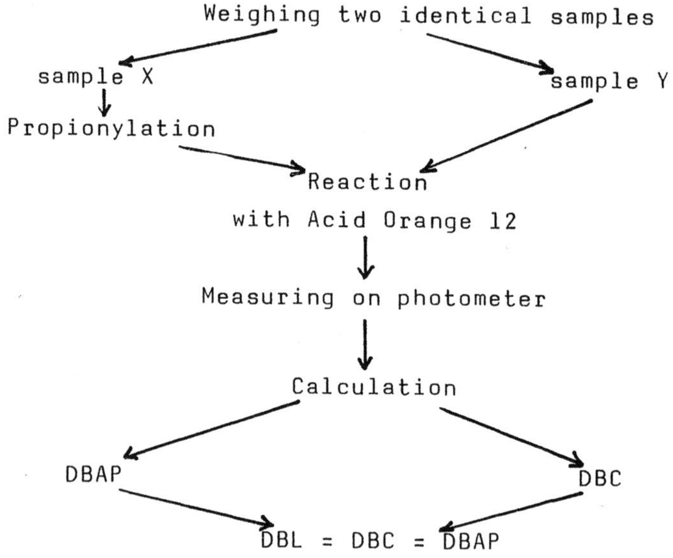

Fig.1

In the realization of the methods the following aspects were taken into consideration:

- it seemed to be necessary that the determination of the optimal sample weight should be taken, being in relation with the protein content of the test sample

- the determination of the suitable concentration range for the plotting of the standard curve from the point of view of reweighing of the dye remainder from the test portion, further in order to reduce the error of extinction measurement to the minimum.

Determinations were carried out according to Fig.1. From two similar test portions a suspension was prepared with 2-2 cm^3 of semi-saturated Na-acetate solution. As a following step, in one of the samples prepared the blockage of ε-amino acid groups was carried out with the addition of 0.2 cm^3 anhydrous propionic acid in a laboratory shaker, by shaking it for 15 minutes at room temperature. Then, the dye-binding reaction was made with the propionylated and unpropionylated probe, with the addition of 40-40 cm^3 Acid Orange 12 dye solution (3.89 $mmol/dm^3$) shaking for 1.5 hours in a laboratory shaker.

Following this procedure, centrifugation took place for 10 minutes with a rotation speed of 3000 min^{-1}. The solution can be filtered, but a special silicon-impregnated filter-paper should be used as a certain dye-binding capacity of the normal filter paper risks the accuracy of measurement. After centrifugation, 1 cm^3 of the supernatant was diluted 100-fold and extinction was measured on a wavelength of 480 nm corresponding to the absorption maximum in a cell of 1 cm pathlenght, using distilled water as reference.

On the basis of resulting extinction values and the calibration curve, the amount of dye not bound by the test sample can be read. Based on this, the dye-binding can be calculated for propionylated and for unpropionylated samples as well. The calibration curve needed was prepared from recrystallized Acid Orange 12 dye in a concentration range between 3.89 $mmol/dm^3$ - 1.11 $mmol/dm^3$ (Fig.2).

Calibration curve of recrystallized Acid Orange 12

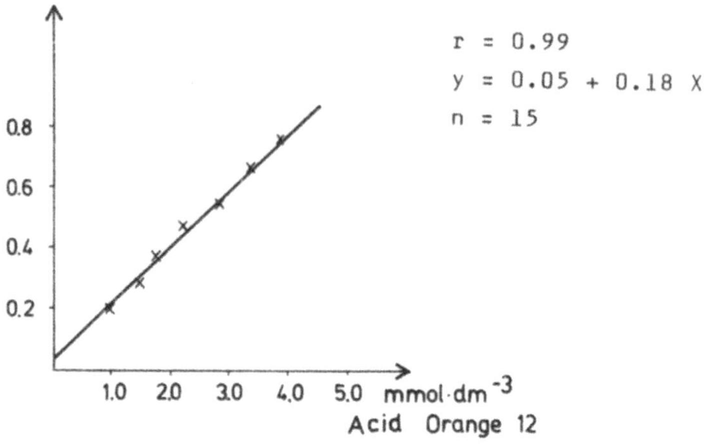

Fig.2

On determining the lysine content by the dye-binding method the test conditions influence the amount of interaction. In order to obtain reproducible results it is recommended to standardize the test conditions.

Studying the reproducibility of the method, several assays were carried out with the same sample under similar test conditions. As a result we found that the parallel values vary between relatively wide boundaries, and 5-20 p.c. variation coefficients were observed.

During our experimentations made with the above procedure, comparison was made with samples of different protein contents between the protein values measured with a Kjel-Foss automatical instrument for nitrogen-determination and the values of dye-binding capacity (DBC). The relation obtained can be seen in Fig.3 and as it is presented on the figure, there is a close regression between values of Kjel-Foss and DBC, the correlation coefficient being 0.96.

Relationship between dye-binding capacity and protein content

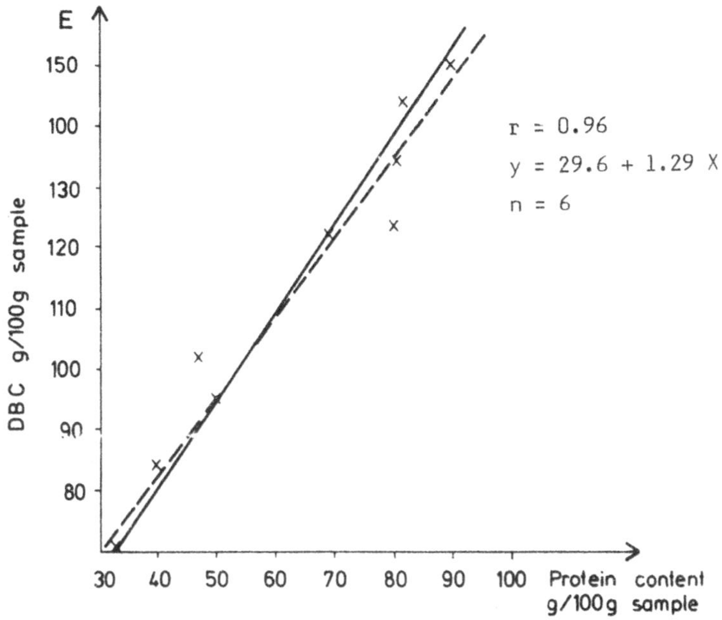

Fig.3

Further, comparative tests were made from samples with various protein contents between the dye-binding lysine content of the samples and their available lysine content determinated by amino acid analyser blocked with fluorodinitrobenzene. The relation between the two available lysine contents determinated by two different methods is presented in Fig.4, where the close correlation between the two methods can be observed.

The method described has been used for the testing of macaroni products prepared of AESTIVUM and DURUM flours (both of them TL-55), and of samples made of these flours among laboratory conditions extruded at three different

The relationship between fluorodinitrobenzene (FDNB) reactive lysine and dye-binding lysine (DBL)

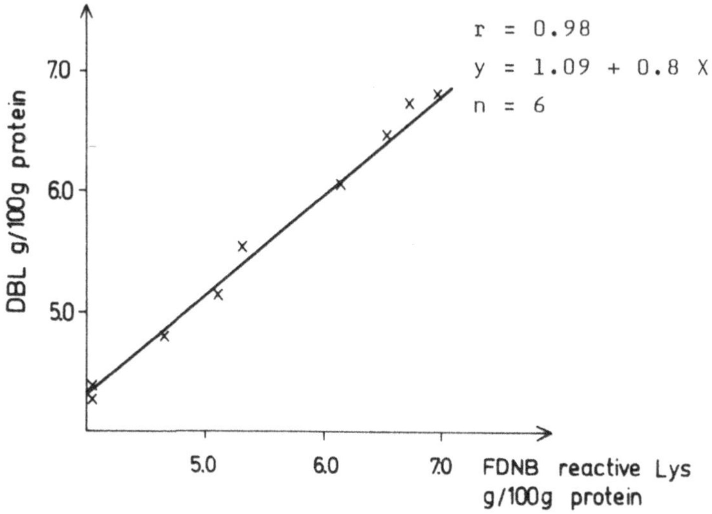

Fig.4

temperatures (40-, 70- and 90°C). The main characteristics of the tested flours were given in Table 1.

Table 1

The main characteristics of the tested flours

	AESTIVUM	DURUM
Moisture content	11.53 %	11.0 %
Ash content	0.34 %	0.75 %
Fat content	0.33 %	0.62 %
Wet gluten	19.5 g/100 g flour	21.4 g/100 g flour
Protein content (Kjel -Foss)	11.9 %	13.8 %

The testing of the flour samples started with the determination of optimal amounts to be weighed in. As the protein content of the test samples is relatively low, large amounts had to be weighed in. In both cases, the work started with sample sizes of 0.8, 1.0 and 1.2 g. In Fig.5, the dye-binding capacity (DBC), dye-binding after the propionylation (DBAP) and the dye-binding lysine content (DBL) were plotted in the function of the sample size.

From the figure it can be seen that for both flour samples an optimum could be observed at a weigh-in of 1 g. For this reason, we used an amount of 1g in case of testing the flour as well as the macaroni samples.

The pasteproducts used as assay models were produced on laboratory extruder type BRABENDER with an extrusion at temperatures of 40-, 70- and 90°C and drying at room temperature.

The effect of sample weight on the amount of dye-bound

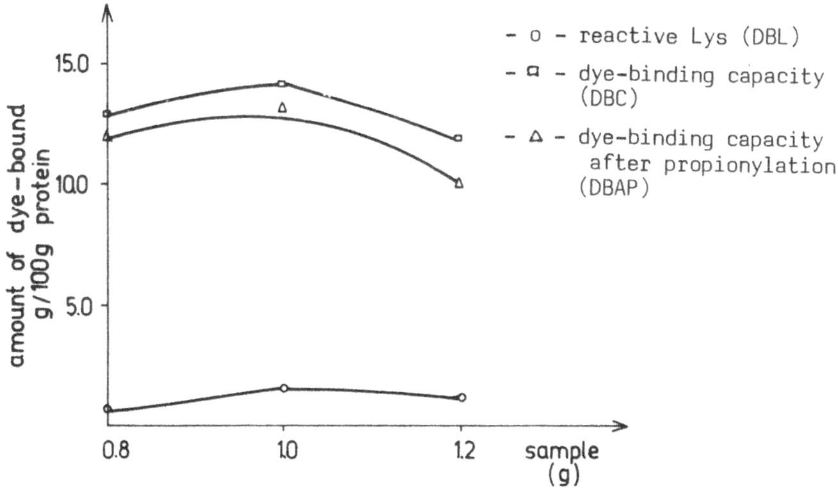

Fig.5

From the samples thus prepared the available lysine content were determined by the method described above and the crude protein content by the Kjel -Foss automatical instrument for nitrogen determination.

In Table 2 the data of macaroni products made of AESTIVUM flour and extruded among laboratory conditions are presented.

Table 2

Reactive lysine content of extruded paste made of AESTIVUM flour

Extrusion temperature °C	Reactive Lys (DBL) g/100 g protein	Protein content (Kjel-Foss) %
o (flour)	1.3	11.9
40	1.3	12.2
70	1.2	12.3
90	1.15	12.2

In Table 3 the data of extruded paste made of DURUM flour are given.

Table 3

Reactive lysine content of extruded pasta made of DURUM flour

Extrusion temperature °C	Reactive Lys (DBL) g/100 g protein	Protein content (Kjel-Foss) %
0 (flour)	1.44	13.8
40	1.40	14.0
70	1.38	14.0
90	1.28	14.0

It can be seen from the data that the change in the measured available lysine content caused by extrusions at increasing temperatures is of similar range as the variation coefficient of the method. Thus finally, the changes due to the tested technological process (heat treatments at different temperatures) cannot be registered by the dye-binding method in the available lysine content.

Nevertheless, the dye-binding method, due to its simple and rapid operational procedure, can be applied favourably for routine examinations, for the analysis of large sample series, thus for the determinations of the available lysine content of various flour samples, pasta products and other cereals.

Finally, we would like to draw attention to the fact- - in relation with this method - that in order to get reliable information on the available lysine content the optimal size of the sample to be weighed in should be determined, a dye solution of permanent concentration should be prepared to be performed generally with the recrystallization of the dye, and last but not least, due to the relatively large variation coefficient of the parallels, assays should be carried out from each sample.

REFERENCES

HURREL,R.F., CARPENTER,K.J. (1976): An approach to the rapid measurement of reactive lysine in foods by dye-binding. The proceedings of the Nutrition Society 35, 23A-24A.

WALKER,A.F. (1979): Determination of protein and reactive lysine in leafprotein concentrates by dye-binding. Br.J.Nutr. 42, 445-454.

WALKER,A.F. (1979): A comparison of the dye-binding and fluorodinitrobenzene methods for determining reactive lysine in leaf protein concentrates. Br.J.Nutr. 42, 455-465.

PART 3

CHEMISTRY (AMINO ACID COMPOSITION) AND BIOCHEMISTRY OF CEREAL PROTEINS

Proc. Int. Assoc. Cereal Chem. Symp. Amino Acid Compn and Biol. Value of Cereal Proteins Budapest, Hungary 1983, R. Lásztity, M. Hidvégi, eds

COMPARATIVE AMINO ACID COMPOSITION OF PROTEINS OF WHEAT, RYE AND TRITICALE GRAIN

GOLENKOV V. F.

All-Union Research Institute for Grain and Grain Products, Dmitrovskoe Chaussee 11, Moscow 127434, USSR

In the paper there is given an analysis of numerous studies of amino acid composition of total proteins of wheat, rye and triticale grain, and also of gluten obtained from these grain crops. Comparison of physico-chemical properties of gluten of wheat, rye and triticale grain and carob beans allows to make an assumption about particular significance of the quantitative content of glutamic acid and proline.

The problem of providing people with nutritious food is growing more and more urgent with every year practically in all countries of the globe.

According to the studies of food consumption on a world-wide scale carried out by FAO and WHO, about 40-50% of the total consumed protein is provided by cereal crops.

In connection with the above mentioned, comparison of amino acid composition of proteins of such crops as wheat, rye and triticale grown on considerable areas, especially in Europe, is of certain interest.

However, it is erroneous to evaluate amino acid composition of proteins of these crops only from the point of view of their nutritive value.

Amino acid composition of protein mainly stipulates its structure and physico-chemical properties and, consequently, it influences technological properties of wheat, rye and triticale grain.

During the last 15-20 years in the laboratories of many countries tnere were carried out quite a few investigations on amino acid composition of proteins of all cereal crops.

In this communication principal attention is given to the analysis of the researches conducted in the USSR.

In recent years in our country amino acid composition of cereal crops was studied in detail with applying most efficient methods of sample preparation and analysis.

The greatest attention was paid to the amino acid composition of wheat proteins depending on different rates of fertilizer application and wheat variety in different regions of the country (1, 14, 15, 20, 21, 23, 26, 27, 30), however, there was also carried out a number of researches of amino acid composition of rye, triticale and other rye-wheat hybrids (4, 5, 7, 9, 16-19, 22, 24, 25, 32).

Summarized mean data of numerous investigations of amino acid composition of wheat, rye and triticale grain grown in the Soviet Union are given in Table 1.

These data are of interest mainly when comparing nutritive value of the mentioned crops since results of the investigations are expressed in grammes of amino acids per 100 g of the product (13) and consequently the content of amino acids is influenced by the protein content of the grain.

The given data show that total content of the essential amino acids of triticale is practically the same compared with that of durum wheat and exceeds that of soft wheat and rye. These data agree well with the results of determination of biological value of triticale grain when feeding laboratory animals (2, 10). However they do not show special features of the total proteins of these crops and their variability depending on variety, agrotechnical and climatic conditions.

Table 2 gives comparative data on amino acid composition of proteins of wheat, rye and triticale.

The results of the analyses show that depending on the content of many amino acids, proteins of triticale of home breeding take intermediate position between proteins of wheat and rye. It is worth to be mentioned that average lysine content in triticale is considerably higher, and variations of lysine content in wheat, even with its maximum value, do not exceed its minimum value of triticale. Rye has a maximum content of lysine and threonine, and its variations of the contents of these amino acids are also higher than those of wheat and triticale.

It is necessary to mention that triticale proteins in comparison with the parental forms have a tendency to higher contents of tyrosine, leucine and isoleucine and to lower contents of proline. Similar data were obtained when analysing triticale in other countries (3). Besides the above mentioned, from the available data it is possible to observe considerable variations in amino acid contents. A special study (7) of variability of amino acid composition of rye to-

Table 1. Amino acid composition (%) of wheat, rye and triticale grain (moisture content 14%)

Amino acids	Wheat		Winter rye	Triticale (hexaploid)
	winter soft	durum		
Essential including:	3,43	3,72	2,95	3,73
lysine	0,36	0,34	0,37	0,41
valine	0,52	0,58	0,48	0,61
isoleucine	0,47	0,52	0,40	0,46
leucine	0,86	0,97	0,62	0,89
methionine	0,18	0,18	0,15	0,18
threonine	0,39	0,37	0,38	0,39
tryptophan	0,15	0,14	0,13	0,14
phenylalanine	0,50	0,62	0,50	0,65
Non-essential including:	8,40	8,63	6,75	8,78
alanine	0,46	0,46	0,42	0,47
arginine	0,61	0,63	0,52	0,62
aspartic acid	0,67	0,68	0,67	0,73
histidine	0,35	0,38	0,20	0,29
glycine	0,47	0,50	0,43	0,49
glutamic acid	3,35	3,68	3,66	3,77
proline	1,29	1,19	0,93	1,32
serine	0,60	0,60	0,42	0,52
tyrosine	0,37	0,42	0,28	0,38
cystine	0,23	0,19	0,16	0,19
Total	11,83	12,35	10,72	12,51

tal proteins has allowed to clear up the influence of the fractional composition.

Changes of amino acid composition of total proteins are influenced, as it is widely known, by changes of relationship between different protein fractions - albumins, globulins, prolamines and glutelins.

Relatively high content of some essential amino acids (lysine and threonine) in rye proteins is the consequence of high quantity of albumins and globulins, and their summed contents can reach 50% while the contents of these fractions in wheat seldom reach 20-25% of the total proteins.

In this rather brief communication it is impossible to

Table 2. Amino acid composition of proteins of wheat, rye and triticale grain in the USSR (% of total protein)

Amino acids	Wheat (26)		Rye (7)		Triticale (25)	
	mean	variations	mean	variations	mean	variations
Lysine	2,64	2,4-2,8	3,91	3,2-5,3	3,06	2,8-3,5
Histidine	2,04	1,7-2,4	2,13	2,6-0,8	2,03	1,8-2,2
Arginine	4,38	3,8-4,9	6,00	4,6-7,7	4,56	4,2-4,9
Aspartic acid	4,87	4,5-5,7	7,32	2,0-9,8	6,56	4,8-9,8
Threonine	2,68	2,5-2,9	3,25	2,5-3,7	2,80	2,5-3,0
Serine	3,98	3,1-4,4	4,61	3,9-5,8	4,26	4,2-4,6
Glutamic acid	32,38	30,0-35,4	30,07	25,6-35,1	34,2	34,0-34,4
Proline	10,32	9,5-12,1	9,93	9,1-12,9	8,76	8,5-9,2
Glycine	3,92	3,4-4,4	4,56	3,7-5,2	4,76	4,0-6,0
Alanine	3,53	3,3-3,8	4,52	4,1-5,3	4,90	3,6-7,5
Cystine	1,91	1,5-2,4	1,80	1,6-1,9	1,83	1,8-1,9
Valine	3,99	3,7-4,8	5,23	5,0-7,2	5,46	4,6-6,7
Methionine	1,50	1,2-2,6	1,51	1,2-1,7	1,56	1,5-1,6
Isoleucine	3,17	2,6-3,9	3,54	3,0-4,3	3,80	3,5-4,1
Leucine	6,61	5,5-7,2	6,72	5,3-7,9	7,26	7,0-7,5
Tyrosine	2,59	2,2-3,3	3,05	2,9-3,7	3,40	3,o-4,2
Phenyl-alanine	4,21	3,9-5,0	4,92	3,7-5,6	4,63	4,2-4,9
Tryptophan	1,21	0,9-1,4	1,42	1,3-1,5	1,33	1,3-1,4

consider in detail amino acid composition of different protein fractions, and that's why I would like to dwell upon the amino acid composition of wheat, rye and triticale gluten.

Importance of gluten for forming baking quality of wheat is widely known. As for its physical properties wheat gluten has, as a rule, higher elasticity compared with rye gluten, and triticale gluten occupies an intermediate position. Besides, it is worth mentioning that while triticale gluten, like wheat gluten, rather easily washed out with water by a wide-spread method, washing out rye gluten, requires special conditions (29).

It is known that many studies of amino acid composition of gluten could not determine relationship between amino acid contents and physical properties of gluten (elasticity, extensibility). Therefore comparison of amino acid composition of gluten of these three crops is of significant interest.

Table 3. Amino acid composition of gluten of wheat, rye and triticale grain (% of total protein)

Amino acids	Wheat (28,31)	Rye (8)	Triticale (34)
Lysine	2,1	2,6	2,8
Histidine	2,3	2,5	2,5
Arginine	4,5	4,0	4,7
Aspartic acid	3,7	4,3	4,2
Threonine	3,5	3,2	3,0
Serine	5,2	6,2	4,7
Glutamic acid	41,0	51,1	39,3
Proline	14,5	17,0	12,4
Glycine	3,9	4,1	3,7
Alanine	3,1	3,1	3,5
Cystine	2,3	2,5	2,4 *
Valine	5,3	5,4	4,4
Methionine	1,7	1,8	1,6 *
Isoleucine	4,9	4,4	4,4
Leucine	8,3	9,1	7,9
Tyrosine	3,8	3,6	3,2
Phenylalanine	6,0	7,1	5,9
Ammonia	3,5	2,8	4,2

* Data obtained in the research (12)

In Table 3 mean data on determination of amino acid composition of wheat gluten (15 samples), rye gluten (12 samples) and triticale gluten (12 samples) of the crops grown in different regions of the USSR are presented (8,12,28,31,34).

Comparison of these mean data allows to note that as to most amino acids, glutens of these three cereals differ very little. Differences in histidine, threonine, alanine, cystine, valine, methionine and tyrosine contents are just within the error of the method. Small differences are observed in lysine, arginine, serine, glycine, leucine, phenyl--alanine contents.

Particularly great difference is observed in glutaminic acid and proline contents. Rye gluten has the highest content of glutamic acid, wheat and rye gluten - practically the same. However triticale has the lowest proline content. Proline, as it is well known, plays a particular role in the structure of protein. In parts of its location, curving of the polypeptide chain and change of the form of the α-spiral of a protein molecule take place. Since gluten proteins of wheat, rye and triticale grain have different proline contents, their structures have significant differences. It is also possible to assume that increased content of glutamic acid in rye gluten is, to a certain extent, responsible for its low elasticity and high extensibility. This assumption agrees well enough with the fact that polyglutaminic acid has increased solubility in weak-alkali water solutions. The same conclusion can be made when comparing amino acid composition of wheat and rye gluten and gluten-like complex of carob beans (Ceratonia siliqua L.) (6). Protein complex of bean germs of C. siliqua, as our investigations have shown, resembles very much wheat gluten as for its physical properties, but differs with its higher elasticity and lower extensibility. Unlike wheat, rye and triticale gluten it has insignificant quantity of alcohol-soluble proteins (only 6%) and contains much less of glutamic acid and proline (20,6 and 2,6%, respectively). Thus, comparison of amino acid composition of wheat, rye and triticale gluten allows to assume that the contents of glutamic acid and proline influence to a certain extent formation of physical properties of this specific cereal complex.

References

1. Batudaev A.P. (1980). Povyshenie urozhainosti i kachestva ozimoi pshenitsy v uslovijakh nechernozjomnoj zony pod deistviem vozrastajushchikh doz mineral'nykh udobrenij. Doklady VASHNIL, 9, 40-42.
2. Boronoeva G.S., Kazakov E.D. (1969). Aminokislotnyj sostav zerna jarovoj rzhi. Prikladnaja biokhimija i mikrobiologija, 5, 3, 314-317.
3. Chen C.H., Bushuk W. (1970). Nature of proteins in triticale and its parental species. 1. Solubility characteristics and amino acid composition of endosperm proteins. Canadian J. Plant Sci. 50, 9.
4. Gil'zin V.M., Golenkov V.F. (1974). K voprosu o statisticheskoj otsenke rezul'tatov aminokislotnogo analiza zerna. Trudy VNIIZ, 79, 113-119.
5. Gil'zin V.M. et al. (1977). Aminokislotnyj sostav i electroforeticheskie osobennosti belkov razlichnykh chastej zernovki rzhi. Bjulleten' Glavnogo botanicheskogo sada, 106, 58-62.
6. Golenkov V.F. (1961). Klejkovina semjan rozhkovogo dereva. Biokhimija zerna. Trudy nauchnoj konferencii VNIIZ, 41, 101.
7. Golenkov V.F., Gil'zin V.M. (1971). Issledovanie aminokislotnogo sostava belkov zerna ozimoj rzhi. Prikladnaja biokhimija i mikrobiologija, 7, 3, 328.
8. Golenkov V.F. et al. (1972). Aminokislotnyj sostav klejkoviny rzhi. Prikladnaja biokhimija i mikrobiologija, 8, 4, 392.
9. Gruzdev L.G., Zhebrak E.A. (1976). Biokhimicheskaja kharakteristika i kachestvo belkov zernovykh tritikale v processe sozrevanija. Sbornik nauchnykh rabot NII sel'skogo khozjajstva Central'no-chernozjomnoj polosy, 13, 1, 115-122.

10. Hulse J.H., Laing E.M. (1974). Nutritive value of triticale protein. International Development Research Centre. Ottawa, Canada.
11. Ivanova V.N. (1980). Vlijanie uslovij vyrashchivanija na aminokislotnyj sostav zerna jachmenja i pshenitsy (v Sverdlovskoj oblasti). Trudy Sverdlovskogo sel'skokhozjajstvennogo instituta, 60, 87-91.
12. Khachaturjan E.E. (1978). Issledovanie biokhimicheskikh i tekhnologicheskikh svojstv muki tritikale kak novogo vida khlebopekarnogo syr'ja. Avtoreferat dissertacii na soiskanie uchjonoj stepeni kandidata tekhnicheskikh nauk, Moskva.
13. Khimicheskij sostav pishchevykh produktov. (1979). Izdatel'stvo "Pishchevaja promyshlennost'", Moskva.
14. Krjuk I.F., Furs I.N. (1981). Aminokislotnyj sostav belkov muki i zerna pshenits BSSR. Sbornik "Tovarovedenie i ljogkaja promyshlennost'", 8, Minsk.
15. Kuz'mina M.V. (1975). Ob aminokislotnom sostave belkov pshenitsy. XI Mendeleevskiy s'ezd po obshche i prikladnoj khimii, Moskva.
16. Kuznetsova N.E., Pleshkov B.P. (1979). Biokhimicheskaja kharakteristika belkov zerna tritikale. Prikladnaja biokhimija i mikrobiologija, 15, 2, 165-171.
17. Lysenkov V.I. et al. (1979). Aminokislotnyj sostav belka zerna mutantov mjagkoj pshenitsy. Doklady VASHNIL, 8, 7-9.
18. Magda Khabib Morsi Allam (1977). Biokhimicheskie osobennosti semjan nekotorykh sortov ozimoj formy tritikale. Sbornik nauchnykh trudov BSHA, 34, 17.
19. Mekhanik F.J., Allam Magda Khabib (1977). Biokhimicheskie osobennosti semjan nekotorykh obraztsov ozimoj formy tritikale. Sbornik nauchnykh trudov BSHA, 34, 109-114.
20. Mineev V.G. et al. (1979). Vlijanie udobrenij pri sistematicheskom primenenii v sevooborotakh na belkovost' i aminokislotnyj sostav zerna pshenitsy. Agrokhimija, 10, 37-46.
21. Nenajdenko G.N. et al. (1978). Vlijanie razlichnykh doz azota, ispol'zuemykh v rannevesennjuju podkormku ozimoj pshenitsy, razmeshchaemoj posle sternevogo predshestvennika, na khimicheskij sostav rastenij i kachestvo urozhaja. Nauchnye trudy Leningradskogo sel'skokhozjajstvennogo instituta, 338, 31-44.
22. Philipas T.B., Bukreeva G.I. (1979). Aminokislotnyj sostav belkov zerna i produktov ego pererabotki u sortov linij pshenitsy i tritikale. Sbornik nauchnykh trudov Krasnodarskogo NIISH, 19, 129-143.
23. Pleshkov B.P. et al. (1978). Aminokislotnyj sostav belkov zerna pshenitsy i pshenichno-pyrejnykh gibridov. Vestnik sel'skokhozjajstvennoj nauki, 2, 12-20.
24. Pleshkov B.P. et al. (1980). Soderzhanie i sostav belkov v zerne pshenichno-pyrejnykh gibridov pri razlichnykh uslovijakh azotnogo pitanija. Izvestija TSHA, 2, 57.
25. Rukosuev A.N., Silant'eva A.G. (1972). Aminokislotnyj sostav zerna rzhi, rzhanoj sejanoj i obdirnoj muki i otrubej. Voprosy pitanija, 31, 5, 42-45.

26. Ryadchikov V.G. (1978). Uluchshenie zernovykh belkov i ikh ocenka. Izdatel'stvo "Kolos", Moskva.
27. Shljonskaja T.V. (1981). Aminokislotnyj sostav zerna pshenitsy. Khlebopekarnaja i konditerskaja promyshlennost', 10, 36.
28. Shorina O.S. et al. (1966). Fiziko-khimicheskie izmenenija klejkoviny pri prorastanii pshenitsy. 2. Aminokislotny sostav. Prikladnaja biokhimija i mikrobiologija, 11, 2, 121.
29. Sirotkin V.V. et al. (1975). Metod vydelenija klejkoviny iz rzhanoj muki. Prikladnaja biokhimija i mikrobiologija, 11, 2, 277.
30. Somin V.I. (1966). Izuchenie aminokislotnogo sostava pshenitsy nekotorykh ozimykh sortov. In: Institut pitanija. Material XYI nauchnoj sessii, Moskva, II, 174.
31. Vakar A.B. (1968). Fiziko-khimicheskie i biokhimicheskie faktory kachestva klejkoviny. Dissertacija na soiskanie uchjonoj stepeni doktora biologicheskikh nauk, AN SSSR, Institut pitanija, Moskva.
32. Zhebrak E.A., Kolchin N.M. (1968). Sostav belkovykh komponentov diploidnoj i tetraploidnoj rzhi. Sel'skokhozjajstvennaja biologija, 3, 3, 439-441.
33. Zhmakina O.A. et al. (1977). Sravnenie biologicheskoj cennosti belkov zerna pshenitsy, rzhi i tritikale. Prikladnaja biokhimija i mikrobiologija, 13, 4, 595-599.
34. Zhmakina O.A. et al. (1977). Aminokislotnyj sostav klejkoviny tritikale. Prikladnaja biokhimija i mikrobiologija, 13, 6, 915-918.

Proc. Int. Assoc. Cereal Chem. Symp. Amino Acid Compn and Biol. Value of Cereal Proteins Budapest, Hungary 1983, R. Lásztity, M. Hidvégi, eds

BIOENERGETIC ASPECTS OF AMINO ACID PRODUCTION IN CEREALS

RUDOLF NEHÉZ

Cereal Research Institute, H-6701 Szeged,
Alsókikötősor 9, Hungary

For assessment of the potential productivity of plants, biochemical mass equivalents were introduced in simple carbohydrate units on the basis of the biosynthetic pathways in the plants. At present energy relations are given for amino acids. Energy data are introduced and applied as enthalpy + input /red/ values, i.e. enthalpy + energy requirements for the reduction of the oxidized forms /nitrate, sulphate/ of nitrogen and sulphur. A considerable proportion of the energy in amino acids is present in the chemical bonds of the reduced N and S forms. The formation of amino acids and proteins is not simply an energy question. Biochemical mass equivalents and energy values have been calculated for the amino acid compositions of proteins in seeds. Calculations have also been performed on the carbohydrate, oil and protein contents of seeds. It is evident that plant productivity can be increased equally via the mass of the crop yield, changes in its chemical composition, and energy production.

As plant cultivation becomes increasingly more intensive, ever greater attention is devoted to achieving the conformity of cultivation and Nature. The natural possibilities tend to be considered primarily as economic factors. This means that efforts are made to increase the biological and agricultural efficiencies of organic matter production, through the agroecological potential /Láng, 1980/, the genetic potential /Vida et al., 1980/, the regional location of cultivation for quality /Szániel, 1980/, the biological aspects of agrotechnology, and a number of other factors.

The effectiveness and productivity of plant cultivation are assessed in most cases in terms of the crop mass yield. Since plants can store solar radiation energy in the form of chemical bonds and their organic matter structures, it is evident that this is output too. The formation of plant organic matter represents the increased, long-lasting and reversible storage of extremely valuable hydrogen energy. Intermediate main carriers for energy are carbohydrates, oils and proteins /Hoffmann, 1978/. Plants provide energy for the whole living kingdom. Profitable plant cultivation can be achieved through a rational energy economy. This is the case for energy produced by all living organisms /Kurnik, 1977/. Plants are renewable sources of energy.

Kurnik /1977/ and others consider that the present age is faced with two great problems: the obtaining of energy and the production of protein. Their existence and insufficiency must be regarded as strategic factors /Baade, 1965/. Unfortunately the increase of protein yield per hectare is not of primary importance in plant cultivation or farming. Genetic, agroecological and other potentials may be important for the increase of the crop yield and for the improvement of its quality /Bálint, 1977/.

The inverse yield-nitrogen law states that the yields of all agrotypes, without any clearly proved exceptions to date, are inversely proportional to the nitrogen content of the total above-ground plant matter under normal conditions /Wilcox, 1954/.

In efforts to elevate productivity in plant cultivation, the aims may be an increased crop mass yield, modification of the chemical composition or the production of more plant energy. The primary importance of one or other of these factors is given by the economic aspects.

In our laboratory screening work on the protein contents of cereals for breeders during the past 15 years, we have achieved very modest results. We have failed to combine in one wheat, maize or other variety a high protein percentage with a high productivity. Breeding programmes throughout the world to attain high protein contents have similarly not attained satisfactory results. The failures have led to a number of breeders giving up such work /Johnson, Mattern, 1980/. It is possible to strive for higher protein contents if the concept of productivity is not limited merely to mass. A biochemical approach to plant productivity and its relations to mass, chemical composition and energy are discussed.

MATERIALS AND METHODS

On the basis of biosynthetic pathways in plant organisms parameters were earlier introduced for the maximal masses, which are equivalent to unit mass of the simple carbohydrate. The effectivity was characterized by the minimal carbohydrate equivalent /ME/ and the production equivalent /1/ME/ /Nehéz, 1971/. The 1/ME values were also termed biochemical minimal mass equivalents. The minimal losses of biosyntheses are derived from the relation 1 - 1/ME.

The substrate-yield correlations of the biosynthesis of plant organic matter were elaborated in the wide-ranging work of Penning de Vries et al. /1974/. They made every effort to define all the mass and energy requirements involved in the plant metabolism. It was believed that the metabolism in higher plants may operate at nearly the maximum efficiency allowed by the biochemical schemes, under fully aerobic conditions and a number of other assumptions.

Their parameters were employed to estimate seed-crop production on the basis of photosynthetate and nitrogen requirements /Sinclair, De Wit, 1975/, in plant breeding for increased protein and oil levels /Bhatia, Rabson, 1976; Mitra, Bhatia, 1979/ and for genetically modified amino acid contents /Mitra et al. 1979/. In practical wheat breeding, negative correlations are interpreted in biochemical terms on the basis of the data of Penning de Vries et al. /1974/ /Kramer, 1980/. Our values for carbohydrate, fibre, oil and protein are in agreement with the data of Penning de Vries et al. /1974/, but our data were obtained in another way. The concept "elemental equivalent" /EE/ denotes the stoichiometric determinacy /according to the law of mass ratios/ of plant organic matter in mass as compared to simple carbohydrate /$-CH_2O-$/x, corresponding to the proportions of the chemical elements. The "minimal equivalent" /ME/ is the equivalent of simple carbohydrate necessary for 1 mass unit of a certain plant organic substance, with regard to the biosynthetic pathways. Minimal equivalents involve elemental equivalents too. These values have been calculated for about 950 plant organic compounds. The meaning of the energy values 1/ME has also been explained /Nehéz, 1971, 1974a, 1975b/.

The protein, protein fraction and amino acid compositions of seeds were investigated by means of minimal equivalents for various forms and endosperm mutants of maize /Nehéz, 1974b, 1975b/, for barley /Nehéz, 1975a/ and for various cereals /Nehéz, 1977b/. From the chemical compositions, minimal equivalents were calculated for fatty acids and sterols of seed oils /Nehéz, 1977a, 1978b/. Energy contents for amino acids relative to oxidized and reduced forms of N and S were calculated, as were the net changes of enzyme energies for various biosynthetic pathways /Nehéz, 1978a, 1980/. A technique was developed to achieve higher productivity than before in plant cultivation, by growing varieties with high oil and protein contents /Nehéz, 1979b, 1984a/.

RESULTS AND DISCUSSION

The results prove that plant production may be increased either by means of the mass yield produced, or by modification of the chemical composition /especially with high oil and/or protein contents/ or through the energy values. The biochemical mass and energy equivalents, and the energy values, are listed in Table 1 /Nehéz, 1983a, 1983b, 1984b/.

Table 1. Biochemical mass and energy equivalents, energy values

Component	1/ME in mass	1/ME in energy	kJ/g
Starch	0.90	1.00	17.362
Plant			
carbohydrate	0.87	0.98	17.675
fibre	0.80	0.95	18.614
oil	0.34	0.86	39.575
protein, from nitrate, sulphate	0.40	0.90	30.685 34.334
proteir, from ammonia, sulphide	0.57	1.22	x

Such detailed values for plant amino acids permit an estimation of their role in vegetal productivity. The importance of the energy of amino acids is measured by means of chemical binding numbers /oxidation numbers or electron equivalents/. These have been taken from the work of Schulek and Kőrös /1955/. The differences between the binding numbers of the oxidized and the reduced forms of C, N and S are 8 in each case, namely +4 - -4, +5 - -3 and +6 - -2, respectively /see Table 2/.

Table 2. Chemical binding numbers /oxidation numbers/

In moles / amino acid mol	From CO_2, NO_3^- and SO_4^{2-}			From CO_2, NH_4^+ and S^{2-}		
	$+IV_C$	$+V_N$	$+VI_S$	$+IV_C$	$-III_N$	$-II_S$
Glycine	6	8		6	0	
Alanine	12	8		12	0	
Serine	10	8		10	0	
Cysteine	10	8	8	10	0	0
Cystine	20	16	14	20	0	-2
Aspartic acid	12	8		12	0	
Asparagine	12	16		12	0	
Threonine	16	8		16	0	
Proline	22	8		22	0	
Glutamic acid	18	8		18	0	
Glutamine	18	16		18	0	
Valine	24	8		24	0	
Methionine	22	8	8	22	0	0
Histidine	20	24		20	0	
Leucine	30	8		30	0	
Isoleucine	30	8		30	0	
Lysine	28	16		28	0	
Arginine	22	32		22	0	
Phenylalanine	40	8		40	0	
Tyrosine	38	8		38	0	
Tryptophan	46	16		46	0	

The energy values for C, N and S are about 109.192, 106.052 and and 91.063 kJ/mol binding number, respectively. The chemical binding numbers are purely formal. They cannot give absolutely reliable energy values. The changes in chemical binding numbers for the amino acids were presented previously /Nehéz, 1978a/. Similar results were reported by McDermitt and Loomis /1981/.

Biochemical mass equivalents and energy values are tabulated from levels of nitrate and sulphate. Enthalpy values have been taken from the handbook of Sober et al. /1970/ /ΔH_0^c, 25 °C/. Values for histidine were calculated from binding numbers. For the reduction of nitrate and sulphate, energies of 960.5 kJ/mol each for N and S /2/6 mol glucose/ were used. These values are in agreement with the observations of Warburg and Negelein /1920/ /cit. Netter, 1969/ and approach well to those of other authors /Penning de Vries et al. 1974/. The enthalpy values taken from energy tables relate to chemical binding numbers of 0 for N and S.

Table 3 contains biochemical mass equivalents, enthalpy + energy values for the reduction of nitrate and sulphate to values of 0 for N and S, and enthalpy - energy values for the reduction from values of 0 for N and S.

Table 3. Biochemical mass equivalents and energy values for amino acids

	1/ME in mass $+V_N$, $+VI_S$	Enthalpy $+input_{red}$ kJ/g	1/ME in energy $-III_N$, $-II_S$	Enthalpy $-input_{red}$ kJ/g
Glycine	0.452	20.666	0.707	7.873
Alanine	0.536	24.661	0.840	13.880
Serine	0.632	19.347	0.991	10.209
Cysteine	0.467	24.137	0.870	8.281
Cystine	0.465	23.212	0.870	8.351
Aspartic acid	0.678	16.375	0.978	9.158
Asparagine	0.485	23.346	0.868	8.807
Threonine	0.607	22.098	0.875	14.033
Proline	0.404	28.738	0.511	20.396
Glutamic acid	0.514	19.204	0.650	12.676
Glutamine	0.403	25.502	0.603	12.359
Valine	0.457	29.890	0.597	21.689
Methionine	0.469	27.181	0.752	14.306
Histidine	0.356	31.397	0.608	12.825
Leucine	0.379	31.728	0.458	24.403
Isoleucine	0.458	31.717	0.580	24.365
Lysine	0.404	33.126	0.603	19.985
Arginine	0.340	34.738	0.640	12.684
Phenylalanine	0.439	31.648	0.522	25.832
Tyrosine	0.481	27.721	0.573	22.420
Tryptophan	0.377	33.235	0.485	23.829

The data demonstrate that the energy values for enthalpy + input /red/ are quite high, while values of enthalpy - input /red/are very much lower. This fact reveals that the reduced forms of N and S contain a considerable proportion of the energy of the amino acids.

Biochemical mass equivalents /from nitrate and sulphate/ and energy values /enthalpy + input /red// have been calculated for the amino acid contents of cereals and other seeds. The basic data were taken from a FAO publication /Anonymous, 1970/, and the values for rape from a handbook /Nesterin, Skurikhin, 1970/. The basic data on the amino acids were calculated for 100 g protein by means of given conversion factors for protein/nitrogen.

The amino acid composition data /see Tables 4a and 4b/ include values relating to aspartic acid and glutamic acid. The biochemical mass equivalents and energy values were calculated for amino acids without amides. In the other case, however, the calculations were made just as if these two amino acids were amides. These calculations were polarized; the real values are within the extremes.

Table 4a. Amino acid compositions of seeds

	Wheat	Maize	Barley	Rye	Oat	Sorghum
Conversion factor	5.83	6.25	5.83	5.83	5.83	6.25
Amino acid g per: g nitrogen	17.15	16.00	17.15	17.15	17.15	16.00
Glycine	4.202	3.920	4.133	4.648	5.042	2.976
Alanine	3.876	3.616	4.236	4.562	4.871	9.344
Serine	4.922	4.592	4.339	4.630	5.042	4.112
Cystine	2.727	2.544	2.435	2.041	2.864	1.504
Aspartic acid	5.282	4.928	6.071	7.666	8.266	6.496
Threonine	3.138	2.928	3.550	3.584	3.550	3.024
Proline	10.650	9.936	11.696	10.050	5.557	8.112
Glutamic acid	32.002	29.856	25.279	25.914	22.449	21.152
Valine	4.733	4.416	5.402	5.094	5.471	5.008
Methionine	1.612	1.504	1.784	1.561	1.801	1.392
Histidine	2.452	2.288	2.264	2.367	2.247	2.144
Leucine	7.152	6.672	7.100	6.603	7.786	13.312
Isoleucine	3.499	3.264	3.842	3.756	4.047	3.920
Lysine	3.070	2.864	3.704	3.636	3.979	2.016
Arginine	4.939	4.608	5.059	4.905	6.740	3.072
Phenylalanine	4.836	4.512	5.505	4.733	5.368	4.896
Tyrosine	3.207	2.992	3.327	2.058	3.533	2.672
Tryptophan	1.166	1.088	1.646	0.789	1.355	1.216

Table 4b. Amino acid compositions of seeds

	Rice	Pea	Soya bean	Rape	Sun-flower	Peanut
Conversion factor	5.95	6.25	5.71	6.25	5.30	5.46
Amino acid g per: g nitrogen	16.81	16.00	17.51	16.00	18.87	18.32
Glycine	5.245	4.048	4.570	4.305	6.378	4.232
Alanine	6.321	4.080	4.658	4.058	4.963	2.986
Serine	5.699	4.336	5.603	3.677	5.095	6.522
Cystine	1.126	1.120	1.453	2.256	1.755	1.429
Aspartic acid	10.775	4.560	12.800	6.188	10.926	7.438
Threonine	4.102	4.064	4.395	3.673	4.340	2.986
Proline	4.925	3.904	6.006	6.502	5.265	5.148
Glutamic acid	21.634	16.144	20.469	16.592	25.720	15.682
Valine	5.783	4.704	5.253	4.605	5.982	4.782
Methionine	2.437	0.912	1.383	2.197	2.246	1.319
Histidine	2.622	2.288	2.767	2.601	2.736	2.528
Leucine	8.640	6.800	7.809	6.502	7.567	7.328
Isoleucine	4.001	4.272	4.973	3.511	5.038	3.866
Lysine	3.984	7.520	6.986	5.233	4.246	4.049
Arginine	8.674	9.520	7.914	6.399	9.416	8.519
Phenylalanine	5.413	4.592	5.411	3.722	5.246	5.698
Tyrosine	3.665	2.736	3.432	3.798	2.227	4.470
Tryptophan	1.311	0.896	1.401	1.614	1.604	1.191

The biochemical mass equivalents and energy values were calculated from the most reliable-seeming analytical data. The conversion factors refer to proteins and not amino acids, and they are not exact. The nitrogen contents are variable, e.g. with the degree of amidation. It is generally believed that the proteins of seeds, especially those of cereals, are almost completely amidated. However, Lásztity /1981/ observed that wheat gluten proteins have an amidation degree of 80–95 %. It is by no means irrelevant whether a nitrogen content of 16 % or some other N level is taken for calculation. In more accurate calculations, many other factors must be taken into consideration.

The amino acids in proteins are linked via peptide bonds. It is believed that the splitting of peptide bonds requires only activation energy. However, about 3 ATP /adenosine triphosphate/ per peptide bond is necessary for the formation of these bonds /Penning de Vries et al. 1974/.

From the basic data on the amino acids, the biochemical mass equivalents and energy values are listed in Tables 5a and 5b.

Table 5a. Biochemical mass equivalents and energy values for amino acids

	Wheat	Maize	Barley	Rye	Oat	Sorghum
Sum of amino acids without amides	103.465	96.528	101.372	98.597	99.968	96.368
1/ME in mass from nitrate, sulphate	0.497	0.464	0.484	0.478	0.484	0.463
Enthalpy + input /red/ kJ/g	25.699	23.976	25.579	24.565	25.285	23.751
Sum of amino acids with amides	103.211	96.284	101.152	98.362	99.753	96.174
1/ME in mass from nitrate, sulphate	0.450	0.420	0.443	0.433	0.442	0.427
Enthalpy + input /red/ kJ/g	28.926	26.144	27.724	26.678	27.226	26.347

Table 5b. Biochemical mass equivalents and energy values for amino acids

	Rice	Pea	Soya bean	Rape	Sun-flower	Peanut
Sum of amino acids without amides	106.357	86.496	107.283	87.433	110.750	90.173
1/ME in mass from nitrate, sulphate	0.518	0.406	0.509	0.416	0.538	0.432
Enthalpy + input /red/ kJ/g	23.110	22.977	27.165	22.682	27.677	23.433
Sum of amino acids with amides	106.130	86.351	107.050	87.264	110.493	90.011
1/ME in mass from nitrate, sulphate	0.472	0.379	0.461	0.385	0.487	0.399
Enthalpy + input /red/ kJ/g	25.173	24.278	29.293	24.122	30.000	24.903

The values of the mass equivalents are low in seeds that have high oil and/or protein contents. The energy values are higher for wheat, barley, oat, rye and sorghum than for maize and rice. The seeds of sunflower and soya bean have high energy values, while peanut pea and rape have low values. Biochemical mass equivalents and energy values have been calculated for the amino acid compositions of gliadin, glutenin and gluten. The basic data were taken from Lásztity /1981/. The values have been calculated for 100 g amino acid /Tables 6a and 6b/.

Table 6a. Amino acid compositions of gliadin, glutenin and gluten

g amino acid in 100 g of amino acids	Gliadin	Glutenin	Gluten
Glycine	5.112	15.026	9.284
Alanine	4.304	5.519	4.994
Serine	5.545	6.879	5.645
Cystine	0.637	0.602	0.865
Aspartic acid	2.305	2.499	2.452
Threonine	2.317	3.155	2.615
Proline	19.715	14.319	17.646
Glutamic acid	33.042	27.323	29.229
Valine	5.629	5.062	5.696
Methionine	1.233	1.163	1.192
Histidine	1.483	1.212	1.434
Leucine	7.248	6.284	6.671
Isoleucine	4.327	3.086	3.732
Lysine	0.524	1.285	0.914
Arginine	1.321	1.660	1.703
Phenylalanine	3.528	2.363	2.873
Tyrosine	1.354	1.996	2.619
Tryptophan	0.376	0.567	0.436

Table 6b. Biochemical mass equivalents and energy values for amino acids

	Gliadin	Glutenin	Gluten
Sum of amino acids without amides	100.000	100.000	100.000
1/ME in mass from nitrate, sulphate	0.447	0.482	0.478
Enthalpy + input /red/ kJ/g	24.595	24.060	24.540
Sum of amino acids with amides	99.765	99.802	99.789
1/ME in mass from nitrate, sulphate	0.435	0.446	0.440
Enthalpy + input /red/ kJ/g	26.783	25.911	26.504

The results point to a high biochemical mass equivalent and a low energy value for glutenin.

The average chemical compositions of seedcrops were taken from handbooks for the calculation of biochemical mass equivalents and energy values. The calculations were performed with joint values for carbohydrate and fibre and are recorded here as carbohydrate /1/ME from nitrate and sulphate: 0.83; energy value: 18.077 kJ/g/. The values refer to air-dry and dry matter /Tables 7a and 7b/.

Table 7a. Compositions of seed crops

	Carbohydrate %	Oil %	Protein %	Ash %	Water %
Wheat	71.2	1.9	12.2	1.7	13.0
Maize	70.5	4.4	8.9	1.2	15.0
Barley	71.0	2.4	10.9	2.6	13.0
Rye	71.7	1.7	11.6	2.0	13.0
Oat	66.7	5.8	11.3	3.2	13.0
Sorghum	73.8	3.5	11.2	1.2	10.0
Rice	77.7	1.7	7.5	1.1	12.0
Pea	59.1	1.9	23.4	2.6	13.0
Soya bean	31.3	19.8	31.3	4.6	13.0
Rape	22.3	43.6	20.4	4.2	9.5
Sunflower	30.7	44.0	14.1	3.2	8.0
Peanut	24.3	42.8	26.2	2.7	4.0

Table 7b. Biochemical mass equivalents and energy values for seed crops

	1/ME in mass	Energy value kJ/g	1/ME in mass	Energy value kJ/g
	in air-dry matter		in dry matter	
Wheat	0.663	17.366	0.762	19.961
Maize	0.648	17.217	0.762	20.255
Barley	0.668	17.129	0.768	19.688
Rye	0.667	17.193	0.767	19.762
Oat	0.651	17.820	0.748	20.483
Sorghum	0.669	18.163	0.744	20.181
Rice	0.692	17.020	0.786	19.341
Pea	0.617	18.616	0.709	21.398
Soya bean	0.498	23.098	0.573	26.549
Rape	0.457	27.546	0.505	30.438
Sunflower	0.493	27.289	0.536	29.662
Peanut	0.633	29.370	0.659	30.594

It is evident from the values that the high oil and protein levels point to low mass equivalents, but the energy values are quite high.

For the relations of chemical composition, biochemical mass equivalent and areal mass output, i.e. of productivity, a model is presented as an example in Table 8. It is very clear that maize B yields higher productivity.

In plant cultivation, the economic expectations in most cases means the areal mass yield /ton/hectare/. The tendencies in the biochemical mass equivalents and energy values seem to be contradictory, but biochemically they are self evident. By means of these numbers, the various forms of plant productivity /i.e. mass, chemical composition and vegetable energy/ can be assessed. The formation of organic matter means energy storage and therefore output too. The various forms of productivity can be calculated together from the energy values.

Table 8. Model for chemical composition, biochemical mass equivalents, energy values, areal mass and energy data

	Maize A	Maize B
Grain yield ton/hectare	5.00	5.00
Chemical composition:		
Carbohydrate %	72.50	66.50
Oil %	4.40	6.40
Protein %	6.90	10.90
Ash %	1.20	1.20
Water %	15.00	15.00
1/ME in mass from nitrate, sulphate	0.656	0.639
Energy value GJ/ton	16.964	17.899
Mass yield ton/hectare	5.00	5.00
Energy value GJ/hectare	84.820	89.495

It is possible to increase the yields /in mass/ more easily than the protein contents by breeding work or in some other manner /Ryadchikov, 1978/. The mass and chemical composition of plant organic matter are determined by inheritance and by environmental factors. These determine which organic compounds in the plants accumulate solar energy and to what extent. Thus, the production of amino acids and proteins is not simply a question of energy. Breeding programmes to increase protein levels in cereals have failed, the combination of high levels of plant mass /ton/hectare/ and protein concentration /%/ in one variety has remained unsuccessful. This fact is not a chance one, but is a consequence of biochemical causes.

Our work gives rise to the practical conclusion that plant productivity can be increased by means of the mass yield, the change of chemical composition and an increased energy efficiency. Such an assessment of the plant processes of production is possible on the basis of calculations relating to varieties, habitats, growing technology and other factors, in the knowledge of the mass yields and chemical compositions.

The author wishes to express his thanks to Professors F.W.T. Penning de Vries and P. Hoffmann for their personal help.

REFERENCES

Anonymous. /1970/. Amino acid content of foods and biological data of proteins. FAO. Nutritional Studies. No. 24. FAO UN, Rome.

Baade, F. /1965/. Versenyfutás a 2000-ik évig. Közgazdasági és Jogi Könyvkiadó, Budapest.

Bálint, A. /1977/. Gazdasági növényeink produkciógenetikája. Akadémiai Kiadó. Budapest.

Bhatia, C.R., Rabson, R. /1976/. Bioenergetic considerations in cereal breeding for protein improvement. Science. 194. 1418-1421.

Hoffmann, P. /1978/. Einheit und Mannigfaltigkeit in Prozess der Photosynthese bei Pro- und Eukaryoten. Biol. Rundsch. 16, 73-78.

Johnson, W.A., Mattern, P.J. /1980/. Genetic improvement of productivity and nutritional quality of wheat. Final Report of Research Findings. Agronomy Department, University of Nebraska, Lincoln. Agency for International Development, Washington. 1-110.

Kralovánszky, U.P. /1983/. A hazai takarmányfehérje-hiány csökkentésének lehetőségei. Tud. Mezőgazd. 21, 2, 35-39.

Kramer, Th. /1980/. Protein content of wheat, crop physiological and breeding aspects. Proc. 3rd Internat. Wheat. Conf., Madrid, Spain. University of Nebraska, Lincoln. Agency for International Development, Washington. 688-696.

Kurnik, E. /1977/. Növénynemesités és energiaszükséglet. I., II. MTA Akadémiai székfoglaló előadás. M. Mezőgazd. 32, 32, 10-11.; 32, 34, 10-11.

Láng, I. /1980/. Az agroökológiai potenciál országos felméréséről. M. Tud. 7, 518-536.

Lásztity, R. /1981/. Gabonafehérjék. Mezőgazdasági Kiadó, Budapest.

McDermitt, D.K., Loomis, R.S. /1981/. Elemental composition of biomass and its relation to energy content, growth efficiency, and growth yield. Ann. Bot. 48, 3, 275-290.

Mitra, R.K., Bhatia, C.R. /1979/. Bioenergetic considerations in the improvement of oil-content and quality in oil-seed crops. Theor. Appl. Genet. 54, 41-47.

Mitra, R.K., Bhatia, C.R., Rabson, R. /1979/. Bioenergetic cost of altering the amino acid composition of cereal grains. Cereal Chem. 56, 4, 249-252.

Nehéz, R. /1971/. Szerves anyagok felhalmozódásának néhány törvényszerüsége kalászos növényekben. MTA Agrártud. Közl. 30, 1-2, 229-234.

Nehéz, R. /1974a/. Szerves anyagok felhalmozódása a növénytermesztésben. Tud. Mezőgazd. 12, 4, 45-49.

Nehéz, R. /1974b/. Adatok kromatográfiás módszerek alkalmazásáról növénynemesitő szelekcióban. 4. Kromatográfiás Vándorgyülés Előadásai. Magyar Kémikusok Egyesülete, Győr. 83-91.

Nehéz, R. /1975a/. Selektionsbemühungen auf die Erhöhung der Eiweissstoffe der Gerste und die minimalische Energie ihrer Bildungen. Koordinationszentrum, Allunionsinstitut für Pflanzengenetik. Odessa. Thema 4. RGW Konferenz. Odessa.

Nehéz, R. /1975b/. Adatok növényi szerves anyagok felhalmozódásáról a kukorica termesztés és nemesités számára. Szeged. Kézirat. MÉM Információs Központja, Budapest /B 11.699/. 1-368.

Nehéz, R. /1976/. Kukoricatermesztésünk jövőjéről. M. Mezőgazd. 31, 17, 3.

Nehéz, R. /1977a/. Some biochemical aspects of the accumulation by weight of vegetable oils. Abstracts of Papers of Conference of Food Biochemistry. 1976. Acta Aliment. 6, 275-276.

Nehéz, R. /1977b/. Einige biochemische Gesetzmässigkeiten für Gewicht-Akkumulation der pflanzlichen Eiweissstoffe. 5th Internat. Conf. of Amino Acids. Budapest. G 14. 1-9.

Nehéz, R. /1978a/. Several plant-energetical relations for use of nitrogenous chemical fertilizers. Proc. 18th Hung. Annu. Meet. Biochem., Biochem. Sect. Hung. Chem. Soc. Salgótarján. 239-240.

Nehéz, R. /1978b/. A szemes kukorica fehérjeszint növelésének néhány energia vonatkozása. MTA Pályázat, Budapest. GKI, Szeged. 1-20.

Nehéz, R. /1979a/. Several energetical relations between the biochemical effectivity of vegetal organic matter production and areal produce. Proc. 19th Hung. Annu. Meet. Biochem., Biochem. Sect. Hung. Chem. Soc. Budapest. 237-238.

Nehéz, R. /1979b/. Nekotorye svyazy biokhimicheskoi effektivnosti produktsii organicheskikh veshchestv zernovykh i ikh otbora. SEV Seminar sostoyalsya aprelya /23-28/ 1979 g. v ISAR, Radzikov. In Razrabotka teoreticheskikh osnov selektsii pshenitsy i yachmenya na vysokoe kachestvo zerna, v tom chisle voprosy uluchsheniya aminokislotnogo sostava. Vypusk. Institut selektsii i akklimatizatsii rastenii, Radzikov. Polska. 71-104.

Nehéz, R. /1980/. Adatok nitrogén- és kén-formák átalakulásának növényi energia vonatkozásairól. Mezőgazdaság Kemizálása. 1980. Keszthely. NEVIKI, KATE, Veszprém, Keszthely. Vol. 1. 139-143.

Nehéz, R. /1981/. Data for biochemical energy effectivity of production of vegetal organic matters. Proc. 21st Hung. Annu. Meet. Biochem., Biochem. Sect. Hung. Chem. Soc. Veszprém. 147-148.

Nehéz, R. /1982a/. A növényi szerves anyagok termelődésének néhány energia hatékonysági vonatkozása a gabonanemesitésben. Magyar Növényélettani Kongresszus. SZBK, Szeged. 1982. Bot. Közl. 69, 3-4, 267.

Nehéz, R. /1982b/. Some theoretical relations between the quality of wheat grain and the processes of formation of organic substances. CEREALS'82. Prague. 7th World Cereal and Bread Congress. Abstracts. No. 82. 124.

Nehéz, R. /1982c/. Organic mass of plants and the conversion of energy. Acta Biochim. biophys., Acad. Sci. Hung. 17, 1-2, 139.

Nehéz, R. /1983a/. Bioenergetic aspects of amino acid production in cereals. ICC Symposium. Amino Acid Composition and Biological Value of Cereal Proteins. Budapest. Abstracts. 26-27.

Nehéz, R. /1983b/. Növényi szerves anyagok termelődésének néhány energia vonatkozása, különös tekintettel a kukoricára. A kukorica termesztésének fejlesztése. Fejlesztőmérnökök Szemináriuma. MÉM Mérnök- és Vezetőképző Intézet. Budapest. 5-24.

Nehéz, R. /1984a/. Data on plant energy relations modifying the mass of organic compounds produced in plants. Acta Aliment. 13, 2, 117-134.

Nehéz, R. /1984b/. A termőképesség növényi energia vonatkozásai. Mezőgazdasági Tudományos Napok. Gödöllő. Előadás kivonatok. 208.

Nesterin, M.F., Skurikhin, I.M. /1979/. Khimicheskii sostav pishchevikh produktov. Pishchevaya promyshlennost', Moskva.

Netter, H. /1969/. Theoretical biochemistry. Oliver and Boyd, Edinburgh.

Penning de Vries F.W.T., Brunsting, A.H.M., van Laar, H.H. /1974/. Products, requirements and efficiency of biosynthesis. A quantitative approach. J. Theor. Biol. 45, 339-377.

Ryadchikov, V.G. /1978/. Uluchshenie zernovykh belkov i ikh otsenka. Kolos, Moskva.

Schulek, E., Kőrös, E. /1955/. A vegyértékről és kötésszámról /oxidációs számról/. M. Kém. F. 61, 11, 321-337.

Sinclair, T.R., De Wit, C.T. /1975/. Photosynthetate and nitrogen requirements for seed production by various crops. Science. 180, 565-567.

Sober, H. A., Harte, R.A., Sober, E. /ed.-s/ /1970/. Handbook of biochemistry. Rubber Company, Cleveland.

Szániel, I. /1980/. A búza- és kukoricatermesztés minőségi-területi kérdései. MTA Doktori értekezés. Budapest.

Vida, G., Gyurján, i., H. Nagy, A., Kassay, L. /1980/. A magyar mezőgazdaság energiastratégiája /A fotoszintétikus energiaátalakitás és a genetikai potenciál/. II. rész. A genetikai potenciál megközelitése. Tud. Mezőgazd. 18, 3, 56-59.

Warburg, O., Negelein, E. /1920/. Über die Reduktion de Salpetersäure in grünen Zellen. Biochem. Zeit. 110, 66.

Wilcox, O.W. /1954/. Quantitative agrobiology: I. The inverse yield-nitrogen law. Agron. J. 46, 315-320.

Proc. Int. Assoc. Cereal Chem. Symp. Amino Acid Compn and Biol. Value of Cereal Proteins Budapest, Hungary 1983, R. Lásztity, M. Hidvégi, eds

VIEWS ON THE AMINO ACID COMPOSITION OF GRAIN AND THE INFLUENCE OF PROCESSING

W. NIERLE

Institut für Biochemie und Analytik, Bundesforschungsanstalt für Getreide- und Kartoffelverarbeitung, Postfach 23, D-4930 Detmold, FRG

There are no differences in the amino acid composition between mineral or biological fertilized wheat and rye. The amount of fertilizing and the different locations are without influence on the distribution of amino acids in triticale varieties and breeding lines, because of their genetic background. Protein fractions of wheat are very different in amino acid composition. Gliadin and glutenin contain relatively high amounts of proline and glutamic acids, lysine and methionine are very low, the globulin fraction is rich in glycine and arginine. A very similar distribution and amino acid composition of these fractions are examined after dough formation, except a remarkable reduction of proline in the glutenin fraction.

During fermentation free amino acids are altered in sour dough, depending on bacterial sources. The drying of wheat up to 75 °C has no influence on the amount of lysine, which is noticeably reduced by extrusion cooking of wheat or oat, depending on the water content and the temperature. Micronizing of corn up to 120 °C did not influence the lysine content.

Processing the grain for breakfast cereals reduces the content of essential amino acids. This loss, however, is balanced out by the milk protein. During cooking of rice different amounts of amino acids are soluble depending on variety and boiling conditions. There is a relatively high amount of glutamic- and aspartic acid in the boiling water. These amino acids are predominant in the rice kernel also.

INTRODUCTION

The amino acid composition of cereal proteins is very important for nutritional quality and for structural characteristics as well as for technological behaviour. Interactions between water and proteins, lipids and carbohydrates for example, are of immense importance for the unique cohesive-elastic properties of hydrated wheat gluten proteins.

Wheat gluten, the most important cereal protein complex, is produced from the endosperm proteins gliadin and glutenin during mixing of flour and water. Endosperm proteins make up about 70 % of the total protein of the kernel, and consists of water soluble albumin, salt soluble globulin, alcohol soluble gliadin, acid soluble glutenin, and insoluble glutenin. The gluten proteins gliadin and glutenin make up about 85 % of endosperm proteins. The yield depends on the extraction procedures. As expected from solubility, the protein fractions differ in amino acid content.

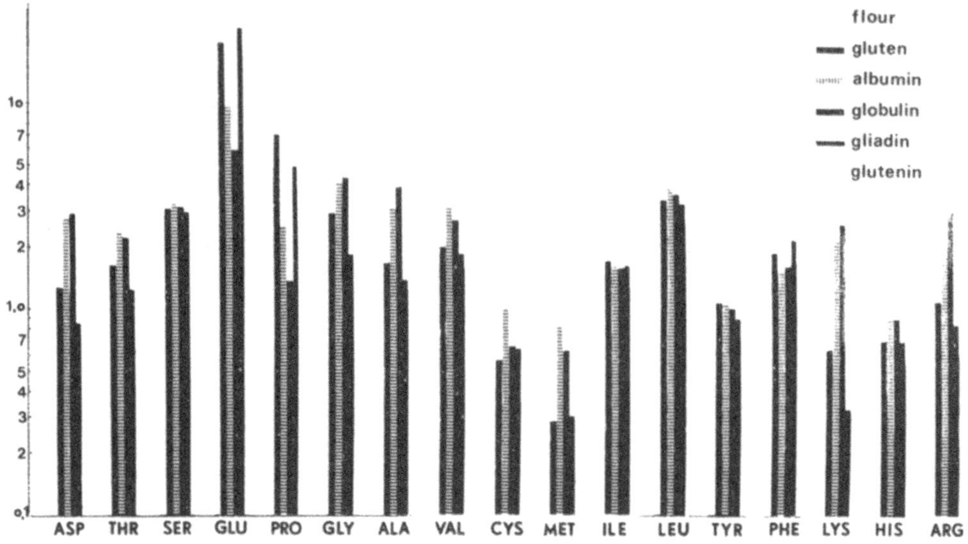

Fig. 1/ Amino acid contents (mmol/gN) of cereal proteins

1. AMINO ACID COMPOSITION OF WHEAT PROTEIN FRACTIONS

The albumins and globulins are rich in ionizable basic amino acids arginine, lysine, and histidine, and in the polar threonine and serine. The amount of sulfur containing amino acids is high, especially in the albumin fractions. Nevertheless, the amount of charged amino acids is smaller than in water insoluble fractions. It is well known that the water soluble fractions have a very high content of amide containing residues such as glutamin and amino acids with long aliphatic side chains, such as leucine. The gliadines and glutenins contain high levels of proline, which disrupt the linear or a-helical structure of the protein chains. It is very plausible that the properties of these fractions may be correlated to the amino acid composition.

Because of the relatively high levels of polar and ionizable amino acids the alcohol soluble wheat gliadin and glutenin can be dissolved in either acetic acid or 3 M urea. The hydration of the gliadin and glutenin is a result of the relatively low content of hydrophobic amino acids such as glycine,alanine, valine, isoleucine and leucine.

In agreement with (Wall, 1969) and (Redman, 1971) we also found a high content of glutamic acid and proline in gliadines and glutenins, which are low in S-containing amino acids, but the amount of aspartic acid is lower than in soluble fractions.

The insolubility of the glutenins is related to their high molecular weights and extended conformation which depends only to a small degree on their amino acid content, which is very similar to that of the gliadines.

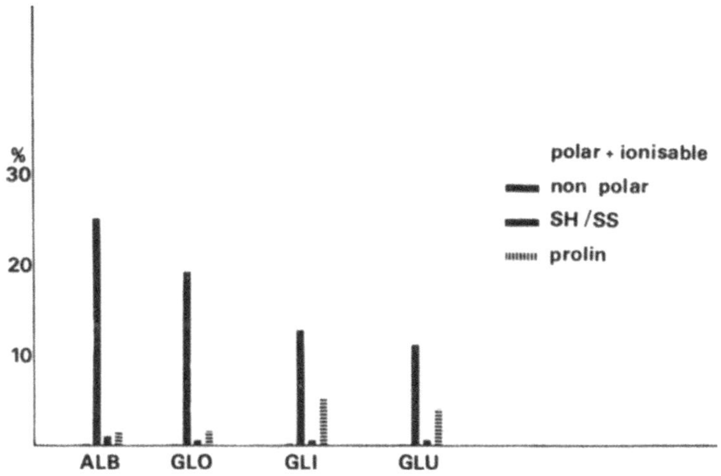

Fig. 2/ Amino acid contents of wheat protein fractions classified according to side chain properties

2. REMARKS ON NUTRITIVE QUALITY OF CEREAL PROTEINS

It is generally known that the relative poor nutritional value of certain cereals is caused by both low quantity and low quality of protein. In all cereal proteins the first limiting essential amino acid is lysine followed by threonine and tryptophan in maize. Regardless of the similar content in lysine and the other essential amino acids except the amounts of isoleucine and phenylalanine, there are remarkable differences in the nutritional value of the proteins.

TABLE 1/ PROTEIN QUALITY OF CEREAL PROTEINS

	BV	PER
Wheat	58 - 67	0.9 - 17
Oat	75	2.0 - 2.5
Barley	74	1.6 - 2.0
Corn	53 - 60	0.9 - 1.3
Rye	74	1.8 - 2.3
Triticale	--	1.2 - 1.5
Egg	95	3.5

BV = biological value(retained N/absorbed N) x 100

PER = Protein efficiency ratio = weight gain/amount of protein fed (Silano 1977)

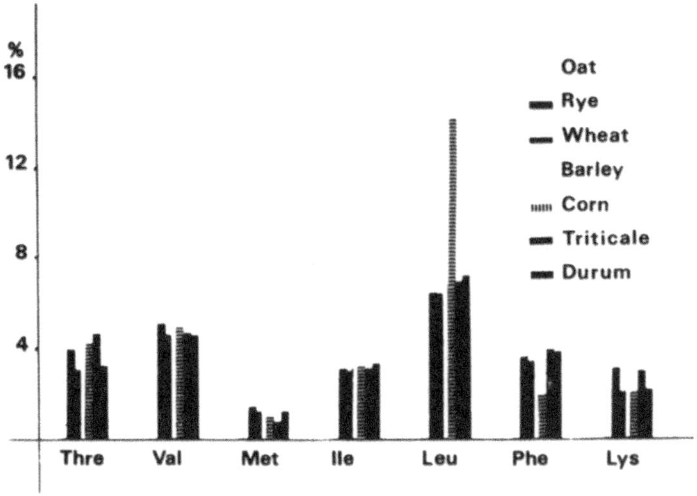

Fig. 3/ Essential amino acids in cereal grain % of amino acids mmol/gN

TABLE 2/ AVAILABILITY OF AMINO ACIDS IN CEREAL PROTEINS ASSESSED BY DIFFERENT METHODS *

Amino acid	Wheat Gluten	Rice Protein	Maize Gluten	Zein
Lysine	83[a] , 99[b]	94[a] , 95[b]	105[a] , 86[b]	
Leucine	102[a]			
Isoleucine		86[a]	63[a]	30[a]
Methionine	94[a] , 99[b]			
Phenylalanine	112[a] , 95[b]			
Threonine	113[a] , 82[b]	100[b]	65[a] , 99[b]	22[a] , 33[b]
Tryptophan	105[a] , 100[b]			
Valine	86[a] , 100[b]	79[a]	68[a] , 84[b]	40[a] , 62[b]

a = Growth and proteins depletion methods *) SILANO

b = Faecal analysis methods

The nutritional efficiency of a protein is often predicted from the amino acid composition. However, there are certain limits in predicting the value for evaluation of protein quality. Nutritional studies revealed by (Silano, 1977) pointed out the lower feeding value of rye, as compared to barley and wheat. This fact could not be explained by differences in protein quantity or amino acid compositions. There are significant differences among the data in the literature for the digestibility of cereal proteins. These data indicate, that the digestibility and availability of amino acids from the same protein source is different, even when present in proteins with similar digestibility coefficients.

Regarding these facts it is very difficult to determine the nutritional quality of cereal products. Nevertheless, wheat bran protein and water soluble proteins have presumably a higher nutritional value than gluten because of the amino acid composition.

TABLE 3/ ESSENTIAL AMINO ACIDS IN WHEAT AND FRACTIONS (μmol/gS) *

	Thr	Val	Met	Ile	Leu	Phe	Lys
Wheat	29	42	26	28	61	32	20
Gluten	18	24	8	17	41	23	7
Bran	40	49	24	26	69	33	36

*) MILADI et al

Under these aspects it is to be questioned, if different agricultural conditions influence the nutritional quality of wheat and rye, even if the amino acid composition related to the amount of protein is almost the same. This question becomes more and more important in FRG, especially in regards to the influence of biological or mineral fertilization on the nutritional quality of food from plant origin.

Triticale, the first man-made cereal is produced by cross-breeding of wheat and rye. Genetic differences between wheat and rye and manifold possibilities for crossing triticale species with each other produce a lot of problems influencing yield and quality. About 350 000 ha are presently under cultivation in the world. Because of the large variety of species triticale becomes in FRG more important too.

Triticale is, because of its high protein and lysine level, well suited for humans and animals. We examined the influence of location of some triticale varieties and species on the amino acid composition. As expected, the content of essential amino acids related to the protein content was about the same in all samples in spite of the fact that the protein content of the triticale ranged between 8.5 and 17.8 % was extremely high. It was shown that one variety of species grown in different locations had almost an identical protein level. Following the different levels of proteins, the amino acid content of triticale ranged between a broad spectrum. There were only little differences in lysine content.

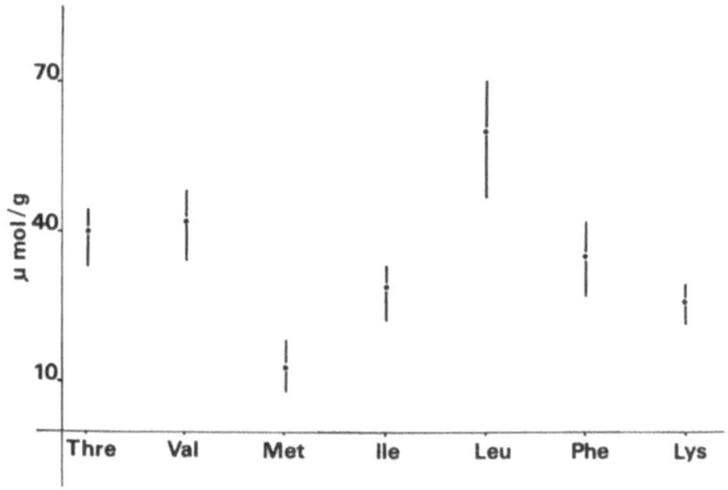

Fig. 4 / Essential amino acids in triticale of different locations

2.1. Heat processing of cereal products

In human diets the proteinous material is usually heated to improve the digestibility. Most heat processes lead to the damage of protein structure and result in several types of reactions. The most severe form of damage is the destruction by the transformation of nitrogen to other non-protein constituents, less destructive reactions that render proteins biologically are more common. In all cases, nevertheless, when proteinous substances remain,they possess a certain nutritional value.

Heating modifies the structure of proteins mainly by disruption of hydrogen bonds and can reduce the nutritional value by degradation of essential amino acids especially lysine or by intramolecular reactions. By several reactions most essential amino acids become indigestible by enzymes.In spite of this fact these fixed amino acids are determinable in acid hydrolysates. Besides destruction and blocking reactions with other non-protein components, e.g. carbohydrates are common. These reactions are well known as Maillard-reactions wherelysine,and to a lower degree arginine,histidine,tyrosine and methionine become more and more unavailable.For the evaluation of the nutritional quality of proteins it is therefore not sufficient only to determine the amount of lysine, but it is also necessary to determine the available lysine. In addition to the determination of the lysine content it is useful to estimate a technological process.

2.1.1. Drying

The effects of heat treatment, drying, extrusion cooking and micronizing were investigated. The amino acid composition, after processing of oat, corn and wheat was compared with the untreated material. Small differences which we found in the lysine content are insignificant, and must be confirmed by further studies. Drying of grain is often necessary because fresh harvested grain contains a high amount of moisture. Moisture contents with about 14 % are too high for storage under normal conditions. Drying of wheat under different drying conditions, e.g. humidity, air stream, drying temperature and time between 40 °C to 75 °C in the kernel, did not influence the amino acid composition. However, some changes in the protein were detectable in that high temperature dried samples by variation of the UV-spectra and by dye binding capacity as well as by reducing the solubility.

2.1.2. Extrusion

As to be expected, during extrusion cooking of oat and wheat up to 160 °C, lysine content deteriorated significantly. It is presumed that a similar reaction takes place during the baking process in the bread crust. Amino acid analysis of raw and heat processed grits point to a loss of lysine to a larger extent in oats than in wheat, depending on the reaction temperatures.

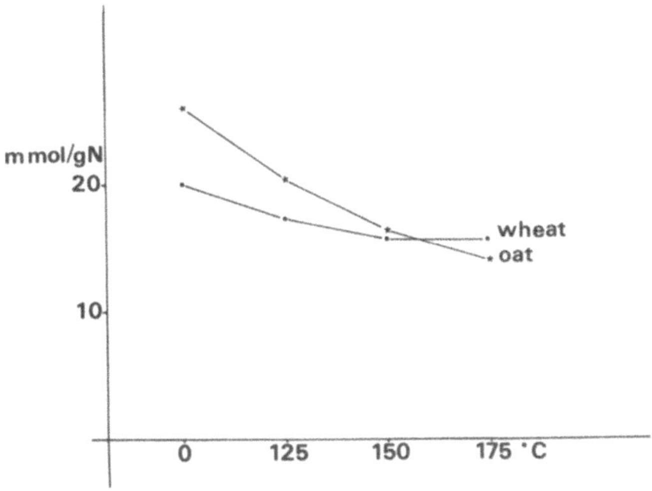

Fig. 5 / Degradation of lysine during extrusion cooking

Therefore, it is concluded that the susceptibility to heat damage varies among different protein sources also. There are some references that in presence of reducing carbohydrates and other food constituents the loss of lysine will be increased.

The extrusion process becomes more important in manufacturing several snack products with additives and in feeding to improve the availability of carbohydrate materials.

2.1.3. Micronizing

Kernel micronizing is a new modern process to improve the feeding quality. The kernels are moistened to 18 - 25 % humidity and irradiated with infrared light of 600 - 1 200 nm for 10 - 60 s. The kernels can reach a temperature up to 120 °C on the surface regions. This temperature does not deteriorate lysine in corn considerably. During this process starch gelatinizes partly, and lipids can be degradated.

Future work must guarantee whether the nutritional quality of such grain protein will be influenced by this process.

2.1.4. Cooking of rice

Rice has one of the highest nutritional values among cereal proteins and is besides wheat the most important food for the world's inhabitants. The rice consumption in FRG is 1.8 kg per person per year. The main methods for cooking rice can be summerized as follows:

1. Rice is cooked in twice its volume of water over a slow fire until the water is completely absorbed,
2. Rice is cooked in large amounts of water and the excess is drained. Naturally with this method part of the nutrients are leached with the water.

It is known that cooking rice does not reduce the availability of the epsilon amino groups of lysine in rice protein and does not result in lysine decomposition or in the binding of its amino groups.

Protein losses during cooking range between 7 % in 5-minute-rice and 0 % in parboiled rice. The amino acid composition of the protein in the cooking liquids is very similar to the protein in the uncooked rice with nearly 30 % of essential amino acids and 4 % of lysine. Additionally,we found different amounts of free amino acids in the cooking liquids.

TABLE 4/ LOSSES ACCOMPANYING COOKING RICE IN EXCESS WATER

Sample	Protein %	Total loss %	Ess.AA µmol/gS	% of total AA	% Lysine
1. Brown rice long grain quality A	9,6	1.3	10.2	10.0	1.3
2. Brown rice medium	9.0	2.0	6.8	13.0	2.0
3. Milled rice long grain quality A	8.7	3.3	1.4	6.2	3.3
4. Milled rice short grain quality A	7,0	4.4	1.3	4.6	4.4
5. Milled rice long grain quality C	9.0	4,3	0.6	3.2	4.3
6. Milled rice,broken kernels	8.2	5.7	0.3	1,9	5,7
7. Parboiled rice,long grain quality A	7.8	3.1	4.6	12.3	3.1
8. Parboiled rice, short grain	7.2	3.5	10,2	8,1	3.5
9. Quick cooking rice	8.5	1.0	0.2	2.3	1.0
10. Five minute rice	8.8	3.2	2.8	4.9	3.2

The content of essential free amino acids in cooking liquid ranges from 10.2 to 0.2 µmol/g dry matter, corresponding with 13 - 1.9 % of total amino acids. The portion of lysine ranges between 1 and 13 %.

These experiments demonstrated that cooking of rice in excess water does not reduce the nutritional quality of rice protein essentially in respect to the amino acid content .

2.1.5. Heat processing

Breakfast cereals are produced mainly from wheat, corn, rice, oats, and sometimes from millet, buckwheat or rye. For example, in USA 6 kg/man/ year cornflakes are consumed, which is ten times more than that of West-German consumption. Because of the nutritional aspects, especially the high level of dietary fiber in breakfast cereals, the consumption increased in West-Europe. The quality of such products depends not only on the ingredients. The processing parameters (drying- and roasting temperatures, moisture, oxygen and ingredients) play an important role. For screening 18 different commercial German cereals were examined for their consumption. The cereal basis of the products were wheat, corn, oat, rice, buckwheat and rye.

Cereals render undoubtedly some important nutrients, for example minerals, vitamins, and essential amino acids. The lysine content of the products seems to be a marker for the grain basis, and to a smaller degree for processing parameters. A relatively high amount of lysine was found in cereals from oat 1 - 3, from rice 4, and wheat and bran 11 - 13. Samples 14 - 17 are whole kernel products consisting of grain mixtures, 18 was based on biological fertilized wheat.

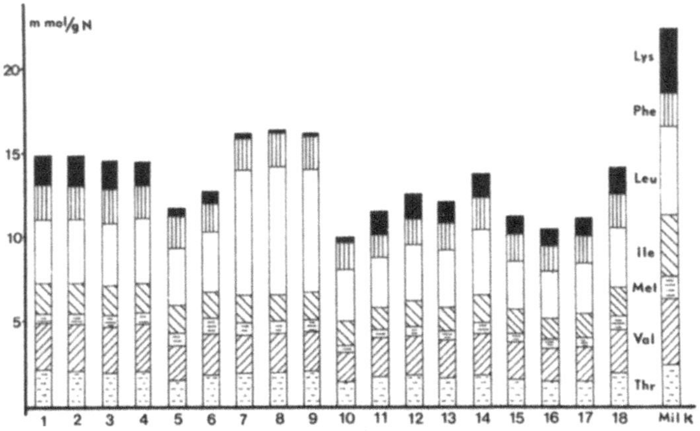

Fig. 6/ Essential amino acids in breakfast cereals

The low lysine content of products 5, 6 and 10 suggests a higher processing temperature, whereas the very low lysine content and the high leucine content of 7 - 9 refer to maize in this cornflakes.

Most of these cereals contain a relatively high amount of sucrose and reducing sugars. Therefore, the amount of essential amino acids was, as expected, lower in comparison with the original grain.

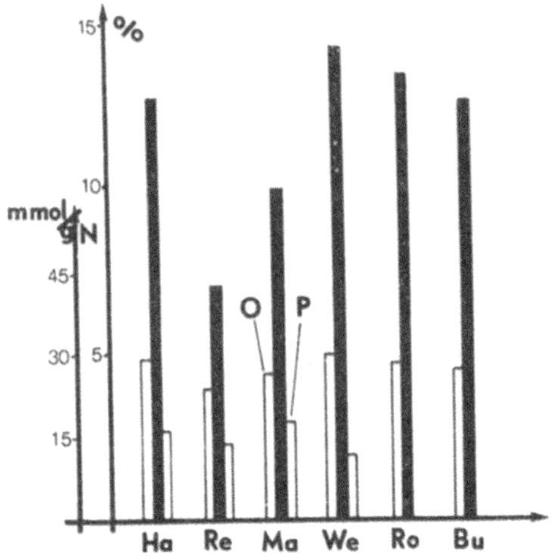

O = content in cereal
P = content in product

Ha = oat
Re = rice
Ma = corn
We = wheat
Ro = rye
Bu = buckwheat

Fig. 7 / Protein content and decrease of amino acids by processing of cereal

Nearly all cereals are heat-treated to improve flavour and digestibility. A relatively high loss of essential amino acids was found in the wheat-based products; these cereals had the highest sugar content. The lower nutritional value of some cereals are improved by the addition of milk to the diet. In regard to other nutritional aspects the consumption of breakfast cereals are well-recommended not only for children but also for adults.

2.2. Fermenting of cereal proteins

The use of rye bread is connected with acidification of the dough by lactic acid bacterials. Fermentation is necessary for the baking performance as well as for improvement of flavour, which is related not only to the bacterials' carbohydrate metabolism, but also to the amount of produced lactic- and acetic acid. It is well known that free amino acids and sugars are precursors in the flavour formation during the bread making process. Sour dough bacterials have a proteolytic activity.

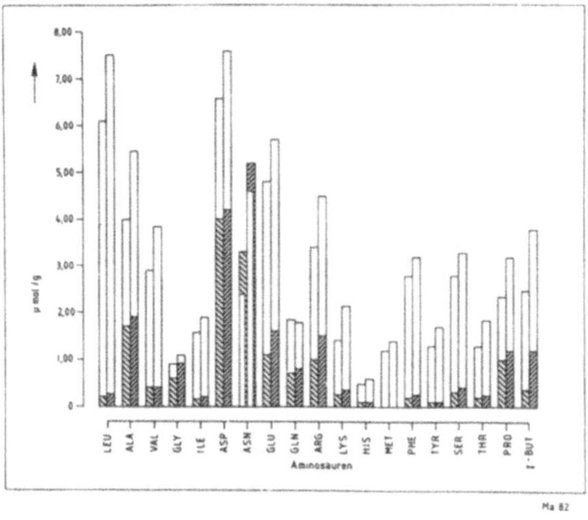

Fig. 8 / Change of amino acids during dough fermentation

□ sour dough

▧ flour, type 815

▨ flour type 1370

During fermentation especially the amounts of essential amino acids, leucine, phenylalanine, methionine, tyrosine, lysine and isoleucine increase to a high degree. There are great differences among the lactobacillus species in the proteolytic activities. The proteolysis depends on several fermenting parameters and on the extraction grade of the flour also. Some species consume amino acids during fermenting for example lactobacillus fructivorans, which consumes glycine, asparagine, and glutamine.

It is doubtful, if parallel to the very important technological efficiency of the sour dough bacterials, whether they will also contribute to improve the availability and the nutritional quality by increasing the level of essential amino acids, because bread with 5 - 8 % protein content contributes only a limited level of the protein requirement for man about 20 % of human's requirement.

3. CONCLUSION

During processing of cereal proteins are changed in many ways; they become more or less available, and the nutritional value may be increased or diminished even by mixing with other food components. Therefore, it is reasonable to look not only at the contents of protein or essential amino acids. The nutritional quality is a complex influenced by several genetic and technological parameters, which are not yet completely understood. Although food manufacturers are producing high quality products, further research is needed for offering foodstuffs with optimal quality for mankind.

REFERENCES

1. Miladi, S. and Hegsted, D.M. /1972/. The relative nutritive value, amino acid content, and digestibility of the proteins of wheat mill fractions. Cer.Chem. 49, 1, 119-127.

2. Redman, D.J. /1971/. Wheat proteins. Chemistry and Industry, 38, 1061-1068.

3. Silano, V. /1977/. Factors affecting digestibility and availability of proteins in cereals. In: Panel proceeding series. - Nutritional evaluation of cereal contents JAEA Vienna 1977.

4. Wall, J.S. and Beckwith, A.C. /1969/. Relationship between structure and rheological properties of gluten proteins. Cereal Science Today, 14, 16-21.

Proc. Int. Assoc. Cereal Chem. Symp. Amino Acid Compn and Biol. Value of Cereal Proteins Budapest, Hungary 1983, R. Lásztity, M. Hidvégi, eds

CONTRIBUTIONS TO THE AMINO ACID COMPOSITION OF PROTEIN FRACTIONS OF WHEAT FLOURS

E. TÖRÖK

College of Food Industry, H-6724 Szeged, Hungary

The amino acid composition of wheat flours of different quality and their protein fractions separated by an acetic acid fractionation method were determined. Flours milled from the following wheats were used: Jubilejnaja 50, Partizanka, GK-F2, Rana 1, Száva. Three protein fractions were separated from the flours: proteins soluble in 1 M NaCl, proteins soluble in 0,1 M acetic acid, and proteins insoluble in 0,1 M acetic acid. The determination of the amino acid composition - except tryptophan - was carried out from the acidic hydrolysate of protein fractions and of the starting flours by means of a Chinoin Lys 75 type automated amino acid analyzer. Some characteristic differences were found in the amino acid composition of protein fractions in comparison with each other and with the composition of the starting flours. The salt-soluble protein fractions show the most considerable differences by their higher asparatic acid, glycine, alanine, leucine, lysine, arginine, and lower glutamic acid and proline values. The amino acid compositions of the acetic acid-soluble and acetic acid-insoluble protein fractions show more similarity, that is the content of basic amino acids is very low, while glutamic acid and proline are present in very high amounts in both. In the latter ones the proportion of glycine is also relatively higher. Similar characteristic differences were not found among the same types of protein fractions of different flours.

INTRODUCTION

The amino acid composition of wheat and wheat fractions has been studied for a long time. A number of works deal with the characteristics of the amino acid composition of wheat flour protein fractions too. A detailed review is given on this topic by Kasarda /1971/. Most of these studies, and the later ones too, are related to the protein fractions separated mainly by the classical fractionation method of Osborne /e.g. Khan, Bushuk 1979/, or to the botanical constituents of wheat /Jensen, Martens 1983/.

In this paper the amino acid composition of wheat flours of different quality and their protein fractions separated by an acetic acid fractionation method were determined. The aim of the work was to compare the amino acid composition of the protein fractions obtained by different solvents, and to investigate what kinds of differences are found among the amino acid composition of the same types of protein fractions of different flours.

MATERIALS AND METHODS

Flours milled from the following wheats were used: Jubilejnaja 50, Partizanka, GK-F2, Rana 1, Száva. The baking quality of these flours determined by the usual testing methods decreases in the order of their mentioning. Three protein fractions were separated from the flours by the method of Bushuk and Orth /1973/: proteins soluble in 1 M NaCl, proteins soluble in 0,1 M acetic acid, proteins insoluble in 0,1 M acetic acid. The protein fractions were purified by dialysis, then were lyophilized.

The determination of the amino acid composition - except tryptophan - was carried out from the 6 N hydrochloric acidic hydrolysate of the lyophilized protein fractions and of the starting flours by means of a Chinoin Lys 75 type automated amino acid analyzer according to Dévényi /1969/. Tryptophan was determined with p-DAB reaction, by spectrophotometrical method.

RESULTS

The results are summarized in tables 1-4.

CONCLUSIONS

On the basis of the data given in tables 1-4 some characteristic differences can be stated in the amino acid composition of protein fractions obtained by different solvents in comparison with each other and with the composition of the starting flours.

In comparison with the starting flours, the salt-soluble protein fractions have very high asparatic acid, glycine, alanine, leucine and arginine values. The increase of the proportion of threonine, serine, valine and lysine is also considerable, whereas the values of glutamic acid, proline and phenylalanine are lower.

The protein fractions soluble in 0,1 M acetic acid in comparison with the starting flours contain less aspartic acid, threonine, glycine, valine, methionine, lysine, arginine and tryptophan, while the amount of proline, leucine and in the fractions of some flours the amount of glutamic acid and isoleucine is higher.

TABLE 1.

The amino acid composition of wheat flours

g/100 g amino acid

	Jubilejnaja 50	Partizanka	GK-F2	Rana 1	Száva
Aspartic acid	3.4	3.7	3.3	3.5	3.7
Threonine	2.7	2.2	2.1	2.7	2.5
Serine	3.2	3.4	3.5	3.1	3.1
Glutamic acid	43.7	46.3	44.2	44.0	42.3
Proline	8.7	9.9	10.6	9.6	9.4
Glycine	2.4	2.5	2.5	2.4	2.5
Alanine	2.4	2.2	2.2	2.1	2.1
Cystine/2	2.0	1.1	0.9	1.0	1.0
Valine	3.4	3.0	2.9	3.3	3.2
Methionine	1.4	1.0	1.9	1.1	1.4
Isoleucine	2.9	2.8	3.3	2.8	2.8
Leucine	5.3	7.2	4.8	4.9	5.6
Tyrosine	2.7	2.7	2.9	2.6	2.5
Phenylalanine	4.3	4.4	3.7	4.1	4.2
Lysine	1.8	2.0	2.0	2.0	1.8
Histidine	2.0	2.0	1.9	1.8	1.7
Arginine	3.3	3.3	3.3	3.0	3.4
Tryptophan	1.0	1.2	1.1	0.7	0.9

TABLE 2.

The amino acid composition of wheat protein fractions soluble in 1 M NaCl

g/100 g amino acid

	Jubilejnaja 50	Partizanka	GK-F2	Rana 1	Száva
Aspartic acid	7.1	7.6	8.1	8.1	8.4
Threonine	4.0	4.2	3.8	4.3	3.8
Serine	4.2	4.6	4.7	5.3	4.4
Glutamic acid	22.9	22.9	23.0	21.3	19.0
Proline	7.7	7.2	8.2	8.4	7.6
Glycine	4.3	4.3	4.9	3.8	4.8
Alanine	5.5	4.6	5.6	7.4	5.9
Cystine/2	3.0	1.7	2.9	1.4	4.0
Valine	6.1	6.6	5.3	5.4	6.0
Methionine	0.4	0.4	0.4	0.4	0.7
Isoleucine	3.0	3.0	3.3	3.0	3.3
Leucine	8.0	6.8	7.9	7.1	8.4
Tyrosine	2.9	3.4	3.0	2.8	3.5
Phenylalanine	3.8	4.4	3.5	2.9	3.6
Lysine	3.7	2.8	4.0	3.4	3.1
Histidine	2.3	2.6	2.2	1.5	1.9
Arginine	7.4	9.5	6.4	10.1	8.0
Tryptophan	1.1	1.0	1.0	1.2	1.2

TABLE 3.

The amino acid composition of wheat protein fractions soluble in 0,1 N acetic acid

g/100 g amino acid

	Jubilejnaja 50	Partizanka	GK-F2	Rana 1	Száva
Aspartic acid	1.8	2.1	1.9	2.0	1.8
Threonine	1.6	1.9	1.5	1.8	1.7
Serine	3.5	4.4	3.5	3.0	3.1
Glutamic acid	44.2	46.6	47.5	50.8	44.9
Proline	13.6	12.4	14.2	10.6	15.9
Glycine	1.7	1.6	1.9	1.7	1.5
Alanine	1.5	1.8	1.8	1.3	1.8
Cystine/2	1.3	1.2	1.2	1.1	0.9
Valine	3.1	3.0	3.4	2.9	2.8
Methionine	0.5	0.5	0.6	1.1	0.6
Isoleucine	4.7	3.0	3.4	2.9	3.6
Leucine	6.6	5.4	6.1	4.7	6.2
Tyrosine	2.0	1.3	1.1	2.7	0.6
Phenylalanine	4.8	4.4	4.4	4.7	5.3
Lysine	0.6	0.6	0.7	0.4	0.6
Histidine	1.7	1.6	1.2	1.9	1.1
Arginine	2.3	3.1	1.8	1.7	1.9
Tryptophan	0.5	1.1	0.8	0.5	1.3

TABLE 4.

The amino acid composition of wheat protein fractions insoluble in 0,1 N acetic acid

g/100 g amino acid

	Jubilejnaja 50	Partizanka	GK-F2	Rana 1	Száva
Aspartic acid	2.2	2.8	3.0	3.1	2.8
Threonine	2.2	2.7	2.9	1.9	2.9
Serine	3.9	4.6	4.9	4.9	4.3
Glutamic acid	41.9	39.8	41.5	43.3	37.6
Proline	11.7	11.2	10.0	9.7	11.1
Glycine	4.1	3.8	4.1	3.9	4.0
Alanine	2.3	2.4	2.5	2.4	2.5
Cystine/2	0.6	1.2	0.8	0.5	1.2
Valine	3.6	3.4	3.5	4.0	3.7
Methionine	0.5	0.8	0.6	0.5	0.6
Isoleucine	2.6	3.1	3.0	3.9	3.2
Leucine	6.8	6.6	5.8	6.5	7.8
Tyrosine	2.7	3.7	2.3	2.3	3.4
Phenylalanine	3.8	3.7	3.6	1.8	4.0
Lysine	1.4	0.9	1.7	0.8	1.6
Histidine	1.9	1.7	2.2	1.7	1.4
Arginine	3.6	2.9	2.8	4.3	4.0
Tryptophan	0.8	1.0	0.9	1.0	1.0

The amino acid composition of the salt-soluble protein fractions show the most characteristic differences in comparison with the acetic acid-soluble and acetic acid-insoluble fractions by their notably higher aspartic acid, threonine, valine, alanine, lysine and arginine values, and much lower glutamic acid and proline values.

The amino acid composition of the acetic acid-soluble and acetic acid-insoluble fractions show more similarity, that is, the content of basic amino acids is very low, while glutamic acid and proline are present in very high amounts in both. In the latter ones the proportion of glycine is also relatively higher.

Similar characteristic differences were not found among the same types of protein fractions of different flours.

REFERENCES

Bushuk, W., Orth, R.A. /1973/. Studies of glutenin. I. Comparison of preparative methods. Cereal Chem. 50, 106-110.

Jensen, S.A., Martens, H. /1983/. The botanical constituents of wheat and wheat milling fractions. II. Quantification by amino acids. Cereal Chem. 60, 172-176.

Kasarda, D.D., Nimmo, C.C., Kohler, G.O. /1971/. Proteins and the amino acid composition of wheat fractions. In: Wheat chemistry and technology, Pomeranz, Y. /ed./ AACC, St Paul Minnesota, pp. 270-280.

Khan, K., Bushuk, W. /1979/. Studies of glutenin. XIV. Gel filtration, isoelectric focusing and amino acid composition studies. Cereal Chem. 56, 505-509.

Proc. Int. Assoc. Cereal Chem. Symp. Amino Acid Compn and Biol. Value of Cereal Proteins
Budapest, Hungary 1983, R. Lásztity, M. Hidvégi, eds

ACTION OF SOME PROTEINASES ON WHEAT GLUTEN ISOLATED FROM MATURE AND DEVELOPING KERNELS

JERZY KAÇZKOWSKI, ELŻBIETA KUROWSKA, MATGORZATA MOSKAL

Department of Biochemistry, Institute of Plant Biology, University of Agriculture, P-02-528 Warsaw, Poland

ABSTRACT

Continuing the investigations on some structural differences of gluten components using proteolytic enzymes, experiments were carried out, concerning the proteolysis rate of gluten isolated from wheats of various development stages, subjected to bromelain action. The results of experiments on three wheat varieties showed that during the course of grain maturation the gluten proteolysis rate decreased. This can suggest that protein molecules become more and more compact and structurally well organised. It was shown also that peptide bonds in proteins isolated from varieties of higher technological value were less accessible for proteinases applied than those of lower quality, already at the earlier maturation stages. These experiments will be continued as concerns the earlier development stages.

INTRODUCTION

Protein systems are of special interest to cereal chemists from both practical and theoretical point of view. Studies with pure enzymes can provide useful information on wheat protein composition and structure, as they split specific and precisely localised peptide bonds. This behaviour made us possible to use those enzymes as a tool in investigations on gluten strenght and quality, as well as concerning more theoretical problems of structural differences of some gluten components.

Some ten years ago we were able to notice that the increase rates of nonprotein nitrogen /npN/ in protein acetic acid extracts obtained from wheat samples differentiated in baking quality and stored at 4°C or 20°C were not uniform and depended somehow on flour technological value. The results of those observations are demonstrated in table 1.

The presented data suggested that the hydrolysis rates of native proteolytic enzyme action could be reversed to gluten quality, or that the activities of those enzymes were higher in samples of lower quality. To exclude the latter suggestion

Table 1

The influence of native proteinases on npN increase in heated and nonheated wheat protein dispersions stored for seven days

Wheat variety	sample	Initial npN mg/g	4°C		20°C	
			mg npN	% incr	mg npN	% incr
Bezenczugska 98	heated	3,62	3,86	7	4,05	12
	nonheated		4,35	20	7,81	116
Saratowska 29	heated	4,13	5,28	28	5,23	26
	nonheated		7,58	83	9,43	128
Polish mixed	heated	4,24	4,60	10	5,49	29
	nonheated		8,62	102	13,40	221
Varigo	heated	4,33	4,96	14	6,33	46
	nonheated		9,02	108	14,46	234

Bezenczugska and Saratowska - high quality, Polish mixed and Varigo - low quality

we determined the activities of native peptidases in samples under investigations, but we could not find among the results differences justifying observations shown in table 1. So the possibility arose that the proteolysis rate of wheat gluten reversly depended on its quality.

Therefore we tried to repeat the same observation using not the native, but added enzyme preparations of bromelain, as well as the wheat malt peptidase purified 21-fold, as compared to the initial extract. Results obtained in those investigations are presented in table 2.

Table 2

The proteolysis rate of gluten components under the action of bromelain and native wheat peptidase in per cents of liberated tyrosine

Wheat variety	bromelain			purified wheat peptidase		
	1	2	3	1	2	3
Saratowska 29	49,6	42,8	36,5	30,4	34,0	31,4
Bezosta 1	59,1	58,2	35,6	29,2	36,4	29,9
Mironowska 808	50,8	60,1	-	30,4	38,5	23,7
Varigo	63,0	50,1	38,3	26,3	30,0	29,9

1 - initial gluten, 2 - glutenin, 3 - gliadin
Saratowska 29 - high quality, Bezosta 1 and Mironowska 808 - medium quality, Varigo - low quality

Those experiments are described also by Liss and Kączkowski /1975/.

On the base of results presented in table 2 it could be concluded that the digestion rates of particular gluten components by some peptidases are different and especially as concerns the glutenin and purified wheat peptidase. This process takes place slower in samples of higher than in those of poorer quality. Of interest should also be the observation of the higher digestion rates of isolated glutenin, than those of initial gluten and even more, than of isolated gliadin, when bromelain or wheat peptidase was applied. Therefore the general suggestion was presented that the comparing of proteolysis rates of wheat gluten components could serve as an index of their structural relationships. We suggested further, that the proteolysis rates of gluten proteins depend on the accessibility of peptide bonds to peptidases, which could indicate, that they should present the different molecule compactness. Our results allowed to assume also that the differences in the molecule compactness concerned particularly the big glutenin complexes, isolated from samples of various quality, rather than gliadin molecules.

We tried also to isolate some glutenin proteolysis products from samples of high and low baking quality. Therefore we subjected glutenin samples to short-term proteolysis using bromelain and then to the Sephadex G 100 column separations, the examples of which are presented in figure 1.

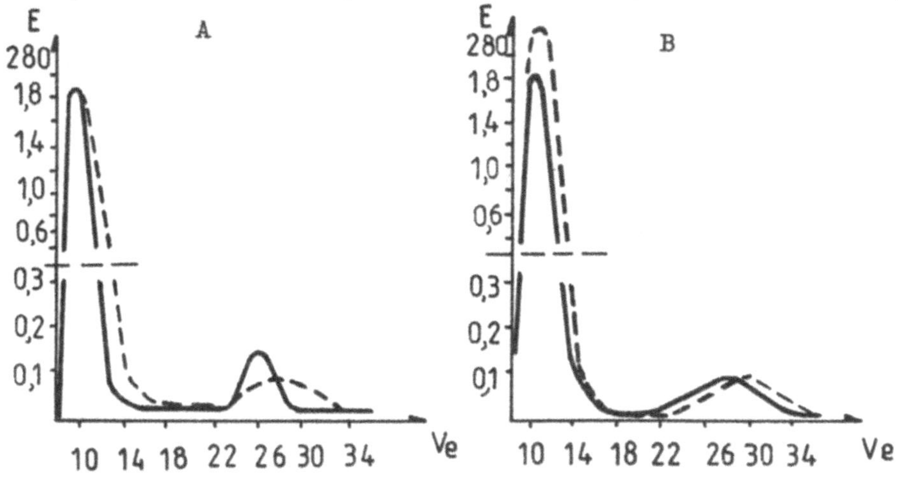

Fig. 1. Sephadex G 100 elution curves of glutenin before /continuous line/ and after 20 min. proteolysis /dashed line/ by 10 /A/ and 16 /B/ µg of bromelain preparation

We were able to demonstrate in those experiments the digestion of low molecular weight protein, but almost no change in that of glutenin, although the new fraction of higher elution volume was formed, probably as a product of glutenin digestion. The only interesting result of those experiments was the much higher loosening of glutenin fractions in samples of poor quality, than in those of higher one, which was manifested by the increase of the E_{280}/total N ratio. We tried to use this last indication as the molecule compactness index /Bernacka et al. 1977/, but it could not be fully confirmed in further experiments. Similar investigations using peptidases were carried out earlier by Bietz and Rothfus /1970/, but they were also unable to demonstrate quality differentiations in proteolysis products.

Parallel to those experiments we subjected glutenin to the moderate bromelain digestion and then to scanning electron microscopy observations for deeper elucidation of the mechanism of this process. Some patterns of digested molecules are presented in figure 2A and B.

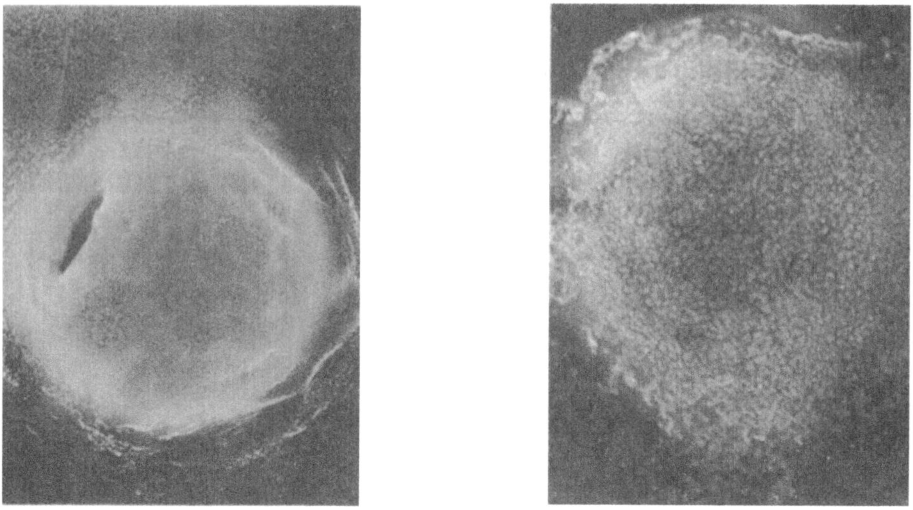

A B

Fig. 2. The scanning electron microscopy patterns of glutenin after 10 /A/ and 60 /B/ min. proteolysis by bromelain

Analysing the presented patterns one could conclude that after the very short proteolysis /10 min./ two kinds of bromelain attack on glutenin complex took place: the very deep penetration inside the complex, as well as the surface attack. In the latter case the detached membrane-like fragments could be observed. But also in those experiments we were unable to demonstrate significant differences between glutenins of various baking quality. Glutenin subjected to the more extended proteolysis showed the general loosening of the whole complex and the formation of many small irregular fragments, which were detached from its surface. Those experiments can probably suggest that in the first step of proteolysis the small joining units of peptide character are removed, which can cause the detachment of big surface membrane-like subunits, but the prolonged enzyme action decomposes all subunits unspecifically.

It should be noticed that the nature and properties of wheat peptidases were investigated by different authors /e.g. Kruger, 1971; Mc Donald, 1969/, but except the paper cited earlier of Bietz and Rothfus /1970/, no other reports of using the proteolytic enzymes for gluten structural investigations, are known. Recently two publications concerning the mechanism of peptidase action on gluten proteins appeared /Gabor et al. 1982a and b/, but in the described experiments enzymes of microbial origin were used.

As we have under investigation wheat samples of differentiated maturation stages, we came back once again to the experiments on gluten proteolysis by means of bromelain and the results obtained in them are the subject of this contribution.

MATERIAL AND METHODS

As the experimental material, three wheat varieties of American origin were used: Justine, Cheyenne and Scout 66. They were grown in the Experimental Farm Wolica near Warsaw on the gray-brown podsolic soil and grains harvested five times during the development, beginning at about 45 per cent of their dry matter - till full maturity. The grains of earlier maturation stages were freeze-dried in the LGA-05 lyophiliser /Janetzki, GDR/ and ground in the laboratory mill, but those being close to full maturity were conditioned to the moisture of 14,5 per cent and ground using the laboratory mill QC 112 of Labor Mim, Hungary. Samples so obtained were stored for analysis under nitrogen at the temp. below $4^{o}C$. They were subjected then to the preliminary analysis and to protein extraction.

The determined amounts of meal dry matter of various maturity were extracted three times by means of 1 h shaking with 3,5 volumes of 0,1M sodium chloride /to remove albumins and globulins/ and then two times with 5 volumes of water to remove the remaining NaCl. The residue was then extracted by two hour shakings with 3,5 volumes /calculated on the initial weight/ of the same portion of 0,05 M acetic acid. In the supernatant /centrifugation for 15 min. at 15 000 rpm/ the total N was determined in the Kjell-Foss equipment /Foss Electric, Kopenhagen/. The incubation mixture contained in the total volume 4,6 cm^3 5 mg of grain nitrogen and 5 mg of bromelain preparation /VEB Arzneimittelwerk, Dresden, GDR/. The proteolysis was carried out for 20 min. at the temp. $35^{o}C$ and the reaction stopped by trichloroacetic acid /TCA/ addition to the final concentration 6 per cent. Samples were allowed to stand at room temp. for 30 min, to precipitate all proteins and then centrifuged for 10 min. at 5 000 rpm. In the supernatant the nonprotein N was determined as above and the protein hydrolysis per cent during the enzymatic reaction was calculated, as related to the control sample, which constituted the same amount of gluten protein and inactivated enzyme treated with TCA.

RESULTS AND DISCUSSION

The results of described experiments, constituting the mean values of at least three repetitions, are presented in table 3

Table 3

Proteolysis per cents of gluten proteins soluble in acetic acid subjected to the bromelain action, isolated from wheat samples of various maturation stages

Stage	Justine		Cheyenne		Scout 66	
	1	2	1	2	1	2
II	-	-	50,0	43,60	-	-
III	45,5	44,44	-	-	61,5	43,26
IV	65,5	43,64	62,0	42,30	66,0	41,17
V	88,0	43,23	70,0	41,18	90,0	37,50
VI	-	-	92,5	40,35	92,4	38,10

1 - dry weight per cent, 2 - proteolysis per cent
Justine - low quality, Cheyenne and Scout 66 - high quality

The data presented in table 3 demonstrate the regular decrease of the proteolysis rates of glutens in the course of grain maturation in all three varieties under investigation. This can suggest that the accessibility of peptide bonds in protein molecules to the peptidase action is higher at the beginning of grain development, than in the latter maturation stages. It can be possible, therefore, that the molecules of gliadin and particularly those of glutenin, which are formed already in the very early maturation stage, are at this time still not fully developed in their final structure, which is continuing to change during the whole grain development.
One of the directions of those conformation changes should be the formation of new bondings of different nature and, may be, the lowering of the molecule asymmetry, and thus - the increasing of their compactness. Of interest should be also the rather small differences between the proteolysis rates of gluten proteins isolated from grains of following maturation stages, amounting 1 till 6 per cent only. Therefore one can suppose also that those changes would concern not the gliadin or glutenin subunits, but rather some albumin-like protein structures, the presence of which we postulated earlier to exist /Dałek-Zawistowska et al. 1975/.
We suggested that those albumin-like subunits could serve in the building up the gluten complex, as the elements sticking together the glutenin and gliadin subunits. This suggestion was confirmed later by Bietz /1981/, who was able to

isolate from gluten complex a protein fraction of such character. The level of albumin-like proteins in gluten complex would be not uniform during the whole maturation period and this could be also one of the reasons of various proteolysis rates of that complex. Nevertheless, the possibility also exists that our observation presented in this contribution could be due to the differentiated compactness of at least some subunits taking part in the building up the gluten complex in the following maturation stages of wheat grains.

Comparing the proteolysis rates of gluten proteins extracted by means of acetic acid from grains of corresponding maturation stages of varieties differing in baking quality, one could notice the direct relationship between those two factors. The variety Justine of poor quality showed the highest proteolysis rates in all compared stages and the Scout 66 of highest one presented the lowest rate of this process. This observation constitutes one more confirmation of the existence of the relationship between the molecule compactness of gluten components and wheat quality, which was demonstrated in our earlier investigations /Liss and Kączkowski, 1975; Bernacka et al. 1977/. Moreover it indicates that such differences can take place already in earlier maturation stages.

The results presented in this contribution may be regarded as being one more example of using the proteolysis rate determination of gluten proteins as a tool of their detailed investigations. We find this approach to be very useful in the elucidation of some structural problems, although bromelain may be possibly not the best proteolytic enzyme to apply, as it is the mixed preparation of peptidases of rather broad specificity. As concerns the quality differences, better results could be probably obtained when the native purified wheat peptidases were used /Liss and Kączkowski, 1975/, but such experiments needed rather complicated enzyme purification procedure, which additionally was not stable enough. Unfortunately, no other investigations of this type were found in literature, except those of Täufel /Gabor, Täufel and Ruttloff, 1982a and b/, but in this case the proteinases of microbial origin were applied and only proteolysis products characterised, as concerns their molecular weight.

Finally, it would be possibly of interest, whether the gluten proteins of various quality, showing different proteolysis rates, would be digested by man or animal with differentiated velocity, and thus - whether those proteins of higher baking quality would be decomposed not fully along the alimentary tract. As one can see from the results presented in tables 2 and 3, the differences in proteolysis rates between gluten proteins of high and poor quality are rather low and do not overcome 10 or 15 per cent. On the other hand, our calculations allow to suggest, that because of the significant excess of the proteolytic enzymes of various specificity in the alimentary tract, there should exist no danger that the former should be digested slower, than the latter.

Acknowledgment: This work was carried out under the partial financial support of the US Department of Agriculture, Grant No J-MOA/USDA-17.

REFERENCES

Bernacka T., Kączkowski J., Liss W. and Serwatowska J. /1977/. The fractional composition of wheat proteins and the possibility of its hereditability in F_1 generation. Acta Agrobotanica 30, 5 - 11.

Bietz J.A. /1981/. Private communication

Bietz J.A. and Rothfus J.A. /1970/. Comparison of peptides from wheat gliadin and glutenin. Cereal Chem. 47, 381 - 392.

Dałek-Zawistowska U., Bartoszewicz K. and Kączkowski J. /1975/. The equilibrium between the high and low molecular fractions of wheat gluten. Bull.Acad.Polon.Sci. ser.sci.biol. 23, 75 - 81.

Gabor R., Täufel A. and Ruttloff H. /1982a/. Veränderungen der Molmassen von Weizenkleberproteinen nach schwacher Proteolyse. Z.Lebensm.Unters.Forsch. 175, 399 - 402.

Gabor R., Täufel A. and Ruttloff H. /1982b/. Zur Wirkungsweise verschiedener mikrobieller Proteasepräparate auf Weizengluten und Mehl. Die Nahrung 26, 37 - 46.

Galińska Z. and Kączkowski J. /1977/. Electrophoretic investigations of proteolysis products of wheat gluten. Acta.Aliment.Polon. 3/27/, 379 - 386.

Kruger J.E. /1971/. Purification and some properties of malted wheat BAPA-ase. Cereal Chem. 48, 512 - 522.

Liss W. and Kączkowski J. /1975/. Proteolysis as the compactness index of wheat gluten molecules. Acta Aliment. Polon. 1/25/, 281 - 288.

Mc Donald E.C. /1969/. Proteolytic enzymes of wheat and their relation to baking quality. Bakers Digest, 43, 26 - 28, 30.

Proc. Int. Assoc. Cereal Chem. Symp. Amino Acid Compn and Biol. Value of Cereal Proteins Budapest, Hungary 1983, R. Lásztity, M. Hidvégi, eds

EFFECTS OF FERTILIZERS ON THE AMINO ACID COMPOSITION OF CEREAL PROTEIN

ISTVÁN NÉMETH

Department of Crop Cultivation, Agricultural University
H-8361 Keszthely, Hungary

ABSTRACT

We tested samples from the experiments conducted by the Crop Cultivation Department of the Keszthely University of Agricultural Sciences on faintly eluviated brown forest soil at Keszthely in 1963, and on highly eluviated pseudogleyed brown forest soil at Szentgyörgyvölgy in 1965 to find out the effect on N P and K fertilizers on yields, crude protein and on amino acid contents of wheat and maize. In wheat protein, methionine and lysine were present in the smallest amount and were decreased by N fertilization, P and K with no N added were found to reduce, 87 kg/ha N, on the other hand, to increase the methionine, lysine, valine, phenylalanine and isoleucine content of wheat protein. As compared to a dressing of 87 kg/ha, 174 kg/ha N proved to decrease the total amino acid amount, while 261 kg/ha N continued reducing the amounts of lysine and arginine. EAAI of the wheat protein was the lowest on application of 174 kg/ha and the highest at 87 kg/ha N. In maize protein, lysine and methionine were found in the lowest amount. In the no-N treatment, with the exception of arginine and methionine, the rest of the amino acids were found to decrease, 87 kg/ha N proved to increase lysine, valine, histidine and phenylalanine and decrease the rest; 174 kg/ha N continued decreasing them, except leucine. On application of 261 kg/ha N, all amino acids tested – except methionine - were found to increase, whereas in response to 348 kg/ha N the amount of amino acids was increased without exception; so the EAAI for the maize protein was at its highest at 348 kg/ha N. K and N fertilization without P proved to decrease, the addition of 120 kg/ha P_2O_5 to increase all essential amino acids of wheat protein, though in response to 180 kg/ha P_2O_5 they were decreased, except leucine. EAAI of maize protein was decreased by both P deficiency and P_2O_5 dressing exceeding 120 kg.

In maize protein, amino acid content was less adversely affected by P deficiency than in wheat protein, it was only methionine that decreased, the rest increased, while the application of 120 kg/ha P_2O_5 involved an increase in the amino acids examined, with the exception of leucine. The EAAI of maize protein was the highest in response to 180 kg/ha P_2O_5.

P and N fertilization without K was found to decrease the amount of essential amino acids except histidine in wheat protein and to increase it in maize protein.

INTRODUCTION

At the present stage of agricultural development, the role of quality is more and more often emphasized. Cereals give most of the vegetable proteins in the human diet, though if we examine cereal protein, it appears that it is poor in several essential amino acids; especially in lysine. Potsubay et al./1966/ found that - from the point of view of feeding - the essential amino acid content of cereals is less favourable as compared to other feeds; mostly because of their low lysine content.

N fertilizers have different effects on the amounts of amino acids. Németh and Keresztes /1969/, Müller /1965/ and Michael /1964/ find that the biological value of protein does not decrease as a result of N fertilizers if supplemented with adequate amounts of P and K. The utilization of proteins, consequently their biological value, depends mostly on the quality and quantity of amino acids they contain /Mitchell 1959, Popov 1961, Nehring and Schröder 1962/.

Examining the protein percentage and amino acid composition of wheat grain, Vincze and Szüts /1978/ found that higher levels resulted in an increase in ASP, GLU, GLY, LYS, to a lesser degree in SER, ALA, ILE, LEU, TYR, PHE, whereas there was no change in the absolute amount of PRO, CYS, MET, HIS, ARG. The maximum amounts of TYR, ILE and ALA were observed when N was applied at 120-160 kg/ha, while the lowest level of methionine and proline could be detected at the same rate of N application.

Stock breeds try to improve protein and amino acid percentage by using feed mixtures. Also, synthetic amino acids can be used as additives.

Methionine is produced in the greatest quantities /200000 t/year/; 95 % is used in chick mash and 5 % in various feeds for swine.

The addition of synthetic amino acids implies extra charges and it calls for an adequate industrial background. The application of fertilizers not only increases the average yields of maize and wheat considerably but also effects the feeding value. Consequently, we must find the ratio of nutrients giving the highest yields with the most favourable feeding value.

MATERIALS AND METHODS

Samples were taken from experiments started at Szentgyörgyvölgy and Keszthely in 1963. The soil in the experimental plots at Keszthely was the Ramann-type, faintly eluviated brown forest soil while at Szentgyörgyvölgy it was highly eluviated pseudogleyed brown forest soil.

RESULTS AND DISCUSSION

The effect of N fertilization on the development of amino acid content of wheat protein and its EAAI is shown in Table 1. In wheat protein, methionine and lysine were present in the smallest amount of the essential amino acids tested; N fertilization decreased the amount of lysine according to data found in literature - there was a similar decrease in methionine, though the extent of decrease depended on the amount of fertilizers applied.

Table 1. Effect of nitrogen fertilization on amino acid content of wheat as expressed in g/16N /Szentgyörgyvölgy/

Amino acid	Fertilizer kg/ha	Treatments					
		1	2	3	4	5	6
	P_2O_5	-	140	140	140	140	140
	K_2O	-	140	140	140	140	140
	N	-	-	87	174	261	348
LYS		2,80	2,66	2,79	2,48	2,32	2,40
MET		1,21	0,92	1,09	0,78	0,92	1,14
VAL		4,30	3,94	4,08	3,96	4,01	4,28
ARG		4,67	4,76	4,68	4,19	4,08	4,54
PHE		4,39	3,94	4,18	3,96	4,58	4,68
ILE		4,11	3,39	3,38	3,34	3,59	3,87
LEU		7,94	6,14	6,67	6,67	6,83	7,15
HIS		1,96	2,01	1,99	1,78	1,83	1,87
EAAI		59,20	54,20	56,60	50,90	53,50	55,90

P and K were found to reduce EAAI by 5 %, 87 kg/ha N, on the other hand, to increase it by 2,4 %, but 174 kg/ha N decreased it to such an extent that it did not reach the level of control in spite of increasing it by 2,6 % /261 kg/ha N/ and, further, by 2,4 % /348 kg/ha N/.

N deficiency /2nd treatment/ increased the histidine and arginine content of wheat protein to a small degree, while it decreased the rest. The highest degree of decrease was found in isoleucine + leucine, phenylalanine, methionine, and lysine.

87 kg/ha N decreased histidine and arginine, while it slightly increased the rest. 174 kg/ha N decreased the amounts of each amino acid; consequently the EAAI of protein was the lowest in this treatment. As a result of 261 kg/ha N application, arginine and lysine further decreased in amount, while the rest was adversely affected; phenylalanine, methionine and threonine showed the highest increase rate, the others did not change considerably.

The effect of N fertilization on amino acids and EAAI of maize protein is demonstrated in Table 2.

Table 2. Effect of N fertilization on amino acid content of maize as expressed in g/16 g N /Keszthely/

Amino acid	Fertilizer kg/ha	Treatments 1	2	3	4	5	6
	P_2O_5	-	140	140	140	140	140
	K_2O	-	140	140	140	140	140
	N	-	-	87	174	261	348
LYS		2,16	2,10	2,29	2,26	2,29	2,63
MET		1,40	1,49	1,26	1,24	1,14	1,37
VAL		4,19	4,08	4,58	4,18	4,58	4,92
ARG		3,94	4,21	4,00	3,95	4,12	4,35
PHE		3,81	3,71	4,12	3,50	4,23	4,69
ILE		3,56	3,22	3,66	3,28	3,32	3,66
LEU		12,33	11,39	10,30	13,22	13,39	13,50
HIS		2,03	1,98	2,29	2,03	2,17	2,63
EAAI		58,60	57,50	59,70	57,50	60,00	66,40

Maize protein - similarly to wheat - contained lysine and methionine in the smallest amounts. The amount of lysine on plots with N deficiency decreased, though, a slight increase was observed as a result of 87 kg/ha N application, which was kept on the same level up to 261 kg/ha, to show an increase again at 348 kg/ha N- due to the lower dry substance percentage at harvest.

In the no-N treatment /treatment No.2/, with the exception of arginine and methionine, the rest of the amino acids were found to decrease. 87 kg/ha N proved to decrease the amount of nitrogen, leucine and methionine, but it increased that of the rest.

Similarly to wheat, 174 kg/ha N as compared with 87 kg/ha, decreased the amino acid content of maize protein with the exception of leucine, while, histidine, phenylalanine, valine showed the greatest rate of decrease. On application of 261 kg/ha N, all amino acids were found to increase, except methionine; 348 kg/ha N increased the amount of all amino acids; histidine, phenylalanine, methionine, lysine and valine showed the highest level of increase.

In the no-N treatment /treatment No.2 /, the EAAI decreased by 1,1 % as compared with the control, though it increased by 2,2 % on the application of 87 kg/ha N, while it again dropped to the level of no-N treatments as a result of 174 kg/ha N application, then it rose again by 2,5-8,9 % following a 261-348 kg/ha N treatment.

The effect of phosphorous fertilization on amino acid content of maize-protein is shown in Table 3.

Table 3.

Effect of phosphorous fertilization on amino acid content of wheat as expressed in g/16 g N /Szentgyörgyvölgy/

Amino acid	Fertilizer kg/ha	Treatments			
		1	2	3	4
	N	-	174	174	174
	K_2O	-	140	140	140
	P_2O_5	-	-	120	180
LYS		2,80	2,29	2,65	2,23
MET		1,21	1,00	1,12	0,91
VAL		4,30	3,86	4,50	4,29
ARG		4,67	4,43	4,98	4,04
PHE		4,39	4,08	4,74	4,62
ILE		4,11	3,65	4,26	4,04
LEU		7,94	6,44	7,47	7,50
HIS		1,96	1,79	2,01	1,65
EAAI		59,20	51,90	59,10	53,80

As compared with the amino acid content of wheat protein grown on plots receiving no fertilizers, K and N fertilization without P decreased all amino acids, whereas 120 kg/ha P increased them all. A further rise in P decreased all the amino acids. Accordingly, P deficiency and amounts of P higher than 120 kg/ha both decreased EAAI.

Table 4 illustrates the effect of P fertilization on the amino acid content of maize protein.

Table 4.

Effect of phosphorous fertilization on amino acid content of maize as expressed in g/16 g N /Keszthely/

Amino acid	Fertilizer kg/ha	Treatments 1	2	3	4
	N	-	174	174	174
	K_2O	-	140	140	140
	P_2O_5	-	-	120	180
LYS		2,16	2,52	2,86	2,90
MET		1,40	1,26	1,49	1,45
VAL		4,19	4,69	4,69	5,02
ARG		3,94	4,23	4,35	4,35
PHE		3,81	4,69	5,03	5,02
ILE		3,56	3,55	3,32	3,68
LEU		12,33	14,30	13,39	15,63
HIS		2,03	2,63	2,75	2,68
EAAI		58,60	65,40	69,10	70,70

N and K fertilization decreased the amount of methionine, but it increased that of the others; histidine, phenylalanine and leucine showed the highest rate of increase.

The amount of isoleucine and leucine was decreased as a result of application of 120 kg/ha P_2O_5; it had no effect on valine, while the rest was increased.

180 kg/ha P_2O_5 increased the percentage of valine and isoleucine + leucine only, as compared with the application of 120 kg/ha, whereas, it slightly decreased the amount of methionine and histidine and had no considerable effect on the rest.

EAAI was found to be rising as a result of rising

fertilizer levels, but the rate of rise was the lowest at 180 kg/ha P_2O_5.

The effect of potassium fertilization on the amino acid content of wheat protein can be seen in Table 5.

Table 5.

Effect of potassium fertilization on amino acid content of wheat as expressed in g/16 g N /Szentgyörgyvölgy/

Amino acid	Fertilizer kg/ha	Treatments 1	2	3	4
	N	-	174	174	174
	P_2O_5	-	140	140	140
	K_2	-	-	160	240
LYS		2,80	2,45	2,31	2,46
MET		1,21	1,18	1,15	0,97
VAL		4,30	3,95	3,96	3,79
ARG		4,67	4,58	4,37	3,79
PHE		4,39	4,10	4,20	3,87
ILE		4,11	3,55	3,63	3,61
LEU		7,94	6,71	6,60	6,51
HIS		1,96	1,97	1,73	1,76
EAAI		59,20	55,10	53,40	51,10

As compared to the amino acid content of wheat grown on plots receiving no fertilization, N and P fertilizers decreased the amino acid content of wheat protein, with the exception of histidine, and, lysine, valine, isoleucine + leucine showed the most marked decrease.

The application of 160 kg/ha K_2O resulted in a decrease in the amount of other amino acids, except phenylalanine, valine, and isoleucine.

A further decrease in methionine, valine, arginine, and phenylalanine percentage was observed at the application of 240 kg/ha K_2O, while no considerable change was found in the amount of isoleucine + leucine, though it slightly increased the amount of lysine and histidine.

The EAAI for maize protein was at its highest with wheat varieties grown on plots without fertilization, P and N fertilizers decreased it by 4,1 %, furthermore 160 kg/ha K_2O by 1,7 %, and 240 kg/ha K_2O by 2,3 %.

The effect of potassium fertilizers on the amino acid content of wheat protein is shown in Table 6.

Table 6. Effect of potassium fertilization on amino acid content of maize as expressed in g/16 g N /Keszthely/

Amino acid	Fertilizer kg/ha	Treatments 1	2	3	4
	N	-	174	174	174
	P_2O_5	-	140	140	140
	K_2	-	-	160	240
LYS		2,16	2,89	2,61	2,61
MET		1,40	1,33	1,20	1,42
VAL		4,19	4,70	4,25	4,14
ARG		3,94	4,70	4,47	4,03
PHE		3,81	4,46	4,58	4,14
ILE		3,56	3,37	3,38	3,81
LEU		12,33	13,61	12,85	13,62
HIS		2,03	2,65	2,72	2,61
EAAI		58,60	69,00	65,40	63,50

While N and P decreased the amino acid percentage with the exception of histidine in wheat as compared to the amino acid levels of wheat yields, collected from plots without fertilization, N and P increased the amount of the other amino acids, except methionine; the highest values were found with histidine, arginine, phenylalanine and valine.

Witn the exception of phenylalanine and histidine, 160 kg/ha K_2O decreased the amount of amino acids, the rate of decrease was most considerable in the case of lysine, methionine, valine and arginine, which are to be found in maize protein in the smallest amounts. The application of 240 kg/ha K_2O brought about an increase in the amounts of methionine and isoleucine + leucine, whereas it had no significant effect on lysine percentage, and it decreased those of the others. The EAAI for maize was increased by the application of N and P fertilizers as opposed to wheat, though it was decreased by potassium fertilizers, but in spite of the decrease, EAAI for maize grown on plots receiving potassium fertilization was higher than in the case of maize receiving no fertilization.

REFERENCES

Michael, G. /1964/. Vlijanie arotnüh udobrenija n kolicsesztvo i kocsesztvo belka u kulturnüh rasztenij. Szelszk. Hoz. Rub. Rosztenievodsztvo, Moscow, 9, 32-34.

Mitchell, H.H. /1959/. Some species and age differences in amino acid requirements. In: Protein and Amino Acid Nutrition. New York, pp. 180-195.

Müller, K. /1965/. Über die Protein- und Kohlenhydratsynthese in der Kartoffel in Verlauf der Vegetation bei unterschiedlicher Kaliversorgung der Pflanze. Der Kartoffelban, Hildesheim. 16, 8-10.

Nehring, K. and Schröder, I. /1962/. Untersuchungen zur enzymatischen Hydrolyse von Eiweissfutterstoffen. I. Mitteil. Zur Methodik der enzymatischen Hydrolyse. Arch. Tierernährung, Berlin. 12, 305-313.

Németh, I. and Keresztes, I. /1969/. A burgonya aminosavtartalmának alakulása különböző mütrágyaadagok hatására. /Effects of fertilization on the amino acid content of potato./ Keszthelyi Agrártudományi Főiskola Közleményei XI, 9, 1-44.

Popov, I.Sz. /1961/. Problema aminokiszlot v kormlenü szel'szkohozjajsztvennüh zsivotnüh. Zsivotnovodsztvo, Moscow, 3, 13-25.

Potsubay, J., Duduk, V. and Vincze, L. /1966/. Baromfitakarmányok aminosavtartalmának vizsgálata. /Investigation of the amino acid content of poultry feeds./ Keszthelyi Agrártudományi Főiskola Kiadványa VIII, 7, 1-28.

Vincze, L. and Szüts, G. /1978/. A buza és a kukorica fehérje aminosavtartalom alapján számitott biológiai értékének alakulása a nitrogén mütrágyaadag változásának függvényében. /Effect of nitrogen fertilization on the biological value of wheat- and maize proteins, calculated from amino acid composition./ In: XX. Georgikon Napok Keszthelyen. pp. 380-397.

Proc. Int. Assoc. Cereal Chem. Symp. Amino Acid Compn and Biol. Value of Cereal Proteins Budapest, Hungary 1983, R. Lásztity, M. Hidvégi, eds

EFFECT OF THERMAL PROCESSING ON THE TRYPTOPHAN CONTENT OF BABY FOODS

FERENC ÖRSI

Department of Biochemistry and Food Technology,
Technical University of Budapest
H-1111 Budapest, Müegyetem rkp. 3, Hungary

Holz's /1972/ method for the determination of tryptophan, adapted to the Contiflo automatic analyzer is optimized for determining the tryptophan content of baby food. The effect of heat treatment /40-100 °C/ and humidity during storage /0-80 % relative humidity/ is studied on the tryptophan content of the baby food "Linolac". The decomposition can be described well by a first order kinetic model. Its activation energy is found to be 105 kJ/mol. The effect of moisture on the activation energy is interpreted as a decreasing factor.

In judging the biological value of baby foods an important role is played by its amino acid composition, especially the amount of essential amino acids is of great importance. The determination of tryptophan cannot be carried out from the acid hydrolysate of the protein, as its sensitive ring decomposes in acidic media. Therefore numerous methods are elaborated for its analysis by its alkaline and enzymatic hydrolysis or modified acidic hydrolysis. We have reported earlier /Örsi and Zsigmond, 1980/ on the adaptation of the method of Holz /1972/ for a Contiflo type analyzer, which method is successfully applied in the determination of tryptophan in alkaline hydrolysates since then.

In the present work the parameters of this method were optimized for the determination of tryptophan in the baby food "Linolac", and changes due to heat treatment as well as the effect of humidity on the tryptophan content during storage of the baby food at 40 °C were studied.

1. MATERIALS AND METHODS

The baby food "Linolac", product of the EGyT Lacta Baby Food Factory /Hungary/ has been used for the investigations. The p-N,N-dimethylaminocinnaldehyde /Koch-Light Ltd./ has been applied as reagent for the determination of tryptophan. For the preparation of the standard tryptophan solutions DL-tryptophan produced by REANAL has been used.

1.1 Hydrolysis of the protein sample

Baby food corresponding to about 60 mg of protein was weighed into a test tube, 10 cm^3 of a 4M NaOH solution was added, the solution freed from air by bubbling N_2 through it, then the test tube was sealed. Hydrolysis was carried out at 105 °C. for 16 h. After that the test tubes were opened and acidified by 10 cm^3 of 4M H_2SO_4 solution, transferred into a 25 cm^3 normal flask and filled up. Determinations were made immediately after filtration.

1.2 Determination of tryptophan by automatic Contiflo analyzer

The modul produced by Labor MIM for total sugar determination /OL-734/ has been modified for the analysis of tryptophan and is shown in Fig. 1.

1.2.1 Reagents needed are the following:

1.2.1.1 Diluting solution: 0.2 cm^3 water solution of detergent Brij 35 in a concentration of 0.3 g/cm^3 /BDH Ltd./ is added to 1 l of distilled water.

1.2.1.2 H_2SO_4 solution: 7 volume unit of concentrated sulfuric acid is diluted with 3 volume unit of distilled water. The concentration of the resulting sulfuric acid solution is about 78 % /m/m/.

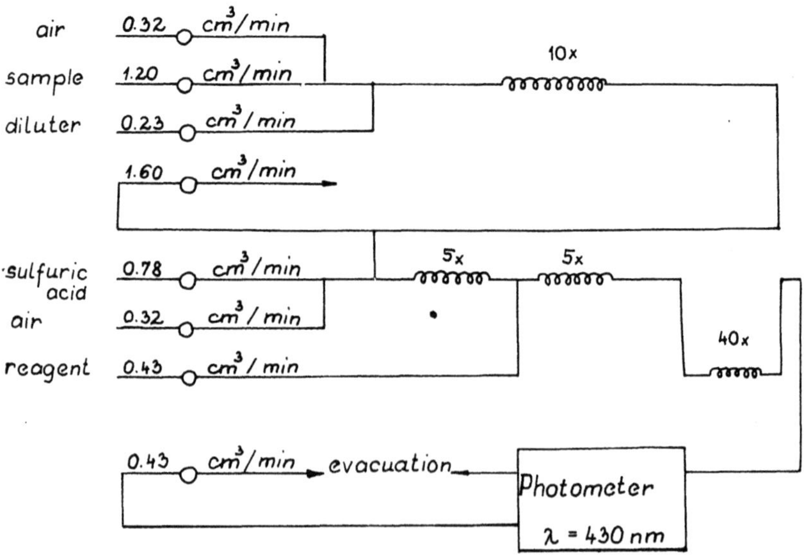

Fig.1. Modul for tryptophan analysis.

1.2.1.3 Reagent solution: 0.5 mg/cm^3 of p-N,N-dimethylamino-cinnaldehyde in a 1M H_2SO_4 solution. The reagent can be stored for 2-3 weeks at ambient temperature.

1.2.2 Operation of the modul

The sample to be studied is diluted with the detergent--containing water, then a small part of it is added to the sulfuric acid solution, and to this mixture is the reagent solution added. The colour is developed at ambient temperature, its intensity is measured photometrically at 430 nm. The measurement is carried out at a speed of 40 sample/h and at a suction/washing ratio of 2:1. For determining the calibration curve, a series of standard solutions was prepared in the concentration range of 0-120 mg/dm^3 from the DL-tryptophan. Significant deviation from linearity was observed only above the concentration of 100 mg/dm^3.

The variance coefficient of parallel measurements is 1.62 %. The minimum tryptophan content which can be determined under the above conditions is 0.05 %.

1.3 Determination of the moisture content of baby food

The moisture content of baby food samples was determined from thermogravimetric curves recorded in the temperature range of 20-250 °C. The curves were obtained with 500 mg samples on plate sample holders at a heating rate of 5°C/min. Water evolved from the samples till 170 °C.

1.4 Heat treatment of samples

500 mg of the baby food was weighed into a test tube and heat-treated at 40,60,80 and 100 °C in a test tube thermostat made of an aluminium block by KUTESz, for 4-7 h, then the necessary amount of the alkaline hydrolyzing solution was added and the tryptophan content determined. In every case, three parallel measurements were made.

1.5 Storage of baby food samples

50 g portions of the baby food were stored in 5 l desiccators in which the relative humidity desired was adjusted by 2 l H_2SO_4 solution /Perry, 1968/. The humidity values studied and the sulfuric acid concentrations needed for their adjustment are summarized in Table 1.

The desiccators with the samples were stored in a water-jacketted biological thermostat /Labor MIM/ at 40 °C. After thorough mixing, three 500 mg samples were taken every other day, and their tryptophan contents were determined according to the method described above.

Table 1. H_2SO_4 concentrations for adjusting given relative humidities

Relative humidity / % /	H_2SO_4 concentration /%, m/m/
0	96
40	48
80	27

2. RESULTS

2.1 Optimization of conditions

As a first step, the critical parameters of the determination /concentrations of the hydrolyzing alkali, the sulfuric acid and reagent, time of hydrolysis/ were investigated.

The effect of the concentration of H_2SO_4 and p-N,N--dimethylaminocinnaldehyde reagent on the peak height obtained by using a standard tryptophan solution of a concentration of 60 mg/dm^3 is shown in Fig. 2. It is seen that H_2SO_4 diluted in a H_2SO_4:H_2O ratio of 7:3, and a concentration of 0.5 mg/cm^3 for the p-N,N-dimethylaminocinnaldehyde proved to be optimum. In further experiments these concentrations have been used.

For determining the optimal alkali concentration, 20 h hydrolyses were carried out with the same baby food sample in the concentration range of 0.1-6 mol/dm^3. The measured tryptophan content is plotted against the alkali concentration in Fig.3. It can be seen that the 4 mol/dm^3 proved to be a suitable concentration.

The effect of the time of hydrolysis was studied in the range of 0-30 h with the same baby food sample, and the tryptophan content obtained is plotted as the function of the time of hydrolysis in Fig.4. The results show that a hydrolysis time of 16 h is sufficient, therefore this was used in further experiments.

2.2 Study of the effect of heat treatment

The change in the tryptophan content of samples heat-treated at 40, 60, 80 and 100°C is shown in Fig.5.

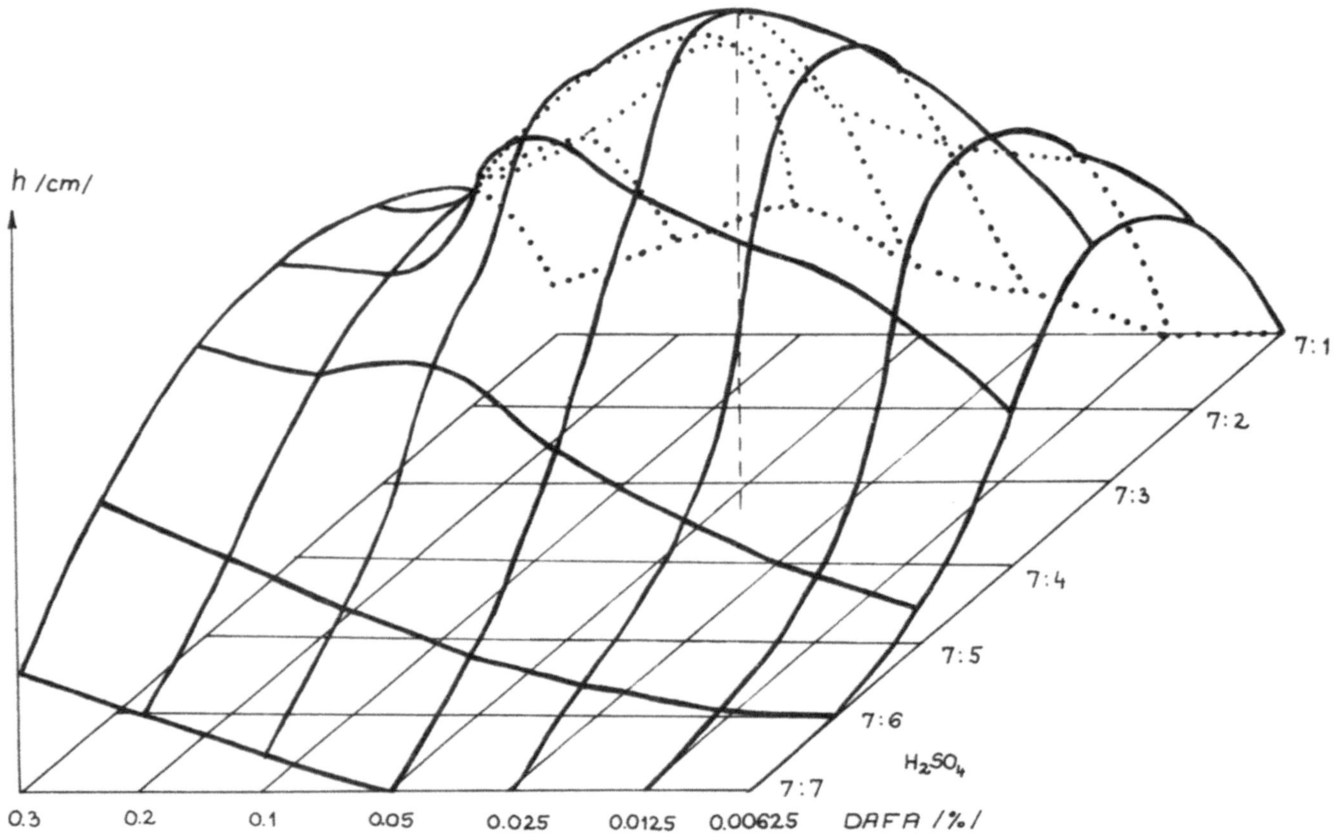

Fig.2. Experimental results of optimization.

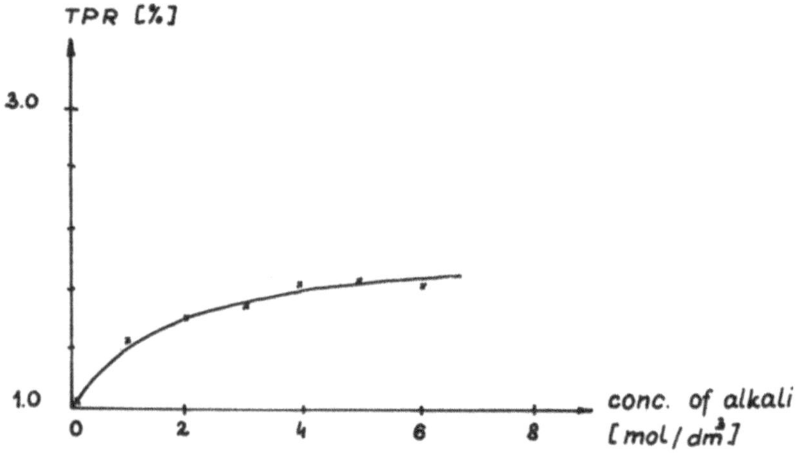

Fig.3. Dependence of the tryptophan content on the concentration of alkali.

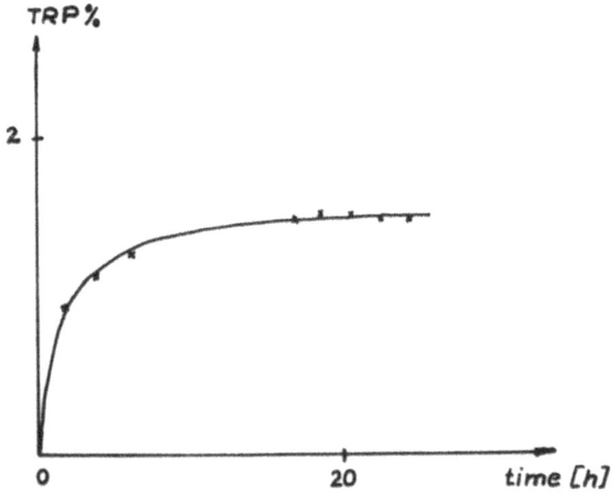

Fig.4. Dependence of the tryptophan content on hydrolysis time.

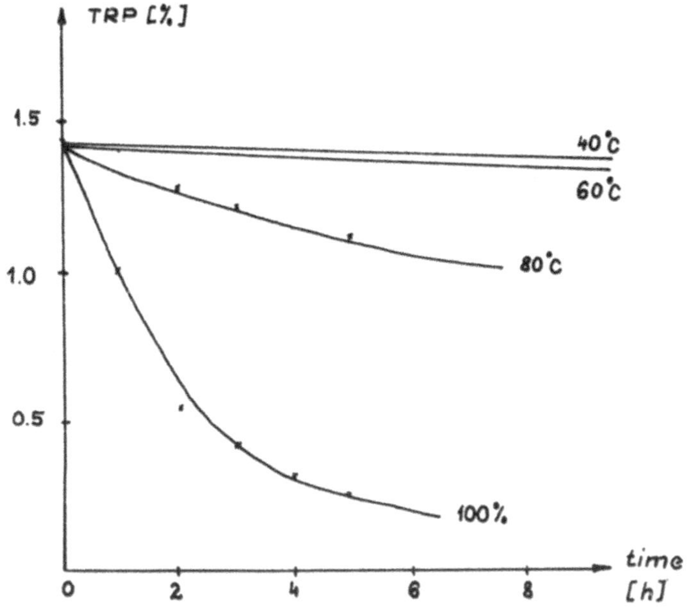

Fig.5. Experimental results of heat treatments.

The decrease in the tryptophan content is unequivocal, and it takes place with an increasing rate with increasing temperature.

Dworschák showed /1976/ that the change in the tryptophan content in baby foods follows a first order kinetics, therefore we also tried to process our data by a first order kinetical model.
The measured data were approximated with the following first order kinetic equation:

$$\ln / C_{TRP} / = \ln C_o - kt \qquad /1/$$

where

- C_{TRP}: concentration of tryptophan,
- C_o : initial concentration of tryptophan,
- k : reaction rate constant /min^{-1}/,
- t : time /min/.

Model parameters were determined by the least squares method.

A very good agreement has been found between the measured and calculated values, the correlation coefficient characterizing the goodness of fit was above 0.94 in every case.

In Fig.6 the logarithm of the calculated rate constant is plotted against the reciprocal temperature measured in K. The values thus obtained lie on a straight line, i.e. the temperature dependence of the reaction can be described by the Arrhenius equation. The straight line best fitted to the experimental points was also determined by the least squares method. From the slope of the straight line the activation energy has been calculated by the following relationship:

$$H = R \times m \qquad /2/$$

where
- m is the slope /K/,
- R is the gas constant / kJ/mol xK/,
- H is the activation energy / kJ/mol/.

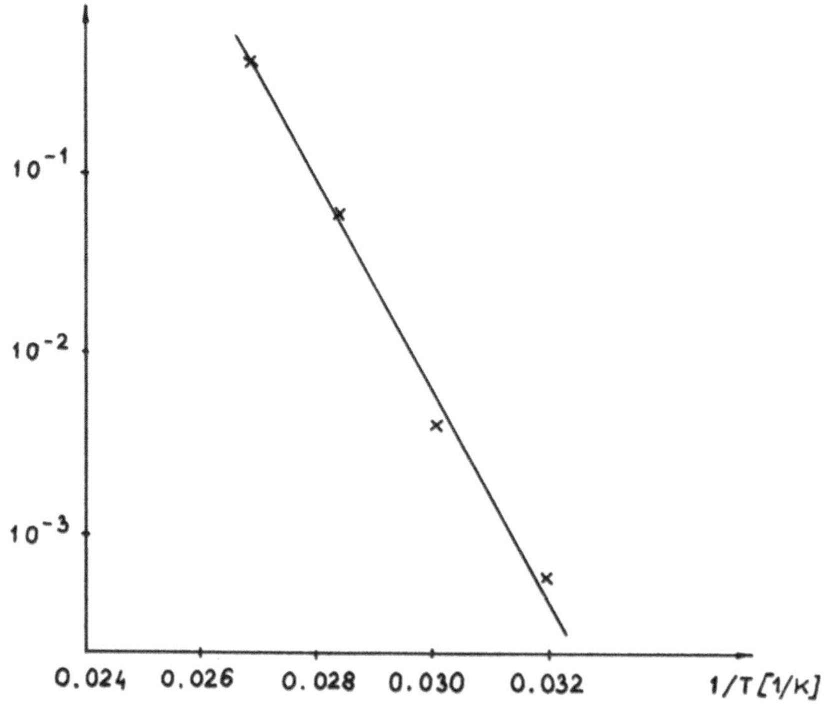

Fig.6. Temperature dependence of the reaction rate constant.

Upon calculation, the activation energy of the decomposition of tryptophan, from this equation 105± 6.88 kJ/mol is obtained.

The reaction kinetic parameters thus obtained allow the estimation of the decomposition of tryptophan at any temperature.

2.3 Study of the effect of moisture content on the effect of tryptophan

Decomposition of tryptophan in baby food "Linolac" at 40 °C was investigated at 0, 40 and 80 % humidity.

In Fig. 7 changes in the tryptophan content are plotted in the function of storage time during the two weeks storage in desiccators with different relative humidities. It is seen that similar curves are obtained as at the heat treatment, corresponding to a first order kinetic model. The rate constant calculated was greater than that for samples only heat treated but not stored.

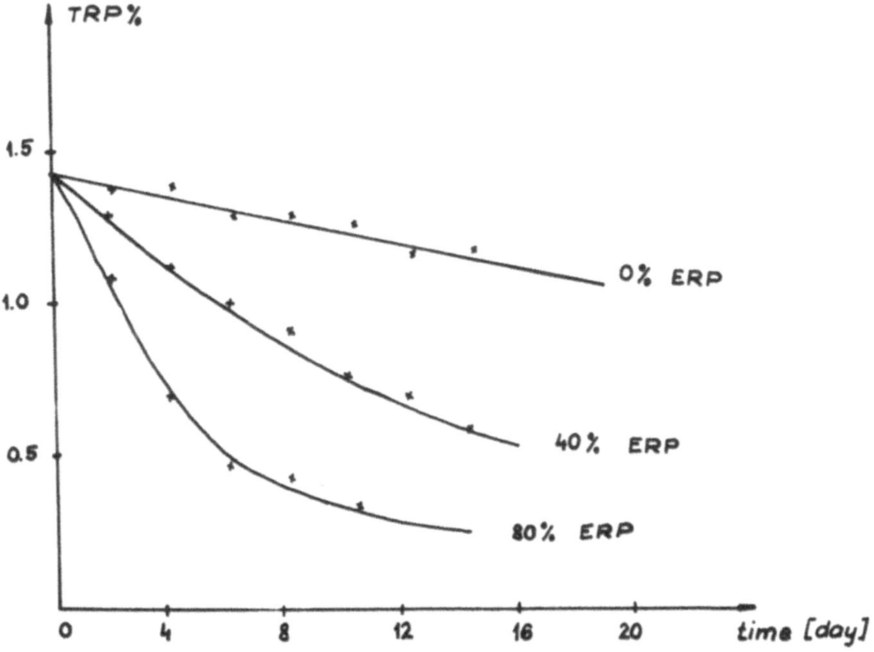

Fig.7. Results of the storage experiments.

In our opinion, the increase of the rate constant can be ascribed to the increased mobility of the reactants in the environment with more humidity due to the water uptake, and as a consequence, the activation energy of the reaction decreases. The decrease in the activation energy can be calculated from the rate constants, measured originally and in the environment with greater humidity by the following relationship:

$$\Delta H = RT \ln k/k_o \qquad /3/$$

where
- k = rate constant measured in the wet environment at 40°C /min^{-1}/,
- k_o = rate constant measured without storage /min^{-1}/,
- R = gas constant,
- T = 313 K.

The degree of the decrease in the activation energy as the function of the relative humidity at storage is shown in Fig. 8. It can be seen that the activation energy decreases with increasing humidity, and that an increase of 10 % in humidity results in a decrease in the activation energy of about 0.8 kJ/mol.

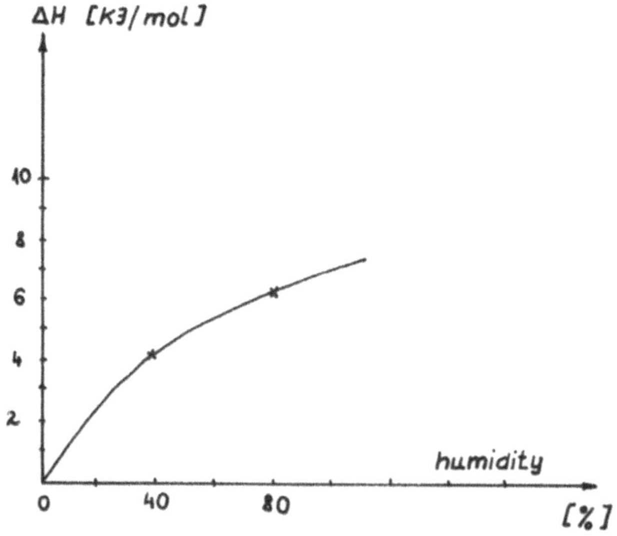

Fig.8. Change of activation energy as a function of humidity of the storage room.

On the basis of literature data it can be expected that with a further increase in humidity the decrease in the activation energy stops and the reaction rate decreases again. Our data show that the decrease in the activation energy is really smaller between 0 and 40 % of humidity than in the range of 40-80 %. As the decomposition of tryptophan in baby foods can be significant even under unfavourable conditions with regard to this reaction, the model of the decomposition process makes an accurate estimation of this phenomenon possible. This is the more significant, as the tryptophan content of the baby food is smaller than that of mother's milk, only 1.4 % instead of 1.9 %, and this can further diminish during storage.

REFERENCES

Dworschák, E.: /1976/ Reactions of carbohydrates and amino acids in foods due to heat treatment. Ph. D. Thesis, Budapest.

Holz, F.: /1972/ Automatische Bestimmung von Tryptophan in Proteinen und proteinhaltigen Pflanzenprodukten mit Dimethylaminozimtaldehyd. Landw. Forsch., 27, 96.

Örsi, F., Zsigmond, A.: /1980/ Determination of tryptophan by Contiflo automatic analyzer. MTA, MÉTE, KÉKI Colloquium.

Perry, J.M.: /1968/ Handbook of Chemistry. Müszaki Kiadó, Budapest, /Hung. translation/.

Proc. Int. Assoc. Cereal Chem. Symp. Amino Acid Compn and Biol. Value of Cereal Proteins Budapest, Hungary 1983, R. Lásztity, M. Hidvégi, eds

AMINO ACID CONTENT AND IN VITRO PROTEIN QUALITY OF DIFFERENT CORN VARIETIES

SAMY FANOUS SHAROBEEM*, RADOMIR LÁSZTITY, MÁTÉ HIDVÉGI, ANDRÁS SALGÓ, LIVIA SIMON-SARKADI

Department of Biochemistry and Food Technology, Technical University of Budapest, H-1111 Budapest, Müegyetem rkp. 3, Hungary
*Permanent address: Department of Biochemistry, Faculty of Agriculture, Zagazig University, Zagazig, Egypt

ABSTRACT

25 different corn varieties from 4 countries were investigated for protein content, amino acid composition and protein quality. The latter was measured by in vitro techniques, i.e. protein digestibility was determined by a multienzymic method and biological value was computed from amino acid data.

INTRODUCTION

Corn is a major, however, low quality source of protein for many people having a small income. These strata of human population can mostly be found in the developing countries. On the other hand, there is a growing interest toward the general use of sweet corn varieties in snack meals, garnishments, etc. In the latter case the essential amino acid content of the crops is not a question of importance. Mainly, it is the undigestable parts (seed coat, hulls, etc.) which can endow the grains with significance. But, from the point of view of the starving millions, the essential amino acid supply provided by dietary corn is of vital importance. The point that corn is a source of essential amino acids has also a great importance in the feeding of monogastric animals because corn constitutes the majority of mixed feeds' components.

There are several papers in the literature concerning the amino acid composition of corn. One of the classics is the work of Bressani and Mertz (1958) where different maize varieties were comparatively investigated. No significant differences in amino acid composition were observed between the varieties of the same countries, although some differences in the amino acid composition of the low and high protein corns of each country were apparent. Similar results were obtained by Vinnichenko and Sytnik (1969). Since the discovery of Mertz et al. (1964) that the opaque-2 mutant gene brings about substantial increases in the lysine and tryptophan contents of maize endosperm proteins, considerable efforts have been devoted to acquire better knowledge on the chemical composition of these and further mutant genotypes (Robutti et al. 1974, Gevers 1975, Ma and Nelson 1975, Tomov 1979, El Kady 1983, El Kady et al. 1983a).

Parallel with the increase of chemical data on corn proteins the nutritional characterization of them has gained more significance. The in vivo biological value of normal corn for albino rats was found to be approximately 63%, however, that of the genetically improved varieties can reach the value of 78% (Eggum et al. 1979). The low biological value of normal corn's protein is due to its reduced lysine and tryptophan content. It was proved that supplementation of maize protein by adding synthetic lysine and tryptophan resulted in better protein quality for rats (Duggal and Sidhu 1970). The relative importance of the level of methionine in corn protein was emphasized by Kies and Fox (1970) who found that methionine rather than tryptophan was the second limiting essential amino acid for humans under conditions of high total nitrogen intake.

In the following, results of a comparative study concerning the amino acid composition, in vitro biological value and in vitro true digestibility of corn proteins from different countries will be presented and discussed.

MATERIALS - METHODS - RESULTS

Varieties

Corn samples grown in four countries were used in the investigation. The 25 varieties selected for analysis are listed in Table 1.

Table 1. Corn varieties from different countries

Country	Variety
Egypt	Pioneer (dent) Giza 2 (dent) Sc 201 (dent) DC 202 (dent)
FRG	Brillant (dent) Nicco (flint) Forte (flint) Dea (flint)
Hungary	BEMA Tc 210 (flint) Mv Sc 394 (flint) Mv Sc 434 (flint) Mv Sc 484 (flint) Pioneer 3732 Sc (dent) Pioneer 3901 Sc (dent) Pioneer 3965A MTC (dent) Mv Sc 550 Wx (dent) Sc 6390 HL opaque-2 (dent) White sweet corn (dent) Sweet corn Mv Sc Ideal (dent)
USA	White flint corn Yellow dent corn K 811 opaque-2 inbredline (dent) K 812 opaque-2 inbredline (flint) K 813 opaque-2 inbredline (dent) K 814 opaque-2 inbredline (flint)

Macro composition of samples

Random samples of the air-dried grains were ground to a fine powder in a laboratory electric mill and these materials were used in the analyses.

Determinations of moisture and nitrogen content were carried out by the standard methods (AOAC 1975). Crude protein content was obtained by multiplying the nitrogen content by the factor of 6.25. The determination of fat content was done by NIR technique using "Infrapid 31" instrument made by Labor Instrument Works, Hungary. These chemical data are demonstrated in Tables 2-5. Values represent the algebraic mean of three analyses.

Table 2. Moisture, protein and fat content of corn varieties from Egypt

Variety	Moisture, %	Protein, %	Fat, %
Pioneer	10.34	9.90	4.40
Giza 2	9.33	10.40	4.06
Sc 201	10.54	9.00	4.20
Dc 202	9.38	9.50	4.05

Table 3. Moisture, protein and fat content of corn varieties from the FRG

Variety	Moisture, %	Protein, %	Fat, %
Brillant	9.89	11.10	4.20
Nicco	10.17	11.10	4.38
Forte	10.06	10.60	4.30
Dea	9.86	10.50	4.25

Table 4. Moisture, protein and fat content of corn varieties from Hungary

Variety	Moisture, %	Protein, %	Fat, %
BEMA Tc 210	10.35	10.50	4.58
Mv Sc 394	10.17	12.31	4.57
Mv Sc 434	10.69	9.13	4.24
Mv Sc 484	10.56	10.88	4.70
Pioneer 3732 Sc	10.83	8.75	4.30
Pioneer 3901 Sc	10.16	9.25	4.20
Pioneer 3965A MTC	10.22	9.88	4.30
Mv Sc 550 Wx	10.54	9.19	4.37
Sc 6390 HL opaque-2	9.98	9.81	3.92
White sweet corn	8.92	13.44	4.30
Sweet corn Mv Sc Ideal	8.89	14.06	4.50

Table 5. Moisture, protein and fat content of corn varieties from the USA

Variety	Moisture, %	Protein, %	Fat, %
White flint corn	9.40	12.20	4.24
Yellow dent corn	9.36	9.80	4.00
K 811 opaque-2	9.05	10.30	3.85
K 812 opaque-2	9.67	10.20	4.00
K 813 opaque-2	9.60	10.70	4.00
K 814 opaque-2	9.13	11.20	3.90

Amino acid analysis

Acid hydrolysis of samples for amino acid analysis was carried out as follows. Samples containing approx. 30 mg protein were measured into heat-resistant test-tubes using an analytical balance.The test-tubes were placed in a boiling water-bath for 15 min for preliminary hydrolysis with 5 cm^3 6 mol per dm^3 hydrochloric acid containing 1% Na-sulphite. Then a further 5 cm^3 6 mol per dm^3 hydrochloric acid containing 0.5% Na-hydrogen sulphite was added and boiling was continued for another 5 min. After this, nitrogen gas was passed through the samples for three minutes to eliminate the air, then the test-tubes were sealed. The hydrolysis was carried out for 24 hours in a test-tube thermostat at 110 °C, after which the test-tubes were opened and the contents washed into 25 cm^3 measuring flasks containing 10 cm^3 neutralizing solution. (1000 cm^3 neutralizing solution contains 39.2 g of Na-citrate, 33.0 cm^3 of cc. HCl, 20.0 cm^3 of thiodiglycol and 0.1 cm^3 of 0.5% pentachlorophenol solution.) The final volume was adjusted using Na-citrate solution with a pH of 2.2. After making up to the mark, the samples were filtered and stored at -18 °C until the analysis was carried out.

The determination of the amino acid composition was carried out using a Mikrotechna AAA 881 automatic amino acid analyser made in Czechoslovakia, where elution takes place on a single column using four buffer solutions. The ninhydrin colour reaction was used for detection. The reagent was produced by mixing two components. The resulting compound was automatically measured photometrically and recorded at 570 and 440 nm with the aid of two flow cuvettes.

The evaluation was carried out manually. The area of the chromatographic peaks was compared to those of standard amino acids chromatographed under identical conditions.

The determination of tryptophan, which is destroyed in the course of hydrochloric acid hydrolysis was carried out after alkali hydrolysis using a Contiflo (Labor Instrument Works, Hungary) automatic analyser with the method developed at the Department of Biochemistry and Food Technology, Technical University, Budapest.)

Samples containing approx. 80 mg protein were measured into heat-resistant test-tubes using an analytical balance. 10 cm^3 4 mol per dm^3 sodium hydroxide were added and preliminary hydrolysis was carried out in a 100 $^{\circ}C$ water-bath for 10 min.

Nitrogen gas was then passed through the samples for 3 min, after which the test-tubes were sealed. The hydrolysis was carried out for 10 hours in a test-tube thermostat at 110 $^{\circ}C$. At the end of this period the test-tubes were opened and the contents were washed into 25 cm^3 measuring flasks containing 10 cm^3 4 mol per dm^3 sulphuric acid. One mol per dm^3 sulphuric acid was used to make up to the mark. The samples were analysed immediately after filtration. The sample passes from the diluting section into a sulphuric acid solution (sulphuric acid: water = 7 : 3) segmented with air in the determination module, then, after mixing, 0.05% p-dimethylamino cinnamic aldehyde reagent dissolved in 20% sulphuric acid is added. The colour reaction takes place at room temperature in a spiral with 40 turns. The coloured product is then measured photometrically at 430 nm. The signals emitted by the photometer are continuously recorded throughout the analysis. Calibration required for evaluation was carried out using standard tryptophan solutions (in the concentration range 0-100 mg per dm^3).

In the course of hydrochloric acid hydrolysis sulphur-containing amino acids suffer a greater or lesser degree of damage, so it is advisable to produce stable oxidation forms of these amino acids for analytical purposes.

Samples containing approx. 60 mg protein were measured into heat-resistant test-tubes using an analytical balance. Four cm^3 performic acid (30% hydrogen peroxide: 98% formic acid = 1 : 9, left to stand for 1 hour before use) were added and the mixture was left to stand in a refrigerator for 20 hours. During this time the sample completely dissolves and oxidation takes place. In order to stop the reaction, 0.6 cm^3 48% hydrogen bromide were added to the sample, after which the material was evaporated to dryness in a vacuum drying cabinet.

Ten cm^3 6 mol per dm^3 hydrochloric acid were added to the oxidized, evaporated samples, which then underwent preliminary hydrolysis on a 100 ^oC water-bath for 15 min. Nitrogen gas was then passed through the samples and the test-tubes were sealed. The hydrolysis was carried out for 24 hours in a test-tube thermostat at 110 ^oC. After hydrolysis the samples were treated as described for the determination of gross amino acid composition.

The amino acid analysis was also carried out in an identical manner, except that in this case the first buffer (pH 3.25) is sufficient for elution.

During the evaluation, the chromatographic peak was compared to a standard cysteic acid peak, after which the values were transformed into cystine assuming a 0.93 degree of conversion for the oxidation.

The amino acid composition of whole grain of corn varieties of different locations are presented in Tables 6-9. Values represent the algebraic mean of three analyses.

In vitro digestibility studies

For the determination of in vitro true digestibility of the corn varieties investigated, the pH-stat procedure followed by linear regression, as modified by Salgó et al. (1984), was used.

The sample containing 200 mg of protein was suspended in 25 cm^3 of bidistilled water, and the pH of the suspension was

Table 6. Amino acid composition of whole grain of corn varieties from Egypt

Amino acid (g per 16 g N)	Dc 202	Giza 2	Sc 201	Pioneer
Aspartic acid	5.43	1.67	7.61	4.95
Threonine	2.50	3.83	4.42	2.63
Serine	3.79	5.99	4.43	3.53
Glutamic acid	17.10	31.73	22.05	18.34
Proline	13.33	5.25	8.96	16.04
Glycine	4.08	4.13	3.99	3.20
Alanine	7.85	9.07	6.36	5.85
Cysteine	1.96	1.25	1.30	1.64
Valine	3.34	2.64	3.92	4.63
Methionine	2.32	2.18	2.29	2.43
Isoleucine	2.54	2.13	2.24	3.52
Leucine	13.40	14.87	12.27	14.73
Tyrosine	4.12	4.00	3.63	3.20
Phenylalanine	5.70	4.20	4.34	5.81
Lysine	2.80	1.89	3.57	2.81
Histidine	3.64	1.88	2.65	2.44
Tryptophan	0.40	0.37	0.38	0.39
Arginine	4.40	2.77	5.72	4.06

Table 7. Amino acid composition of whole grain of corn varieties from the FRG

Amino acid (g per 16 g N)	Brillant	Nicco	Forte	Dea
Aspartic acid	5.82	6.09	7.20	5.95
Threonine	2.36	2.80	3.19	3.12
Serine	4.12	6.09	4.93	4.52
Glutamic acid	21.58	29.76	28.77	30.04
Proline	16.44	5.64	7.14	6.67
Glycine	3.47	2.23	3.14	3.79
Alanine	7.35	9.82	6.95	6.84
Cysteine	1.33	1.85	1.48	1.49
Valine	2.26	2.34	2.63	2.79
Methionine	2.43	1.51	1.46	1.60
Isoleucine	2.43	2.07	1.66	2.15
Leucine	14.76	14.13	14.61	13.62
Tyrosine	3.58	3.82	3.57	3.55
Phenylalanine	3.97	3.87	3.92	4.05
Lysine	3.84	2.31	2.65	2.90
Histidine	1.36	2.71	2.66	2.33
Tryptophan	0.31	0.32	0.29	0.27
Arginine	2.48	3.02	3.69	3.79

Table 8a. Amino acid composition of whole grain of corn varieties from Hungary

Amino acid (g per 16 g N)	BEMA Tc 210	Mv Sc 394	Mv Sc 434	Mv Sc 484	Pioneer 3732 Sc	Pioneer 3901 Sc
Aspartic acid	7.18	6.80	7.43	7.85	6.71	7.09
Threonine	4.32	3.86	4.16	4.64	3.92	3.61
Serine	4.99	5.17	4.57	5.92	3.84	4.21
Glutamic acid	26.70	27.55	29.44	27.50	18.23	22.71
Proline	9.63	7.39	10.63	5.65	17.48	11.99
Glycine	3.28	2.85	3.68	3.54	4.26	3.52
Alanine	5.10	5.92	5.38	6.66	4.29	6.03
Cysteine	1.14	1.46	1.42	1.56	1.04	1.06
Valine	3.64	4.12	3.75	4.46	5.00	5.02
Methionine	1.36	1.51	2.12	1.93	1.95	1.53
Isoleucine	2.45	2.23	3.07	2.02	3.68	3.08
Leucine	13.58	15.75	12.33	15.33	13.61	12.59
Tyrosine	2.86	3.11	2.66	3.26	3.14	2.92
Phenylalanine	4.53	4.62	4.43	5.14	4.43	4.70
Lysine	3.02	2.85	2.12	1.74	2.26	2.39
Histidine	1.30	0.88	0.82	0.73	0.84	0.71
Tryptophan	0.30	0.36	0.29	0.30	0.41	0.32
Arginine	5.15	4.33	2.18	2.62	3.41	5.58

Table 8b. Amino acid composition of whole grain of corn varieties from Hungary

Amino acid (g per 16 g N)	Pioneer 3965A MTC	Mv Sc 550 Wx	Sc 6390 HL opaque-2	White sweet corn	Sweet corn Mv Sc Ideal
Aspartic acid	7.21	7.71	9.33	6.21	7.21
Threonine	4.16	4.14	3.80	3.53	4.39
Serine	3.89	3.80	4.53	4.31	4.01
Glutamic acid	18.94	18.28	21.64	24.80	21.77
Proline	15.43	12.35	10.54	10.13	15.33
Glycine	4.53	4.89	4.43	3.71	1.17
Alanine	5.18	5.55	5.73	6.59	5.65
Cysteine	0.67	0.61	0.70	0.85	0.44
Valine	5.80	6.57	5.74	5.29	5.28
Methionine	1.61	1.82	1.60	1.60	1.26
Isoleucine	2.78	3.34	3.41	3.23	2.94
Leucine	12.30	11.65	8.52	13.05	13.41
Tyrosine	3.19	2.88	2.90	2.61	2.80
Phenylalanine	4.25	4.45	4.22	3.97	4.40
Lysine	2.44	3.17	3.89	2.68	2.72
Histidine	1.50	1.76	1.67	1.94	2.64
Tryptophan	0.29	0.33	0.40	0.28	0.27
Arginine	5.07	5.74	6.25	4.92	3.79

Table 9. Amino acid composition of whole grain of corn varieties from the USA

Amino acid (g per 16 g N)	White flint corn	Yellow dent corn	K 811 opaque-2	K 812 opaque-2	K 813 opaque-2	K 814 opaque-2
Aspartic acid	6.90	5.89	7.59	11.73	13.88	18.98
Threonine	2.56	2.90	4.58	4.58	3.71	3.68
Serine	5.19	3.95	4.62	4.92	5.67	5.24
Glutamic acid	32.07	21.90	20.31	20.23	25.37	25.55
Proline	6.53	12.20	7.45	6.97	4.37	3.41
Glycine	2.72	4.22	5.74	4.03	3.14	3.51
Alanine	6.28	7.01	5.68	7.05	8.55	7.06
Cysteine	1.80	1.65	1.61	1.64	2.13	1.28
Valine	2.75	4.14	3.76	2.68	2.40	2.92
Methionine	1.66	2.25	1.23	1.62	1.40	1.49
Isoleucine	1.77	2.77	2.30	2.07	1.96	2.01
Leucine	11.44	14.77	8.68	7.10	8.65	6.69
Tyrosine	3.60	3.37	3.38	3.11	2.87	2.85
Phenylalanine	4.24	4.71	4.16	3.08	2.45	3.30
Lysine	2.77	2.17	5.96	6.21	4.69	4.81
Histidine	2.83	2.38	3.40	4.12	3.17	2.34
Tryptophan	0.23	0.31	0.36	0.43	0.43	0.41
Arginine	4.40	3.63	8.68	7.73	5.40	4.70

adjusted to 8.00 at a temperature of 37 $\pm$ 0.1 °C, while mixing continously. Simultaneously, 0.5 cm^3 of porcine trypsin (Merck 24579) solution of 8.0 mg per cm^3 concentration and 0.5 cm^3 of porcine pancreatin (Sigma P-1750) solution of 20 mg per cm^3 concentration - freshly prepared and kept in ice - exactly adjusted to pH 8.00, were injected into the test solution. The pH of the suspension was kept at the value of 8.00 by an automatic titrator (Radiometer, Copenhagen) using 0.05 N NaOH as titrant. The quantity (µl) of the alkali consumed was measured from the moment of injection for ten minutes. The in vitro true digestibility can then be calculated by the equation:

$$\text{in vitro TD \%} = 52.00 + 0.0223 \times A, \qquad (1)$$

where A is the µl-s of the titrant added during ten minutes of digestion. Results are shown in Tables 10-13. Values represent the algebraic mean of three analyses.

Table 10. In vitro true digestibility of corn varieties from Egypt

Variety	TD, %
Dc 202	86.1
Giza 2	85.3
Sc 201	88.2
Pioneer	87.0

Table 11. In vitro true digestibility of corn varieties from the FRG

Variety	TD, %
Brillant	93.3
Nicco	87.6
Forte	84.0
Dea	88.7

Table 12. In vitro true digestibility of corn varieties from Hungary

Variety	TD, %
BEMA Tc 210	91.9
Mv Sc 394	87.7
Mv Sc 434	85.1
Mv Sc 484	86.4
Pioneer 3732 Sc	84.8
Pioneer 3901 Sc	84.8
Pioneer 3965A MTC	93.3
Mv Sc 550 Wx	89.8
Sc 6390 HL opaque-2	84.5
White sweet corn	86.1
Sweet corn Mv Sc Ideal	94.8

Table 13. In vitro true digestibility of corn varieties from the USA

Variety	TD, %
White flint corn	86.1
Yellow dent corn	86.0
K 811 opaque-2	88.3
K 812 opaque-2	83.4
K 813 opaque-2	87.7
K 814 opaque-2	83.7

Computation of in vitro biological value

For determining the in vitro biological value of the corn varieties, three methods were used. The first one was the determination of the first and second limiting essential amino acids according to the standard FAO/WHO procedure. This was as follows: the contents of each of the essential amino acids in the sample proteins were divided by those of the reference pattern. The concentration of the essential amino acids were expressed in milligrams of the individual amino acid per gram of total essential amino acids. The amino acid with the smallest value of the above-mentioned ratios was the first limiting essential amino acid. The amino acid with the second smallest value was the second limiting essential amino acid. The reference pattern is presented in Table 14.

Table 14. FAO/WHO (1973) reference pattern (FAO (1973))

Essential amino acid (mg per g of total essential amino acids)	FAO/WHO (1973)
Isoleucine	111
Leucine	196
Lysine	151
Phenylalanine + tyrosine	169
Methionine + cystine	98
Threonine	111
Tryptophan	27
Valine	138

The second method used in this investigation was the computation of the so-called Transformed Gaussian Index by the procedure of Békés et al. (1984), (also, see Hidvégi and Békés 1984). The mathematical expression of the method is the following.

$$\mathrm{TGI}\ (\%) = 100 \times (q_{LYS}^{0.28} \times q_{PHE+TYR}^{0.72} \times q_{MET+CYS}^{0.67} \times q_{THR}^{3.32} \times q_{TRP}^{0.19})^{0.125} \qquad (2)$$

where

$$q_i = \exp\left[(-4.5) \cdot \left(\frac{A_i - A_{i,ref}}{A_{i,ref}}\right)^2\right] \qquad (3)$$

where

A_i and $A_{i,ref}$ are the concentration of the i-th essential amino acid in the sample and the reference protein, respectively. These are expressed in mg per g of total essential amino acids. Reference values are shown in Table 15.

Table 15. Reference pattern for the calculation of the Gaussian Index

Essential amino acid (mg per g of total essential amino acids)	A_{ref}
Isoleucine	(110)
Leucine	(179)
Lysine	141
Phenylalanine + tyrosine	212
Methionine + cystine	89
Threonine	99
Tryptophan	30
Valine	(140)

The third method used was the taking into account of in vitro digestibility in computing protein quality. That is, the Transformed Gaussian Index Corrected for Digestibility was,

$$\text{TGICD (\%)} = \text{TGI (\%)} \times \frac{\text{in vitro TD (\%)}}{100} \qquad (4)$$

Results of in vitro protein quality studies are demonstrated in Table 16.

Table 16. In vitro biological value of the corn varieties investigated

Variety	First limiting essential amino acid	Second limiting essential amino acid	TGI, %	TGICD, %
BEMA Tc 210	TRP	LYS	84.77	77.90
Mv Sc 394	TRP	LYS	90.09	79.01
Mv Sc 434	TRP	LYS	84.95	72.29
Mv Sc 484	TRP	LYS	83.10	71.80
Pioneer 3732 Sc	LYS	TRP	89.31	75.73
Pioneer 3901 Sc	TRP	LYS	88.67	75.19
Pioneer 3965A MTC	TRP	LYS	84.26	78.61
Mv Sc 550 Wx	TRP	LYS	87.62	78.68
Sc 6390 HL opaque-2	TRP	LYS	91.27	77.12
White sweet corn	TRP	LYS	87.29	75.16
Sweet corn Mv Sc Ideal	TRP	LYS	77.80	73.75
White flint corn	TRP	ILE	82.57	71.35
Yellow dent corn	TRP	LYS	78.83	67.79
K 811 opaque-2	TRP	ILE	81.20	71.70
K 812 opaque-2	TRP	ILE	67.24	56.08
K 813 opaque-2	TRP	VAL	84.50	74.11
K 814 opaque-2	TRP	ILE	84.81	70.99
Brillant	TRP	VAL	72.81	67.93
Nicco	TRP	LYS	84.52	74.04
Forte	TRP	ILE	89.71	75.36
Dea	TRP	ILE	89.43	79.32
Dc 202	TRP	LYS	70.31	60.54
Giza 2	LYS	TRP	89.13	76.03
Sc 201	TRP	ILE	88.92	78.43
Pioneer	TRP	LYS	70.81	61.60

CONCLUSION

From the point of view of crude protein content the maize varieties investigated can be divided into three classes, that is, into varieties with normal, high and very high protein content. The "normal" range is approx. 9-10%. While, the "high" and "very high" ranges are approx. 10-12% and 12-14%, respectively. Sweet corn Mv Sc Ideal, White sweet corn, Mv Sc 394 and White flint corn have the highest levels of protein.

Furthermore, as a group, the K 811-814 opaque-2 line, as well as the corns from the FRG are the richest protein sources.

As it was expected, the most characteristic features of the amino acid patterns are the low tryptophan and lysine contents; however, the latter is replaced by isoleucine at the high lysine mutants. It is valine which is - in two cases - the second limiting essential amino acid. The leucine : isoleucine ratios are high, except the opaque-2 mutants. It may be due to the reduced zein content.

If we accept a value of 85% for "normal" corn protein digestibility, which, in turn, confirms the FAO recommendation, or if we consider the digestibility of Yellow dent corn (86%) for comparisons, the following conclusions can be drawn. Sweet corn Mv Sc Ideal, Pioneer 3965A MTC, Brillant and BEMA Tc 210 have very well digestible proteins. The relatively "normal" digestibility of opaque-2 corns is significantly lower than that of the formers, however, K811 and K813 have better digestibility than an average corn.

There are remarkable differences in the TGI values of the varieties, too. Varieties: Pioneer (Egypt), Dc 202 (Egypt) and K 812 opaque-2 (USA) have rather poor quality, however, the Sc 201 and Giza 2 corns from Egypt and the K 811, 813, 814 opaque-2 mutants from the USA have significantly good protein quality. The more sophisticated mutants (Sc 6390 HL opaque-2, Pioneer 3732, 3901 Sc, Mv Sc 394, Mv Sc 550 Wx) from Hungary, as well as the Forte and Dea varieties from the FRG also have very good quality proteins.

A similar trend can be observed in the TGICD, the "in vitro net protein utilization", values.

In a previous paper (El Kady et al. 1983b) where corn varieties from Egypt, Hungary, Poland and Yugoslavia were compared in a similar manner as here, we found that combined single cross X opaque-2 mutants showed the best nutritional charachteristics. This conclusion seemes to be corroborated now, too.

REFERENCES

AOAC (1975). Official methods of analysis. Washington, D.C.

Békés, F., Hidvégi, M., Zsigmond, A. and Lásztity, R. (1984). Studies on the evaluation of the in vitro biological value of food proteins. Acta Alim. 13, 135-158.

Bressani, R. and Mertz, E.T. (1958). Studies on corn proteins. IV. Protein and amino acid content of different corn varieties. Cereal Chem. 35, 227-235.

Duggal, S.K. and Sidhu, G.S. (1970). Effect of amino acid supplementation on PER (protein efficiency ratio) values of some varieties of maize and groundnut. J. Res., Punjab Agr. Univ. 7, 62-68.

El Kady, A. (1983). Investigation of corn proteins and of their nutritive value. Ph.D. Thesis. Technical University Budapest.

El Kady, A., Lásztity, R., Örsi F. and Simon-Sarkadi, L. (1983a). Studies on corn proteins. IV. Amino acid content of different corn varieties. Gabonaipar 30, 53-58.

El Kady, A., Hidvégi, M., Lásztity, R. and Simon-Sarkadi, L. (1983b). Studies on corn proteins. V. Digestibility and biological value of corn proteins. Gabonaipar 30, 107-111.

Eggum, B.O., Villegas, E.M. and Vasal, S.K. (1979). Progress in protein quality of maize. J. Sci. Food Agric. 30, 1148-1153.

FAO (1973). Energy and protein requirements. Rome.

Gevers, H.O. (1975). A note on the correlation between lysine and tryptophan content in maize kernel endosperms. Cereal Chem. 52, 115-118.

Hidvégi, M. and Békés, F. (1984). Mathematical modeling of protein nutritional quality from amino acid composition. (In this book.)

Kies, C. and Fox, H.M. (1970). Effect of level of total nitrogen intake on second limiting amino acid in corn for humans. J. Nutr. 100, 1275-1286.

Ma, Y. and Nelson, O.E. (1975). Amino acid composition and storage proteins in two new high-lysine mutants in maize. Cereal Chem. 52, 412-419.

Mertz, E.T., Bates, L.S. and Nelson, O.E. (1964). Mutant gene that changes protein compositions and increases lysine content of maize endosperm. Science 145, 279-280.

Salgó, A., Ganzler, K. and Jécsai, J. (1984). Simple enzymic methods for prediction of plant protein digestibility. (In this book.)

Robutti, J.L., Hoseney, R.C. and Deyoe, C.W. (1974). Modified opaque-2 corn endosperms. I. Protein distribution and amino acid composition.Cereal Chem. 51, 163-172.

Tomov, N. (1979). Corn as a source of essential amino acids. Priroda 28, 40-45.

Vinnichenko, O.M. and Sytnik, K.M. (1969). Amino acid composition of grain of some subspecies of corn. Ukr. Bot. Zh. 26, 65-71.

Proc. Int. Assoc. Cereal Chem. Symp. Amino Acid Compn and Biol. Value of Cereal Proteins Budapest, Hungary 1983, R. Lásztity, M. Hidvégi, eds

THE AMINO ACID COMPOSITION OF WHEAT GRAIN AS RELATED TO ITS PROTEIN CONTENT

JACQUES BAUDET, JEAN-CLAUDE HUET, JACQUES MOSSÉ

Laboratoire d'Etude des Protéines, Département de Physiologie et Biochimie Végétales, INRA, 78000 Versailles, France

ABSTRACT

Basic amino acids and protein content of 59 mature grain samples of wheat (Triticum aestivum) have been determined. The samples were obtained in different environmental conditions (fertilization, year of harvesting, location and conditions of wheat growth). Several of them also differed genetically : 12 varieties or cultivars have been studied. The protein content ranged from 9.1 to 20.6 per cent (in g of nitrogen x 6.25 per 100 g of grain dry matter). Whatever the cause of variation of protein content for each amino acid may be, linear relations are pointed out between amino acid percentages of the grain and crude protein content. Thus knowing only the protein content of a wheat grain sample enables to infer its basic amino acid composition. As for the amino acid levels of crude proteins, they are related to protein content by hyperbolic laws. When grain protein content increases, the whole protein of grain becomes much poorer in lysine, their arginine level also drops, whereas their histidine level remains constant.

I. INTRODUCTION

It is generally agreed that amino acid composition of mature wheat grain is changed according to protein level. For instance Lawrence et al. (1958) noticed very early that low protein wheats exhibit an inverse relationship between protein content and lysine in the protein. Many studies have been reported in the literature on a single cultivar (or a small number of cultivars) with which a more or less wide range of protein level was obtained by use of different conditions of fertilization or climate or also different locations and years of harvesting (Byers and Bolton, 1979 ; Eppendorfer, 1975 and 1978 ; McElroy et al., 1949 ; Sihlbom, 1962). Other studies deal with genetic differences and their possible interactions with amino acid composition of wheat grains (Diehl et al., 1978 ; Hepburn and Bradley, 1965 ; Johnson et al., 1979 ; Mattern et al., 1968 ; Müntz et al., 1979 ; Villegas et al., 1970 ; Vogel et al., 1976). This has been reviewed for wheat by Konzak (1977) and Porceddu et al. (1983), and also for several different species by Frey (1973), Mossé and Baudet (1983), Nelson (1979) and Röbbelen (1976).

Many of these results are confined to lysine which is indeed the most limiting essential amino acid for human beings and for cattle. For analytical reasons, they are sometimes confined to basic amino acids. Whatever amino acids may be determined, the general conclusion is that amino acid composition is related to protein level in wheat grain. However, several questions such as the magnitude of amino acid variations with protein level, the nature of the relationships involved, the respective weight of genome and of environment in such changes remain debated or unclear. With other species like barley it has been shown that basic amino acids obeyed a very simple law (Mossé and Baudet, 1969 and 1977b) : the amino acid contents of the barley grain are linear functions of protein level. Similar relationships have been found in an oilseed like sunflower (Baudet et al., 1971) and in a legume seed like broad bean (Mossé and Baudet, 1977a and Baudet and Mossé, 1980). Thus homologous results could be expected in any species, particularly in cereals other than barley. The aim of the present work was to investigate this question in wheat grain.

II. MATERIAL AND METHODS

Initially, the choice of wheat samples was not really programmed in order to result in the present study. As a matter of fact, year after year, different samples happened to be analysed for their amino acids, either for checking the composition of samples used in plant breeding, or more frequently in order to know the composition of wheats after very different conditions of growth.

The 59 samples which have been analysed belong to 12 different varieties or cultivars. Two sets of samples were obtained from greenhouse grown wheats : the 11 samples of variety Aronde were obtained with the aim to cover a range of protein content as wide as possible and the 6 samples of variety Bastion in order to produce the highest possible protein content. All the others were harvested from field grown wheats during seven different years. Among the 9 samples of variety Cappelle, one was submitted to subsampling. Fractionation of the sample was first made according to the individual grain weight (from 20 to 25, 25 to 30, and so on up to 60 mg). This resulted in 8 different weight classes the grains of which were then distributed into 2 subclasses depending on their more or less mealy aspect, at least when the amount of grain was still sufficient (i.e. for 6 of the 8 weight classes). Hence it led to 14 subsamples differing by their protein level.

Analytical samples of 30 g were obtained by several successive uses of Prometer static divider. The weight of grains submitted to analyses was still much weaker for some of the 14 subsamples obtained from one Cappelle sample as described above. Samples were poured in liquid nitrogen just before grinding in a Prometer knife mill. After air equilibration, all aliquots for analysis were taken at the same time.

The dry matter content was determined by heating at 105° C for 24 hours. Nitrogen content was determined by a micro-kjeldahl procedure and data are the average of duplicate analyses. For basic amino acids, 300 mg of milled samples were hydrolysed for 24 and 48 hours in 300 ml of boiling HCl under reflux. For the 11 samples of variety Aronde, only one 24 hour-hydrolysis was carried out. Determinations were performed on short columns

Table 1

Basic amino acid and protein content of wheat grain samples

Variety	ARONDE											CLEMENT			
P	9.1	9.15	9.3	9.45	9.5	10.7	10.75	11.75	14.4	15.35	16.55	10.0	12.0	12.5	14.05
Lysine	3.3	3.4	3.25	3.3	3.3	3.2	3.25	3.0	2.9	2.6	2.8	3.05	2.9	2.8	2.7
Histidine	1.95	2.3	2.2	2.2	2.2	2.3	2.35	2.05	2.35	2.2	2.15	2.2	2.05	2.05	2.05
Arginine	6.0	4.7	5.15	5.4	5.25	5.5	4.45	5.2	5.35	5.0	5.1	5.25	4.75	4.8	4.8

Variety	CAPPELLE									BASTION					
P	11.4	13.15	14.85	15.2	15.35	16.2	17.45	17.75	18.7	19.4	19.5	19.6	20.45	20.45	20.6
Lysine	3.05	2.85	2.75	2.7	2.7	2.55	2.5	2.55	2.5	2.4	2.4	2.45	2.4	2.4	2.4
Histidine	2.3	2.3	2.35	2.3	2.3	2.05	2.2	2.2	2.25	2.25	2.15	2.15	2.25	2.2	2.25
Arginine	5.2	5.0	4.95	4.85	4.9	4.75	4.75	4.8	4.7	4.8	4.8	4.7	4.75	4.65	4.65

Variety	ETOILE DE CHOISY					CAPITOLE		HARDI		MARIS HUNT.		HYBR.	CHAM.	MAGD.	REM.
P	10.5	10.55	14.4	14.55	14.65	12.6	14.35	10.55	11.65	12.6	13.45	15.3	14.5	16.2	13.7
Lysine	3.05	3.25	2.7	2.65	2.6	2.9	2.85	3.05	2.9	2.85	2.8	2.85	2.85	2.6	2.8
Histidine	2.2	2.35	2.25	2.0	2.2	2.25	2.3	2.45	2.35	2.3	2.25	2.05	2.3	2.05	2.3
Arginine	5.15	5.35	4.9	4.8	4.9	5.4	4.95	5.1	4.95	5.05	4.85	4.85	4.85	4.7	4.85

Amino acid content is expressed in g per 16 g of nitrogen and protein content in g of nitrogen x 6.25 per 100 g of seed dry matter.
MARIS HUNT = Maris Huntsman ; CHAM = Champlein ; MAGD = Magdalena ; HYBR = Hybrid B17 x V81 ; REM = Remois.

of a Phoenix Precision Instrument Company autoanalyser for the oldest samples and on a Kontron Liquimat III instrument for the most recent samples. Commercial standard solutions containing aminoguanidinopropionic acid in addition to the basic amino acids were used for standardisation.

III. RESULTS

For amino acid compositions of seeds and their possible relation with protein content, it is interesting to take into account the content of each amino acid both on a protein basis (C, in g of amino acid per 16 g of nitrogen) and on a grain dry matter basis (A, in g of amino acid per 100 g of grain dry matter). The results of protein percentage P on a grain dry matter basis have been calculated by using 6.25 as a nitrogen to protein conversion factor. They are given in Table 1 with levels C of basic amino acids (in g per 16 g of nitrogen) for the first 45 samples which were studied in a first step. They allow to calculate the basic amino acid content A of grain dry matter and to plot it against P, as shown in Figures 1 to 3.

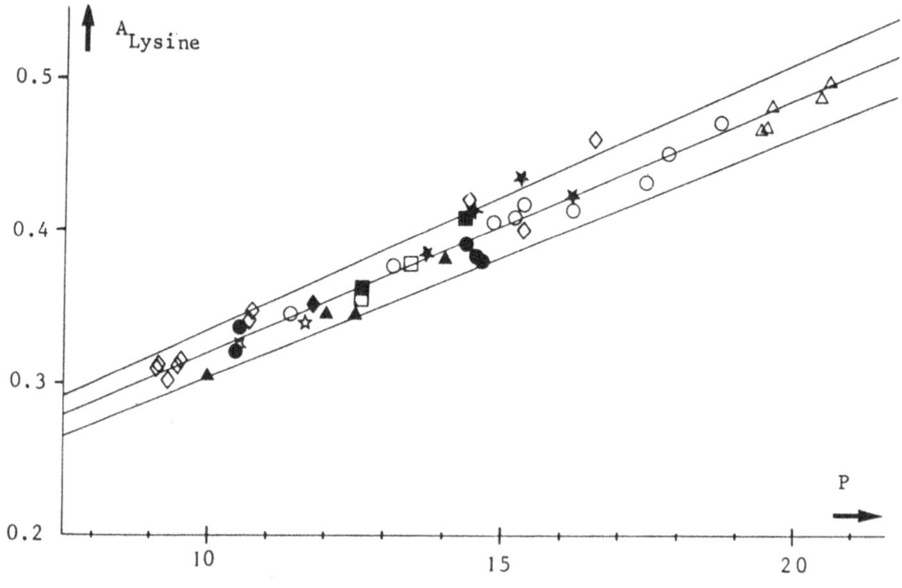

Fig. 1 : Relationship between lysine percentage A on a grain dry matter basis and protein content P in 45 grain samples from wheat of 12 varieties : Aronde ◇ ; Clement ▲ ; Cappelle ○ ; Bastion △ ; Etoile de Choisy ●; Capitole ■ ; Hardi ☆ ; Maris Huntsman □ ; Hybrid ★ ; Champlein ★ ; Magadalena ★ ; Remois ★. On each side of the regression line are drawn lines which correspond to relative deviations of ± 5 %.

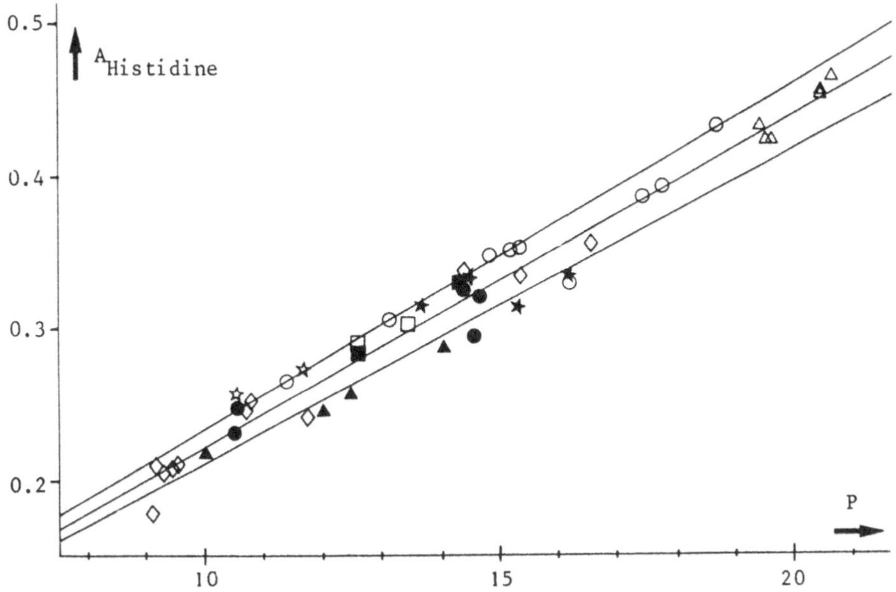

Fig. 2 : Relationship between histidine percentage A on a grain dry matter basis and protein content P in 45 grain samples from wheat of 12 varieties : see legend of Figure 1.

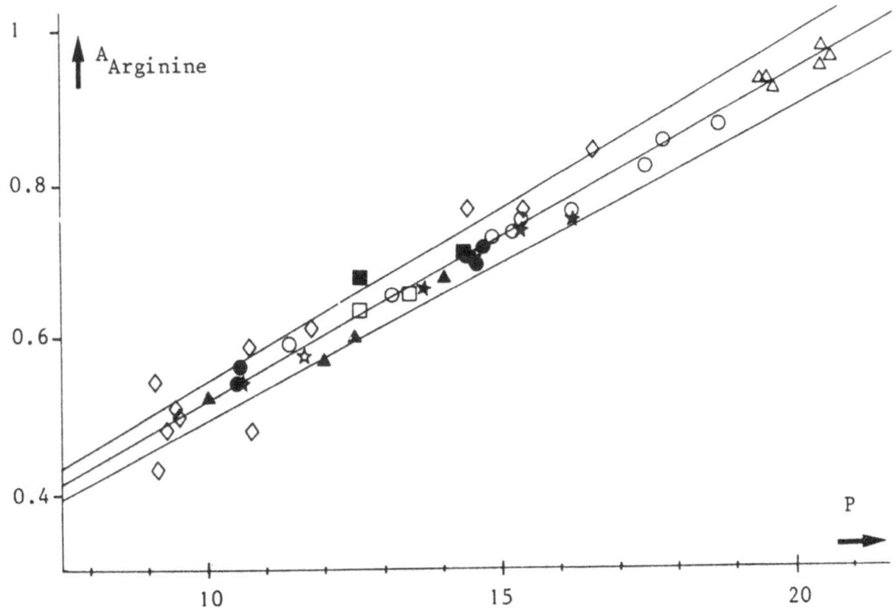

Fig. 3 : Relationship between arginine percentage A on a grain dry matter basis and protein content P in 45 grain samples from wheat of 12 varieties : see legend of Figure 1.

The two varieties which correspond to the highest number of samples show a rather wide range of protein content : from 9.1 to 16.55 for the 11 Aronde samples and from 11.4 to 18.7 for the 9 Cappelle samples. They are represented by white rhombs and open circles respectively.

It can be first noticed that the different points corresponding to one variety are relatively well aligned on the three figures. This shows that there is a linear relationship between P and A inside of a given variety. The second chief point is that this law is obeyed by all the other varieties investigated, whatever they may be.

On Figures 1 to 3, two straight lines have been drawn on both sides of the regression lines. They correspond to a relative variation of ± 5 % of A. The figures show that almost all of the points which represent the 45 samples are within a strip limited by the two straight lines. In other words A obeys the equation :

$$A = \alpha P + \beta \qquad (1)$$

in which the coefficients α and β are constant for each basic amino acid

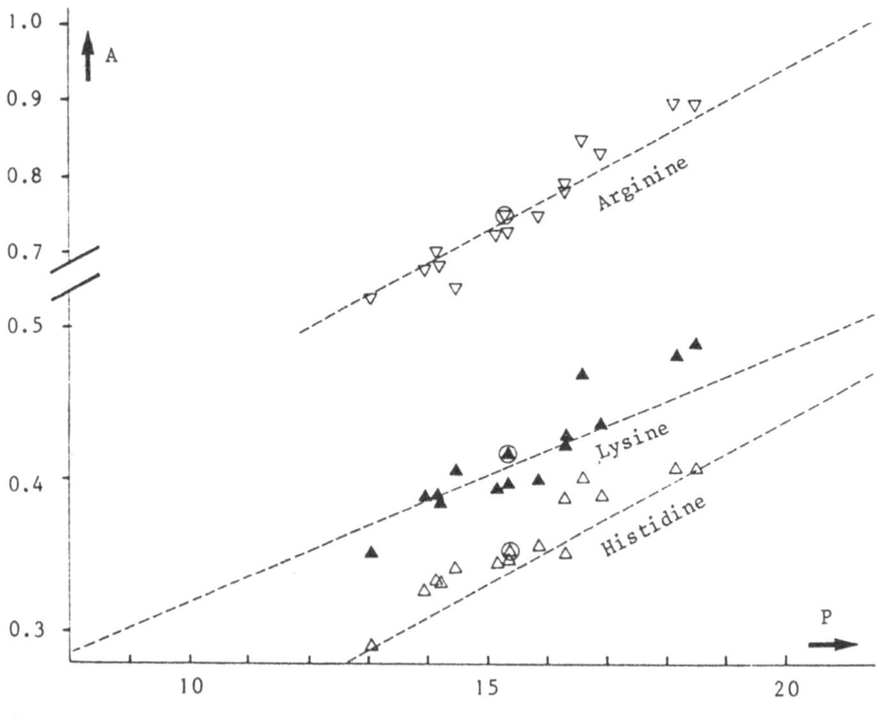

Fig. 4 Relationship between basic amino acid percentage A on a grain dry matter basis and protein content P in 14 subsamples separated according to individual grain weight and vitreousness from a Cappelle sample. Triangles surrounded by a circle correspond to this initial sample. Dotted lines recall the regression lines from Fig. 1 to 3.

Table 2

Basic amino acid and protein content of Cappelle wheat subsamples according to grain weight and vitreousness

grain weight (mg)	20-25	25-30		30-35	35-40		40-45		45-50		50-55		55-60	
Aspect([1])	I	I	V	I	M	V	M	V	M	V	M	V	M	I
P	18.5	16.6	18.15	16.3	14.15	16.9	13.95	16.3	14.45	15.35	14.2	15.85	13.05	15.15
Lysine	2.65	2.85	2.65	2.6	2.75	2.6	2.8	2.65	2.8	2.6	2.7	2.55	2.7	2.6
Histidine	2.2	2.4	2.25	2.3	2.35	2.3	2.35	2.4	2.4	2.25	2.35	2.25	2.25	2.3
Arginine	4.85	5.15	4.95	4.9	5.0	4.95	4.9	4.85	4.75	4.85	4.85	4.75	4.9	4.8

([1])M = mealy ; V = vitrous ; I = intermediary

Amino acid content is expressed in g per 16 g of nitrogen and protein content in g of nitrogen x 6.25 per 100 g of seed dry matter.

but differ from one to another. The three figures (or the data deduced from Table 1) allow to determine that :

$\alpha = 16.6 \times 10^{-3}$ and $\beta = 0.154$ for lysine
$\alpha = 21.8 \times 10^{-3}$ $\beta = 0.005$ for histidine
$\alpha = 42.6 \times 10^{-3}$ $\beta = 0.094$ for arginine

with correlation coefficients which are equal to 0.98 for each of these three amino acids. Thus, when P increases from 9.1 to 20.6 % in grain, the levels of lysine, histidine and arginine rise from 0.3 to 0.5, 0.2 to 0.45 and 0.48 to 0.97 g per 100 g of grain respectively.

The coefficients α (the slope of the plotted regression straight lines) indicate the increments of A per unit of protein percentage in wheat grain. When P increases by one percentage unit, the amino acid level of wheat grain increases by 16.6 mg for lysine, 21.8 mg for histidine and 42.6 mg for arginine. The coefficients β correspond to the intercepts of the regression straight lines. They are positive for lysine and arginine. For histidine, β is virtually equal to zero ($A_{His} \sim \alpha_{His} P$), which means that the increase of wheat grain histidine is roughly proportional to protein content.

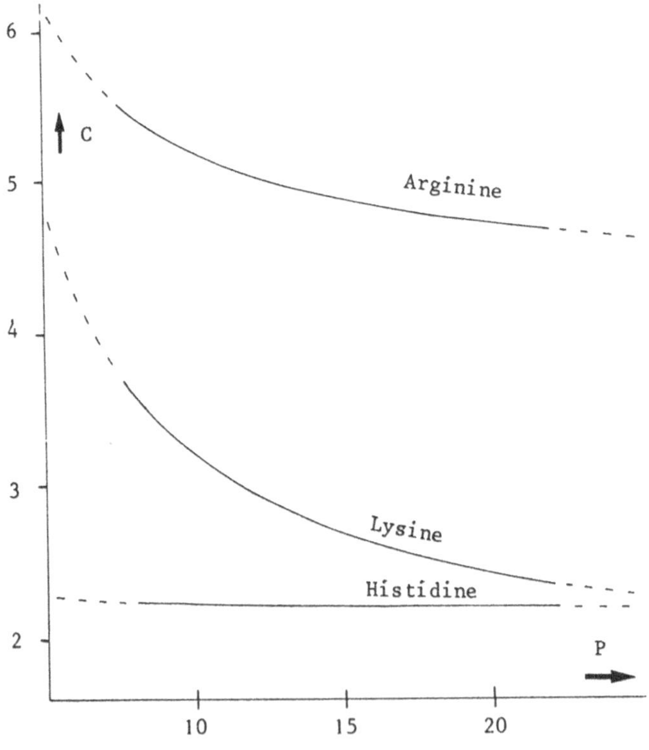

Fig. 5 : Relationship between basic amino acid content C on a crude protein basis (g per 16 g nitrogen) and protein content P.

Table 2 gives the results which concern the 14 subsets of the sample of variety Cappelle which has a protein content of 15.35 % as indicated in Table 1. It appears that the smallest grains are generally the highest in protein. Within the same class of grain size, it is confirmed that vitrous grains are richer in protein than mealy ones, as could be expected.

The subsampling results into protein contents ranging from 13 to 18.5 %. The corresponding amino acid levels per grain weight have been plotted against P in Figure 4. This figure shows again that the representative points are distributed near and along straight lines determined from Figures 1 to 3.

It is also interesting to study the variations of C in function of P. As a matter of fact, C is related to A by the equation :

$$C = 100\ A/P \qquad (2)$$

Elimination of A between equations (1) and (2) gives :

$$C = 100\,\alpha + 100\,\beta/P \qquad (3)$$

and indicates that the level C of each amino acid on a protein basis is a hyperbolic function of P, as shown on Figure 5. When β is positive, C decreases in function of P more strongly as the value of β is high. Figure 5 shows that the lysine level decreases rather rapidly in low protein wheats (from 3.6 to 2.85 per 16 g nitrogen when P goes up from 8 to 13 %) and more slowly in high protein wheats (only from 2.55 to 2.45 when P goes up from 17 to 22 %). With arginine which has a coefficient weaker than that one of lysine, the decrease is lower, although still significant. For histidine, the level is nearly constant :

$$C_{His} \sim 100\,\alpha_{His} = 2.2 \text{ g per 16 g of nitrogen.}$$

IV. DISCUSSION

The first question with which we are faced is the validity of the linear relations found between A and P for the three basic amino acids. Are the deviations from the regression straight lines due to a possible biological variation, or do they arise from analytical errors ? It can be noted that many of the points which are outside of the strips drawn for lysine (Fig. 1) and arginine (Fig. 3) correspond to variety Aronde, i.e., to the only samples which were analysed after only one 24 hour-hydrolysis. With histidine (Fig. 2), several points are still under the strip. For instance it is the case for 3 of the 4 samples of variety Clément. Such discrepancies are likely to arise from the imperfect calibration of analysers. Though the occurrence of some slight biological variations cannot be discarded, we suggest that the observed deviations are essentially due to analytical errors, more especially as only some of the 20 protein amino acids were determined.

Regarding the nature of relations obeyed by amino acids as function of grain protein content, the results allow to claim that A is a linear function of P. Preliminary unpublished results suggest that the same kind of relations are valid for each of the 20 protein amino acids. This is in agreement with homologous results found with broad bean (Baudet and Mossé, 1980). However, for amino acids which exhibit a very low coefficient β, C remains practically constant and independent of P so that its variations are also represented by a straight line.

This could explain why literature is so confusing about the nature of these relations. Many authors indeed claim that it is C which is linearly correlated with P. This kind of conclusion often results from an insufficient width of the range of protein content among samples investigated. The probability to fit a curve to a straight line obviously increases with the narrowness of the range of variation. Figure 5 shows that even for arginine but not for lysine, the segment of hyperbola we have found could be assimilated to a straight line especially for protein content higher than 12 %. The strong variations of lysine for low protein wheats had already been noticed by Lawrence et al. (1958) and Müntz et al. (1979). Data of Sihlbom (1962), Vogel et al. (1976) and Eppendorfer (1978) also support the conclusion that A is a linear function of P though these authors did not explicitly formulate it.

The variations of the three basic amino acids on a protein basis are very similar to those ones observed in barley by Mossé and Baudet (1977b). For arginine, both curves of variation of C in wheat and barley are practically superposable. It is almost the samething for histidine which remains also constant in barley proteins, with a slightly lower level than in wheat (2.1 instead of 2.2 g. per 16 g nitrogen). There is still a significant difference for barley lysine the curve of which is significantly above the curve of wheat lysine. For grains containing 10 % of protein, barley proteins contain 3.9 g of lysine per 16 g nitrogen instead of 3.2 in wheat. For 20 % of protein, barley proteins contain 3.2 g of lysine instead of 2.25 in wheat. This illustrates with more accuracy the well known fact that lysine is a more limiting assential amino acid in wheat than in barley.

It can be also noticed that lysine and histidine levels on a protein basis show a similar behaviour in wheat and in broad bean (Baudet and Mossé, 1980). It is the contrary for arginine which strongly increases in protein of broad bean for increasing protein content. The decreasing lysine and arginine in wheat proteins result from the composition of the storage proteins. The latter which are accumulated mainly in high protein wheats are poorer in the above two amino acids than the proteins of low protein wheats. By obvious compensation, storage proteins of wheat are richer in other amino acids like glutamine and proline than the proteins of low protein wheats. Unfortunately, from a nutritional point of view these amino acids the level of which increases in proteins with protein content of grain are not essential amino acids.

V. CONCLUSION

As could be expected from results reported on other species, it can already be claimed that basic amino acids exhibit linear variations as a function of grain protein content. This conclusion appears to be valid on a wide range of protein content whatever the origin or the cause of variation of protein content may be. A similar result can be expected for the other amino acids so that this work needs to be extended to the 20 protein amino acids with maximal analytical fiability. The corresponding study is in progress. It should provide tables (or graphs) giving amino acid composition of any wheat grain sample (of the species Triticum aestivum, provided its protein content is known. It may also confirm that, from a basic point of view, proteosynthesis in wheat grain is controlled by very strictly regulated mechanisms.

REFERENCES

Baudet, J., Leclercq, P. and Mossé, J. (1971). Sur la richesse en lysine des graines de Tournesol en fonction de leur teneur en protéines. C.R. Acad. Sci. Paris 273D, 1112-1113.

Baudet, J., and Mossé, J. (1980). Amino acid composition of different cultivars of broad beans (Vicia faba). Comparison with other legume seeds. In: "World Crops : Production, Utilization and Description. Vol. 3, Vicia faba : feeding value, processing and viruses - EEC seminar, Cambridge, 1979, D.A. Bond (ed.), Martinus Nijhoff Publishers, The Hague, pp. 67-82.

Byers, M., and Bolton, J. (1979). Effects of nitrogen and sulphur fertilisers on the yield, N and S content, and amino acid composition of the grain of spring wheat. J. Sci. Food Agric. 30, 251-263.

Diehl, A.L., Johnson, V.A. and Mattern, P.J. (1978). Inheritance of protein and lysine in 3 wheat crosses. Crop Sci. 18, 391-395.

Eppendorfer, W.H. (1975). Effects of fertilizers on quality and nutrition value of grain protein. In: Fertilizer Use and Protein Production, Proceedings of the 11th Colloquium of the International Potash Institute, Bornholm, Denmark, pp. 249-263.

Eppendorfer, W.H. (1978). Effects of nitrogen, phosphorus and potassium on amino acid composition and on relationships between nitrogen and amino acids in wheat and oat grain. J. Sci. Fd Agric. 29, 995-1001.

Frey, K.J. (1973). Improvement of the quantity and quality of cereal grain protein. In: Alternate Sources of Protein for Animal Production. Natl. Acad. Sci. Washington D.C., pp. 9-41.

Hepburn, F.N. and Bradley, W.B. (1965). The amino acid composition of hard vheat varieties as a function of nitrogen content. Cereal Chem. 42, 140-148.

Johnson, V.A., Mattern, P.J. and Kuhr, S.L. (1979). Genetic improvement of wheat protein. In: Seed Protein Improvement in Cereals and Grain Legumes - IAEA-FAO Symposium, Neuherberg, 1978 - IAEA, Vienna, pp. 165-169.

Konzac, C.F. (1977). Genetic control of the content, amino acid composition and processing properties of proteins in wheat. Adv. Genetics 19, 408-546.

Lawrence, J.M., Day, M.K., Huey, E. and Lee, B. (1958). Lysine content of wheat varieties, species, and related genera. Cereal Chem. 35, 169-178.

McElroy, L.W., Clandinin, D.R., Lobay, W. and Pethybridge, S.I. (1949). Nine essential amino acids in pure varieties of wheat, barley and oats. J. Nutr. 37, 329-336.

Mattern, P.J., Salem, A., Johnson, V.A. and Schmidt, J.W. (1968). Amino acid composition of selected high-protein wheats. Cereal Chem. 45, 437-444.

Mossé, J. and Baudet, J. (1969). Etude intervariétale de la qualité protéique des Orges : taux d'azote, composition en acides aminés et richesse en lysine. Ann. Physiol. Vég. 11, 51-66.

Mossé, J. and Baudet, J. (1977a). Relationship between amino acid composition and nitrogen contents of broad bean seed. In: Protein Quality from Leguminous Crops - EEC seminar, Dijon, 1977 - pp. 48-56.

Mossé, J. and Baudet J. (1977b). Relations entre la composition en acides aminés basiques et la teneur en azote des grains d'Orge. In: European Brewery Convention, Proceedings of the 16th Congress, Amsterdam, 1977, pp 27-34.

Mossé, J. and Baudet, J. (1983). Crude protein content and amino acid composition of seeds : variability and correlations. In: Plant Proteins for Human Food, C.E. Bodwell and L. Petit (ed.), Martinus Nijhoff/Dr W. Junk Publishers, The Hague, pp. 21-42.
Müntz, K., Hammer, K., Lehmann, C., Meister, A., Rudolph, A., Scholz, F. (1979). Variability of protein and lysine content in barley and wheat specimens from the world collection of cultivated plants at Gatersleben. in: Seed Protein Improvement in Cereals and Grain Legumes Vol. II - IAEA-FAO symposium, Neuherberg, 1978 - IAEA, Vienna, pp. 183-200.
Nelson, O.E. (1979). Inheritance of amino acid content in cereals. In: Seed Protein Improvement in Cereals and Grain Legumes Vol. I - IAEA-FAO symposium, Neuherberg, 1978 - IAEA, Vienna, pp. 79-87.
Porceddu, E., Lafiandra, D. and Scarascia-Mugnozza, G.T. (1983). Genetics of seed proteins in wheat. In: Seed Proteins, Biochemistry, Genetics, Nutritive value, W. Gottschalk and H.P. Müller (ed.), Martinus Nijhoff/Dr W. Junk, The Hague, pp. 77-141.
Röbbelen, G. (1976). Beeinflüssung von Qualitätsmerkmalen durch Pflanzenzüchtung - Möglichkeiten und Probleme. Qual. Plant Pl. Fds 26, 149-166.
Sihlbom, E. (1962). Amino acid composition of Swedish wheat protein. Acta Chem. Scand. 12, 148-156.
Villegas, E., McDonald, C.E., Gilles, K.A. (1970). Variability in the lysine content of wheat, rye and triticale proteins. Cereal Chem. 47, 746-757.
Vogel, K.P., Johnson, V.A. and Mattern, P.J. (1976). Protein and lysine content of grain, endosperm, and bran of wheats from the USDA world wheat collection. Crop Sci. 16, 655-660.

PART 4

PROTEIN PREPARATIONS AND CEREALS — COMPOSITION AND NUTRITIVE VALUE

Proc. Int. Assoc. Cereal Chem. Symp. Amino Acid Compn and Biol. Value of Cereal Proteins Budapest, Hungary 1983, R. Lásztity, M. Hidvégi, eds

AMINO ACID COMPOSITION AND BIOLOGICAL VALUE OF CEREAL GERMS

CHO C. TSEN

Department of Grain Science and Industry, Kansas State University, Manhattan, KS 66506, USA

ABSTRACT

Cereal germs, rich in protein, fat, vitamins, minerals and fiber, are well known for their nutritional contributions to foods and feeds. They are readily available in large quantities as a by-product of the huge yearly crop of cereals.

The composition of different cereal germs varies greatly. Rye and wheat germs have more protein and less fat than corn, rice and sorghum germs.

Cereal germs contain an adequate level of lysine. Since most cereal products are deficient in lysine, cereal germs are ideally suited to be used as nutrient fortifiers for cereal foods. So far as the protein composition is concerned, cereal germs are generally low in isoleucine, cystine, and methionine as compared to cereal endosperms. The nutritive value of proteins in cereal germs is approximately equivalent to that of animal proteins, as demonstrated by feeding studies.

The protein digestibility is reported in wheat germ to vary from 79.5 to 92.8%, in rice germ to range from 81.4 to 86.9%, and in corn germ to fluctuate from 76 to 85% by different investigators with in vitro or in vivo procedure.

Wheat and rice germs contain antinutritional factors including hemiagglutinin and trypsin inhibitors. However, corn germ does not show to have such factors to affect its protein digestibility.

Acceptable bakery foods and other cereal products have been successfully developed with cereal germs as one of their ingredients. Additional research and development work is needed to explore fully the potential use of cereal germs in foods to divert more germs from the feed lot to the food market to enhance their nutritional contribution and marketing value.

INTRODUCTION

Cereal germs have long been known for their nutritive values because of their high content in protein, minerals, fat and vitamins. The

Table 1. World Production of Cereals /FAO, 1982/ and Cereal Germs in 1981

Cereal		Germ	
Name	Production /unit x 1000 MT/	% Kernel	Yield /unit X 1000 MT/
Barley	158488	1.7/Kent, 1966/	2694
Corn	451704	11.9/Earle et al., 1946/	53753
Millet	39653	-	-
Oats	44024	1.2/Youngs, 1972/	528
Rice, paddy	413785	1.5/Juliano, 1980/	6207
Rye	24473	1.8/Tsen, 1984/	441
Sorghum	71984	9.8/Hubbard et al. 1950/	7054
Wheat	459195	2.5/MacMasters et al. 1971/	11455

proportion of germ in each cereal kernel is generally small. However, the huge cereal crops do bring forth a substantial supply of germs each year. As shown in Table 1, the world production of wheat, rice, corn, and sorghum germs could reach 11.5, 6.2, 53.8, and 7.1 million tons, respectively, if all the germs could be separated from the cereal grains in 1981. Obviously, cereal germs, with their high nutritional qualities and huge yearly productions, play an important role in raising the nutritive value of cereal foods and feeds.

COMPOSITION OF CEREAL GERMS

It is well known that the composition of different fractions in a cereal kernel varies greatly. The endosperm is abundant in starch; the bran and hulls are high in fiber and ash; and the germ is rich in protein, oil, vitamins, and sugars. Although there is a great number of studies concerning the compositon of cereal endosperm, particularly its milled products such as wheat and rice flours, only a small number of studies are found in literature dealing with the composition of cereal germs.

Table 2 shows the composition of corn, rice, rye, sorghum, and wheat germs. Of the germs, rye and wheat germs contain more protein and less fat than the others; while the reverse is true for corn and sorghum germs. The high content of protein, fat, ash and fiber of these cereal germs certainly make cereal germs unique in their nutritional contributions.

Table 2. Composition of Cereal Germs /Dry Basis/

Germ	Protein /N x 6.25/ %	Fat %	Ash %	Crude fiber %	Reference
Corn	18.8	34.5	10.1	-	Earle et al., 1946
Rice	23.4	25.7	8.8	4.9	Fong, 1980
Rye	40.7	11.4	5.1	3.2	Tsen, 1980
Sorghum	18.9	28.1	10.4	-	Hubbard et al., 1950
Wheat	27.5	7.2	4.8	3.4	Farrell et al., 1967

Table 3. Amino Acid Compsition of Cereal Germs (g Amino Acid/100g Amino Acid Recovered)

Amino acid	Oats /Emb. axis/ /Pomeranz et al. 1973/	Wheat /Pomeranz et al. 1980/	Rice /Fong, 1980/	Corn /Tsen et al. 1974/	Rye /Tsen, 1980/
Lysine	8.2	7.76	5.89	5.7	7.4
Histidine	3.9	2.65	3.25	2.70	-
Arginine	8.3	8.86	8.68	8.25	-
Aspartic acid	10.2	10 21	8.45	7.09	-
Threonine	5.0	4.82	3.84	3.37	4.7
Serine	4.8	4.62	4.60	4.13	-
Glutamic acid	14.2	15.45	14.02	12.12	-
Proline	3.3	4.37	4.15	4.74	-
Cystine	0.5	0.66	1.08	1.88	0.3
Glycine	6.3	6.54	5.74	5.10	-
Alanine	7.2	7.00	6.28	5.64	-
Valine	6.0	5.65	4.54	4.38	4.3
Methionine	2.2	1.88	2.02	1.26	2.0
Isoleucine	3.9	3.91	3.55	2.53	2.6
Leucine	7.1	6.79	6.39	5.84	6.9
Tyrosine	2.9	3.12	3.05	2.59	2.8
Phenylalanine	4.2	4.07	3.95	3.17	3.8

AMINO ACID COMPOSITION OF CEREAL GERMS

The nutritional quality of protein depends on its amino acid composition and availability (digestibility). Table 3 presents the amino acid composition of corn, oats, rice, rye, and wheat germs.

Comparing their compositions with the World Health Organization's requirement pattern for essential amino acids reveals that cereal germs, in general, contain an adequate amount of lysine. Since most cereal products are deficient in lysine, cereal germs are ideally suited to be used as a lysine supplement or fortifier for cereal foods. The comparison also shows that isoleucine, cystine and methionine are limiting amino acids for the cereal germs /Tsen, 1980/. Miladi et al. /1972/, based on their work on the amino acid composition of wheat milled fractions, showed that isoleucine and methionine were the first and second limiting amino acids for wheat germ. /Fong, 1980/ found that isoleucine, methionine and cysteine are the most limiting amino acids for rice germ. Moran et al. /1968/, using various combinations of amino acid supplements in their chick feeding test, found that isoleucine, methionine and tryptophan were respectively the first, second, and third limiting amino acids in wheat germ.

The protein content and amino acid composition of cereal germs differ greatly from those of cereal endosperms. Table 4 compares the amino acid composition of proteins in rice and wheat milled products to that of proteins in rice and wheat germs. Rice and wheat germs contain more lysine,

Table 4. Amino Acid Composition of Rice[a] and Wheat[b] Milled Products and Germs

Amino Acid	Rice /Cagampang et al. 1976/ Brown	Milled	Germ	Wheat /Miladi et al. 1972/ Clear flour	Patent flour	Germ
Lysine	4.4	4.0	6.8	1.9	2.0	4.9
Histidine	2.6	2.7	3.8	2.1	2.1	2.4
Ammonia	2.8	3.3	3.4	4.1	4.2	2.4
Arginine	9.0	8.5	9.6	3.7	3.6	6.9
Tryptophan	1.2	1.3	1.4	1.1	1.1	1.3
Aspartic acid	9.0	9.0	9.1	3.8	3.9	7.3
Threonine	3.9	3.9	4.5	2.6	2.7	3.5
Serine	5.8	5.9	5.3	4.5	4.6	4.2
Glutamic acid	16.8	18.3	15.1	35.2	35.4	17.1
Proline	4.9	5.3	4.5	11.6	11.2	5.2
Glycine	4.8	4.7	6.0	3.4	3.4	5.4
Alanine	4.8	5.8	6.6	2.9	2.8	5.2
Valine	6.6	6.8	6.3	4.5	4.6	5.2
Isoleucine	4.5	4.7	3.8	4.1	4.3	3.7
Leucine	8.3	8.5	6.8	6.8	6.8	6.0
Tyrosine	4.0	3.8	3.3	3.1	3.1	2.6
Phenylalanine	5.3	5.5	4.2	5.1	5.1	3.8
Cystine	2.4	2.6	2.0	2.6	2.6	1.9
Methionine	2.6	2.6	1.9	2.0	2.0	1.9

[a]g. amino acid/16.8g. N
[b]g. amino acid/16.0g. N

threonine and tryptophan but less isoleucine, leucine, methionine and phenylalanine than rice and wheat milled products. It is understood that the milled products mainly represent the endosperm fraction of rice and wheat.

NUTRITIVE VALUE OF CEREAL GERMS

In a cereal kernel, most nutrients with the exception of starch, are concentrated in the germ. Accordingly, the germ becomes more nutritious than the other fractions. As early as in 1943, Hove and Harrel /1943/ did studies on the nutritive value of raw and heated wheat germs with young chicks and found the protein efficiency ratio /PER/ of wheat germ to be 2.76 - a growth promoting value equivalent to that of animal protein. Later Hove et al. /1945/ reported that low fat wheat germ produced a PER of 2.86. In the same report, 97% flour supplemented with 3% low-fat wheat germ gave a PER of 1.10. Increasing supplementation to 6% and 20% further increased PER to 1.36 and 1.99 respectively. The PER of wheat germ in a study by Jones and Widness /1946/ was 2.54. Maladi et al. /1972/ stated that the relative nutritive value /RNV/ of wheat germ approached that of many animal proteins. They found the RNV of wheat germ to be 80% - a value compared very favorably with 74% for casein determined by Hegsted and Chang /1965/. All of these indicate the high nutritional quality of wheat germ.

Only a few studies have been conducted to evaluate the nutritive value of rice germ. The PER of rice germ, determined with young rats over a 70 day test period, without a casein standard, was found to be 2.59 at a 5.7 dietary protein level by Kik /1954/. The biological value and the net protein utilization were found to be 78 and 67.8, respectively, at a 9% dietary protein level /Kik, 1954/.

Wall et al. /1971/ reported that the PER value of solvent-extracted corn germ varies from 2.04 to 2.29. Rat feeding studies showed differences in protein quality between air-dried and oven-dried corn germs.

The relative protein value of defatted corn germ flour has been studied by Canolty et al. /1977/. Isocaloric diets containing various levels of protein supplied as commercially prepared defatted corn germ flour /CGF/, CGF supplemented with 0.07% methionine and 0.02% leucine /SCGF/, casein /C/ or lactoalbumin /LA/ were compared in their study. Weight gains of weanling rats fed various growth-limiting amounts of protein were used to determine a protein value /PV/ defined as the slope of the regression line relating weight gain to protein intake, for each of the protein sources. The PV of CGF was significantly different from that of LA, but did not differ significantly from the PV of SCGF and C. The relative protein value /RPV/ of CGF, the ratio of the PV of CGF to the PV of LA is 0.62 ± 0.06. Their data indicate the protein in commercially prepared CGF is of good quality and could be a valuable source for human diet.

The excellent protein quality of cereal germs is also shown by their high PER values, as found by Tsen /1980/.

flour	PER
corn germ	2.60
wheat germ	2.62
wheat	0.93
soy	2.32
casein	2.50

The PERs of corn and wheat germs are slightly higher than that of casein, and significantly higher than 0.93 and 2.32, respectively for wheat and soy flours.

DIGESTIBILITY OF CEREAL GERMS

The nutritional quality of protein also depends on the availability of amino acids. Thus it becomes important to evaluate the protein digestibility of a protein when it is considered to be used in foods and feeds. There are, unfortunately, not many studies dealing with the protein digestibility of cereal germs.

Saunders and Kohler/1972/ measured the protein digestibility in wheat milled products by in vitro and in vivo procedures. Their results are presented in Table 5. They reported that the protein in the branny layers was of limited digestibility in wheat milled products. As the amount of these layers in the milled products decreased /bran > shorts > germ > red dog > flour/, there was a corresponding increase in the amount of protein which was available. The low digestibility of bran, shorts or germ is mostly due to the presence of the fiber matrix /aleurone cells/ in these milled products. They also found that the protein digestibility in wheat germ varied from 85.5 to 92.8% as measured by difference in vitro procedures.

Summers et al. /1969/, from their rat-feeding tests, found the protein digestibility values ranging from 79.5 to 85.6%. Miladi and Hegsted /1972/ reported the protein digestibility in wheat germ to be 91.6%.

The protein digestibility in vitro of rice germ fraction varied from 81.4 to 84.6 from different rice germ products, according to Fong's finding /1980/. Her data on the digestibility of whole rice germ stored under

Table 5. Protein Digestibility in Wheat Milled Products Measured by In Vitro and In Vivo Procedures /Saunders and Kohler, 1972/

Milled product	Protein digestibility, %	
	In Vitro	In Vivo
Casein control	98.5	99.3
Patent flour	96.7+1.3	93.2
Red dog	89.5±0.6	84.6
Germ	85.5±0.4	86.7
Shorts	79.1±0.3	77.4
Bran	71.5±0.6	73.0

Table 6. Protein Digestibility In Vitro of Whole Rice Germ After 12-week Storage Under Various Conditions /Fong, 1980/

Storage condition	Protein digestibility % 0	12 wks
Frozen (-28.9°C)	83.0+0.6	85.0+1.5
Refrigerated (2.2°C)		82.3+1.2
Ambient temp. (19-25°C)		84.6+0.8
High temp. and Humidity (35-36.7°C, 85% R.H.)		83.1+2.7

various conditions are presented in Table 6. Her digestibility figures are not far off from the early reported digestibility of 86.9% for rice germ by Kirk /1954/.

Mitchell and Beadles /1944/ studied the digestibility and biological value /BV/ of defatted corn germ flour which contained 21.2% protein on a 7% moisture basis. The digestibility of defatted corn germ was 85% compared to 99.5% for beef round steak. The BV of defatted corn germ was 77.6, against 76.9 for beef round steak.

Using human subjects, Murlin et al. /1946/ reported the BV of corn germ to be 75.5 and its digestibility to be 77%.

Schulz and Thomas /1949ab/ did two studies on the digestibility and BV of defatted corn germ. The first study utilized experimentally milled ether-extracted corn germ. Its digestibility and BV were found to be 79% to 85% and 65 to 72, respectively. Storage effects were evaluated in their second study with commercially milled ether-extracted corn germ. The corn germ stored three months did not change its digestibility or BV at 72% or 83. However, after two years of storage, corn germ increased its digestibility to 81% but decreased its BV to 79.

Tsen /1984/ recently reported the apparent digestibility in defatted wheat and corn germs to be 86 and 76%, respectively, with rat-feeding tests. The low digestibility of defatted corn germ was presumably due to its high fiber and pentosan content. It was noted that rats on the defatted corn germ diet ate approximately the same amount as those on the casein diet, but the amount of feces was more than twice as much.

ANTI-NUTRITIONAL FACTORS OF CEREAL GERMS

The nutritive quality of proteins in cereal germs can be influenced by the other components such as anti-nutritional factors and fiber.

In the early 1960s, reports began to appear stating that raw wheat germ contains anti-nutritional factors. Creek et al. /1961, 1962ab/, and Attia and Creek /1965/, reported that raw wheat germ contained hemi-agglutinin, a thermolable factor responsible for depressing growth and fat utilization in chicks. Autoclaving destroyed hemi-agglutinin. Moran et al.

/1968/ found hemi-agglutinin and anti-trypsin activities to be high in raw wheat germ. Ewart /1975/ characterized hemi-agglutinin in wheat germ. However, no factors toxic to rats were found in raw wheat germ by Olsen /1967/. In fact, he reported that wheat germ contained high-quality protein and any heat treatment or autoclaving reduced its PER value and digestibility. The conflicting opinions about the improving effect of heat treatment or autoclaving on the nutritive value of wheat germ are still waiting for further clarification.

Rice germ is known to contain trypsin inhibitors and hemi-agglutinins. Acid-extractable trypsin inhibitors caused growth depression and pancreatic hypertrophy in chicks. The inhibitors were found by Tsai /1976/ to be quite stable to dry heat but not to autoclaving or steaming. Rice germ hemi-agglutinin was reported by Barber et al. /1977/ to account for 95% of the activity in rice kernel. It agglutinated rabbit /Benedito de Barber and Barber, 1978/ and human /Bog-Hansen et al., 1976/ red blood cells. However, it was much weaker than that found in castor seed. There appears to be more than one hemagglutinating agent. Takahashi et al. /1973/ obtained a hemagglutinin of molecular weight of 10,000 from rice by aqueous extraction at pH 40. The isolated hemagglutinin consisted of protein, carbohydrate and calcium which was essential for hemagglutination. Tsuda /1979/, extracted a proteinaceous hemagglutinin with phosphate-buffered saline. The extracted compound, existed as a dimer with a molecular weight of 19,000, could be dissociated into two non-identical and inactive subunits.

Little information is available from the literature to show that corn germ contains anti-nutritional factors as are found in other cereal germs. Wall et al. /1971/ found no evidence for heat-labile anti-nutritional factors in corn germ when they compared the nutritive value of air-dried and heat-dried solvent-extracted corn germs.

FOOD USES OF CEREAL GERMS

Cereal germs have long been used in foods and feeds. In view of their large supply and high contents of nutrients together with an adequate amount of fiber, the value of cereal germs can be greatly raised if their uses in foods can be expanded.

Working on wheat germ for breadmaking, Sullivan et al. /1936, 1937/ noticed first that glutathionine in wheat germ had some harmful effects exhibited through decreased loaf volume and poor crumb structure. Grewe and LeClerc /1943/ reported the steeping of wheat germ or the addition of bromate improved loaf volume and crumb gain. Pomeranz /1970/ and Pomeranz et al. /1970/ reported that heat treatment of wheat germ and the addition of lecithin or other phospholipids increased loaf volume and crumb grain. Bolling et al. /1973/ demonstrated that the increasing levels of wheat germ added brought about a decrease in loaf volume, and addition of wheat germ oil at optimum levels improved it. They concluded that wheat germ oil played a positive role in improving the baking quality of wheat flour.

Zaitsev et al. /1974/ found that bread made from flour enriched with 5% wheat germ contained more protein, lysine, and other essential amino acids. The enriched bread had better taste with pronounced flavor than regular bread.

Boero and Tsen /1984/ have recently found that acceptable 12% wheat germ bread can be prepared with the addition of surfactants such as sodium stearoyl lactylate, polysorbate 60, and ethoxylated monoglycerides. The flavor and texture of 12% wheat germ bread was also found to be acceptable to consumers.

The use of wheat germs as an ingredient for making biscuits, cakes and pasta products such as noodle and macaroni, in addition to breads, has been reviewed by Shurpalekar and Rao /1977/.

Rice germ has been proposed by Primo et al., /1970/, and Vasan et al., /1979/ to be used in biscuits, chocolates, puddings, and infant and other special foods. However, few rice germ foods have been commercialized. One major obstacle to the food use of rice germ as a food ingredient is the rapid development of off-flavors as a result of oil rancidity /Desikachar, 1977/.

Fong /1980/ recently demonstrated that whole or broken germs were rather stable during storage at ambient /19-25°C/ or refrigerated /2°C/ temperatures. However, storage of whole germ of high moisture content /15-17%/ at 37°C provoked a rapid increase in titratable acidity and development of odor and visible microbial growth. Her finding of the storage stability of rice germ certainly encourages the food use of rice germs. Fong prepared breads and cakes from wheat flour fortified with 11% rice germ, and granola containing 12% rice germ; she reported that sensory panels reacted favorably to the order of rice germ as well as the taste of the germ fortified bread, cake, and granola.

Of all cereal germs, corn germ has recently received the most attention in research and development to explore its potential food uses. A pilot plant for producing defatted corn germ has been established by Lauhoff Grain Co., and substantial research carried out at the Northern Regional Research Laboratory, USDA and the Department of Grain Science and Industry, Kansas State University in this country.

Defatted corn germ flour has been examined as a nutritive supplement for a number of foods including, muffins, and patties by Gardner et al. /1971/ and Blessin et al. /1972, 1973, and 1974/. Tsen et al. /1974, 1975/ found that acceptable bread could be made from wheat flour fortified with 12% defatted corn germ with the addition of a dough conditioner such as sodium stearoyl lactylate /SSL/, as shown in Table 7. In many countries where loaf volume is not emphasized, the fortified level could be raised to 24%. They have also found that defatted corn germ contains fewer sulfhydryl compounds than wheat germ. Accordingly, heat treatment and high dosage of oxidant were not required to improve the baking performance of corn germ-fortified wheat flour, as did for wheat germ-fortified flour.

Tsen and Weber /1977/ have found that corn germ flour is particularly suitable for deposit or wire-cut cookie such as chocolate chip and oatmeal cookies. It may be incorporated at up to 48% /on wheat flour basis/ without detrimental quality effects, as shown in Table 8. At this level, corn germ cookies are effective in supplying children with dietary protein.

Table 7. Baking Quality of Wheat Flour Fortified With Indicated Levels of Corn-Germ Flour (Tsen et al. 1974)

Corn-Germ flour %	SSL %	Bromate p.p.m.	Abs. %	Mix min.	Avg. Sp. Loaf Vol. cc./g.	Grain score
0	0	50	68	9:30	6.65	9
0	0.5	50	68	9:30	7.17	10
12	0	70	84	4:30	4.16	4
12	0.5	70	84	4:30	6.69	8
16	0	76	88	3:30	3.63	3
16	0.5	76	88	3:30	5.58	7
20	0	82	92	3:00	3.19	3
20	0.5	82	92	3:00	5.11	6
24	0	88	96	3:00	2.81	2
24	0.5	88	96	3:00	4.66	5
28	0	94	100	2:30	2.76	2
28	0.5	94	100	2:30	3.65	4

Table 8. Sensory Evaluation of Fortified Chocolate Chip Cookies (MEAN± SEM)[b] /Tsen and Weber, 1977/

Corn germ flour, %	Texture	Flavor	Taste
0 (Control)	4.4±0.2^{A}	4.2±0.2^{A,B}	4.2±0.2^{A}
12	4.4±0.1^{A}	4.5±0.2^{A}	4.3±0.3^{A}
24	4.4±0.1^{A}	4.4±0.2^{A}	4.4±0.2^{A}
36	3.7±0.2^{B}	3.9±0.2^{B}	3.3±0.3^{B}
48	3.3±0.3^{B}	3.8±0.4^{B}	3.2±0.3^{B}

[b]Means without a superscript letter in common differ significantly (LSD 0.05).

REFERENCES

Attia, F. and Creek, R. D. /1965/. Studies on raw and heated wheat germ for young chicks. Cereal Chem. 42, 494.

Barber, S., Benedito de Barber, C. and Tortosa, E. /1977/. Process for the stabilization of rice bran. Effects of the heat treatment of bran on: a) protein extractability, and b) toxic constituents. In Rice Report 1976. Ed. Barber, S., Mitsuda, H., Desikachar, H. S. R. and Tortosa, E. p. 97. Instituto de Agroquimica y Tecologia de Alimentos, Valencia, Spain.

Beeson, W. M., Lehrer, W. P. and Woods, E. /1947/. Peas, supplemented with wheat germ or corn germ, as a source of protein for growth. J. Nutri. 34, 587.

Benedito de Barber, C. and Barber, S. /1978/. Constituyentes toxicos del salva do de arroz. II. Actividad hemaglutinante del salvado crudo y tratado termicamente. Rev. Agroquim. Tec. Alim. 18, 89.

Blessin, C. W., Inglett, G. E., Garcia, W. J. and Deatherage, W. L. /1972/. Defatted germ flour - Food ingredient from corn. Food Prod. Development 6(3):34.

Blessin, C. W., Garcia, W. J., Deatherage, W. L., Cavins, J. F., and Inglett, G. E. /1973/. Composition of three food products containing defatted corn germ flour. J. Food Sci. 38, 3326.

Blessin, C. W., Garcia, W. J., Deatherage, W. L., and Inglett, G. E. /1974/. An edible defatted germ flour from a dry-milled corn fraction. Cereal Sci. Today 19, 224.

Bog-Hansen, T. C., Ory, R. L. and Mod, R. R. /1976/. Analysis of rice proteins and hemagglutins by crossed immunoelectrophoresis. Proc. 16th Rice Technical Working Group Meeting, March 2-4, 1976, Lake Charles, LA (Abstracts), p. 80.

Bolling, H., El Baya, A. W., and Zwingelberg, H. /1973/. Germ fat and baking quality of wheat. Getreide, Mehl Brot. 27, 92.

Boero, S. and Tsen, C. C. /1984/. Unpublished data.

Cagampang, G. B., Perdon, A. A. and Juliano, B. O. /1976/. Changes in salt-soluble proteins of rice during grain development. Phytochem. 15, 1425.

Canolty, N. L., Schoenborne, M., Gregg, V. A. and Haring, R. V. /1977/. Relative protein value of defatted corn germ flour. J. of Food Sci. 42, 269.

Creek, R. D., Vasaitis, V., Pollard, W. O. and Schumaier, G. /1962a/. Evidence for the presence of a thermolabile growth inhibitor in raw wheat germ. Poultry Sci. 41, 901.

Creek, R. D. and Vasaitis, V. /1962b/. Detection of an anti-proteolytic substance in raw wheat germ. Poultry Sci. 41, 1351.

Creek, R. D., Vasaitis, V. and Schumaier, G. /1961/. The improvement of the nutritive value of raw wheat germ meal by autoclaving. Poultry Sci. 40, 822.

Desikachar, H. S. R. /1977/. Status report: Preservation of by-products of rice milling. Proc. Rice By-prod. Util. Int. Conf. Valencia, Spain 1974, 2, 1.

Earle, F. R., Curtis, J. J. and Hubbard, J. E. /1946/. The composition of the component parts of the corn kernel. Cereal Chem. 23, 504.

Ewart, J. A. D. /1975/. Partial characterization of a wheat germ agglutinin and an albumin. J. Food Sci. Agric. 26, 5.

FAO, U.N., /1982/. FAO production yearbook. Italy 35.

Farrell, E. P., Ward, A., Miller, G. D. and Lovett, L. A. /1967/.

Extensive analyses of flour and millfeeds made from nine different wheat mixes. 1. Amounts and analyses. Cereal Chem. 44, 39.

Fong, R. Y. T. /1980/. Rice germ: Its potential as a food. MS Thesis, University of California, Berkeley, CA.

Gardner, H. W., Inglett, G. E., Deatherage, W. L., Kwolek, W. F. and Anderson, R. A. /1971/. Food products from corn germ: Evaluation as a good supplement after roll-cooking. J. Food Sci. 36, 4.

Grewe, E. and LeClerc, J. A. /1943/. Wheat germ in breadmaking. Cereal Chem. 20, 434.

Hegsted, D. M. and Chang, Y. /1965/. Protein utilization in growing rats at differnt levels of intake. J. Nutri. 87, 19.

Hove, E. L., Carpenter, L. E. and Harrel, C. G. /1945/. The nutritive quality of some plant proteins and the supplemental effect of some protein concentrates on patent flour and whole wheat. Cereal Chem. 22, 287.

Hove, E. L. and Harrel, C. G. /1943/. Studies on raw and heated wheat germ for young chicks. Cereal Chem. 42, 141.

Hubbard, J. E., Hall, H. H. and Earle, F. R. /1950/. Composition of the component parts of the sorghum kernel. Cereal Chem. 27, 415.

Jones, D. B. and Widness, K. D. /1946/. The comparative growth promoting value of the proteins of wheat germ, corn germ and of some other protein foods and plant origin. J. Nutr. 31, 675.

Juliano, B. O. /1980/. Properties of rice caryopsis. In: Rice: production and utiization. Bor S. Luh /ed./ AVI, Westport, CT, p. 403.

Kent, N. L. /1966/. Technology of cereals with special reference to wheat. Pergamon Press, Oxford.

Kik, M. C. /1954/. Nutritive value of rice germ. J. Agr. Food Chem. 2 /23/, 1179.

MacMasters, M. M., Hinton, J. J. C. and Bradbury, D. /1971/. Microscopic structure and composition of the wheat kernel. In: Wheat chemistry and technology. Y. Pomeranz /ed./ St. Paul, MN, p. 51.

Miladi, S., Hegsted, D. M., Saunders, R. M. and Kohler, G. O. /1972/. The relative nutritive value, amino acid content, and digestibility of the proteins of wheat mill fractions. Cereal Chem. 49, 119.

Mitchell, H. H. and J. R. Beadles /1944/. Corn germ: a valuable protein food. Science 99, 129.

Moran, E. T., Summers, J. D. and Bass, E. J. /1968/. Heat processing of wheat germ meal and its effect on utilization and protein quality for the growing chick-toasting and autoclaving. Cereal Chem. 45, 304.

Murlin, J. R., Edwards, L. E., Fried, S., Szymanski, T. A. /1946/. Biological value of proteins in relation to the essential amino acids which they contain. II. Comparison of proteins with mixtures of amino acids. J. Nutr. 31, 715.

Olsen, E. M. /1967/. Effect of heat treatment on the quality and utilization by the rat of protein in wheat germ meal. Can. J. Biochem. 45, 673.

Primo, E., Barber, S., Tortosa, E., Camacho, J., Ulldemolins, J., Jimenez, A. and Vega, R. /1970/. Composicion quimica del arroz. V. Subproductos Obtenidos en las differentes etapas del deagrama de elaboracion. Rev. Agroquim. Tec. Alim. 10(2), 244,

Pomeranz, Y. /1970/. Germ bread. Bakers Dig. 44, 30.

Pomeranz, Y., Carvajal, M. J., Shogren, M. D., Hoseney, R. C. and Finney, K. F. /1970/. Wheat germ in breadmaking. II. Improving breadmaking properties by physical and chemical methods. Cereal Chem. 47, 429.

Pomeranz, Y., Carvajal, M. J., Hoseney, R. C. and Ward, A. B. /1970/. Wheat germ in breadmaking I. Composition of germ lipids and germ protein fraction. Cereal Chem. 47, 373.

Pomeranz, Y., Young, V. L. and Robbins, G. S. /1973/. Protein content and amino acid composition of oat species and tissues. Cereal Chem. 50, 702.

Schulz, J. A. and Thomas, B. H./1949a/. The biological value of the proteins of corn germ and endosperm wet milled experimentally. Cereal Chem. 26, 67

Schulz, J. A. and Thomas, B. H./1949b/. The biological value of some commercial corn protein fractions. Cereal Chem. 26, 60.

Saunders, R. M. and Kohler, G. O. /1972/. In vitro determination of protein digestibility in wheat millfeeds for monogastric animals. Cereal Chem. 49, 98.

Shurpalekar, S. R. and Rao, H. P. /1977/. Wheat Germ. In: Adv. Food Res. C. O. Chichester et al. /ed./ New York, AP p. 187.

Sullivan, B., Howe, M. and Schmaly, F. D. /1936/. On the presence of glutathione in wheat germ. Cereal Chem. 13, 665.

Sullivan, B., Howe, M. and Schmaly, F. D. /1937/. An explanation of the effect of heat treatment on wheat germ. Cereal Chem. 14, 489.

Summers, J. D., Moran, E. T., and Pepper, W. F. /1969/. Nitrogen digestibility of various selected wheat fractions. Can. J. Anim. Sci. 49, 105.

Takahashi, T., Yamada, N., Iwamoto, K., Shimabayashi, Y. and Izutsu, K. /1973/. Some properties and characterization of rice seed hemagglutinin. Agr. Biol. Chem. 37, 29.

Tsai, Yuh-Chi. /1976/. Contribution of protease inhibitors to the deleterious effects of fractions and heat-treated rice bran fed to chicken. J. Chin. Agr. Chem. Soc. 14 (3-4), 187.

Tsen, C. C. /1975/. Defatted corn germ flour - A nutritive ingredient for breadmaking. Bakers Dig. 49(5), 42.

Tsen, C. C. /1984/. Unpublished data.

Tsen, C. C., Mojibican, C. N. and Inglet, G. E. /1974/. Defatted corn-germ flour as a nutrient fortifier for bread. Cereal Chem. 51, 262.

Tsen, C. C. /1980/. Cereal germs used in bakery products: chemistry and nutrition. In: Cereals in food and beverages. G. E. Inglett and Lars Munch /ed./ AP New York.

Tsen, C. C. and Weber, J. /1977/. Corn germ flour as a nutritive ingredient for cookies. Food Product Development 11(4), 75.

Tsuda, M. /1979/. Purification and characterization of a lectin from rice bran. J. Bioch. (Tokyo) 86, 1451 (seen in Chem. Abstr. 92, 1954).

Vasan, B. S., Venkatesan, V., Kousalya, K. and Ganesan, G. /1979/. Separation, procesing and utilization of rice germ. J. Food Sci. Tech. (Mysore) 16(3), 116.

Wall, J. S., James, C. and Cavins, J. F. /1971/. Nutritive value of protein in hominy feed fractions. Cereal Chem. 48, 456.

Youngs /1972/. Protein distribution in out kernel. Cereal Chem. 49, 407.

Zaitsev, V. I., Shaskina, N. Z., and Tyuterov, S. L. /1974/. Improvement of nutritive value of bread by adding wheat germ. Khlibopekarnaya i Kondit. Prom. 7, 7.

Proc. Int. Assoc. Cereal Chem. Symp. Amino Acid Compn and Biol. Value of Cereal Proteins Budapest, Hungary 1983, R. Lásztity, M. Hidvégi, eds

MAIZE GERM PROTEINS, THEIR COMPOSITION, NUTRITIVE VALUE AND FUNCTIONAL PROPERTIES

PAOLO CERLETTI, PATRIZIA RESTANI

Department of General Biochemistry, University of Milan,
Via Celoria, 2, I-20133 Milano, Italy

ABSTRACT - Maize germ is potentially a copious source of protein for human uses. Moreover it is the source of oil of good quality. The protein composition of maize germ is examined. The amino acid composition of germ albumins and globulins is nutritionally more favourable than that of similar proteins of the endosperm and of the envelops.

Nutritional and functional properties of maize germ proteins are generally referred to defatted maize germ, residual from oil extraction. The properties of these proteins are partially modified as compared to the native protein and residual endosperm may contaminate the germ. However, this material represents the most handy and economically favourable source of maize germ protein.

The "in vitro" digestibilities of proteins from germ flour from the wet extraction line or from the dry line are comparable.

For what concerns functional properties, solubility, emulsifying properties and fat adsorption were studied. Extrusion-cooking experiments carried out on maize germ meal, operating at different temperatures and moisture, have shown that this process does not determine a significant decrease of nutritional value.

The increasing impact of world undernourishment and malnutrition has stimulated research into new food sources. These must be able to eliminate the protein deficit both quantitatively and qualitatively, namely for what concerns aminoacid composition and digestibility.

More than 70% of proteins consumed in the world are plant proteins and 71% of them are cereal proteins. In the cereal kernel, the germ contains about 20% of total proteins. Germs have high nutritional value, since they are rich in proteins, minerals, oil and vitamins. Maize germ contains 20-32% of oil and is already used in the food industry as an oil source. In the germ cake residual after oil extraction the proteins range from 15 to 30% in weight: it is therefore a good potential protein source.

Maize used in Italy yearly is 10 million metric tons of which 6 million come from national production and 4 million from imports. Nine million tons are used, as such, for feed, 550,000 tons in the starch industries and 450,000 tons in the meal industry.

Oil extraction is performed on 70,000 metric tons of maize germ, 42,500 of them coming from the meal industry (dry milling) and 27,500 from the starch industry (wet milling). In all, 22,000 metric tons of maize germ oil are produced in Italy: the cakes obtained are about 48,000 tons, corresponding to 9,600 tons of proteins (Peri and Barbieri, 1980).

At present these proteins are used for animal feed but they could profitably be employed for human food because of their nutritional quality. The available amount might easily be increased. Indeed, a greater use of maize for oil extraction is desirable since its oil contains valuable fatty acids from the nutritional point of view. If maize is consumed by animals, its fats are transformed into saturated fats with loss of nutritional quality.

1) Protein composition.

Maize proteins represent about 10% of the kernel, as dry weight; more than 80% of them are in the endosperm. The germ contains 15% of total protein, its protein concentration being twice as high as that of the endosperm (20% vs 10%). In the Opaque-2 variety, the amount of germ relative to total kernel increases and it contains more proteins. The protein distribution is detailed in table 1 (Landry and Moureaux 1980).

Proteins of kernel pertain for what their solubility is concerned to four major classes: albumins, soluble in water, globulins, soluble in dilute neutral salt solution, zein, a prolamine, soluble in 70% ethanol and glutelins G1, G2, G3, soluble in dilute alkali.

In normal grains, albumins and globulins represent 70% of germ proteins, while, they are less than 10% of endosperm proteins. Starch gel electrophoresis demonstrated differences between the albumin and the globulin fraction both in endosperm and germ; however, patterns of fractions from the endosperm and the germ were similar (Paulis and Wall 1969). The Opaque-2 variety contains in the endosperm more albumins and globulins as compared to normal grain while zein is considerably less. Glutelins G1, G2 and specially G3 and insoluble proteins are increased (Landry and Moureaux 1980). Percentages in the germ are unmodified, but in Opaque-2 the germ represents a larger part of kernel weight. As shown in table 1, this results in a significant increase of albumin and globulin content in the seed. The total yield of protein per ha of Opaque-2 is 75-80% of that of normal varieties, but the decrease involves mainly the proteins of the endosperm.

2) Aminoacid composition and nutritional properties.

Proteins of the various groups differ considerably in content of essential aminoacids. Therefore differences in relative proportion of the main protein fractions in each kernel portion result in differences in aminoacid composition of germ and endosperm.

As shown in table 2, lysine, the first limiting aminoacid of cereal kernel is very scarce in zein and is considerably higher in glutelins. The nutritional quality of total grain is improved by using the Opaque-2

TABLE 1

PROTEIN DISTRIBUTION IN WHOLE MAIZE KERNEL AND ITS PORTIONS[1]

Component	Whole grain		Endosperm		Germ		Envelopes	
	normal	Op-2	normal	Op-2	normal	Op-2	normal	Op-2
Weight, % of kernel	100	100	84.0	61.0	8.1	35.0	7.9	4.0
Protein %, w:w	10.5	12.0	10.2	9.7	19.7	26.9	6.2	5.6
Protein, % of total	100	100	80.5	60.7	14.9	35.0	4.6	4.2
Protein classes, % of total proteins								
Albumins	9.0	34.7 (Albumins + Globulins)	2.8	14.4 (Albumins + Globulins)	52.1	69.8 (Albumins + Globulins)		
Globulins	5.0		3.2		16.4			
Zein (prolamin)	15.4	11.8	54.2	13.6	3.3	2.5		
Glutelins G1 + G2	16.3	20.8	18.9	23.5	3.6	5.3		
Glutelin G3	16.2	23.3	16.2	30.8	19.7	19.7		
Insoluble proteins	8.1	9.4	4.6	17.7	4.9	2.7		

[1] Landry and Moureaux (1980)

TABLE 2

ESSENTIAL AMINOACID CONTENT AND CHEMICAL SCORE OF CORN PROTEIN[1]

Aminoacids	Endosperm		Germ		Germ, mg/g			
	mg/g	chemical score	mg/g	chemical score	Alb.+ Glob.	Zein	Gl + G2	G3
Lysine	16	29	26	102	63	5	40	55
Threonine	39	97	42	105	50	33	44	53
Methionine	13	37	18	71	14	9	14	9
Cysteine	n.d.		7		n.d.	3	n.d.	7
Leucine	116	116	73	104	72	165	72	99
Isoleucine	31	78	21	53	35	25	23	44
Valine	48	96	38	76	64	39	51	73
Phenylalanine	42	125	39	112	40	39	29	40
Tyrosine	33		28		23	32	21	26
Tryptophan	n.d.		13	130	n.d.	n.d.	n.d.	n.d.
EAA INDEX (vs WHO Pattern)			90.4					

[1] Tsen 1980, Landry and Moureaux 1980.

variety which has less endosperm in the kernel and lower zein in the endosperm. As already stated the isolated germ has a similar protein composition in Opaque-2 and normal grain. There is therefore no advantage in using Opaque-2 (Landry and Moureaux 1980, Paulis and Wall 1969, Tsen 1980). In the germ lysine is no limiting and the chemical scores of the limiting species (isoleucine and sulphurated aminoacids) are higher than values measured in the endosperm. The essential aminoacid index (EAA index) for the germ, calculated on all essential aminoacids is quite satisfactory, giving a value of 90 or compared to WHO request pattern made equal to 100.

The biological utilization of proteins depends on protein digestibility as well as on protein content. The digestibility of protein is reduced by the presence of peptide bonds resistent to the proteases of the stomach and the intestine. Most investigators conclude that digestibility of all classes of native maize proteins is not a limiting factor on their nutritional performance. Osborne and Mendel (1914) found that zein digestibility for rats ranged from 71 to 84% and these values were somewhat lower than those found in other protein classes. Zein can therefore not be considered a limiting protein for maize flour digestibility; for the germ, where zein is less than 5%, this is even more true (Wall and Paulis 1977).

"In vitro" protein digestibility, according to a modified Satterlee's multi-enzyme procedure (trypsin, chimotrypsin and intestinal peptidase) (Hsu et al. 1977) was about 78% in the separated germ (Peri and Barbieri 1980). These "in vitro" findings are supported by "in vivo" tests: in fact, the very good nutritional quality of germ proteins is confirmed by their high PER values. As shown in table 3, maize germ PER values range between

TABLE 3

PROTEIN EFFICIENCY RATIO (PER) OF CEREAL FLOURS AND CASEIN[1]

Flour	PER*
Whole maize	1.26
Maize germ	2.64
	2.55
Whole weat	0.93
Wheat germ	2.62
Soybean	2.10
Casein	2.50

$$^{*}\mathrm{PER} = \frac{\text{weight gain (g)}}{\text{protein consumed (g)}}$$

[1]Tsen 1980

2.55 and 2.64, very close to the one of wheat germ and slightly higher than the PER of casein. These values are remarkably higher than those of flour from whole wheat or maize kernel. Soybean flour is intermediate with a PER value of 2.10 (Tsen 1980).

3) Oil extraction processes on maize germ.

Maize germ is obtained by wet milling in the starch industry and by dry milling in the flour industry. The germ prepared by the first process is less contaminated by starch. The yield is 5% of the kernel weight in normal grains. The germ preparation, obtained by dry milling is richer in starch and the yield is 10% of starting material. Both the above preparations are used for oil extraction.

Germ cakes obtained have different content of proteins: 25-30% in that form wet-milling and 15-20% in the one from dry milling (fig. 1). These differences come from residual starch in the starting preparations (Peri and Barbieri 1980). Figure 1 gives a summarized scheme of the wet and the dry process. Germ and oil average yields refer to 100 kg of starting maize. Protein and lipid content of different products are also given.

The treatments applied for oil extraction differ: pressing is more easily performed on the product of wet milling, but the germ obtained is defatted only partially and further oil extraction with solvent is required to remove the residual lipid. Moreover, the temperature during conditioning and pressing reaches higher levels. As discussed later, this modifies the nutritional peroperties of the proteins. Table 4 compares the nutritional characteristics of the different products. The "in vitro" digestibility is only slightly changed in the defatted germ deriving from either processes of oil extraction. On the other hand, the PER value, which

TABLE 4

NUTRITIONAL VALUES OF DEFATTED CAKES OBTAINED FROM DRY AND WET MILLING[1]

Product	Proteins %	Lipid	"In vitro" digestibility	PER
Germ from dry milling:				
untreated	13.7	19.9	77.1	2.60
defatted with solvents	17.8	1.5	75.1	2.29
Germ from wet milling:				
untreated	18	40	79.4	2.60
defatted by pressing	27	10	74.0	1.54

[1] Peri et al. (1980), Wall (1977).

is an "in vivo" assay, remains high in the germ treated with solvents but decreases considerably in the product from pressing. The most denaturing

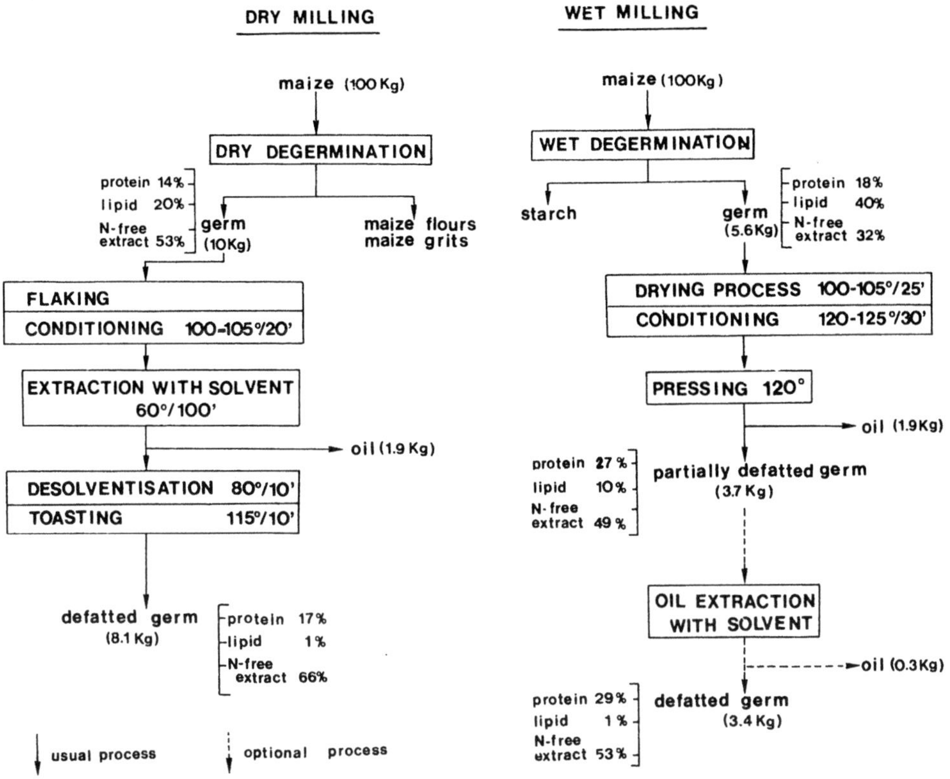

Fig.1 - Oil extraction processes of maize germ.

step in the wet process is conditioning at 120-125°C. In the dry process, desolventisation, performed at only slightly lower temperature, has not the same damaging effect. Probably this behaviour depends on the different degree of moisture, which is high in the wet process and very low in the other one (Peri and Barbieri 1980).

Proteins are indeed modified by applied heat: during maize drying with air at 143°C, intermolecular disulfide bonds are formed. The number of sulphydryl groups decreases during heating of whole grain; a parallel decrease occurs in grain viability. Lysine and available lysine contents are slightly reduced (Wall et al. 1975).

4) Functional properties.

In our laboratory, we studied the functional properties of the protein concentrate separated from the germ cake prepared by the dry process (Restani et al.1980, 1983). Proteins were extracted by a modified Concon procedure (Concon 1973): the cake was treated at room temperature with 70% ethanol (3:1, w:w), after one hour we added 0.7% NaOH (11:1, w:w) which diluted ethanol to 15%. These conditions are not typical for solubilization of albumins and globulins: indeed, only scarce protein was extracted in aqueous medium at neutral pH, whereas the treatment used solubilized 75% of total protein. On a dry basis the concentrate contained 58% proteins, 30% carbohydrate and 9% ashes.

Proteins obtained were soluble in water at a final ionic strength of I = 0.02. A minimum of 20% dissolved at pH 5.0, while at more acidic pH and in alkaline medium solubility was close to 100%. Increasing the ionic strength at the pH of minimum solubility enhanced only by 5% the amount of protein dissolved: the greatest effect was at ionic strength between 0.1 and 0.4, the same where globulins from other sources become solubilized. This behaviour suggests that the structure of cake residual after oil extraction may be limiting to protein solubilization. The proteins may also be in part modified by the treatment they undergo during oil extraction (table 5).

The amount of water absorbed is very high reaching 1 g per g protein at 95% relative humidity. As shown in fig. 2 the sorption capacity of maize germ proteins largely overcomes that of other food proteins. The data quoted for Promine D and whey proteins refer to 15°C and it is known that less water is adsorbed when temperature increases. Comparison of sorption and desorption curves indicates that hysteresis is quite small, hence the process is reversible.

The amount of emulsion produced and the stability of emulsions are quite good in all the pH range assayed except for a minimum at pH 5.5 (table 6). This minimum is slightly displaced towards neutrality with respect to the pH of lowest solubility and is quite sharp, good emulsifying properties being displayed at pH values where solubility is reduced. This indicates that the emulsion behaviour is not directly related to the solubility properties of the proteins.

The ability of part of the proteins to disperse at the interface between oil and water phase stabilizing the emulsion suggests that these

TABLE 5

EFFECT OF pH (A) AND OF IONIC STRENGTH (B) ON THE SOLUBILITY OF PROTEINS FROM MAIZE GERM CAKE

Proteins (100 mg) were suspended: A) in 10 ml water at the desired pH, the final ionic strength being made 0.02 with NaCl or B) in 10 ml water at pH 5.0, the ionic strength being adjusted at the desired value with NaCl. The suspensions were shaken 2 hours at 25°C the pH being controlled and the undissolved material was then centrifuged off at 7,800 x g for 45 min. Total nitrogen was determined in the supernatant.

A		B	
pH	protein solubilized (%)	I	protein solubilized (%)
2	85.2	0.01	21.9
3	39.9	0.05	22.9
4	27.8	0.10	24.3
5	22.1	0.40	27.8
6	50.0	0.50	28.1
7	68.2	0.80	28.2
8	84.1		
9	92.8		
10	97.5		
11	99.8		

TABLE 6

EMULSION PROPERTIES OF PROTEINS FROM MAIZE GERM CAKE

Proteins (140 mg) suspended in water and adjusted to the desired pH and to final volume of 2 ml were shaken for 1 min at 710 revolutions per min with 2 ml soy oil, then were centrifuged for 5 min at 1,200 x g. The height of emulsion layer, as percent of the total content of the tube, measures the emulsion activity. An equivalent measure made after keeping the tube 30 min at 80°C and 15 min at 15°C before centrifuging gives the stability of emulsion.

pH	Emulsion activity	Stability of emulsion
2.0	45.9	48.1
4.0	50.0	55.4
5.0	49.5	56.9
5.5	9.3	12.3
6.0	49.5	53.9
8.0	52.6	49.5
11.0	49.2	50.5

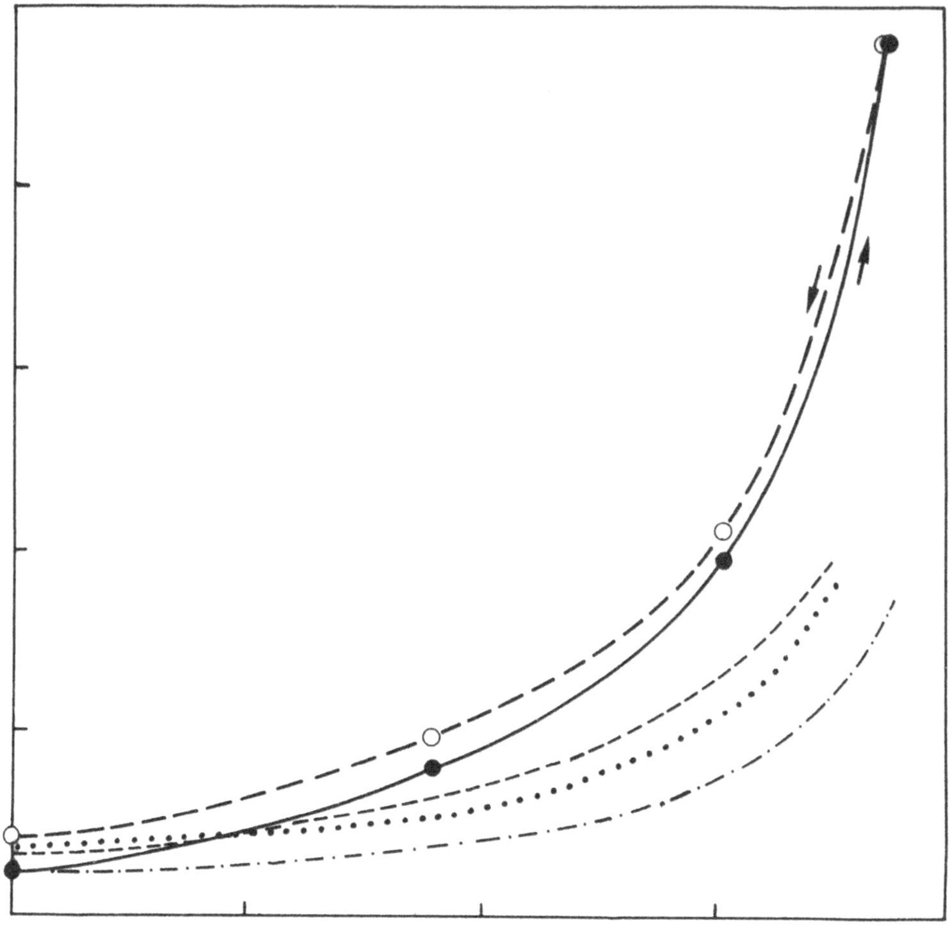

Fig. 2 - Sorption and desorption behaviour of maize germ proteins

Germ proteins were dried at 50°C for four days and then equilibrated at 20°C in a dessicator in presence of saturated salt sulutions of known relative humidity. The relative humidity was checked throughout with an hygrometer. The data on germ proteins are compared with those on other proteins, obtained in our laboratory (lupine globulins, -·-·) or reported in the literature: Promine D ....., Whey protein concentrate -----, both measured at 15°C. (Restani et al. 1980) molecules dissociate and unfold and that part of peptide has hydrophobic character.

Fat absorption is remarkably high and better than that of several food proteins (soybean, sunflower, alfa alfa leaf, etc.) (Hermansson 1977) (table 7). Protein isolated from solvent extracted dry milled maize germ contains little free lipid but contains 7-11% of bound lipid, the presence of which results in flavours describable as stale and rancid (Nielsen et al. 1977). Removal of bound lipid improves both flavour and odour however the flavour of the improved product is still not as that of caseinate. The two best methods developed for removing bound lipid were:

1) extract maize germ meal three times with 5 vol of 80% ethanol before protein isolation or
2) rigorously extract the still wet, freshly precipitated protein three times with 10 vol of 80% ethanol (Nielsen et al.1973).

TABLE 7
FAT ADSORPTION OF PROTEINS FROM MAIZE GERM CAKE

Proteins (500 mg) were shaken for 1 min in a centrifuge tube on a Vortex vibrator with 3 ml soy oil. They were than kept at 24°C for 30 min. After centrifuging for 25 min at 1,610 x g the volume of free oil was measured. Fat adsorbed is expressed as ml oil bound (gm sample)$^{-1}$. 100.

	Fat adsorption
Corn germ proteins	549
Lupine globulins	190
Soy concentrates and isolates (10)	From 92 to 154
Sunflower concentrates and isolates (10)	From 227 to 256
Alfa alfa leaf protein preparations (7)	From 180 to 430

5) Food applications.

Defatted maize germ is used almost exclusively for animal feed: although cakes obtained by present processes are rich in fiber which decreases their digestibility. The functional properties described above allow the use of cake in several foods, as protein fortifier.

Loaves with different content of maize germ have been prepared. The fortification can adversely affect on dough properties and baking quality. However, modifying the bread making process and adding a surfactant effectively improve the quality of germ-fortified bread and biscuits (Table 8) (Tsen 1980). In vivo and in vitro assays showed that supplementation significantly improves the PER value of bread, while its digestibility is only slightly increased.

Extrusion-cooking experiments were carried out on maize germ meal from dry milling, operating at different temperatures (130°, 150°, 170°, 190° C) and moisture (16, 18, 20, 22%) of the product. The extruded products can be used as protein fortifiers or as meat product substitutes. The

TABLE 8

PROTEIN EFFICIENCY RATIOS OF GERM FORTIFIED BREAD DIET FED RATS, AND "IN VITRO" DIGESTIBILITY[1]

Bread		PER[+]	Digestibility %
Wheat, no addition		0.90	82
Maize germ added	12%	1.16	88
	24%	1.43	86
	36%	1.73	85

[+] In rats, during 28 days.
[1] Tsen (1980).

extrusion-cooking process does not determine a significant decrease in the nutritional value, while improving the hygienic and organoleptic quality of the product (Peri et al.1980) (table 9).

TABLE 9

DIGESTIBILITY OF EXTRUDED GERM CAKE OBTAINED AT DIFFERENT TEMPERATURE AND MOISTURE CONDITIONS[*,1]

Extrusion temperature °C	Starting cake moisture %	"In vitro" digestibility %
130	18	77.3
150	18	75.4
170	18	73.3
190	18	72.3
150	16	81.4
150	18	76.0
150	20	75.2
150	22	73.2
Starting cake, untreated	12	77.7

[*] Extrusion was performed on solvent defatted maize germ meal obtained from dry milling.

[1] Peri et al. (1980).

6) Conclusion

As previously indicated, some steps in the oil extraction processes cause protein damage and hence a decrease of nutritional value.

In the wet milling industry protein damage could be eliminated if pressing at 120°C is substituted by extraction with solvents, operating at 60°C. To the same purpose, desolventisation under vacuum could be applied (Peri and Barbieri 1980).

As the findings reported above indicate, maize germ shows a good protein composition with nutritional value very close to casein and remarkably higher than that of several other food proteins (including the soybean). Of all foods, bread, in various forms, is the most popular. Its high consumption, wide acceptability, and low price make it an ideal staple to be fortified, for various feeding programs and for general public use. Biscuits and cakes are particularly popular snack items for children. All can be fortified to increase their nutritional values.

For its functional properties the protein concentrate from maize germ oil cake is a good binder and emulsifying agent for food formulations (frankfurters, sausages, creams, etc.). In particular its very high fat adsorption capacity indicates its use in hypercaloric formulations, with high fat contents. Being soluble at low pH, it can be added to acid beverages.

ACKNOWLEDGEMENT

The partecipation of dr. P.Restani to the Meeting in Budapest was supported by Chiari e Forti of Silea (Treviso) to which grateful acknowledgment is made.

Research work was partially supported by C.N.R., Italy, Special grant I.P.R.A., Subproject 3.

REFERENCES

CONCON,J.N. (1973) Rapid and simple method for the quantitative extraction of corn endosperm proteins. Anal. Biochem. 55, 563-572.

HERMANSSON, A.M. (1977) Functional properties of proteins for foods-water vapor sorption. J. Food Technol. 12, 177-187.

HSU, H.W., VAVAK, D.L., SATTERLEE, L.D. and MILLER, G.A. (1977) A multienzyme technique for estimating protein digestibility. J. Food Sci. 42, 1269-1273.

LANDRY, J. and MOUREAUX, T. (1980) Distribution and amino acid composition of protein groups located in different histological parts of maize grain. J. Agric. Food Chem. 28, 1186-1191.

NIELSEN, H.C., INGLETT, G.E., WALL, J.S. and DONALDSON, G.L. (1973) Corn germ protein isolate. Preliminary studies on preparation and properties. Cereal Chem. 50, 435-443.

OSBORNE, T.B. and MENDEL, L.B. (1914) Nutritive properties of proteins of the maize kernel. J. Biol. Chem. 18, 1-6.

PAULIS, J.W. and WALL, J.S. (1969) Albumins and globulins in extracts of corn grain parts. Cereal Chem. 46, 263-273.

PERI, C. and BARBIERI, R. (1980) Utilizzazione del panello di germe di mais come fonte proteica. I-qualità proteica e tecnologie di produzione. Riv. Ital. Sost. Grasse 57, 185-191.

PERI, C., BARBIERI, R., BRAMBILLA, C. and TOMMASONE, G. (1980) Utilizzazione del panello di germe di mais come fonte proteica. II-studio delle condizioni di estrusione e della qualità degli estrusi. Riv. Ital. Sost. Grasse 57, 240-247.

RESTANI, P., RICCARDI, A. and CERLETTI, P. (1980) Functional properties of corn germ protein related to the interaction with water and with fats. Ann.Technol. Agric. 29, 409-414.

RESTANI, P., RICCARDI A., DURANTI, M. and CERLETTI, P. (1983) Corn germ protein concentrate and its functional properties. In: Progress in Food Engineering - Proceedings of a European Symposium of the Food Working Party of the E.F.C.E., 1981, Milan, Italy, C.Cantarelli and C.Peri (eds.) Forster-Verlag AG/Forster Publishing Ltd., Küsnacht, Zurigo, p.737-739.

TSEN, C.C. (1980) Cereal germs used in bakery products: chemistry and nutrition. In: Cereal for food beverages - Recent progress in cereal chemistry and technology. G.E. Inglett and L.Munck (eds.) Academic Press Inc., New York p. 245-253.

WALL, J.S., JAMES, C. and DONALDSON, G.L. (1975) Corn proteins: chemical and physical changes during drying of grain. Cereal Chem. 52, 779-790.

WALL, J.S. and PAULIS, J.W. (1977) Corn and sorghum grain proteins. In: Advances in cereal science and technology, vol. II, American Assoc. of Cereal Chemists, St.Paul, p.132-219.

Proc. Int. Assoc. Cereal Chem. Symp. Amino Acid Compn and Biol. Value of Cereal Proteins Budapest, Hungary 1983, R. Lásztity, M. Hidvégi, eds

CHEMICAL AND BIOLOGICAL DATA OF RICE PROTEINS FOR NUTRITION AND FEEDING

S. BARBER, C. BENEDITO de BARBER

Laboratorio de Cereales y Proteaginosas, Instituto de Agroquimica y Tecnología de Alimentos, CSIC, Jaime Roig 11, VALENCIA-10, Spain

ABSTRACT

Husks, bran, brokens and milled rice, the four major products from rice milling, differ in the quantity and the quality of the protein they contain. The protein content and the protein quality of these milling fractions is critically reviewed in the ligth of available data on: total protein (P), true protein (TP), non-protein nitrogen (NPN), individual amino acids (AA), essential amino acids (EAA), available amino acids (AAA), limiting amino acid (LAA), amino acid score, protein efficiency ratio (PER), net protein ratio (NPR), net protein utilization (NPU), biological value (BV), true digestibility (TD), and other indices.

1. CHEMICAL DATA OF PROTEIN QUALITY OF RICE

Paddy gives upon milling white milled rice (40-55%) plus three major byproducts: Husks (20%), bran (10%) and brokens (10-22%) (Barber et al., 1981). Protein content of commercial milling fractions of paddy can be placed as follows: milled rice, 8%; husks, 3%; bran, 17%; brokens, 8.5%. Brown rice contains a little bit more proteins than milled rice - 9.5% as compared to 8%. Rice germ, a minor but valuable byproduct can reach 20-25% protein (Barber and Benedito de Barber, 1977; Barber and Benedito de Barber, 1980).

About 3% of the total nitrogen of brown rice (Palmiano et al., 1968) and 2% of milled rice is non-protein nitrogen (Kester et al., 1963). Approximately 0.7% of the protein of brown rice, 0.7% of milled rice, 1.35% of bran-polish and 4.6% of embryo are free amino acids (Tamura and Kenmochi, 1963).

Although brokens are regularly used in food manufacture - flour, semolina, nooddles and extrusion-cooked products (Barber et al., 1981) - published data on the nutritional value of their specific protein are meager. Brokens protein are in between brown and milled rice proteins.

Data on amino acid composition of rice and rice byproducts are abundant in the literature - data on husks are meager (Houston et al., 1969; Baldi et al., 1976; Juliano, 1980). Variability of results from different sources, frequently influenced by analytical techniques, makes difficult to assess the most reasonable average levels of amino acids in each milling fraction, specifying actual differences, if any, among them. However, there is a demand for such figures for practical purposes.

Based on a critical analysis of published data available to us we have developed "our best estimate" of the typical amino acid composition of brown rice, milled rice, husks, bran, polish and germ (Table 1). "Our best estimate" for every mill stream is presented separately (Tables 2 through 7) showing expected range of variation of each amino acid. Non-essential amino acids range within 5-10 percent. So do essential amino acids, although cystine, triptophan and tyrosine, and sometimes methionine and isoleucine, may show bigger variation according to the source of data.

Rough rice and its milling fractions differ in amino acid composition (Tables 8 through 11) (Baldi et al., 1976) (Bradbury et al., 1980 a and b) (Eggum et al., 1982) (Cagampang et al., 1976) (Houston and Kohler, 1970). Studies on the amino acid distribution among the different milling fractions of rice have shown that: a) as essential amino acids are concerned (Tables 8 and 9): leucine is lowest in germ; lysine is highest in germ and intermediate in bran, husk and polish; brown-rice protein contains more lysine than milled-rice protein; cystine + methionine is lowest in husks; phenylalanine + tyrosine is lowest in husks and germ; threonine is highest in husks and intermediate in bran, polish and germ; and other amino acids do not show great differences. b) As non-essential amino acids are concerned (Tables 10 and 11): arginine and histidine are highest in germ; arginine, glutamic acid and histidine are lowest in husks; and proline is highest in husks.

"Our proposed best estimate", given in Table 1, shows an amino acid distribution pattern among the various milling fractions of rice which is in close agreement with the general tendency observed in individual sources of data discussed above.

TABLE 1

TYPICAL AMINO ACID COMPOSITION OF RICE AND RICE BY-PRODUCTS

	Brown rice g/16.8 g N	Milled rice g/16.8 g N	Husks g/16.0 g N	Bran g/16.0 g N	Polish g/16.0 g N	Germ g/16.0 g N
1. Alanine	5.6	5.5	7.0	6.6	5.8	6.2
2. Arginine	8.4	8.5	5.0	7.7	8.5	9.2
3. Aspartic acid ...	9.6	9.0	10.2	9.2	9.4	8.8
4. Cystine	1.7	1.8	2.0	2.2	2.2	2.2
5. Glutamic acid ..	19.2	17.0	12.4	14.3	16.5	15.2
6. Glycine	4.6	4.5	6.3	5.5	5.0	5.5
7. Histidine	2.4	2.3	1.5	2.8	2.7	3.5
8. Isoleucine	4.1	4.5	3.8	3.9	3.7	3.6
9. Leucine	8.2	8.2	7.9	7.2	7.8	6.8
10. Lysine	3.9	3.7	4.5	4.9	4.3	6.5
11. Methionine	2.2	2.7	1.8	2.2	2.4	1.9
12. Phenylalanine ..	5.2	5.5	4.9	4.4	4.7	4.5
13. Proline........	4.8	5.0	8.6	4.5	5.0	4.7
14. Serine	5.2	5.0	5.4	4.6	5.0	4.6
15. Threonine	3.8	3.7	5.0	3.8	3.6	3.8
16. Tryptophan....	1.3	1.2	–	1.4	1.5	1.5
17. Tyrosine	4.0	5.2	2.4	3.3	4.5	3.2
18. Valine	5.8	6.0	6.2	5.7	5.4	4.9

TABLE 2

TYPICAL AMINO ACID COMPOSITION
OF RICE AND RICE BY-PRODUCTS

1. Brown rice

Non essential amino acids			Essential amino acids		
Amino acid	g/16.8 g N	Range	Amino acid	g/16.8 g N	Range
1. Ala	5.6	± 0.5	4. Cys	1.7	± 0.5
2. Arg	8.4	± 0.8	8. Ile	4.1	± 0.4
3. Asp	9.6	± 0.8	9. Leu	8.2	± 0.7
5. Glu	19.2	± 3.0	10. Lys	3.9	± 0.4
6. Gly	4.6	± 0.5	11. Met	2.2	± 0.3
7. His.	2.4	± 0.3	12. Phe	5.2	± 0.5
13. Pro	4.8	± 0.5	15. Thr	3.8	± 0.3
14. Ser.	5.2	± 0.6	16. Trp	1.3	± 0.3
			17. Tyr	4.0	± 0.8
			18. Val	5.8	± 0.5

TABLE 3

TYPICAL AMINO ACID COMPOSITION
OF RICE AND RICE BY-PRODUCTS

2. Milled rice

Non essential amino acids			Essential amino acids		
Amino acid	g/16.8 g N	Range	Amino acid	g/16.8 g N	Range
1. Ala	5.5	± 0.4	4. Cys	1.8	± 0.4
2. Arg	8.5	± 0.7	8. Ile	4.5	± 0.6
3. Asp	9.0	± 0.5	9. Leu	8.2	± 0.9
5. Glu	17.0	± 1.5	10. Lys	3.7	± 0.5
6. Gly	4.5	± 0.5	11. Met	2.7	± 0.7
7. His.	2.3	± 0.3	12. Phe	5.5	± 0.6
13. Pro	5.0	± 0.6	15. Thr	3.7	± 0.4
14. Ser.	5.0	± 0.5	16. Trp	1.2	± 0.3
			17. Tyr	5.2	± 0.9
			18. Val	6.0	± 0.5

TABLE 4

TYPICAL AMINO ACID COMPOSITION
OF RICE AND RICE BY-PRODUCTS

3. Husks

Non essential amino acids			Essential amino acids		
Amino acid	g/16.0 g N	Range	Amino acid	g/16.0 g N	Range
1. Ala	7.0	± 0.5	4. Cys	2.0	± 0.3
2. Arg	5.0	± 0.3	8. Ile	3.8	± 0.6
3. Asp	10.2	± 0.4	9. Leu	7.9	± 0.4
5. Glu	12.4	± 0.4	10. Lys	4.5	± 0.3
6. Gly	6.3	± 0.3	11. Met	1.8	± 0.3
7. His.	1.5	± 0.2	12. Phe	4.9	± 0.4
13. Pro	8.6	± 0.8	15. Thr	5.0	∓ 0.3
14. Ser.	5.4	± 0.3	16. Trp	—	—
			17. Tyr	2.4	± 0.2
			18. Val	6.2	± 0.7

TABLE 5

TYPICAL AMINO ACID COMPOSITION
OF RICE AND RICE BY-PRODUCTS

4. Bran

Non essential amino acids			Essential amino acids		
Amino acid	g/16.0 g N	Range	Amino acid	g/16.0 g N	Range
1. Ala	6.6	± 0.5	4. Cys	2.2	± 0.4
2. Arg	7.7	± 0.6	8. Ile	3.9	± 0.4
3. Asp	9.2	± 0.7	9. Leu	7.2	± 0.7
5. Glu	14.3	± 1.7	10. Lys	4.9	± 0.5
6. Gly	5.5	± 0.4	11. Met	2.2	± 0.3
7. His.	2.8	± 0.3	12. Phe	4.4	± 0.4
13. Pro	4.5	± 0.7	15. Thr	3.8	± 0.4
14. Ser.	4.6	± 0.5	16. Trp	1.4	± 0.3
			17. Tyr	3.3	± 0.5
			18. Val	5.7	± 0.7

TABLE 6

TYPICAL AMINO ACID COMPOSITION OF RICE AND RICE BY-PRODUCTS

5. Polish

Non essential amino acids			Essential amino acids		
Amino acid	g/16.0 g N	Range	Amino acid	g/16.0 g N	Range
1. Ala	5.8	± 0.3	4. Cys	2.2	± 0.4
2. Arg	8.5	± 0.5	8. Ile	3.7	± 0.8
3. Asp	9.4	± 0.5	9. Leu	7.8	± 0.3
5. Glu	16.5	± 1.5	10. Lys	4.3	± 0.7
6. Gly	5.0	± 0.6	11. Met	2.4	± 0.3
7. His.	2.7	± 0.2	12. Phe	4.7	± 0.5
13. Pro	5.0	± 0.7	15. Thr	3.6	± 0.4
14. Ser.	5.0	± 0.5	16. Trp	1.5	± 0.2
			17. Tyr	4.5	± 1.0
			18. Val	5.4	± 1.0

TABLE 7

TYPICAL AMINO ACID COMPOSITION OF RICE AND RICE BY-PRODUCTS

6. Germ

Non essential amino acids			Essential amino acids		
Amino acid	g/16.0 g N	Range	Amino acid	g/16.0 g N	Range
1. Ala	6.2	± 0.9	4. Cys	2.2	± 1.0
2. Arg	9.2	± 0.5	8. Ile	3.6	± 0.6
3. Asp	8.8	± 0.7	9. Leu	6.8	± 0.9
5. Glu	15.2	± 1.4	10. Lys	6.5	± 1.0
6. Gly	5.5	± 0.7	11. Met	1.9	± 0.5
7. His.	3.5	± 0.7	12. Phe	4.5	± 1.0
13. Pro	4.7	± 1.0	15. Thr	3.8	± 0.5
14. Ser.	4.6	± 0.9	16. Trp	1.5	± 0.4
			17. Tyr	3.2	± 1.0
			18. Val	4.9	± 0.4

TABLE 8

COMPARISON OF AMINO ACID COMPOSITION OF ROUGH RICE AND ITS MILLING FRACTIONS

a) Essential amino acids (g/16.0 g N)

	Ile	Leu	Lys	Cys + Met	Phe + Tyr	Thr	Trp	Val
1. Rough rice. . .	3.0	7.9	3.6	5.0	8.8	3.7	–	4.4
2. Brown rice. . .	3.5	7.9	3.5	4.6	9.1	3.7	–	5.1
3. Milled rice . . .	3.5	8.1	3.0	4.9	9.2	3.6	–	5.1
4. Husks	3.2	8.0	4.7	3.6	6.8	4.9	–	5.5
5. Bran	2.8	7.6	4.9	4.8	7.9	4.3	–	4.5
6. Polish	2.9	7.7	4.2	4.9	8.5	4.1	–	4.4
7. Germ.......	3.1	6.6	7.5	4.5	6.9	4.2	–	4.9

Source: Baldi et al., 1976.

TABLE 9

COMPARISON OF AMINO ACID COMPOSITION OF RICE CARYOPSIS AND ITS HISTOLOGICAL COMPONENTS

Essential amino acids (residues of AA/100 residues)

	Ile	Leu	Lys	Cys + Met	Phe + Tyr	Thr	Trp	Val
Rice caryopsis	4.6	8.7	4.1	2.1	6.8	3.7	–	7.4
Grain coat[(a)]	4.9	9.2	4.8	0.8	7.0	4.3	–	7.6
Grain coat[(a)] + aleurone cells.........	4.5	8.3	4.9	1.3	6.7	3.9	–	7.8
Embryo..........................	4.1	6.8	6.4	1.7	5.5	4.6	–	7.3
Starchy endosperm	4.8	9.0	3.7	1.8	6.8	3.5	–	7.4

(a) Pericarp, seed coat and nucella.
Source: Bradbury et al., 1980..

Amino acid scores calculated using "our best estimate" of typical amino acid composition (Table 1) and the FAO amino acid scoring pattern (Table 12), are: milled rice 0.65; brown rice 0.68; polish 0.79; husks 0.83; bran and germ 0.90 (Table 13). Lysine and threonine are first and second limiting amino acids for brown rice and its milling fractions with only two exceptions: isoleucine is the first limiting amino acid in germ protein and the second one in husks protein. Amino acid scores calculated from "our best estimate" amino acid composition also are in close agreement with corresponding experimental results from individual sources of data.

When amino acid scores are referred to the requirement pattern for child (Table 12), limiting amino acids are those cited above (Table 15) but for infant (Table 12) threonine in bran and polish and leucine in germ and bran gain greater importance (Table 14).

2. BIOLOGICAL DATA OF PROTEIN QUALITY OF RICE

In 1972 Juliano reported "few comparative nutritional studies on brown rice and its milling fractions ... have been made. The data are difficult to compare because the protein levels, age, sex, and number of rats and feeding periods used differ". Today, eleven years later, no satisfactory solution has been achieved.Reliable typical values are difficult to ascertain.

We have compiled available data on quality indexes for rice proteins and, after disregarding discordant results, their expected range of variation and eventually "our best estimate" for typical values have been summarized in Table 16. Protein efficiency ratio (PER) has been the quality index most widely used. Generally it has been obtained at the level of 5-6 percent dietary protein for milled rice, 5-8 per cent for brown rice, 8-10 percent for bran, 9-15 per cent for polish, and 9 per cent for germ. Observed values for milled rice, bran and polish vary between 1.5 and 2.0, 1.6 and 2.2, and 1.8 and 2.0 respectively. PER values for brown rice and germ are very close to 1.8 and 1.9 respectively (Table 16). Variability of results make difficult comparative evaluation of milling fractions.

The repeatedly cited faults and disadvantages of the PER assay (Pellet and Young, 1980) (Hegsted, 1968) (Bender and Doell, 1957) seem to be considered with increasing interest. Consequently, other protein quality indexes based either on changes in body weight or on nitrogen balance, using rats, are determined preferentially. So NPR (net protein ratio) values ranging 3.31 to 4.02 at 6 per cent dietary protein (Vaugham et al., 1980) and 3.07 to 3.71 at 5 per cent protein (Bressani et al., 1971) have been reported for milled rice (Table 17) and 4.15 to 4.39 at 8 percent protein for brown rice (Mitra and Das, 1971).

Evaluation of true digestibility (TD), biological value (BV) and net protein utilization (NPU) of the protein utilization (NPU) of the protein of brown rice and its milling fractions has been carried out by several authors. "Our best estimate" of typical values of these indexes is given in Table 16. All sources of data give high (90%) digestibility values, within a narrow range of variation, for brown rice (Kik, 1952 and 1962) (Eggum and Juliano, 1973) (Khan and Eggum, 1978) (Chavan and Duggal, 1978) (Eggum et al., 1982) and milled rice (Kik, 1952 and 1962) (Bressani and Valiente, 1962) (Eggum and Juliano, 1973 and 1975) (Miyazaki and Horii,1975) (Eggum, 1977) (Eggum et al., 1982) protein. Amino acid digestibility is

TABLE 10

COMPARISON OF AMINO ACID COMPOSITION OF ROUGH RICE AND ITS MILLING FRACTIONS

b) Non essential amino acids (g/16.0 g N)

	Ala	Arg	Asp	Glu	Gly	His	Pro	Ser
1. Rough rice...	5.7	7.8	9.2	16.8	4.7	2.3	5.1	5.3
2. Brown rice...	5.5	8.0	8.8	17.1	4.6	2.3	4.9	5.1
3. Milled rice...	5.2	7.8	8.7	17.7	4.2	2.1	4.9	5.2
4. Husks	6.4	4.9	9.9	12.5	5.9	1.7	9.4	4.9
5. Bran	6.6	7.6	10.3	14.2	5.8	2.6	5.6	5.4
6. Polish	6.0	8.1	9.5	15.8	5.1	2.6	5.1	5.2
7. Germ.......	6.3	9.5	8.7	14.8	5.8	3.4	4.8	4.6

Source: Baldi et al., 1976.

TABLE 12

PATTERNS OF AMINO ACID REQUIREMENTS AND AMINO ACID SCORING PATTERNS FOR EVALUATION OF PROTEINS (mg/g N)

Amino acid	Requirement pattern			Scoring pattern
	Infant	Child	Adult	
Isoleucine	220	230	113	250
Leucine..................	500	350	156	440
Lysine..................	325	469	138	340
Methionine + cystine	180	213	150	220
Phenylalanine + tyrosine	394	213	156	380
Threonine	275	275	81	250
Tryptophan...............	56	30	44	60
Valine	294	256	113	310

Source: Pellet and Young, 1980.

TABLE 11

COMPARISON OF AMINO ACID COMPOSITION OF RICE CARYOPSIS AND ITS HISTOLOGICAL COMPONENTS

Non essential amino acids (residues of AA/100 residues)

	Ala	Arg	Asp	Glu	Gly	His	Pro	Ser
Rice caryopsis..............	8.6	6.1	9.2	16.4	9.0	2.5	6.3	4.5
Grain coat(a)...............	11.5	4.4	11.7	8.5	10.8	1.9	7.8	4.5
Grain coat(a) + aleurone cells...	10.2	5.8	10.5	13.2	10.4	2.7	6.1	3.9
Embryo....................	9.8	8.2	8.9	13.8	11.4	3.0	4.9	3.6
Starchy endosperm	8.9	5.5	9.2	17.1	8.4	2.3	6.9	4.7

(a) Pericarp, seed coat and nucella.
Source: Bradbury et al., 1980.

TABLE 13

AMINO ACIDS SCORES AND LIMITING AMINO ACIDS OF RICE AND RICE BY-PRODUCTS

1. FAO Scoring pattern

	1rst limiting AA		2nd limiting AA	
	AA	Score	AA	Score
1. Brown rice...	Lys	0.68	Thr	0.90
2. Milled rice...	Lys	0.65	Thr	0.88
3. Husks	Lys	0.83	Ile	0.95
4. Bran	Lys	0.90	Thr	0.95
5. Polish	Lys	0.79	Thr	0.90
			Ile	0.92
6. Germ.......	Ile	0.90	Thr	0.95
			Leu	0.96

TABLE 14

AMINO ACIDS SCORES AND LIMITING AMINO ACID OF RICE AND RICE BY-PRODUCTS

	2. Infant (FAO, 1973)			
	1srt limiting AA		2nd limiting AA	
	AA	Score	AA	Score
1. Brown rice...	Lys	0'71	Thr	0.82
2. Milled rice...	Lys	0.68	Thr	0.80
3. Husks	Lys	0.86	Leu	0.99
4. Bran	Thr	0.86	Leu	0.90
5. Polish	Thr	0.82	Lys	0.83
6. Germ.......	Leu	0.85	Thr	0.86

TABLE 15

AMINO ACIDS SCORES AND LIMITING AMINO ACIDS OF RICE AND RICE BY-PRODUCTS

	3. Child (FAO, 1973)			
	1rst limiting AA		2nd limiting AA	
	AA	Score	AA	Score
1. Brown rice...	Lys	0.49	Thr	0.82
2. Milled rice...	Lys	0.47	Thr	0.80
3. Husks	Lys	0.60		
4. Bran	Lys	0.65	Thr	0.86
5. Polish	Lys	0.57	Thr	0.82
6. Germ.......	Thr	0.86	Lys	0.87

TABLE 16

PROPOSED TYPICAL VALUES FOR TD, BV, NPU AND PER OF RICE AND RICE BY-PRODUCTS PROTEINS

Rice product	TD (%)	BV (%)	NPU (%)	PER
Brown rice......	91	70	64	1.8
Milled rice......	93	68	63	1.5-2.0
Bran	78	83	65	1.6-2.2
Polish	80	85	68	1.8-2.0
Germ..........	87	78	68	1.9

TABLE 17

REPORTED VALUES FOR NET PROTEIN RATIO (NPR) OF MILLED RICE PROTEIN

Milled rice		Casein	
Protein (%) (N × 5.95)	NPR	NPR	Reference
6.31-9.40	3.31-4.02(a)	4.63	Vaugham et al., 1980
5.68-9.73	3.07-3.71(b)	3.36	Bressani et al., 1971

(a) 6 % protein dietary level; (b) id. 5 %.

also very high (94 - 100%) (Eggum and Juliano, 1973) (Eggum, 1977). Results for BV of both brown-rice (Kik, 1952) (Houston and Kohler, 1970) (Mitra and Das, 1971) (Eggum and Juliano, 1973) (Khan and Eggum, 1978) (Eggum et al., 1982) and milled rice (Kik, 1952 and 1962) (Eggum and Juliano, 1973 and 1975) (Eggum, 1977) (Eggum et al., 1982) protein show greater variability, ranging 65 to 80% and 67 to 89%, respectively; notwithstanding, "our best estimates" 5 percentage units include the majority of reported individual data. Data for bran (Connor et al., 1976) (Varela and Escriva, 1977) (Kratzer et al., 1977) (Eggum et al., 1982) (Table 18), polish (Wakefield and Rowlands, 1973) (Kik, 1957) (Kennedy and Schelstraete, 1974) (Eggum et al., 1982) (Table 19), and germ (Kik, 1954) are very scarce.

Recently, Eggum et al., (1982) have carried out a comparative study of the protein utilization of rice milling fractions by rats, showing that: a) brown rice has lower TD, but similar BV and NPU as milled rice; and b) bran and polish have lower TD, but higher BV than brown and milled rice, but polish has higher NPU than bran and brown and milled rice (Table 20).

Our best estimate" for TD, BV, and NPU of brown rice and its milling fractions (Table 16) compares fairly well with reported data. Differences in NPU among brown rice, milled rice and bran are not great.

Surprisingly, the only available complete evaluation of TD, BV, and NPU of rice germ is that by Kik (1954). On this basis, rice germ has the highest nutritive value of all rice products.

3. SOURCES OF VARIATION OF THE NUTRITIONAL VALUE OF RICE PROTEIN

The proposed "best estimates" of typical amino acid composition (including corresponding chemical scores) and biological indexes of quality of rice protein may vary with the protein content of the grain, and can be affected by heating and other treatments of rice. Then, judicious use of typical values demand careful consideration of possible sources of variation.

The levels of lysine, threonine, methionine + cystine, and triptophan decrease in rice protein as protein content of milled rice increases (Bressani et al., 1971). The lysine content of milled rice had a 0.9 points range among varieties. Screening 10,493 varieties from the world rice collection for lysine content showed that lysine content of rice protein varied only by at most 0.5: point at any protein level (Juliano et al., 1973). Available amino acid contents of protein from different deepness layers in the ricecaryopsis also varies (Table 21) (Benedito de Barber et al., 1977).

Protein quality - as estimated by PER, NPR and NGI - of four milled rices differing in protein content (range 5.68% - 14.3%) tended to decrease as protein content increased (Table 22) (Bressani et al., 1971).

Nitrogen balance studies in rats of milled rices differing from 5.9% to 14.7% protein showed that NPU and TD decreased little and irregularly as protein content increased (Table 23) (Eggum and Juliano, 1973). Utilizable protein was higher in rices of increased protein content.

It has been shown that N fertilizer application (0 - 180 Kg/ha) increases N content of rice (up to 3 percentage units) (Table 24) but has no significant effect on the lysine content of the protein, PER and NPR

TABLE 18

REPORTED VALUES FOR TD, BV AND NPU OF RICE BRAN PROTEIN

	TD (%)	BV (%)	NPU (%)	Reference
Bran	58.5			Connors et al., 1976
Casein	100.1			"
Casein + 14 % fat	100.9			"
Bran	68.0	79.2	53.9	Varela and Escrivá, 1977
Bran	73.0			Kratzer et al., 1977
Casein	99.4			
Bran(a)	78.8	86.6	68.3	Eggum et al., 1982

(a) Egg protein completely utilized by rats.

TABLE 19

REPORTED VALUES FOR TD, BV AND NPU OF RICE POLISH PROTEIN

	TD (%)	BV (%)	NPU (%)	Reference
Polish	74.88	77.5	58.1	Wakefield and Rowland, 1973
Casein	96.59	89.88		"
Polish adjusted to a casein value of 100	77.5	86.2	66.8	"
Polish	85.5	86.3	71.2	Eggum et al., 1982

TABLE 20

COMPARISON OF TD, BV AND NPU VALUES OF PROTEINS OF DIFFERENT MILLING FRACTIONS OF RICE

Rice product	TD (%)	BV (%)	NPU (%)
Brown rice	96.9	68.9	66.7
Milled rice	98.4	67.5	66.4
Rice bran	78.8	86.6	68.3
Rice polish	82.5	86.3	71.2

Source: Eggum et al., 1982.

TABLE 21

AVAILABLE AMINO ACIDS IN LAYERS OF DIFFERENT DEEPNESS OF THE RICE CARYOPSIS

Percent layer	Available amino acid (g/16.8 g N)		
	Lysine	Tryptophan	Methionine
0-4.39	4.21	0.51	2.64
4.39-9.32	3.81	0.39	2.45
9.32-14.77	3.31	0.37	2.74
85.23 (nucleus)	2.95	0.27	2.17

TABLE 22

PROTEIN QUALITY OF FOUR MILLED RICES DIFFERING IN PROTEIN CONTENT

Protein content (N X 5.95)	PER (5 % protein diet)	NPR	NGI
5.68	2.56	3.71	3.49
7.73	2.20	3.36	3.25
9.73	1.94	3.07	3.04
14.30	1.53	2.50	2.47

Adapted from: Bressani et al., 1971.

TABLE 23

PROTEIN QUALITY OF MILLED RICES DIFFERING IN PROTEIN CONTENT

N (%)	TD (%)	BV (%)	NPU (%)	Utilizable N (%)
1.10	100	75	75	0.83
1.36	96	73	70	0.96
1.77	95	68	65	1.15
1.88	98	70	69	1.29
2.10	96	74	71	1.49
2.17	94	68	64	1.39
2.73	94	70	66	1.81

Adapted from: Eggum and Juliano, 1973.

TABLE 24

EFFECT OF FERTILIZER LEVEL ON MILLED RICE YIELD AND PROTEIN CONTENT (3 RICE VARIETIES)

Fertilizer (Kg/Ha)	Milled yield (Kg/Ha)	Protein % of milled rice
0	3,853	7.50
90	4,658	8.21
180	5,280	8.92
0	5,365	5.59
90	6,998	5.83
180	7,538	6.84
0	5,744	6.19
90	6,836	6.31
180	7,232	7.74

Adapted from: Vaugham et al., 1980.

TABLE 25

EFFECT OF HIGHER PROTEIN CONTENT FROM FERTILIZER LEVEL ON THE NUTRITIONAL QUALITY OF MILLED-RICE PROTEIN

Rice variety	A		B	
Fertilizer (Kg/Ha) . .	0	120	0	90
Protein (N X 6.25) .	8.14	9.90	9.90	13.0
TD, %	99	98	100	100
BV, %	69	69	71	68
NPU, %	69	68	71	68
Utilizable protein . .	5.61	6.71	7.03	8.81

Adapted from: Eggum and Juliano, 1975.

(Vaugham et al., 1980) and has little effect on the TD, BV and NPU of the protein (Table 25) (Eggum and Juliano, 1975).

Cooking of milled rice has no effect on amino acid composition, reduces TD (From 99.7% to 88.6 % - mean values) and increases BV (from 67.7% to 78.2% - mean values), resulting in a small increase in NPU (Table 26) (Eggum et al., 1977).

Parboiling of rough rice has no effect on amino acid composition of parboiled milled rice (Table 27) (Eggum et al., 1977) but decreases amino acid availability (Table 28) (Benedito de Barber et al., 1977). Cystine had the highest decrease in digestibility (Eggum et al., 1977). Parboiling also results in slightly lower TD and a bit higher BV, changes being compensated and leading to similar NPU in raw and parboiled rices (Table 29) (Eggum et al., 1977).

Thermal stabilization of rice bran (Barber et al., 1977) has been reported to cause no loss of nutritional value, changes in TD, BV, and NPU being non-significant (Varela and Escriva, 1977).

Baking (220º - 230ºC for 7 - 10 minutes) of a rice flour dough had no effect on either TD or BV (Khan and Eggum, 1978).

TABLE 26

EFFECT OF COOKING ON THE NUTRITIONAL VALUE OF MILLED RICE PROTEIN

	Raw	Cooked
TD	100.7	91.5
BV	66.3	76.4
NPU	66.7	69.9
Utilizable protein (w.b.)	5.40	5.84

Source: Eggum *et al.*, 1977.

TABLE 28

EFFECTS OF PARBOILING ON AVAILABLE AMINO ACIDS OF RICE

Treatment conditions	Percent layer	Available amino acid (g/16.8 g N) Lysine	Methionine
Raw	0-4	4.21	2.64
Parboiled	"	3.81	1.12
Raw	4-9	3.81	2.45
Parboiled	"	3.22	1.50
Raw	9-15	3.31	2.74
Parboiled	"	3.17	1.54
Raw	Nucleus	2.95	2.17
Parboiled	"	2.91	0.45

TABLE 27

EFFECTS OF PARBOILING ON AMINO ACID COMPOSITION OF MILLED RICE PROTEIN

Amino acid (g/16.0 g N)	Raw	Parboiled
Lys	3.42	3.60
Thr	3.76	3.73
Ile	4.09	4.55
Leu	8.64	8.46
Cys + Met	3.87	3.52

Source: Eggum *et al.*, 1977.

TABLE 29

EFFECT OF PARBOILING ON THE NUTRITIONAL QUALITY OF MILLED RICE PROTEIN

	Raw	Parboiled
TD	100.4	94.7
BV	66.8	70.4
NPU	67.1	66.7
Utilizable protein (w.b.)	7.53	6.94

Source: Eggum *et al.*, 1977.

REFERENCES

BALDI,G., FOSSATI,G. and FANTONE,G.C. 1976. Sottoprodotti della laborazione del riso. II. Frazoni proteiche e composizione amminoacidica. Il Riso, 25/4, 347.

BARBER,S. and BENEDITO DE BARBER,C. 1977. Basic and applied research needs for optimizing rice bran utilization as food and feed. In:Proc. of the Rice By-products Util. Int. Conf., 1974. Valencia, Spain. Vol. IV, pg. 1-99. S.Barber and E.Tortosa (Editors). Inst. Agric. Chem. and Food Technol., Valencia, Spain.

BARBER,S. and BENEDITO de BARBER, C. 1980. Rice bran: chemistry and technology. Chapter 24 in Rice: Production and Utilization. B.S.Luh, editor. Pub. by Avi Pub. Co., Inc, Westport, Conn., USA.

BARBER,S., CAMACHO,J.M., CERNI,R., TORTOSA,E. and PRIMO, E. 1977. Process for the stabilization of rice bran. I. Basic research studies. In: Proc. of the Rice By-products Util. Int. Conf., 1974, Valencia, Spain. Vol. II, pg. 49-62. S.Barber and E.Tortosa (Editors). Inst. Agric. Chem. and Food Technol., Valencia, Spain.

BARBER,S., BENEDITO de BARBER,C. and TORTOSA,E. 1981. Theory and practice of rice by-products utilization. In: Cereals, a renewable resource. Pg.471-488. Y.Pomeranz and L.Munck, editors. Pub. by The American Association of Cereal Chemists. St.Paul, Minn., USA.

BENDER,A.E. and DOELL,B.H. 1957. Brit. J. Nutr., 11, 140.Cited by Mitra and Das, 1971.

BENEDITO de BARBER,C., MARTINEZ,J. and BARBER,S. 1977. Effects of parboiling processes on the chemical composition and nutritional characteristics an rice bran. In: Proc. of the Rice By-products Util. Int. Conf., 1974, Valencia, Spain. Vol. IV, pg. 121-130, S.Barber and E.Tortosa, editors. Inst. Agric. Chem. and Food Technol., Valencia,Spain.

BRADBURY,J.H., COLLINS,J.G., and PYLIOTIS, N,A. 1980a. Methods of separation of the major histological components of rice and characterization of their proteins by amino acid analysis. Cereal Chem., 57/2, 133-137.

BRADBURY,J.H., COLLINS,J.G., and PYLIOTIS,N.A. 1980b. Amino acid analyses of the proteins on the major histological components of a high-protein rice. Cereal Chem., 57/5, 343-346.

BRESSANI,R. and VALIENTE,T. 1962. All-vegetable protein mixtures for human feeding. VII. Protein complementation between polished rice and cooked black beans. J. Food Sci., 21: 401-406.

BRESSANI,R., ELIAS,L.G. and JULIANO,B.O. 1971. Evaluation of the protein quality and milled rices differing in protein content. J. Agr. Food Chem., 19/5, 1028-1034.

CAGAMPANG,G.B., PERDON,A.A. and JULIANO,B.O. 1976. Changes in salt-soluble proteins of rice during grain development. Phytochem. 15, 1425-1430. Cited by Juliano, 1980.

CHAVAN,J.K. and DUGGAL,S.K. 1978. Studies on the essential amino acid composition, protein fractions and biological value (BV) of some new varieties of rice. J. Sci. Food Agric. 29, 225-229.

CONNOR,M.A., SAUNDERS,R.M., and KOHLER,G.O. 1976. Rice bran protein concentrates obtained by wet alkaline extraction. Cereal Chem., 53/4, 488-496.

EGGUM,B.O. 1977. Nutritional aspects of cereal proteins. In:Genetic diversity in plants. Ed. by A.Muhammed, R. Aksel and R.C.Borstel. Pub by Plemm Pub. Corp.

EGGUM,B.O. and JULIANO,B.O. 1973. Nitrogen balance in rats fed rices differing in protein content. J. Sci. Fd. Agric., 24, 921-927.

EGGUM,B.O. and JULIANO,B.O. 1975. Higher protein content from nitrogen fertilizer application and nutritive value of milled rice protein. J. Sci. Fd. Agric., 26, 425-427

EGGUM, B.O., RESURRECCION,A.P. and JULIANO,B.O. 1977. Effect of cooking on nutritional value of milled rice in rats. Nutrition Reports International, 16/5, 649-655.

EGGUM,B.O., JULIANO,B.O. and MANIÑGAT,C.C. 1982. Protein and energy utilization of rice milling fractions by rats. Qualitas Plantarum,32

HEGSTED,D.M. 1968. Nutritional value of cereal proteins. Cereal Sci.Today 13/3: Abst. No. 185. Cited by Houston and Kohler, 1970.

HOUSTON,D.F. and KOHLER,G.O. 1970. Nutritional properties of rices. Pub. by National Academy of Sciences, Washington, D.C.

HOUSTON,D.F., ALLIS,M.E., and KOHLER,G.O. 1969. Amino acid composition of rice and rice by-products. Cereal Chem., 46/5, 527-537.

JULIANO,B.O., 1972. Studies on protein quality and quantity of rice. In Symposium: Seed proteins. G.E. Inglett, editor. Pub. by Avi Pub.Co., Inc., Wesport, Conn., USA.

JULIANO,B.O. 1980. Properties of the rice caryopsis. Chapter 10, in: Rice, Production and Utilization. B.S.Luh, editor. pub. by Avi Pub. Co.,Inc., Westport, Conn., USA.

JULIANO,B.O., ANTONIO,A.A., and ESMANA,B.V. 1973. Effects of protein content on the distribution and properties of rice protein. J.Sci.Fd. Agric., 24, 295-306.

KENNEDY,B.M. and SCHELSTRAETE,M. 1974. Chemical, physical, and nutritional properties of high-protein flours and residual kernel from the overmilling of uncoated milled rice. II. Amino acid composition and biological evaluation of the protein.Cereal Chem.,51/4, 448-457.

KESTER,E.B., LUKENS,H.C., FERREL,R.E., MOHAMMAD,A., and FINROCK,D.C. 1963. Influence of maturity on properties of western rices. Cereal Chem., 40, 323.

KHAN,M.A., and EGGUM,B.O. 1978. Effect of baking on the nutritive value of Pakistani bread. J. Sci. Fd. Agric., 29, 1069-1075.

KIK,M.C. 1952. The nutritive value of rice and rice byproducts. Ark. Agr. Exp. Station Bulletin No. 589, Fayetteville. Cited by Houston and Kohler, 1970.

KIK,M.C. 1954. Nutritive value of rice germ. J. Agr. Food Chem., 2(23), 1179-1181.

KIK,M.C. 1957. The nutritive value of rice and its by-products, B. Ark. Agr. Expt. Sta. 589, 24p.

KIK,M.C. 1962. J. Agr. Food Chem., 10: 59. Cited by Houeston and Kohler, 1970.

KRATZER,F.H., BETSCHART;A.A., and SAUNDERS,R.M., 1977. Evaluation of heat treated rice bran. J. Sci. Food Agric.

MITRA,G.N. and DAS,N.B. 1971. Protein quality of the high yielding varieties of rice. J. Agr. Food Chem., 19/5, 927-929.

MIYAZAKI,M. and HORII,M. 1975. Nutritional availability of rice proteins. Xth Int. Congress of Nutrition, Kyoto, Japan.

PALMIANO,E.P., ALMAZAN,A.M., and JULIANO,B.O. 1968. Physicochemical properties of protein of development and mature rice grain. Cereal Chem., 45, 1.

PELLETT,P.L. and YOUNG,V.R. 1980. Evaluación nutricional de alimentos proteínicos. Pub. by Universidad de las Naciones Unidas.

TAMURA,S., and KENMOCHI,K. 1963. Nippon Nogeikagaku Kaishi, 37: 753. Cited by Houston and Kohler, 1970.

VARELA,G., and ESCRIVA,J. 1977. Process for the stabilization of rice bran. IV. Nutritional quality of the protein of raw and stabilized bran. In: Proc. of the Rice Byproducts Util.Int. Conf., 1974, Valencia, Spain. Vol. IV, pg. 131-138. S. Barber and E.Tortosa, editors, Ins. Agric. Chem. and Food Technol., Valencia, Spain.

VAUGHAM,D.A., WOMACK,M., SMITH,R.T., and WISER,W.J. 1980. Protein quality of rice as affected by application of nitrogen fertilizer. J. Agric. Food Chem. 28, 894-896.

WAKEFIELD,L.M., and ROWLANDS,R. 1973. Protein quality of rice polish and combinations with peanut flour, fish protein concentrate, and lysine. Cereal chem., 50/2, 428-434.

Proc. Int. Assoc. Cereal Chem. Symp. Amino Acid Compn and Biol. Value of Cereal Proteins Budapest, Hungary 1983, R. Lásztity, M. Hidvégi, eds

THE INFLUENCE OF HOME PROCESSING ON THE QUALITY OF CEREAL AND MILLET PROTEINS

P. GEERVANI

Department of Foods and Nutrition, College of Home Science, Andhra Pradesh Agricultural University, Hyderabad 500004, India

Cereals and millets constitute the bulk of the diet for the majority of world population. Rice, wheat, sorghum, bajra (Pearl millet), maize and ragi (Finger millet) are the common grains consumed by a large section. They are chief sources of protein and energy. Processing of food is of great importance, as it improves palatability, digestibility and, to some extent, nutritional quality. The word processing means in a general sense the treatment to which food is subjected to before consumption. The conditions of processing are important in understanding the changes that take place in nutritional quality. The medium of heat transfer and the amount of heat applied may differ in each process. There are some processes where no heat is applied, like germination and fermentation. Among the nutrients that are likely to be influenced by processing are vitamins and proteins.

The changes in the protein nutritional quality of cereals and millets are especially important for populations deriving most of the proteins from these grains. Generally other protein foods are recommended on the basis of the quantity and quality of cereal/millet protein, in order to enhance the overall quality of the diet. By and large, the cost of protein derived from cereals/millets is less than other plant proteins. Improvement in the income among the low-income population has shown, the world over, immediate increase in the cereal/millet consumption. In view of the bulk consumption of processed cereals and millets it is of great relevance to study the influence of processing on protein quality.

PROCESSING METHODS AND CONSEQUENT CHANGES

Methods of processing

The general methods of processing cereals and millets can be broadly divided into five categories: application of moist heat, e.g. boiling, steaming; application of dry heat, e.g. baking, roasting; application of heat through fats and oils; fermentation and germination. Certain recipes require more than one method of processing.

The temperature of moist heat processing ranges from simmering temperature of 60°C to pressure cooking temperatures of 120°C, although many recipes suggest cooking at boiling temperature. The termperature for dry heat processes ranges from 100°C to 275°C. It can be done in open pans or closed containers (ovens). The frying temperature ranges from 120°C for shallow frying, to 180-200°C for deep frying. For fermented products, the period of fermentation extends from 4 hours to 24 hours, depending on room temperature and the final product. The period of germination varies from 12 to 36 hours, depending on the grains and viability and the ultimate use. Both fermented and germinated products are processed subsequently by some other method before consumption.

Changes in processing

Changes in the overall nutrient composition and quality take place when any food is subjected to processing. Processing causes a chain of interactions between several components of food. The changes in protein chiefly depend upon reactions with carbohydrates, lipid oxidation products, and are due to inter- and intra-reactions within the protein molecule in the presence or absence of oxygen. The extent of damage is a function of time, temperature, moisture content of the product, presence of reducing substances and pH. The interaction of all these factors is, in essence, the alteration that will affect the protein.

The important factors influencing changes in cereal proteins on processing are, presence of reducing sugar, temperature of processing and level of moisture. The Maillard reaction that causes browning in cereal foods at high temperature is a classical example of the reaction between carbohydrates and amino acids. The reaction is more severe at high temperature. The reaction between the reducing sugar and the epsilon amino group of lysine has been shown to cause considerable reduction in protein quality of cereal preparations into which sugar has been added. It has been demonstrated by Carpenter et al. (1962) that greater loss of available lysine takes place at a moisture range of 5-14%. The damage to protein quality is greater at high temperature and low moisture level, and if it is coupled with longer exposure to heat, the reduction in quality will be drastic.

Methods of assessment of protein quality

Amino acid composition

The amino acid compositions of whole grains and milled grains have been thoroughly investigated. Cereal and millet proteins are all deficient in lysine. Rice protein is deficient in threonine, wheat protein in valine, corn protein in tryptophan, threonine and methionine. Sorghum protein has an imbalance of leucine and isoleucine. The absence of any essential amino acid in right amounts causes an imbalance and produces negative nitrogen balance.

Availability of amino acids

The rate and the amount of the amino acids that are liberated from a source of protein is important because the utilization of protein depends upon availability of amino acids. In the process of acid hydrolysis, used for estimating amino acids, enzyme-resistant bonds are also broken. Therefore, the estimation of amino acids by such procedures does not give a true picture of available amino acids. Variation in availability can be due to linkage and incomplete digestion, particularly in the case of coarse grains. For optimum utilization complete digestion and absorption of the proteins are necessary.Processing can alter the linkages in the protein and thus improve availability, or lead to the formation of linkages which are resistant to digestion and reduce availability.

Biological methods

The ability of a protein to promote growth and maintenance has been discussed extensively by Pellet and Young (1980). Protein efficiency ratio (PER), true digestibility (TD), biological value (BV) and net protein utilization (NPU) are the usual parameters used for assessment of biological quality. The quality of vegetable protein is assessed in comparison with a reference protein that is either milk or egg protein.

INFLUENCE OF PROCESSING ON THE QUALITY OF CEREAL AND MILLET PROTEINS

Moist heat processing

The proteins in cereals range from 6 to 13 per cent and the first limiting amino acid in all cereals is lysine, the second being threonine. Any process that results in the loss of these two amino acids is likely to influence the protein quality. Since lysine is highly heat sensitive, most workers have tried to estimate the loss of available lysine to determine the protein quality.

Boiling, steaming at atmospheric pressure or under pressure are three principal moist heat processes followed in cereal cooking. Nutrient loss in boiling of rice may vary, depending upon the way how rice is cooked. While some use just sufficient water to cook, some cook in excess water and throw away the left-over water. The leaching losses can be higher if the water used for cooking is more.

The loss of both lysine and threonine is negligible in cooking rice (Tara & Bains, 1971). They reported 3.4% lysine and 6.2% threonine lost from milled and parboiled rice, respectively. Losses in cooking of parboiled rice, which took almost the double time for cooking than milled rice, was not different, indicating that the time of cooking is not such an important factor. Tabekhia et al. (1981) reported no loss of protein from three California rice varieties on cooking, as the per cent of protein in the uncooked rice was 6.48, 6.85 and 6.83 and the corresponding values for cooked product was 6.30, 6.75 and 6.45.

Slight differences are observed in the loss of protein from short (6.79 to 7.36%) and long grain (7.79 to 8.95%) varieties, after 30 minutes of cooking. Reduction in amino acid content of cooked rice is attributed to reduced extraction efficiency after cooking, and not to cooking (Said et al. 1980).

The per cent loss of lysine, threonine, methionine and tryptophan has been found to be considerable in cereal and millet recipes consumed in Andhra Pradesh (india) (Pushpamma et al., 1982). The loss of amino acids reported are presented in Table 1.

Table 1. Per cent loss of limiting amino acids on boiling

Process	Number of recipes	Lysine	Threonine	Methionine	Tryptophan
Boiling	14	16.9	12.4	14.4	26.2

The influence of boiling on the amino acid composition and biological quality of wheat and millets after grinding with water at 1:3 ratio and boiling for 30 minutes is presented in Tables 2 and 3 (Eggum, 1973). Lysine, methionine and tryptophan decreased considerably on boiling. A significant reduction in BV of barley and rye is noticed. Boiling increased Td, but was significant only in oats.

Information on the biological quality of rice is limited. One of the recent studies of Eggum (1977) revealed a reduction in TD of protein from 99.7 to 88.6% in three varieties of rice, namely IR-29, IR-32 and IR-480-5, and a corresponding increase in BV from 67.7 to 78.2

Table 2. The influence of boiling on protein quality in barley, oats and wheat

Sample	Barley		Oats		Wheat	
Boiled (min)	0	30	0	30	0	30
Urease activity (meq/g)	0.04	0.03	0.04	0.04	0.06	0.04
	(g/16gN)	(g/16gN)	(g/16gN)	(g/16gN)	(g/16gN)	(g/16gN)
Lysine	3.36	3.25	4.25	3.97	2.98	2.88
Methionine	1.88	1.45	2.00	1.75	1.88	1.70
Cystine	2.10	1.90	2.59	2.29	2.49	2.10
Aspartic acid	6.18	5.56	8.12	8.01	5.24	5.19
Threonine	3.16	3.17	3.41	3.38	2.99	2.88
Serine	4.16	4.01	4.52	4.45	4.57	4.22
Glutamic acid	25.19	26.69	21.54	21.24	32.36	29.73
Proline	10.86	10.92	4.96	4.72	9.55	8.60
Glycine	4.02	3.65	4.80	4.71	4.02	3.85
Alanine	4.11	3.74	4.61	4.49	3.79	3.61
Valine	4.91	4.97	5.39	5.00	4.69	4.39
Isoleucine	3.56	3.54	3.82	3.68	3.63	3.54
Leucine	7.01	6.85	7.34	7.21	7.08	6.76
Tyrosine	3.21	3.33	3.35	3.63	3.04	2.56
Phenylalanine	5.00	5.14	5.24	4.98	4.56	4.47
Histidine	2.06	1.99	2.32	2.16	2.32	2.21
Arginine	5.08	4.66	6.49	6.47	4.86	4.75
Tryptophan	1.28	1.05	1.21	1.17	1.36	0.98
Protein value expressed in percentage:						
TD	84.6	84.8	89.9	94.4	90.7	93.2
BV	77.5	72.4	77.5	79.1	68.2	66.5
NPU	65.3	61.4	69.7	74.4	61.8	63.7

The nutritive value with regard to the total protein, lysine, threonine, methionine and tryptophan contents of some of the common Indian recipes made with cereals and millets

Table 3. The influence of boiling on protein quality in rye, maize and sorghum

Sample	Rye		Maize		Sorghum	
Boiled (min)	0	30	0	30	0	30
Urease activity (meq/g)	0.06	0.04	0.07	0.04	0.09	0.05
	(g/16gN)	(g/16gN)	(g/16gN)	(g/16gN)	(g/16gN)	(g/16gN)
Lysine	3.96	4.00	2.96	2.69	1.81	1.73
Methionine	1.79	1.70	2.26	2.17	1.73	1.68
Cystine	2.00	1.97	2.05	1.76	1.28	1.21
Aspartic acid	7.61	7.52	6.39	6.38	7.68	7.93
Threonine	3.42	3.36	3.64	3.63	3.48	3.49
Serine	4.11	4.18	4.72	4.78	4.73	4.81
Glutamic acid	23.58	23.65	20.67	21.98	22.00	22.06
Proline	8.51	8.16	8.99	9.19	8.21	8.41
Glycine	4.40	4.30	3.72	3.74	3.11	3.18
Alanine	4.34	4.35	7.27	7.29	9.56	9.48
Valine	4.67	4.77	4.89	4.82	5.38	5.46
Isoleucine	3.53	3.43	3.56	3.39	4.36	4.29
Leucine	6.34	6.37	12.61	12.75	11.83	11.64
Tyrosine	2.73	2.91	4.42	4.28	4.03	4.16
Phenylalanine	4.33	4.46	5.01	4.89	5.31	5.19
Histidine	3.03	2.27	2.97	2.88	2.05	2.10
Arginine	5.26	5.35	4.54	4.66	3.47	3.39
Tryptophan	1.51	1.14	0.87	0.71	0.94	0.87
Protein value expressed in percentage:						
TD	79.4	78.3	95.7	93.8	87.3	88.1
BV	74.3	78.7	62.4	61.4	48.4	48.1
NPU	58.9	61.6	59.7	57.6	42.5	42.4

by boiling process revealed 10-20% reduction in all the four amino acids (Pushpamma and Geervani, 1982).

From the data available it is seen that 10 to 25% loss of limiting amino acids occurs in boiling of cereals and millets. These are the amino acids which are likely to be inadequately consumed by the population in developing countries. Of these amino acids, the loss of tryptophan and lysine seems to be higher. The data on the changes in digestibility and biological value of boiled grains is not considerable, which implies that changes which take place in the biological quality of protein subjected to heat in the presence of high moisture are not appreciable.

Dry heat processing

Two popular dry heat methods are baking and roasting. Of the two baking methods, open baking is more popular in home processing, whereas baking in a closed oven is also done at home level occasionally. Cereal and millet preparations made simply by roasting are rare and it is only an intermediary step or finishing step in cooking. Other dry heat methods such as parching, puffing and flaking are commercial processes with the exception of puffed maize, which is done at home since the introduction of puffing pans into the market.

Owing to the low gluten content of rice flour, it is not used for baked products. Wheat and sometimes millet flours are used for baked products. Baked products are of three categories. Biscuits leavened by baking powders, breads leavened by yeast and unleavened bread popularly known as Roti and Chapati in India.

Biscuits represent a large group of baked products. As early as 1946, Block et al. had reported that baking reduced the quality of protein, but comparatively less than roasting. Storage of dough had no effect on the concentration of lysine in biscuits (Clark et al. 1959). However, loss of available lysine was observed to be higher, with increased thickness of biscuits (NIN, 1970). Geetha and Pushpamma (1970) found a considerable loss of total and available lysine due to baking of wheat biscuits, and particularly so in the presence of sugar and jaggery (Table 4). A similar observation of higher loss of

Table 4. Per cent loss of total and available lysine in salt and sweet biscuits

Products	Baking temperature	Time in minutes	Lysine	Available lysine	Tryptophan
Salt biscuits	220°C	15	1.18	33.5	-
Sugar biscuits	220°C	15	17.4	21.2	-
Jaggery biscuits	220°C	15	24.7	21.2	-
Salt biscuits	150°C	20	-	14.6	15.0
Sweet biscuits	150°C	20	-	17.1	20.0

available lysine and tryptophan was reported by Yasoda Devi and Geervani (1973) in wheat biscuits (Table 4).

Clark (1959) examined the effect of baking time and conditions, on the available lysine content in biscuits. He found the per cent loss to be 9.3 in 20 minutes, 18.1 in 25 minutes and 27 in 30 minutes of baking. Neither the type nor the proportion of baking powder used seem to alter the quantity of lysine in biscuits. Addition of sugar up to 14.5% of the weight of the flour was not found to reduce the available lysine content, but higher amounts caused a sharp decline.

The loss of lysine in biscuits made of wheat flour (70% extraction) and wheat flour partly substituted by maize or sorghum (10 to 20%), baked at 230°C for 15 minutes and at 350°C for 5 minutes, showed 7% increase in the loss of total lysine and 3% loss of available lysine (Table 5). This could be due to increase in temperature (Usha and Khader, 1983). High temperature had more damaging effect on lysine than time, and the losses increased further, due to the incorporation of sugar in the biscuits.

Breads constitute a second large group of baked products. It is customary to use wheat flour (70% extraction) for breads. Bread is largely a commercial product, although in some homes it is prepared occasionally. Studies carried out almost 3 decades back by Rosenberg and Rohdenberg (1951) revealed a loss of 15% lysine during baking of bread fortified with DL-lysine,

Table 5. Influence of baking temperature on the per cent range and loss of lysine and available lysine

	Total lysine (g/16gN)	Loss, %	Available lysine	Loss, %
Dough	2.078-2.146	-	1.27-1.99	-
Baked at 230°C for 15 minutes	1.721-1.773	16.5-17.3	1.02	15.3-17.3
Baked at 350°C for 5 minutes	1.616-1.696	24.0-25.2	0.6-0.98	18.11-20.5

and in commercial baking the loss was 11%. The same team in another study in 1952, reported that the availability of lysine was the same both in fortified and unfortified bread and that no detectable change was observed by biological methods of evaluation. Baking of bread or allowing it to become stale and dry reduced the lysine content further by 5 to 10%. Ericson et al. (1961) observed 10-15% loss of lysine and threonine as estimated by the rat growth method and 5-10% when estimated microbiologically, due to baking of wheat bread.

Jansen et al. (1974) had observed higher losses of lysine with increasing the baking time from 0, to 10, 20, 30, 40 and 50 minutes, as assessed by the rat growth method.

The findings of Yasoda Devi and Geervani (1973) on the protein quality of plain and milk bread showed considerable loss of lysine and tryptophan (Table 6) and losses were significantly ($P<0.01$) higher in milk bread.

Table 6. Per cent loss of available lysine and tryptophan in plain and milk bread

Product	Baking		Protein Nx6.26	Moisture, %	Available lysine	Trypto-phan
	Tempe-rature	Time				
Plain bread	250°C	40	12.25	30	9.8	12.0
Milk bread	250°C	40	16.04	30	20.9	16.0

Unleavened breads are popular among all income groups in India. Chapati is a common form of unleavened product made with wheat flour (90% extraction) and Roti is the common form of unleavened product made out of millet flour. One of the early studies on Chapati carried out by Mathews et al. (1969) had shown that the destruction of lysine was comparatively less (25%) in Chapati than in bread.

Studies carried out by Chawla and Kapoor (1982) on wheat triticale Chapatis revealed that in 4 varieties of triticale lysine ranged from 2.94 to 3.46 g, and in wheat it was 250 g. The available lysine ranged from 2.44 to 2.84 in 4 varieties of triticale and 2.07 g in wheat. Chemical scores were 53-64 and 45. Losses of other amino acids in Chapatis were negligible. In biological studies the PER of wheat Chapati was found to be 1.6 as against 1.63-1.95 for Chapatis made out of mixed flour (30-50% triticale flour). The PER was found to increase with increasing amount of triticale flour.

The loss of available lysine and tryptophan in Pulka similar to Chapati, except that it is slightly thinner) was 10% and 9%, respectively (Yasoda Devi and Geervani, 1973). The PER of Iranian flat breads (which are closer to Indian Chapatis) increased with flour extraction rate as shown below. They found that baking decreased PER (Faridi et al. 1982).

Flat breads	PER	Flour extraction rates, %
Barbari	1.13	78
Lavash	1.14	82
Tafoon	1.29	84
Sangak	1.29	87
Village	1.39	97

Frying

Fried preparations of cereals and millets are consumed only occasionally. This is perhaps the reason for limited studies on the nutritional evaluation of fried products. In

Table 7. Per cent loss of available lysine and tryptophan in Poori

	PER	Available lysine	Tryptophan
Plain Poori	0.64	34.6	-
Sugar Poori	0.70	22.7	-
Jaggery Poori	0.46	47.7	-
Plain Poori	-	35.2	22.0

India Poori is one of the common deep fried foods made with wheat flour. Data of Geetha and Pushpamma (1970) and Yasoda Devi and Geervani (1973) on the protein quality of different types of Poori is shown in Table 7.

The per cent loss of lysine, threonine, methionine and tryptophan in some of the deep and shallow fried millet recipes commonly consumed in Andhra Pradesh (India) observed by Pushpamma et al. (1982) is shown in Table 8.

Table 8. Per cent loss of limiting amino acids due to deep frying and shallow frying

Process	Number of recipes	Lysine	Threonine	Methionine	Tryptophan
Deep frying (180-200°C)	9	26.5	19.5	31.1	32.1
Shallow frying (100°C)	3	1.22	8.1	19.5	24.7

The temperature of frying seems to have a more destructive effect on amino acids, like in the baking process. Deep frying, which is done at much higher temperature than boiling, has resulted in greater loss of amino acids in spite of a short cooking time. Hence temperature seems to be a critical factor, followed by the level of moisture. The presence of sugars and fats has an adverse effect on the quality of cereal and millet protein.

Fermentation

Fermentation of foods is useful in preservation and in improvement of flavour and enhancement of the nutritive value of food. Chemical changes that take place in fermentation include increase in amino nitrogen, partial breakdown of protein to peptides and amino acids. When microbes act on amino acids, deamination takes place. Sulphur-containing amino acids decompose in the process. The extent of breakdown depends on the pH, presence of moisture and growth of microorganisms. Once fermentation sets in, it continues to produce a series of changes. As a consequence of the breakdown of proteins, the products are readily absorbed and utilized. Trypsin inhibitors are also destroyed in the process and digestibility increases. Hence there is scope for better digestion and efficient absorption of protein due to fermentation. The stage at which fermentation is checked will determine the quality of the protein and the palatability of the product.

Fermentation is a traditional method of processing cereals, millets and legumes, particularly in tropical countries. Only a few fermented foods are exclusively prepared with cereals and millets, but many are prepared in combination with a legume. The agents used for fermentation are microorganisms, that are naturally trapped into the food, and yeast. Curds and sugar are added into the batter to promote fermentation.

Studies on fermented foods largely concentrated on changes in B-vitamins rather than proteins. Because of the cereal and pulse combination in some fermented foods, attention was paid to evaluate the quality of protein. Idli is one of the common breakfast foods prepared by steaming, fermented batter of rice and black gram dhal (P. Mungo). Observations of Desikachar et al. (1960) on the quality of protein in Idli showed an increase in non-protein nitrogen (NPN) with the increase in fermentation time. The TD of Idli increased by 4%, but BV was reduced from

79 to 69 on fermentation (Khandwala et al. 1962). Changes in TD and BV were significant. Similarly, in the growth studies conducted by Ananthachar and Desikachar (1962) no improvement was noticed in PER due to fermentation.

Contrary to these earlier findings, Rajalaxmi and Vanaja (1967) reported beneficial effects in the protein quality of Idli. They fermented the Idli batter with L. mesenteroides, and found an increase in the PER from 1.5 to 2.0. In the same year another group of workers (Van Veen et al. 1967) reported that PER and DC were not affected by fermentation. The proportion of cereal to legume used by them was 1:1 and the period of fermentation was 24 hours. The range of PER was 1.7 to 1.99 for unfermented raw, unfermented steamed and fermented steamed batter. The overall DC was also very close, ranging from 88.7 to 92.7. The same team in a subsequent study (Van Veen, 1972) observed that in fermented rice (Sierra rice) there was no improvement in the PER, and the apparent digestibility decreased from 86.8 to 72.6.

Contradicting reports on fermentation can be partly due to the different proportions of cereal to legume and the differences in the conditions of fermentation, and partly to the specific organism. Fermented food similar to Idli when made with rice and Bengal gram dhal (Cicer arietinum) is known as Khaman and it is a popular recipe in the central and western parts of India. The only difference between Idli and Khaman is that curds or yeast are added to the batter to promote fermentation. Observation of Khader (1982) on Khaman, showed no significant difference in PER and digestibility due to fermentation. But yeast-fermented batters had significantly higher PER (2.63-2.72) compared to batters fermented by curds only (2.25-2.41).

Among the millets, most fermented products of sorghum are more extensively investigated. A significant ($P<0.001$) increase in available lysine, leucine, isoleucine and methionine was observed due to lactic fermentation of sorghum products (Kazanas and Fields, 1981). It is generally believed that sorghum proteins are less digestible than rice, maize and wheat protein. Axtell et al. (1981) found Kisra and Abrey, two fermented products of sorghum, to be more digestible (65 to 86%) compared to unfermented (44-56%) products. The RNV of fermented sorghum (55.1 to 56.2) is found to be higher than the unfermented (45.6) (Au and Fields, 1981). Kazanas and Fields (1981) indicated an increase in the availability of amino acids and protein as a result of fermentation as shown below.

	Unfermented mg/gN	Fermented mg/gN
Lysine	40	23
Leucine	59	28
Isoleucine	82	39
Methionine	33	16
RNV	84	70
Protein availability	83	14

Hamad and Fields (1979) observed natural lactic acid fermentation over a period of 6 days to increase the RNV (3 to 22%) of wheat, barley and rice. However, the total protein content was reduced by 1 to 2% due to fermentation. Even the available lysine had increased significantly in fermented oats, rice, millet, maize and wheat. The increase in available lysine varied between grains as seen from the following data.

	Available lysine mg/gN
Wheat control	23.3
Fermented at 22-25°C	64.2
Fermented at 37°C	79.8
Barley control	19.0
Fermented at 22-25°C	75.6
Fermented at 37°C	96.3
Oats control	15.0
Fermented at 22-25°C	104.6
Fermented at 37°C	113.0
Rice control	5.0
Fermented at 22-25°C	46.0
Fermented at 37°C	61.0

	Available lysine mg/gN
Millet control	3.0
Fermented at 22-25°C	36.0
Fermented at 37°C	45.0
Maize control	17.4
Fermented at 22-25°C	47.4
Fermented at 37°C	51.8

Although fermentation increased the available lysine considerably, whether the product is palatable after six days of fermentation is of practical importance. Normally fermentation for longer than 24 hours leaves the product sour and less platable as food.

A comparative assessment of fermented millet products (Ambali) of sorghum, Bajra (Pearl millet) and Ragi (Finger millet) revealed that TD of only sorghum increased significantly, but not of Bajra and Ragi. But BV and NPU of sorghum and Ragi increased on fermentation. No change was noticed in the PER due to fermentation (Aliya, and Geervani, 1981). The data on changes in protein quality due to fermentation are presented in Table 9.

Table 9. PER, TD, BV and NPU of unfermented and fermented millet products

Product	PER	TD	BV	NPU
Bajra Ambali				
Unfermented	1.43	84.4	72.6	61.4
Fermented	1.54	87.4	76.0	66.2
Sorghum Ambali				
Unfermented	1.50	82.0	64.6	53.4
Fermented	1.56	85.6	72.5	62.3
Ragi Ambali				
Unfermented	1.48	84.3	68.0	57.5
Fermented	1.79	86.9	76.7	66.6

In spite of the improvement observed in BV of sorghum and Ragi, the PER did not improve significantly. These findings are similar to that of Ananthachar and Desikachar (1962), Ven Veen et al. (1967) and Khandwala et al. (1962). Fermentation on the whole seems to improve digestibility and not the growth promoting quality of coarse grains.

In Sudan, sorghum products, particularly fermented products are popular. Eggum et al. (1983) investigated the protein quality of a number of sorghum products. In Kisra, a fermented product of sorghum, only small changes were noticed. Cooked, fermented and cooked, unfermented, acid-adjusted Aceda (gruel) had lower digestibility of protein but higher BV than uncooked, fermented Aceda. Marissa, a beer made with sorghum had a higher BV after sieving than before, but in this product the protein digestibility was adversely affected by the beer preparation. Data on several parameters used for assessment of protein quality are given in Table 10.

Table 10. Protein quality of several varieties of sorghum products

	Ugali (Porridge)	Kisra (fermented cooked) pan cake	Aceda (fermented cooked	Aceda (fermented uncooked)	Aceda (unfermented cooked)
Lysine	1.9-2.1	2.3	1.7	1.6	1.5
Threonine	3.0	3-3.2	3.0	3.0	3.0
Methionine + cystine	3.4-3.5	3.5-3.7	3.5	3.5	3.4
Proline	7.8-7.9	8.1-8.9	8.5	8.3	8.7
Glutamic acid	21.3-22.4	22.2-25.3	23.3	23.0	24.2
TD	82.4-94.4	92.8-96.9	95.9	99.5	95.4
BV	54.4-60.8	50.8-55.3	52.2	46.1	52.7
NPU	51.4-53.2	47.3-53.4	50.1	45.9	50.3
Utilisable protein	6 - 6.8	3.8-6.7	6.6	6.1	6.7

The low lysine content of sorghum is perhaps responsible for the low biological value. In spite of digestibility having been improved by fermentation, growth promotion was not improved because of the limiting amino acids.

The relative nutritive value of fermented corn meal is closer to casein thus suggesting that there is a feasibility to improve the protein quality of corn by fermentation (Wang and Fields, 1978).

Unlike in the wet and dry heat processes, no loss of lysine and threonine is seen due to fermentation. Fermentation has a positive influence on digestibility but not an BV and PER. Perhaps this is so because unless the deficiency in lysine and threonine is made up, significant alteration in the BV and PER might not take place. The increase in the amino acids that takes place during fermentation is perhaps insufficient to make up for the gap.

Germination

The process of germination alone and germination followed by roasting have been traditional methods of processing, practised in the tropics for millets. Germinated grain is consumed as it is, and sometimes after roasting and powdering. These are termed malts. Malted foods are specially liked for their flavour; they are used in beverages and also as weaning foods.

The effect of germination on the protein quality of wheat, barley, oats and rice showed significant increase in available lysine and RNV in all grains but oats. The PER of germinated grains also increased in case of barley and wheat (Hamad and Field, 1979). A more extensive study on germination was carried out by Tsai and Dalley (1975) on several grains, and changes in tryptophan, lysine and prolamine were assessed five days after germination (Table 11).

In general, for all cereal proteins there is an increase in the lysine and tryptophan and a decrease in prolamine during germination. The increase in lysine and tryptophan appears to be inversely correlated with the decrease in prolamine and its

Table 11. Changes in tryptophan, lysine and prolamine due to germination of cereals and millets (% dry weight)

Cereal	Amino acids	Before germination	After 5 days of germination
Wheat	Tryptophan	0.18	0.25
	Lysine	0.60	0.88
	Prolamine	3.5	0.5
Triticale	Tryptophan	0.16	0.22
	Lysine	0.66	0.90
	Prolamine	3.0	1.9
Barley	Tryptophan	0.12	0.16
	Lysine	0.62	0.78
	Prolamine	3.8	0.4
Oats	Tryptophan	0.15	0.18
	Lysine	0.62	0.81
	Prolamine	2.1	1.0
Rye	Tryptophan	0.11	0.16
	Lysine	0.48	0.74
	Prolamine	2.2	0.80
Rice	Tryptophan	0.07	0.1
	Lysine	0.28	0.3
	Prolamine	0.0	0.0
Maize	Tryptophan	0.08	0.14
	Lysine	0.38	0.71
	Prolamine	7.0	1.1

rate of mobility. In case of rice and oats, which have the lowest prolamine content, the reduction is also less and the increase in lysine is also less. Contrary to this, in wheat, which showed sharp increase in lysine and tryptophan, reduction in prolamine is also drastic. The protein expressed on dry matter basis also increased on germination. Therefore, germinated grain, on a unit basis, will contain a greater number of grain and therefore more nitrogen compared to ungerminated grains. The increased total protein cannot be accounted for by the increase in lysine and tryptophan levels (Tsai and Dalley, 1975).

The total protein tends to decrease as the period of germination increases in Ragi and sorghum, but correspondingly there is an increase in free amino nitrogen. This is a consequence of changes in the reserve protein of the grain. Another important change is the increase in tryptophan and available lysine. In cereal-based diets these are the amino acids that are limiting. Hence it is advantageous to convert poor quality protein to better quality by germination process (Chandra and Reddy, 1977). The lysine content increased due to germination from 2.2-3.2 g to 3.0-7.8 g/16gN and this increase is due to increase in albumin, which is also an important change in germination (Wu & Wall, 1980). Similar improvement is seen in triticale also, due to germination, in the lysine content but the amount of protein/kernel decreased (Wu, 1982). Dry matter loss is an inevitable feature of germination, and hence the absolute amount of protein per kernel is not increased.

Studies carried out in some of the maize varieties in India also revealed significant increases in lysine and tryptophan and slight but distinct improvement in BV and utilizable nitrogen (Ram et al. 1979). Even the RNV of germinated maize is significantly higher (80.8) than of ungerminated one (64.6; Lay and Fields, 1982).

In Ragi the protein content decreased from 7.7 to 3.9% by sprouting followed by roasting and sieving, and the biological quality is not altered by germination (Hemamalini et al., 1980). Germination, in general, decreased the total protein expressed on fresh weight basis but improved protein quality by increasing lysine and tryptophan levels. If germinated grains are roasted subsequently for malting purpose, part of the amino acids may be again lost.

Each method of processing has different influence on the quality of protein. By and large, application of heat causes reduction in the limiting amino acids and available amino acids. In methods involving no application of heat, an increase in some of the essential amino acids take place. All processing methods increase the digestibility of cereals and millets, but it is only in millets that the improvement is considerable. Slight changes in biological values take place due to processing, but the effect is not uniform in all grains. The chief factor influencing the protein quality is the intensity of heat rather than the period of exposure to heat. Presence of moisture reduces the impact of heat, but the presence of sugars increases the deterioration in quality. In recipes where germination and fermentation is followed by heating, the beneficial effects of the earlier processes may be lost. Foods are processed keeping the palatability in mind and not the qualitative changes in protein. However, as cereals constitute the staple food, the preparations most frequently consumed should be processed such that the protein quality should not be adversely affected. Millets considered to be less digestable can be consumed as fermented and germinated products, to get the full advantage of the proteins.

REFERENCES

Aliya, S. and Geervani, P. (1981). An assessment of the protein quality and vitamin B content of commonly used fermented products of legumes and millets. J. Sci. Food Agric. 32, 837-842.

Ananthachar, T.K. and Desikachar, H.S.R. (1962). Effect of fermentation on the nutritive value of Idli. J. Sci. Ind. Res. 21C, 191-192.

Au, P.M. and Fields, M.L. (1981). Nutritive value of fermented sorghum. J. Food. Sci. 46, 652-654.

Axtell, J.D., Kirleis, A.W., Hassen, H.M., Manson, N.D., Mertz, E.T. and Munck, L. (1981). Digestibility of sorghum proteins. Proc. of National Academy of Sciences of USA.78, 1333-1335.

Block, R.J. Cannon, P.R., Wissler, R.W., Steffee, C.H., Straube, R.L., Fraizer, L.E. and Woodridge, R.L. (1946). The effect of baking on the nutritional value of proteins. Arch. Bio. Chem. Bio. Phys. 10, 295-298.

Carpenter, K.J., Morgan, L.B., Lea, C.H. and Parr, I.J. (1962). Chemical and nutritional changes in stored herring meal, 3. Effect of heating at controlled moisture contents on the binding of amino acids in freeze dried herring press cake and in related model system. Brit. J. Nutrition, 16, 451-455.

Chandra, R. and Reddy, U. (1977). Changes in protein, tryptophan and lysine content of some millets and legumes. Thesis submitted to A.P. Agric. Univ., Hyderabad, India.

Chawla, V.K., Kapoor, A.C. (1982). Chemical composition and protein quality of wheat triticale capatis. J. Food. Sci. 47, 2015-2017.

Clarke, H.E., Howe, J.M., Mertz, E.T. and Reitz, L.L. (1959). Lysine in baking powder biscuits. J. Amer. Diet. Assoc. 38, 469-472.

Desikachar, H.S.R., Radhakrishnan, R.M. and Rama Rao, G. (1960). Studies on Idli Fermentation, Part-I. Some accompanying changes in batter. J. Sci. Ind. Res. 19C, 168-171.

Eggum, B.O. (1973). A study of certain factors influencing protein utilization in rats and pigs. Pub. Dept. of Animal Phys. and Chem. Copenhagen, p. 123-132.

Eggum, B.O. (1977). Effect of cooking on nutritional value of milled rice in rats. Nutr. Reports International. 16, 649-655.

Eggum, B.O., Monowar, L., Bach Knudsen, K.E., Munck and Axtell, J. (1983). Nutritional quality of sorghum and sorghum foods from Sudan. Journal of Cereal Sci. 1, 127-137.

Ericson, L.E., Larson, S. and Lid, G. (1961). The loss of added lysine and thiamine during baking of wheat meal. Acta. Phy. Scand. 53, 85-89.

Faridi, H.A., Ranhotra, G.S., Finney, P.L. and Rubenthaler, G.L. (1982). Protein quality characteristics of Iranian flat breads. J. Food. Sci. 47, 676-677.

Geetha, K. and Pushpamma, P. (1970). Effect of baking and deep fat frying with sugar and jaggery on the available lysine of wheat. Thesis submitted to A.P. Agric. Univ., Hyderabad, India.

Hamad, A.M. and Fields, M.L. (1979). Evaluation of the protein quality and available lysine of germinated and fermented cereals. J. Food. Sci. 44, 456-460.

Hemamalini, G., Umapathy, K.P., Rao, J.R. and Saraswathi, G. (1980). Nutritional evaluation of sprouted Ragi. Nutr. Reports International, 22, 271-277.

Jansen, C.R., Ehle, S.R. and House, N.L. (1974). Studies on the nutritional loss of supplemented lysine in baking. Food Technol. 18, 367-371.

Khader, V. (1982). Preparation and nutritional evaluation of fermentation of foods similar to Miso. Nutr. Reports International, 26, 17-24.

Khandwala, P.K., Ambegaokar, S.D., Patel, S.M. and Radhakrishnan, M.V. (1962). Studies on fermented foods. Part-I. Nutritional value of Idli. J. Sci. Ind. Res. 21C, 275-278.

Khazanas, N. and Fields, M.L. (1981). Nutritional improvement of sorghum by fermentation. J. Food Sci. 46, 819-821.

Lay, M.M.G. and Fields, M.L. (1982). Nutritive value of germinated corn and corn fermented after germination. J. Food Sci. 46, 1069-1073.

Mathews, R.H., Richardson, G. and Lictenstein, H. (1969). Effect of fortification on quality of chapatis and yeast bread cereal. Chem. 46, 14-18.

National Institute of Nutrition, Annual Report (1970). pp. 22-23.

Pellett, P.L. and Young. V.R. (1980). Nutritional Evaluation of Protein Foods. The United Nations University.

Pushpamma, P., Geervani, P. and Krishna Kumari (1982). Losses of some nutrients in cereal, millet and legume recipes commonly consumed in Andhra Pradesh. The Ind. Nutr. Dietet. 19, 342-349.

Pushpamma, P. and Geervani, P. (1982). The nutritive value of traditional recipes of Andhra Pradesh. Publ. Andhra Pradesh Agric. Univ., Hyderabad (India). pp. 122-123.

Rajalaxmi, R. and Vanaja, V. (1967). Chemical and Biological evaluation of fermentation on the nutritive value of foods from rice and Bengal gram. Brit. J. Nutr. 21, 467-472.

Ram, P.C., Lodha, M.L., Srivatsva, K., Tyagi, J. and Mehta, S.L. (1979). Improving nutritive value of maize by germination. J. Food. Sci. and Tech. 16, 258-260.

Rosenberg, H.R. and Rohdenberg, E.L. (1951). The fortification of bread with lysine. J. Nutr. 45, 593-598.

Said, H.H., Ahmed, E.A., Shirbeeny, N.E., Attar, W.M. (1980). Composition of starch and protein of milled rice as related to cooking. Food Sci. Tech. Abstract. 35, 162-164.

Tabekhia, M.M., Toma, R.B. and Luh, B.S. (1981). Crude protein and amino acid composition of 3 California rice varieties. Nutr. Rep. International. 23, 805-811.

Tara, K.A. and Bains, G.S. (1971). Effect of cooking rice on the stability of lysine and threonine in model system. The Ind. J. Nutr. Dietet. 8, 186-191.

Tsai, C.Y. and Dalley, A. (1975). Lysine and tryptophan increase during germination of cereal grains. Cereal Chem. 52, 356-360.

Usha, S. and Khader, V. (1983). Effect of baking on the protein quality and retention of thiamine and niacin in maize and sorghum incorporated biscuits. Thesis submitted to A.P. Agric. Univ., Hyderabad (India).

Van Veen, A.G., Hackler, R.L. and Steinkraus, K.H. (1967). Nutritive quality of Idli, a fermented food of India. J. Food Sci. 32, 339-341.

Van Veen, A.G. (1972). Rice chemistry and Technology. Fermented rice foods, Monograph series. AACC Pub. IV P. 428-430.

Wang, Y.Y. and Fields, M.L. (1978). Feasibility of home fermentation to improve the amino acid balance of corn meal. J. Food Sci. 43, 1104-1105.

Wu, Y.U. and Wall, J.S. (1980). Lysine content of protein increased by germination of normal and high lysine sorghum. J. Agric. Food Chem. 28, 455-458.

Wu, Y.U. (1982). Lysine content of triticale protein increased by germination. J. Agric. Food Chem. 30, 820-823.

Yasoda Devi, M. and Geervani, P. (1973). Study on loss of lysine and tryptophan in plain and fortified wheat products cooked by different methods. Thesis submitted to A.P. Agric. Univ., Hyderabad (India).

Proc. Int. Assoc. Cereal Chem. Symp. Amino Acid Compn and Biol. Value of Cereal Proteins Budapest, Hungary 1983, R. Lásztity, M. Hidvégi, eds

COMPARATIVE STUDY OF YIELD AND BIOLOGICAL VALUE OF DIFFERENT CORN VARIETIES

BALÁZS JUHÁSZ, MARIANNE SZELÉNYI-GALÁNTAI, JOLÁN JÉCSAI, ISTVÁN SOMSSICH

Department of Physiology, Institute for Animal Nutrition, Research-Center for Animal Nutrition, H-2053 Herceghalom, Hungary

ABSTRACT

Normal and opaque hybrid corn varieties were compared. The most important data obtained are summarized as follows:

	normal	opaque
yield, t/ha	8-11	7-1o
crude protein content %	8-1o	9-12
lysine /d.m./, %	o,23-o,26	o,32-o,48
BV, %	52-75	54-85
TD, %	72-8o	74-86

Both in normal and opaque varieties the mid-maturity types had the highest protein quality while the late-maturity types yielded more.

In our opinion the mid-maturity type opaque corn varieties /FAO 4oo/ are the most suitable in our circumstances.

There was a rapid growth in world pig and chicken stocks and in corn production in the seventies. The number of chickens increased by 27 % /to 6,7 million/ and that of pigs by 22 % /to 763 million/. The production of corn increased in Hungary too and it is the most important component of our compound feeds. In our country, corn constitutes 7o % of feed cereals and this supplies 4o % of the protein requirement of farm animals.

The corn seed contains relatively little protein and half of this protein is zein which is poor in lysine and tryptophan. With appropriate selection, plant breeders increased the proportion of non-zein proteins and developed the breed opaque-2. This and other opaque mutants contain 3o % more lysine and 25 % more crude fat than the varieties with normal endospermium. Therefore, the opaque varieties are grown more and more widely and this is why we have compared their value as feedstuffs with that of the traditional varieties.

MATERIAL AND METHODS

Fifty normal and opaque varieties grown in Hungary were compared. The samples were dried in an oven at 60°C. Analyses were made according to the Hungarian standard /MSZ 683o/: dry matter, crude protein, crude fat, crude fiber, ash and N-free extract.

Amino acid pattern of corn samples was determined with type BC-200 amino acid analyzer and available lysine was assayed with the method of Carpenter and Booth /1973/.

N-balance and growth experiments were made with male albino rats and biological value /BV/, net protein utilization /NPU/ and true digestibility /TD/ were calculated /Szelényiné, 1969/.

At the end of the studies the rats were sacrificed and dry matter, crude protein and crude fat contents of the total bodies were determined. For sake of brevity only the most interesting analytical and biological results are described here.

RESULTS

In the sixties, hybrid corn became widely grown in Hungary. The use of hybrids almost doubled the corn yield /from 38oo to 68oo kg per ha/ between 1969 and 1982 /Fig.1/.

Table 1 shows the area, yield and protein yield of the most popular SC and TC hybrids based on the data of 1982. Yield, crude protein content, total lysine content as well as BV, NPU, and TD values of normal and opaque hybrids are shown in Table 2 and 3, respectively.

TABLE 1. Area and yield of the most important corn hybrids /Hungary, 1982/

	Area		Total yield	Protein yield
	ha	%	/1ooo t/	kg/ha
3965 A MTC	139,335	1o,6	87o,3	58,77
39o1 SC	1o8,69o	8,3	712,1	55,88
Pioneer 37o9 MSC	195,o3o	14,9	1226,4	54,26
Pioneer 3732 SC	1o4,88o	8,o	687,8	54,62
Pioneer 378o MSC	131,84o	1o,1	844,o	65,42

Total corn area in Hungary 1.3o7.125; hybrid is grown on 51 % of the area /679.775 ha/.
Total protein yield: 75.179 t.

BV of normal corn varieties was 68 % in average which may be considered as good protein quality /Table 2/. BV of Szegedi MSC 378o and of Pioneer 37o9 MSC surpassed the average, being

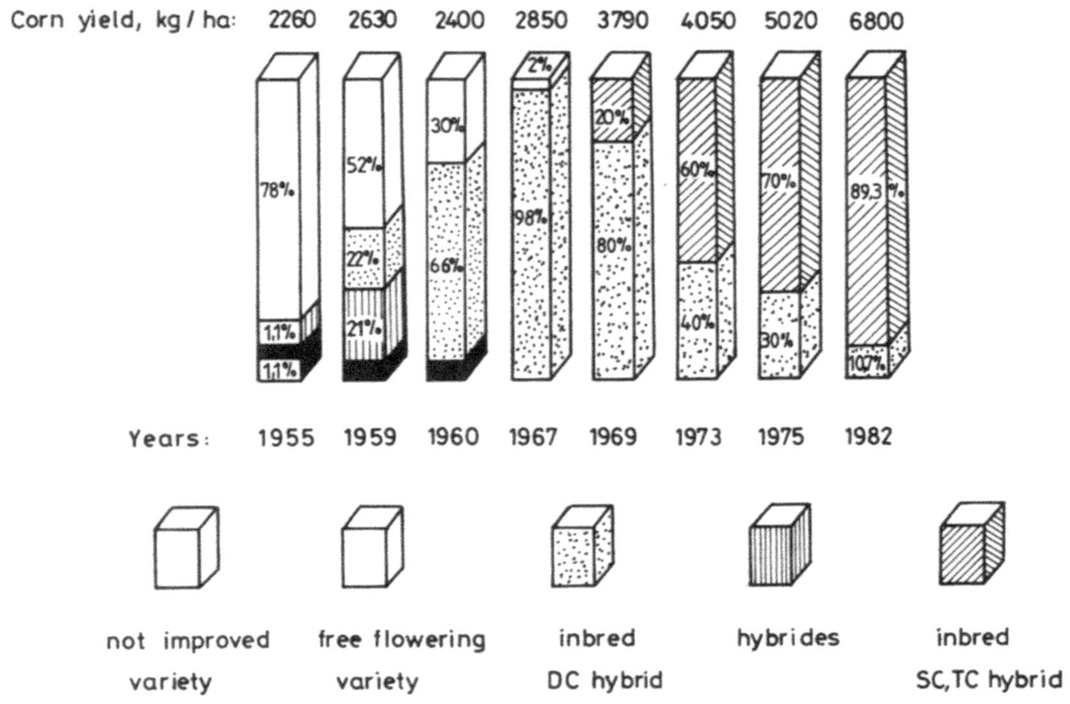

FIGURE 1. Yields of different corn varieties in Hungary

75 and 74 %, respectively. NPU showed similar tendencies. The average TD value was 79 %, the lowest value was obtained with Pioneer 3965 MTC /77 %/.

TABLE 2. Yield and evaluation of normal hybrids

	Pioneer 3965 A MTC FAO 2oo	Szegedi MSC 378o FAO 3oo	Pioneer 37o9 MSC FAO 4oo
Yield t/ha	9,62	1o,45	11,o2
Crude protein %	1o,4o	1o,3o	1o,4o
Total lysine /d.m./%	o,23	o,24	o,25
BV	68±2,6	75±2,5	74±2,7
NPU	62±3,2	69±3,7	67±2,9
TD	77±2,3	79±3,2	79±2,2

Most of the opaque hybrids had high BV-s /Table 3./. The highest BV was obtained with SC 5443 /85 %/ and the lowest with TC 356o /54 %/. NPU values showed similar tendencies. The highest TD was found with SC 3365 /86 %/ and the lowest with TC 356o /74 %/.

TABLE 3. Yield and evaluation of opaque hybrids

	SC 3365 FAO 4oo	SC 5443 FAO 4oo	TC 356o FAO 5oo
Yield t/ha	7,2o	8,25	8,18
Crude protein %	9,8o	8,9o	8,2o
Total lysine /d.m./%	o,37	o,31	o,25
	/SC 3385; o,45/		
BV	78±3,6	85±2,5	54±3,6
NPU	78±3,2	83±1,7	49±3,8
TD	86±o,8	82±3,9	74±4,o

Dry matter, crude protein and crude fat contents of total bodies varied between 27 and 3o %, 14,8 and 17,o % and 5,2 and 7,7 %, respectively. In rats fed on corn varieties of higher biological value the deposition of fat increased with a correlation coefficient of o,45.

Amino acid composition of some corn varieties are summarized in Table 4. The opaque SC 3385 and 3365 corn varieties had almost twice so much total lysine between o.37 and o.45 % than other varieties /between o.23 and o.26 %/. Methionine contents varied between o.13 and o.22 % and that of cystine between o,14 and o,25 %. Arginine contents of corn proteins are relatively high.

FIGURE 2. Relation between the lysine content and BV of corn varieties

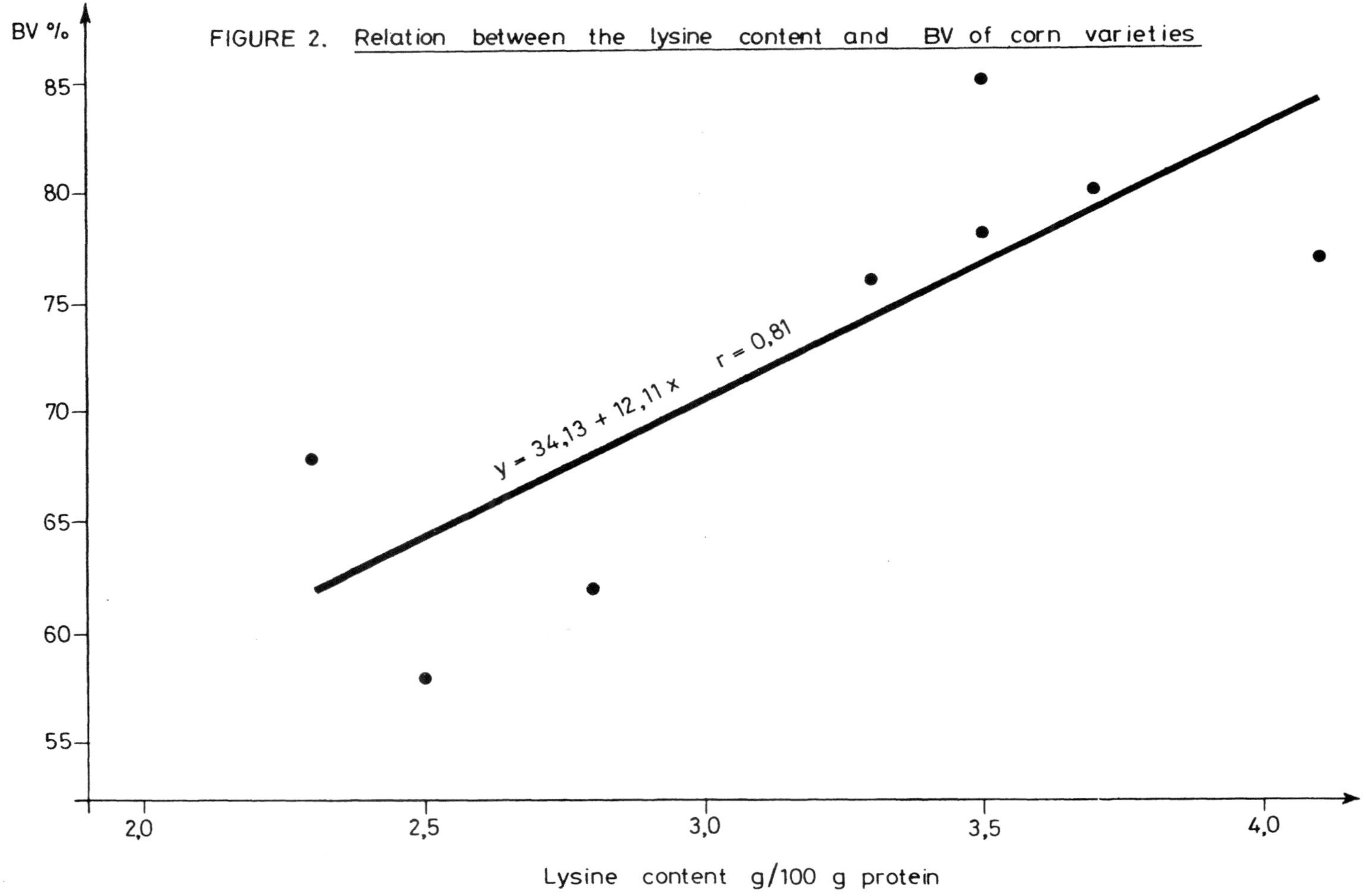

TABLE 4. Amino acid composition of hybrid corn varieties calculated to d.m.

Amino acid	Variety				
	PX 2o	SC 3386	H 4o4	SC 3365	MV 58o
Threonine	o,39	o,47	o,38	o,39	o,37
Cystine	o,19	o,22	o,14	o,25	o,18
Valine	o,44	o,76	o,53	o,64	o,48
Methionine	o,17	o,22	o,16	o,13	o,19
Isoleucine	o,39	o,4o	o,36	o,34	o,3o
Leucine	1,o4	1,35	1,39	o,94	1,2o
Tyrosine	o,35	o,41	o,38	o,27	o,33
Phenylalanine	o,41	o,56	o,61	o,46	o,46
Lysine	o,23	o,45	o,23	o,37	o,26
Histidine	o,22	o,33	o,23	o,29	o,26
Arginine	o,37	o,59	o,34	o,64	o,47

DISCUSSION

In the present studies the normal corn varieties contained approximately lo % crude protein /86 % dry matter/, whereas the opaque varieties had less than this.

Cromwell et al. /1967/, Harpstead /1971/, Rosa et al. /1977, and Rivera /1978/ found o,23 to o,38 % lysine in normal hybrids and a markedly higher content in the opaque varieties /Pick and Meade, 1971; Wahlstrom et al. 1977; Anastasijevic et al. 1978/. Our own data range between o,25 and o,45 %. /Jécsai et al. 1981; Szelényiné et al. 1981/. So the lysine content shows wide variations in the different opaque hybrids /Klein et al. 1971; Eggum et al. 1979; Table 4/. Both in normal and opaque varieties the early- and mid-maturity hybrids had significantly more available lysine than the late-maturity breeds. The length of the vegetation period negatively correlated with the available lysine content. We found the biological value of the early- and mid-maturity normal hybrids generally to be quite good, although they do not reach that of the opaque varieties. Both in the normal and opaque varieties the protein of the late-maturity hybrids /FAO 5oo/ have significantly /$P < o,ool$/ lower BV than that of other maturity types. Hybrid varieties of good quality contain lo,6 to 12,3 % crude protein /N x 6,25/, approximately 5,o crude fat and less than 3 % crude fiber.

SC 3385 and SC 3365 opaque hybrids contained 3o % more lysine and tryptophan, 25 % more cystine and 2o % less methionine than the TC 356o opaque hybrid. A close correlation was found between the BV and lysine content /$r = o,81$; Fig. 2/.

From the corn production experiments it is concluded that Pioneer 37o9, which has a good yield and firm stalk, can be grown securely on a large corn area in Hungary. Szegedi MSC 378o variety also yields well, but its cold resistance is lower. Pioneer 3965 A MTC has an excellent yield, firm stalk and it loses moisture rapidly.

The yield of some of the opaque hybrids approached that of the normal hybrid Szeged SC 369o /8,4 per ha/ used as a control. However, we should also remember of the disadvantages of the opaque hybrids: in cool, wet years the yields decrease.

Initially the farms disliked the opaque hybrids because they yield 8 to lo % less. However, about 15 to 18 kg lysine can be produced per ha with the normal corn varieties and 22 to 23 kg with the opaque hybrids. Therefore, the emphasis should be changed from total corn yield to the quality of protein produced. The economic evaluation of the present results depends on the economic circumstances of the different countries. It is also important that opaque varieties contain 25 % more fat than other hybrids.

Based on the results of the present study, we composed a ration containing corn /opaque/, wheat, barley, synthetic lysine etc. and the proportion of import soybean meal in the ration could be reduced from 16 to 4 %.

REFERENCES

Anastasijevic, V. - Milekic, M. - Pejic, D. /1978/: Stocarstvo, 32. lo9-115.

Carpenter, K.J. - Booth, U.H. /1973/: Nutr.Abstr. Revs. 43. 423-451.

Cromwell, G.L. - Pickett, R.A. - Beeson, M.W. /1967/: J. Anim. Sci. 26 1325-1331.

Eggum, B.O. - Villegas, E.M. - Vasal, S.K. /1979/: Progress in quality of maize. J.Sci. Food Agric. 3o. 1148-1153.

Jécsai Gy.né-Szelényiné, Galántai, M. - Juhász, B. - Kóta, B. - Haraszti, L. /1981/: Állattenyésztés és Takarmányozás 3o. 473-479

Harpstead, D.D. /1971/: Scientific American, 225. 33-42.

Klein, R.G. - Beeson, W.M. - Cline, T.R. - Mertz, E.T. /1971/: J. Anim. Sci. 32. 256-261.

Notheisz, K. - Maráz, L. /1977/: 5th International Amino Acid Symposium H. 3. Budapest.

Pick, R.T. - Meade, R.J. /1971/: J.Nutr. lol. 1241-1248.

Rivera, P.H. - Peo, E.R. - Flowerday, D. - Crenshaw, T.D. - Moser, B.D. - Cunnigham, P.J. /1978/: J.Anim. Sci. 46. lo24-lo36

Rosa, J.G. - Forsyth, D.M. - Glover, D.V. - Cline, T.R. /1977/: J. Anim. Sci. 44. loll-lo2o.

Szelényiné, Galántai Marianna /1969/: Állattenyésztés 18. 189-191.

Szelényiné, Galántai, M. - Jécsai Gyné - Juhász, B. - Somssich, I. /1981/: Állattenyésztés és Takarmányozás, 3o. 467-471.

Wahlstrom, R.C. - Merrill, R.C. - Reiner, L.J. - Libal, G.W. /1977/: J. Anim. Sci., 45. 747-753.

Proc. Int. Assoc. Cereal Chem. Symp. Amino Acid Compn and Biol. Value of Cereal Proteins Budapest, Hungary 1983, R. Lásztity, M. Hidvégi, eds

WHEAT GLUTEN - A NATURAL PROTEIN FOR THE FUTURE - TODAY

J. M. HESSER

International Wheat Gluten Association
10100 Santa Fe Drive, Suite 206, Overland Park, KS 66212 USA

INTRODUCTION

Wheat gluten is the natural protein derived from wheat or wheat flour. In its freshly extracted wet form, it is known as "gum gluten" which when dried yields a cream-to-tan colored, free flowing powder of high protein content and bland taste. When rehydrated, it regains its original characteristics. So unique is the functionality of wheat gluten and so persistent is the structural integrity after cooking, it appears to have no functional competitor.

COMPOSITION AND GENERAL PROPERTIES

Wheat gluten is the water-insoluble complex protein fraction separated from wheat flours. The separation process is accomplished by physical means from aqueous flour suspensions without additives of any kind and the product is thus a natural food protein (Figure 1). Wheat gluten is marketed as a

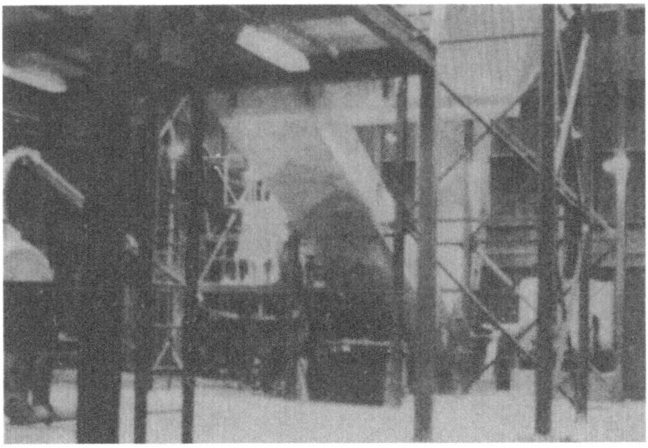

Figure 1.

cream colored, free flowing powder. When rehydrated, it regains virtually all of its instrinsic functionality. Typical analysis of vital wheat gluten appear in Table I.

TABLE I. Typical Analysis of Vital Wheat Gluten

Protein (N x 5.7) dry basis (d.b.)	75.0%-80.0%
Moisture	5.0%-8.0%
Ether extractable fat (d.b.)	0.5%-1.5%
Ash (d.b.)	0.8%-1.2%
Water absorption capacity	150%-200%

VISCOELASTICITY

The ability of wheat gluten to form a viscoelastic mass when fully hydrated sets it apart from all other commercially available vegetable proteins Glutenin and gliadin, the two major protein components of wheat gluten, interact in an aqueous system to produce this viscoelastic property. Glutenin, the high molecular weight protein fraction, contributes elasticity. Gliadin, of lower molecular weight, provides extensibility (Figure 2). These properties are summarized in Table II.

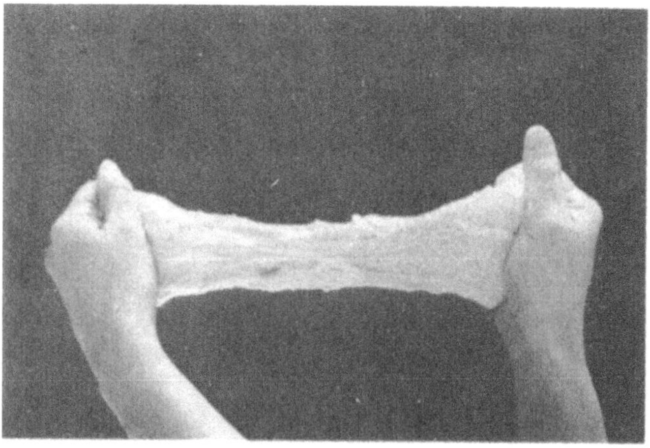

Figure 2.

TABLE II. Fractionation of Wheat Gluten.

Gluten	
Gliadin	**Glutenin**
Highly extensible	Less extensible
Less elastic	Highly elastic
Soluble in alcohols	Insoluble in alcohols
Low molecular weight (less than 100,000)	High molecular weight (greater than 100,000)
Intramolecular bonds	Intra & intermolecular bonds

The viscoelastic behavior of hydrated wheat gluten persists even in the presence of excess water because of the physico-chemical status of these molecular structures in aqueous systems. The dramatic difference in properties of wheat gluten in comparison with almost all other food proteins is largely due to the low level of polarity of the total amino acid structure. Polar grouping levels of 30-45% are normal for most food proteins and impart a net negative electrostatic charge. Wheat gluten, by contrast, has a polar group level of about 10%, with a resultant net positive charge.

The practical result of this reduced polarity is that excess water is repelled and the wheat gluten molecules associate closely together and resist dispersion. Such behavior is crucial to baking technology in that it results in the ability to form adhesive and cohesive masses, films and three dimensional film networks.

Product development scientists contemplating the use of wheat gluten in food systems will recognize that the low positive electrostatic charge is modified by interaction with ionic ingredients. Relatively minor changes in charge magnitude may have functionally significant effects. Indeed, much of bakery technology is oriented to prevent this from occurring. Functional sensitivity to ionic impact thus becomes a challenge and an opportunity for the food scientist in controlling and adjusting wheat gluten behavior in a specific product environment.

FILM FORMING

The film forming property of hydrated wheat gluten is a direct consequence of its viscoelasticity. Whenever carbon dioxide or water vapor forms internally in a gluten mass with sufficient pressure to partially overcome the elasticity, the gluten expands to a spongy or cellular structure. In such structures, pockets or voids are created which are surrounded by a continuous protein phase to entrap and contain the gas or vapor (Figure 3).

This new shape and structure can be rendered dimensionally stable by applying sufficient heat to cause the protein to denature or devitalize and set up irreversibly into a fixed moist gel structure or to a crisp fragile state, depending on final moisture content. The open texture of leavened breads, the suspension of solid particles such as fruit pieces or grains,

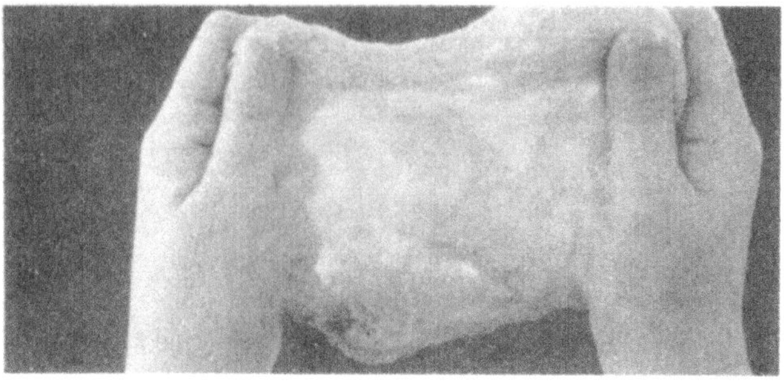

Figure 3.

and high fiber bread are examples of success due to the continuous phase of the strength possible from the flour used, "cripples" result. This is easily correctible by addition of wheat gluten to the flour base (Figure I). Food

Figure I. Effect of Increasing Increments of Vital Wheat Gluten on the Loaf Volume of Raisin Bread Containing 75% Raisins Based on Flour.

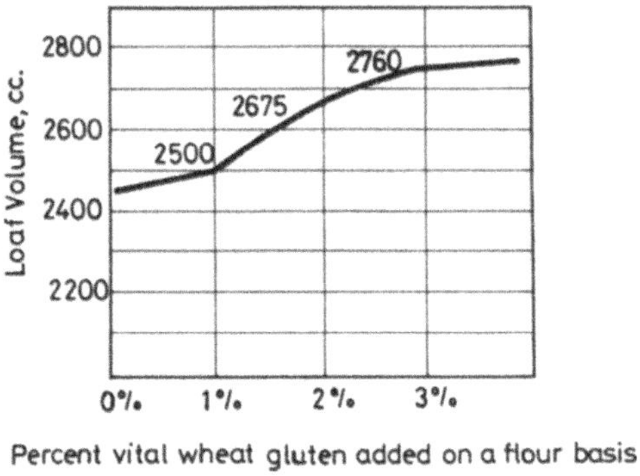

scientists can harness these attributes to create new food structures. (Microwave technology also opens new horizons for exploration.)

In addition to its film forming potential in food systems, cast or floated films of wheat gluten can be made. Glazing of meat paties is possible, and wheat gluten films in the form of sausage casing, tubes or shreds are recorded in the patent literature as the product of gluten "hot melt" techniques

THERMOSETTING PROPERTIES

Although there are obvious exceptions such as gelatin, most hydratable proteins undergo irreversible denaturation and insolubilization when heated to critical temperatures. When protein percentages are high enough and the coagulative insolubilization tendency exists, elegant structures of high dimensional stability can result. Such hydrated wheat gluten is 25-30% protein and heat coagulates at roughly 85 degrees C, thus, its utility in meat binding, canning, meat extenders and analogs, as well as in pastas and various other binding and shaping situations is obvious (Figure 4). Resistance to mushiness in steam table food service is a further benefit.

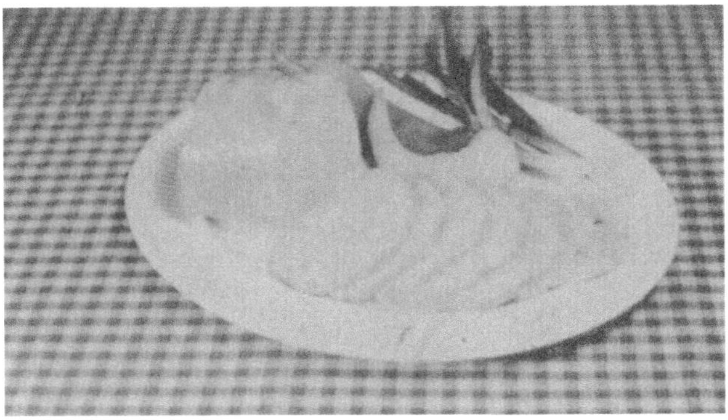

Figure 4.

WATER ABSORPTION

Good quality powdered vital wheat gluten rapidly absorbs about twice its weight of water. Since powdered vital wheat gluten has a protein content of 75-80% (dry basis), the hydrated version will drop to 25-27% protein at full hydration of about 65% moisture. Wheat gluten's capacity for holding water results in increased yield and extended shelf life in food systems into which it is incorporated.

The combination of speed of water absorption and the degree of visco-elasticity produced are evidence of "vitality". Vital wheat gluten is a commonly used term. Deliberate cooking of wet wheat gluten prior to drying results in "devitalized" wheat gluten. This product has undergone irreversible denaturation and does not revitalize or absorb water. It merely absorbs water in an amount related to its particle size distribution. Devitalized wheat gluten is a popular substrate for hydrolysis in vegetable protein hydrolysate flavor manufacture.

Dispersibility and speed of hydration of wheat gluten can vary with different processes of manufacture and are controllable. Suppliers should be consulted for special requirements.

pH EFFECTS

Since wheat gluten is a complex of proteins, it has no sharp isoelectric (minimum solubility and dissociation) point. There is thus no readily discernible point at which the positive and negative charges exactly balance. Because glutenin is essentially insoluble in water over normal pH ranges, wheat gluten tends to reflect the isoelectric behavior of gliadin in its pH/solubility properties.

When gliadin is separately examined for pH/solubility criteria, it displays minimum solubility over the pH range 6.0-9.0 (Figure II). It is in this range that the cohesive, extensible network of wheat gluten is strongest. It is important to note that wheat gluten becomes more soluble in acid or alkaline dispersion. (Some manufacturers utilize this effect to produce spray dried wheat gluten. The aqueous acetic acid or ammonia used is flashed off during the drying step, and the powdered material retains typical vital gluten characteristics.) pH manipulation may thus provide interesting property variations in foods containing wheat gluten.

FIGURE II. Solubility Profile for 1% Gliadin in Distilled Water

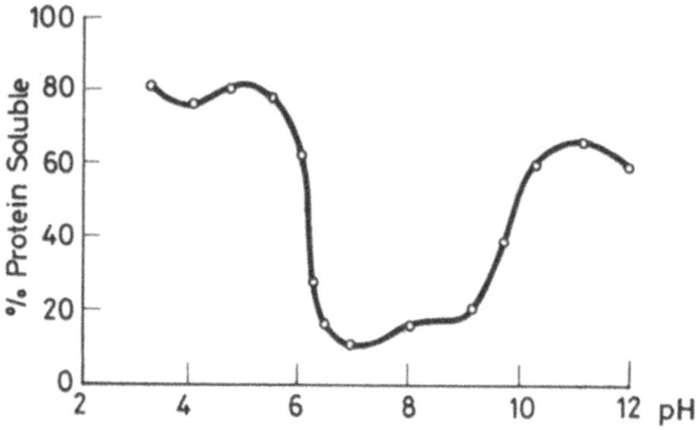

Source: Private study, John Labatt Limited, London, Ontario, Canada. 1976

FLAVOR

Properly produced and given reasonable care in storage, wheat gluten exhibits a flavor note variously described as "bland" or "slight cereal". Wheat flavors enjoy wide acceptance and wheat gluten merges perfectly into all cereal based products. Blending with meats in various binding, adhesive and extension roles need not result in off-flavor notes, even at high percentage use levels (Figure 5).

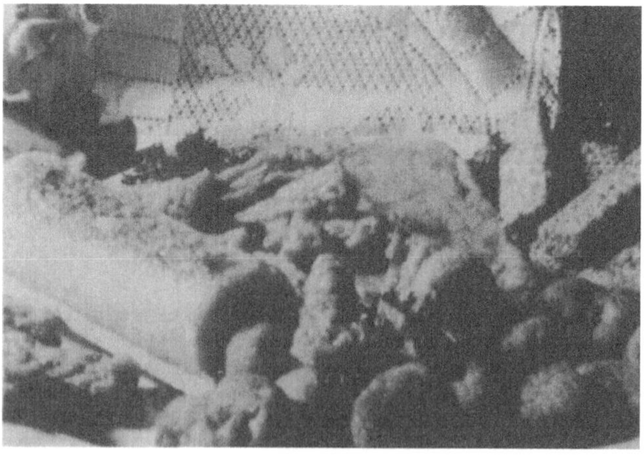

Figure 5.

Blending of wheat gluten with other food proteins which do possess characteristic flavor notes can result in improved total flavor as, for example, when soy/wheat gluten blends are used for textured vegetable protein manufacture. Low and acceptable flavor levels of wheat gluten are the result of careful selection of flours, good manufacturing procedures and proper storage at normal ambient temperatures.

NUTRITIONAL PROPERTIES

Wheat gluten alone, when measured against this standard casein reference in rat bioassay, rates rather low on the Protein Efficiency Ratio (P.E.R.) scale. Vegetable proteins in general rate low on the P.E.R. scale due to low contents of one or more essential amino acids. Blends of different vegetable proteins often result in higher P.E.R. values than the arithmetic average of the components (Table III). Such is the case with the wheat gluten, low in lysine but high in methionine and cystine, when blended with soy flour.

Table III: Typical Essential Amino Acid Profile of Wheat Gluten.
(grams amino acid/100 grams protein)

Amino Acid	FAO/WHO Provisional Pattern[1]	Wheat Gluten[2]	Profile of 40/60% Gluten/Soy Flour[3]
Isoleucine	4.0	4.2	4.4
Leucine	7.0	6.9	7.4
Lysine	5.5	1.6	4.1
Methionine & cystine	3.5	3.4	2.9
Phenylalanine & tyrosine	6.0	7.7	8.3
Threonine	4.0	2.4	3.3
Tryptophan	1.0	1.0	1.2
Valine	5.0	4.3	4.5

[1] *Energy and Protein Requirements*. Report of a Joint FAO/WHO Ad Hoc Expert Committee, 1973. FAO Nutrition Meetings Rep. Series 52, WHO Tech. Rep. Series 522.

[2] Wookey, N. *Journal of the American Oil Chemists Society*, vol. 56, March 1979, p. 307.

[3] Arithmetic projection using typical values for soy flour.

Soy flour, high in lysine but low in methionine, has a P.E.R. value of about 2.0. Table IV demonstrates the synergistic result of blending soy flour and wheat gluten. At a wheat gluten/soy flour protein ratio of 30:70, a P.E.R. value of 2.4 is achieved, or roughly three times the rating of wheat gluten alone. Similar effects are predictable for other food systems, wherein excess lysine is available from meat, milk solids or other sources. Wheat gluten in combination with other proteins can have solid nutritional impact.

Table IV. Protein Efficiency Ratio (P. E.R.) of Wheat Gluten Protein/Soy Flour Protein Blends (Relative to Casein P. E.R. of 2.5)

	WHEAT GLUTEN PROTEIN/SOY FLOUR PROTEIN BLEND RATIO				
	100/0	55/45	45/55	30/70	0/100
P. E.R.	0.8	2.1	2.3	2.4	2.0

Source: Private study, Industrial Grain Products, Montreal, Quebec, Canada (1975).

APPLICATIONS

Milling and Baking

Probably no area of food processing enjoys greater benefit from wheat gluten than does the baking industry. To the baker the most valuable properties of wheat gluten are: (1) dough strengthening; (2) gas retention and controlled expansion resulting in uniform shaped products; (3) structural enhancement due to thermosetting; (4) water absorption and retention allowing improved yield, product softness and extended shelf life; and (5) natural flavor enhancement (Figure 6).

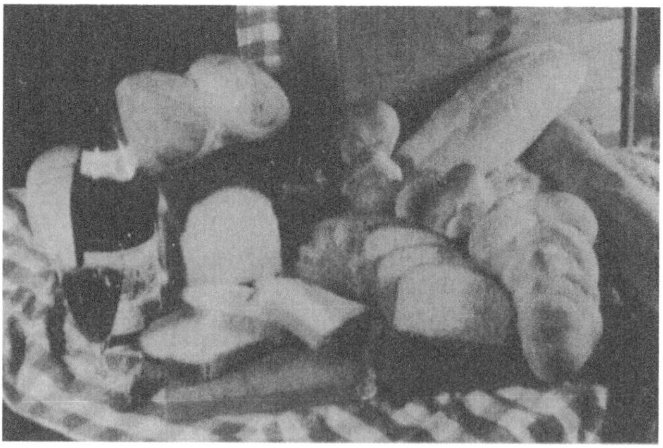

Figure 6.

From the beginning when gluten was used to produce a high protein, low carbohydrate product for diabetics, the industry has grown to where virtually every large manufacturer of yeast raised bakery products uses this ingredient *in order to provide added strength and tolerance to his doughs. It is estimated that about 60 million pounds (27,000 MT) of gluten is used in the United States in various types of bakery foods.*

It is possible to streamline flour inventories by addition of wheat gluten to the level dictated by baking requirements. As a natural additive, there are no limits to the amounts that can be used in achieving product quality objectives. In recent years the baking industry has experienced rapid growth of variety bread products. Added fiber and other "dead weight" ingredients, in most applications, mandate the use of wheat gluten for added strength and necessary water absorption.

Recent studies at the Flour Milling and Baking Research Association at Chorleywood in the U. K. have shown that wheat gluten as a substitute for imported high-protein wheats in the bread grist is technically possible and financially attractive. Both short and long term investigations designed to improve methods for assessing gluten quality in this application and to define optimum conditions of use are in progress.

Considerable research continues to be devoted to composite flour creation in third world countries. Millet, cassava and maize are some foods which can be used with wheat gluten to produce satisfactory bakery products.

Breakfast Cereals, Breadings and Batter Mixes

The mild flavor, adhesive, textural and cooked appearance qualities have encouraged the use of wheat gluten in cereals, breadings and batter mixers. Wheat gluten fortified breakfast cereals enjoy wide consumer acceptance. When consumed with milk, such products offer excellent flavor and high nutritional impact.

Adhesion of batter crusts to fried foods have always been a quality problem, particularly in frozen products. Predusting of such food portions with wheat gluten reduces cooking loss, improves yield and increases hot and cold adhesion scores to levels comparable to those obtained with expensive dried egg albumen (Table V). When wheat gluten is added to a batter mix, the film formation reduces liquid loss and also produces crisp, appetizing surfaces.

Table V: Effect of Various Predusts on the Adhesion of Breading to Fried Chicken Parts.

Predust	Adhesion Scores[1] Cold	Hot
Dried Egg Albumen	8.0	8.0
Vital Wheat Gluten	7.0	6.6
Soy Concentrate	6.2	6.6
Wheat Flour	4.5	5.4
Nonfat Milk Solids	4.2	3.5
Modified Waxy Corn Starch	3.8	3.9
Sodium Caseinate	2.8	2.8
Unmodified Corn Starch	2.4	2.3

[1]*On a scale of 9 to 1, 9 denotes perfect adhesion, 1 denotes no adhesion. Evaluations were made after deep fried chicken had been cooled to room temperature; and after other parts had been frozen for 1-2 weeks and then reheated.*

Excerpted from: Baker, R. C., Darfler, J. M. and Vadehra, D. V., ***Poultry Science 51****, pp. 1220-1222, 1972.*

Pasta

Although reliance on durum wheats to aid in pasta production is less universal than in the past, satisfactory pasta product production from many regionally available flours is strongly assisted by addition of wheat gluten. Improvements in such crucial end product qualities as resistance to breakage, cooking loss, extra heat tolerance, bite characteristics and tolerance to canning and retorting stresses are possible with the addition of wheat gluten.

Nutritional Snacks

The change of "junk" foods or "empty" calories often leveled at snack foods should prompt fabricators of snacks to examine wheat gluten closely as a worthwhile ingredient. Many international examples of such wheat gluten based snacks are now being marketed, including gluten balls in Europe, vegetarian items in the United States, Yachi-fu cakes in Japan, fried gluten items in China (Figure 7) and wafers of 30-45% wheat gluten content in Australia (Figure 8).

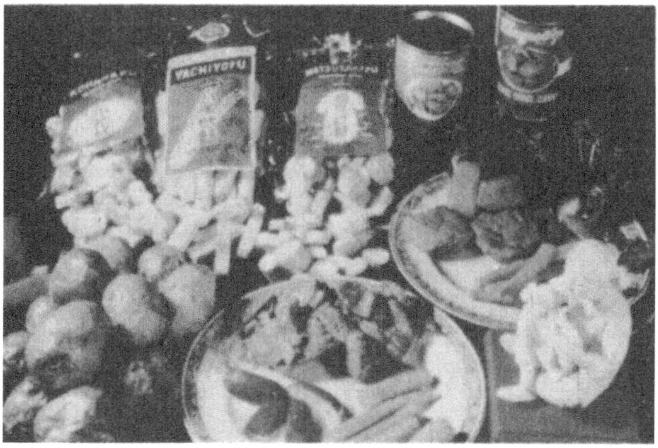

Figure 7.

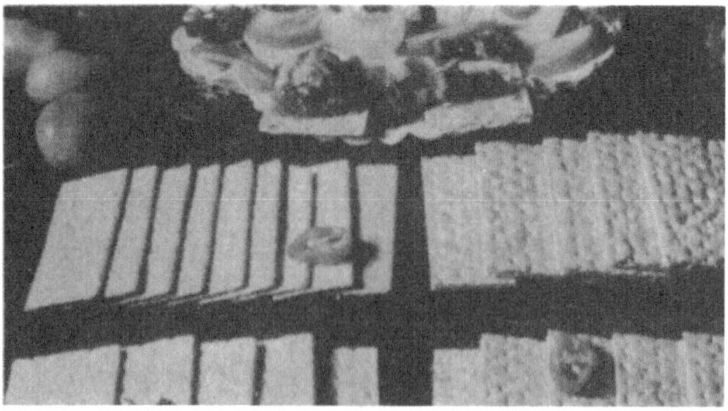

Figure 8.

Aquaculture

As a rapidly growing industry, aquaculture faces problems of feed logistics associated with surface or bottom feeding, oxygen drain due to biodegraduation by solubilization of pellet feeds and associated difficulties. Wheat gluten can bind such feeds for greater aqueous stability while contributing as well to nutritional balance.

Meat, Fish and Poultry Products

The meat industry is becoming increasingly aware of the valuable binding and adhesion properties of wheat gluten. Actual applications utilizing gluten range across the meat, poultry, fish and crustacean spectrum (Table VI). Other examples are:

Extended Ground Meats
Textured Protein Meat Extension
Meat Analogs
Fabricated Steaks
Canned "Intergal" Hams
Poultry Rolls
Various Beef, Pork, Chicken and Fish Sausage Products
Pizza Toppings
Pet Foods

Textured protein products fabricated from soy/wheat gluten blends have the triple virtues of P.E.R. values above 2.0, highly acceptable flavor and structural integrity in hot, moist environments such as canning or institutional food service. A soy/wheat gluten textured meat extender has approval for school lunch programs in the U. S.

Table VI: Performance of Different Protein Materials as Turkey Roll Binders

Binding Agent	Condition of Roll	Sliceability of Ready-to-Serve Roll
Vital Wheat Gluten	Intact	Excellent
Egg White Powder	Intact	Very Good
Casein	Intact	Poor
Milk Solids	Intact	Poor
Isolated Soy Protein	Intact	None
Gelatin	Disintegrated	None

Excerpted from: Aref, M. M. and Tape, N. W. **"A New Method for Processing Turkey Rolls,"** *Can. Food Ind., Dec. 1966.*

A two-phased application research program sponsored by the IWGA at North Carolina State University in Raleigh, North Carolina, under the direction of Dr. J. T. Keeton, has demonstrated the functionality of wheat gluten as a binder and functional protein additive in various types of comminuted meat products. The results of this work will be published within the next year.

Cheese Substitutes and Cheese Analogs

The first segment of an applications research program, also sponsored by the IWGA at the W. L. Clayton Research Center in Dallas, Texas, has shown that it is feasible to use wheat gluten to replace 30% of the caseinate in various cheese substitutes and cheese analogs. Results of this study have been published by the IWGA in the form of a product application bulletin.

New Applications

Other applications include: Gluten glue, icing stabilizer, fish substitutes and analogs and others.

Standard Testing Procedures

Many factors determine gluten baking quality and its suitability for other applications. These factors include raw materials and, probably most important, drying. One of the primary needs of this industry is the standardization of quality assurance and development of new methods of analysis. This need is being addressed to many groups at research centers around the world. Today, the most dependable method of evaluating vital wheat gluten is the bake test.

The Farinograph method has been suggested and is fairly good measure of the absorption requirements and, to a lesser extent, the relative mixing requirement, but it is no measure of the baking quality of that gluten.

One test which is fairly reliable to the nitrogen solubility test developed by Roy Anderson at the U.S.D.A.'s Northern Regional Research Laboratory.

At the 1982 AACC meeting in San Antonio, Texas, a French author presented a paper on a new method for evaluating the baking quality of gluten for research programs.

The Alveograph has been used extensively in Europe for evaluation of gluten quality, and a recent article published in a French journal stated - "Gluten powders vary in characteristics, and choice of appropriate quality gluten for different bakery applications is considered with reference to four commercial glutens of widely differing Alveograph characteristics".

Raw Material Section

In many instances the type of raw material used in gluten production is dictated strictly by economics; but, by knowing a little more about this raw material, we can use both our scientific knowledge and economics to improve our raw material selection.

Use Information

The dough mixing processes vary throughout the world. For example, in the United States, the standard mixer is the horizontal type mixer which processes a dough in 10 to 15 minutes. The future trend may be to spiral high speed mixers or the ultra high speed Tweedy or Stephen mixers which mix doughs in four minutes or less. In still other parts of the world, such as

Southeast Asia, doughs are mixed by hand or with a slow speed mixer of some type.

Modified Glutens

Can the properties of glutens be modified to improve baking characteristics? One modification suggested by Australian workers is treatment of gluten with a reducing agent, such as sodium metabisulfite. They found that the total mixing requirement of five different glutens can be normalized by adding from 250 to 625 ppm of sodium metabisulfite. When an appropriate amount of sodium metabisulfite was added and the doughs mixed in a medium speed mixer, all apparent differences in baking quality between the glutens were removed. It, thus, appeared that the addition of a reducing agent enabled all five gluten samples to be brought to a similar state with regard to both dough and baking properties. It was further found that when the sodium metabisulfite treated glutens were added to a dough, the gluten enriched doughs had no tolerance to nor required a floor time, suggesting that the reducing agent had brought the final dough to a suitable state for immediate processing.

ACKNOWLEDGEMENT

The author serves as Executive Director of the International Wheat Gluten Association (IWGA) to which he extends his gratitude for assistance in preparing this paper. The IWGA, chartered in 1979, presently consists of eighteen members in eight countries (Figure 9). The primary objective of the IWGA is to promote the common interests of its members and the general welfare of the international wheat gluten industry.

INTERNATIONAL WHEAT GLUTEN ASSOCIATION

10100 Santa Fe Drive, Suite 206 • Overland Park, Kansas 66212 USA
Tel: (913) 341-1155 • Telex: 42335 ROANOKE OLPK • Cable: GLUTEN

MEMBER COMPANIES

ABR Chemicals Ltd.
52 Mark Lane
London EC3R 7PE
United Kingdom
Tel: (44) 01/488-1593
Tlx: 888115 MPC G

Allied Mills Industries Pty. Ltd.
A.M.I. — Flour & Starch Division
P. O. Box 1
Summer Hill, N.S.W. 2130
Australia
Tel: (61) 2/797-8333
Tlx: AA 26320 AMILL

Bunge (Australia) Pty. Ltd.
32nd Floor, B.H.P. House
140 Williams Street
Melbourne, Victoria 3000
Australia
Tel: (61) 3/67 81 71
Tlx: AA 30208 BUNGECO

Crespel & Deiters GmbH
Groner Allee 76
Postfach 1661
4530 Ibbenbueren
Federal Republic of Germany
Tel: (49) 05451-4054
Tlx: 94545 CEDE D

Fielder Gillespie Ltd.
55 Clarence Street
Sydney, N.S.W. 2000
Australia
Tel: (61) 2/290-2088
Tlx: AA 26618 FGLTD

George Weston Foods Ltd.
N. B. Love Starches
Braidwood Street
Enfield, N.S.W. 2136
Australia
Tel: (61) 2/764-8222
Tlx: AA 26634 NLOVE

G. R. Amylum N.V.
Van Wambekekaai 13
B-9300 Aalst
Belgium
Tel: (32) 053/21 57 05
Tlx: 12363 AMYLUM B

Henkel Corporation
4620 West 77th Street
Minneapolis, Minnesota 55435
USA
Tel: 612/828-8000
Tlx: 290472 HENKEL MPS

Manildra Milling Corporation
4220 Johnson Drive, Suite 404B
Shawnee Mission, Kansas 66205
USA
Tel: 913/362-0777
Twx: 910-743-4123 MANILDRA SWMS

Manildra Starches Pty. Ltd.
P. O. Box 72
Auburn, N.S.W. 2144
Australia
Tel: (61) 2/649-1444
Tlx: AA 25887 MILLS

Midwest Solvents Co., Inc.
1300 Main Street
Atchison, Kansas 66002
USA
Tel: 913/367-1480
Tlx: 426335 MCCORMICK WSOT

Molinos Juan Semino
Casilla de Correo No. 2
2138 Carcarana (Santa Fe)
Argentina
Tel: (54) 42/941201 or 941233
Tlx: 9900 BTH SD AR
Cbl: SEMINO

Ogilvie Mills Ltd.
1 Place Ville Marie, Suite 2100
Montreal, Quebec H3B 2X2
Canada
Tel: 514/866-1838
Tlx: 055-60489 OGILVIE MTL

Raision Tehtaat
SF 21200 Raisio
Finland
Tel: (358) 21/780311
Tlx: 62236 RATE SF

Roquette Freres, S.A.
4, Rue Patou
59022 Lille Cedex
France
Tel: (33) 20/30 77 97
Tlx: 810858 FECULOR LILLE

Tenstar Aquitaine
36, Quai de Brazza, B.P. 48
33015 Bordeaux-Cedex
France
Tel: (33) 56/86 68 49
Tlx: 540229 TENSTAR

Tenstar Products Ltd.
Tufton Road, Hythe Road
Ashford, Kent TN24 8BH
United Kingdom
Tel: (44) 0233/29231
Tlx: 965219 RHMASH G

Wheat Industries Limited
Factory Cross,
Raheens East,
Carrigaline,
Co. Cork,
Ireland
Tel: (353) 21/921101
Tlx: 75518 WIL EI

Figure 9.

During the last two years, we have submitted a definitional standard for wheat gluten to the Food Chemicals Codex; developed standard methods of analysis and standard test methods for wheat gluten; developed product application bulletins for various uses of wheat gluten; conducted two application research programs for wheat gluten, which have already been discussed and initiated a comprehensive statistical program to define the worldwide market and production of wheat gluten.

The Association also has standing executive, technical, legal, publicit and statistical committees composed of members from the individual companies within the Association.

Finally, to accomplish the objective and purposes of the Association, one of our primary goals is to help food technologists and cereal chemists identify those areas where wheat gluten can play an important role in new protein-based product development. Today's consumers require products with excellent appearance, flavor, nutrition and price value. The foods of tomor row likely will require combinations of complementary proteins and compatibl additives, optimizing on the functional attributes of each concurrent with practical economics.

As a natural food, the increasing awareness of the unique functional properties of wheat gluten coupled with the growing use of all vegetable pro teins augers well for significant market growth in the years ahead. With the evolution from relatively small by-product operations to world-scale sophisticated facilities providing reliable service and quality, the gluten industry is positioned to meet the market challenge of the future. Therefore, wheat protein (gluten) is a natural food for the future - TODAY.

Proc. Int. Assoc. Cereal Chem. Symp. Amino Acid Compn and Biol. Value of Cereal Proteins Budapest, Hungary 1983, R. Lásztity, M. Hidvégi, eds

WHEAT PROTEIN PRODUCTS IN NUTRITION

MARJA-LEENA SARKKI, EIJA-RIITTA SAARINEN

RAISION TEHTAAT, SF-21200 Raisio, Finland

1. INTRODUCTION

Wheat is one of the most important sources for human beings because almost one fifth of our protein need is supplied by wheat protein. The use of grain protein is very common in developing countries and for this reason the nutritive value of wheat and knowledge of its advantages and disadvantages are highly important.

Wheat generally contains 10-17 % protein. The main part of this protein is known as wheat gluten. This is the storage protein in wheat embryo. (Figure 1.) Proteins in bran fraction mainly in aleurone layer and some of the proteins in embryo (enzymes) are mainly soluble albumins and globulins.

Wheat gluten produced with wet starch gluten separation process has been known as a commercial product for many years but the product which contains the soluble proteins of wheat in a heat coagulated form (SWP) has only been on market for a couple of years.

The nutritive value of wheat protein products is discussed mainly by comparing them to whole wheat. This comparison shows the effects of processing on wheat proteins in a starch-protein separation process called Raisio Process. (Figure 2.)

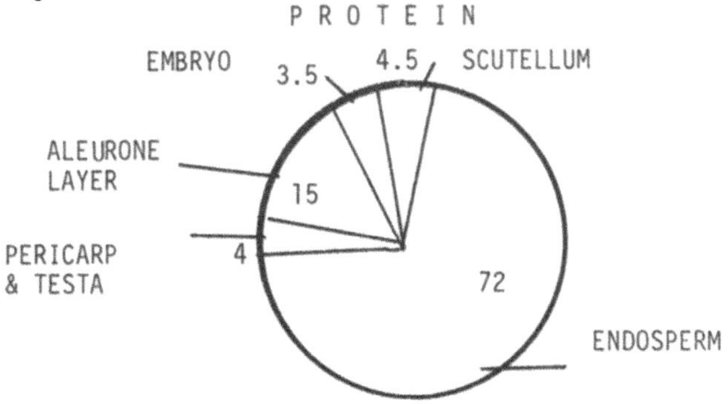

Figure 1. Diagram showing percentage of protein in different parts of the wheat kernel(MacMaster et al., 1971)

2. NUTRITIVE QUALITY

2.1 Quality of protein composition

The quality of protein composition of wheat protein products could be evaluated in many ways. The protein content of wheat gluten is very high 75-80 % and thus valuable as a protein source. Like almost all the grains, wheat has some deficiencies in protein quality. Typically lysine is the most limiting amino acid. The deficiency of lysine is even more clear in wheat gluten, as seen in Table 1, in amino acid pattern. In the same table it is shown that lysine is very heavily concentrated in the SWP product. The protein content of SWP is only 40 % but it is much richer in essential amino acids than gluten. Comparison of the amino acid patterns of wheat protein products with FAO/WHO recommended values demonstrates clearly the advantages of SWP over whole wheat and wheat gluten.

If necessary to compensate the deficiency of lysine in wheat, proteins latter are supplemented with lysine or are used with or supplemented by legume proteins, mainly soy proteins. This supplementation is excellent for both proteins because soy proteins are lacking in methionine while wheat proteins are comparatively rich in methionine and cystine.

Table 1. Typical essential amino acid profiles of wheat proteins. (Grams amino acid/100 grams protein)

	FAO/WHO[1] provisional pattern	Wheat[2]	Wheat[3] Gluten	SWP[4]
ISOLEUCINE	4.0	3.5	4.2	3.8
LEUCINE	7.0	3.5	6.9	7.5
LYSINE	5.5	3.1	1.6	3.7
METHIONINE & CYSTINE	6.0	8.1	7.7	5.6
PHENYLALANINE & TYROSINE	6.0	8.1	7.7	5.6
THREONINE	4.0	3.1	2.4	3.9
TRYPTOPHAN	1.0	1.1	1.0	1.0
VALINE	5.0	4.7	4.3	4.9

1 Energy and Protein Requirements. FAO/WHO, (1973).
2 Hulse & Lang, (1974).
3 Wookey, N., (1979).
4 Private Study, Raision Tehtaat, (1982).

2.2 Rat bioassays for protein quality

Theoretically amino acid composition is the best and most accurate method of evaluating protein quality. However, chemical analysis made by releasing amino acids by hot acid hydrolysis produces higher results than the actual availability of individual amino acids. This is especially true for Maillard reaction bound lysine. For this reason several rat bioassays have been developed to describe the quality of proteins. Wheat protein products are typically exposed to Maillard reaction although at the reasonable temperature, being dried at 80° C.

Several rat bioassays are used to compare wheat proteins and in this paper we are referring to the following: P.E.R., BV, and N.P.U. (See Table 2.)

P.E.R. (Protein Efficiency Ratio) = weight gain/protein consumed
BV (Biological Value) = the proportion of absorbed and N retained
N.P.U. (Net Protein Utilization) = the proportion of nitrogen intake retained

Table 2. Comparison of wheat proteins with reference protein casein and some other proteins with P.E.R., BV, and N.P.U.

	P.E.R.	BV[1]	N.P.U.[1]
REFERENCE CASEIN	2.5	100	100
WHEAT	1.5	64	40
WHEAT GLUTEN	0.7-1.0[2]	58	38
SOY FLOUR	2.2		
SOY ISOLATE	1.6	66	52
SWP	2.2[3]		

1 Amino Acid Content of Foods and Biological Data on Proteins. FAO Rome (1970).
2 Woerman et al., (1974).
3 Private Study, Raision Tehtaat (1973).

Wheat gluten alone, when measured against standard case in reference to rat bioassay, rates rather low in the P.E.R. scale. Values from 0.7 to 1.0 have been recorded. These values reflect a deficiency of the essential amino acid, lysine, a characteristic shared by most cereal grains. The addition of optimal amounts of lysine raised wheat gluten to P.E.R. level of 1.7. The tendency that wheat gluten is less valuable than wheat or SWP from nutritional viewpoint, can be seen in all rat bioassays. Unfortunately only the P.E.R. figure of SWP was available but in future assaying BV and N.P.U. gives more information about the quality of SWP.

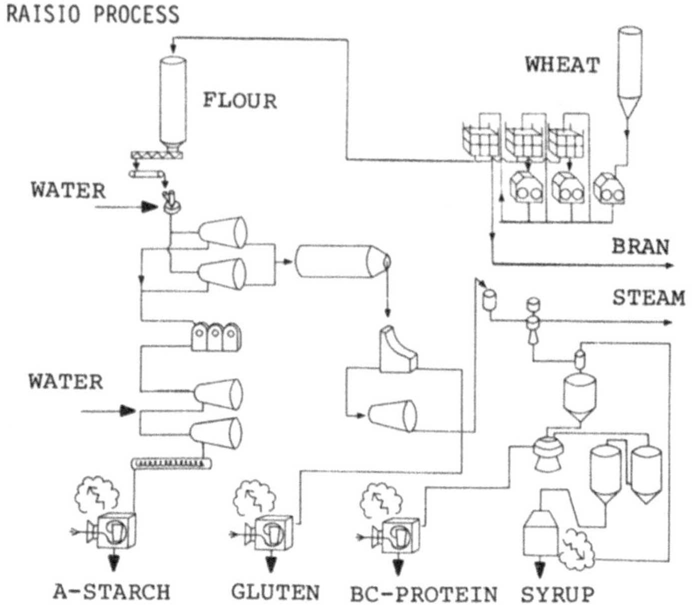

Figure 2. The Raisio Process

3. MINERALS

For human beings, minerals are essential as structural components and in many vital processes. The mineral composition of wheat varies greatly depending on soil, fertilization and climate. Minerals in wheat are to be found principally in the bran fraction (Figure 3) in the aleurone layer as shown in Table 3. Wheat gluten, as part of wheat embryo, contains much fewer minerals than whole wheat and SWP.

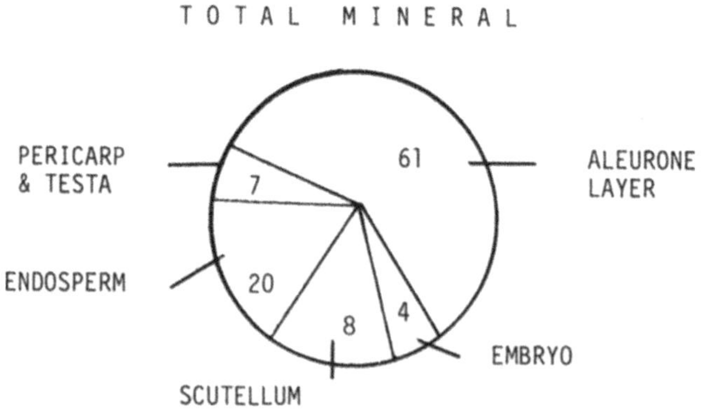

Figure 3. Diagram showing percentages of total mineral in different parts of the wheat kernel (MacMaster et al., 1971)

Table 3. Mineral content of wheat protein products and wheat

		Wheat[3]	Wheat[1] Gluten	SWP[1]	RDA[2]
	total ash, %	1.5	0.6-1.0	2-3	
*	Calcium,mg/100 g	30-41	20-50	180	1.0 g/day
*	Iron, mg/100 g	3.3	3.0	11	18 mg/day
**	Phosphorous, mg/100 g	350-370	100-200	420	1.0 g/day
**	Magnesium, mg/100 g	140	20-35	130	0.4 mg/day
**	Zinc, mg/100 g		2.9	7	15 mg/day
	Selenium[1], mg/100 g (HRW Wheat)	600	1100	580	(50 µg/day)

* minerals which are highly required in nutrition
** minerals which are required in nutrition

1 Private Study, Raision Tehtaat,(1982)
2 Food and Nutrition Board (1974)
3 Feed Uses of Wheat and Its Products, Sanders et al., (1974)

US-RDA (Recommended Daily Allowance) figures have been given to compare wheat protein products with daily human demands.

Wheat is naturally rich in earth metals, such as phosphorous, potassium, magnesium and calcium, but is extremely low in iron, the most important mineral for humans. Because of this, wheat flour in many countries is supplemented with iron. The iron in gluten is on the same level as in wheat. SWP has a little higher figure.

One individual mineral, namely selenium, seems to behave exceptionally by being heavily concentrated in the wheat gluten fraction (see Table 3). This phenomenon might be important in countries where the soil is poor in selenium as for example in Finland. Therefore, as shown in Table 4., if gluten made from selenium rich wheat is added to the Finnish wheat flour at the level of 2-5 %, the selenium content is increased two to three times.

4. VITAMINS

Wheat typically contains vitamins from B-group in addition to small amounts of vitamin E and K. Wheat is totally lacking in vitamins C and D. During the processing of wheat, wheat gluten and SWP are exposed to heat, being dried at 80° C. Consequently the heat sensitive vitamins, thiamine and panthotenic acid lose their activity. This can be seen in Table 5, where the vitamin content of wheat and wheat protein products are shown.

Wheat flour is enriched in many countries in order to obtain quantities of riboflavin, niacin and thiamine in amounts equal to or exceeding those of whole wheat because during milling these vitamins are decreased with separation of bran fraction.

Table 4. The effect of addition of high selenium gluten to the low selenium flour[1]

	Selenium µg/kg
AMERICAN HARD RED WINTER WHEAT (=HRWW)	600
WHEAT GLUTEN MADE FROM HRWW	1100
FINNISH WINTER WHEAT (=FWW)	30
FWW + 2 % GLUTEN HRWW	50
FWW + 5 % GLUTEN HRWW	85

[1] Private Study, Raision Tehtaat, (1982)

Table 5. The average vitamin content of wheat, wheat gluten and SWP

	Wheat[1]	Wheat[2] Gluten	SWP[2]	RDA[3]
* THIAMINE, mg/kg	3.7-5.5	1.0-2.1	2.6	1.4 mg/day
* RIBOFLAVIN, "	1.3-1.7	1.0-1.2	1.0	1.7 "
* NIACIN, "	55-63	27-34	18	20 "
** PANTHOTENIC ACID, mg/kg	9.0-14	1-3	6	5-10 mg/day
** B_6, mg/kg	1.9-2.4	0.9-1.4	1.7	2.0 "

* minerals which are highly required in nutrition
** vitamins which are required in nutrition

1 Feed Uses of Wheat and Its Products, Sanders et al.,(1974)
2 Private Study, Raision Tehtaat, (1983)
3 Food and Nutrition Board, (1974)

5. WHEAT PROTEIN PRODUCTS AND THEIR NUTRITIVE VALUE IN PRACTICAL APPLICATIONS

The production of wheat gluten and SWP is so small that their importance in nutrition remains minimal compared to the use of wheat flour. Only 2 % of the whole wheat production globally is processed into gluten and even smaller amounts into SWP.

Wheat gluten is a typical ingredient of more advanced food products and its use is based on gluten´s functional properties, such as viscoelasticity, water and fat binding properties, film forming and thermosetting properties, rather than on its nutritive value.

The main usage of wheat gluten, constituting 80 % of the gluten market, is to be found in the baking industry. This is because of gluten´s viscoelasticity which improves the baking properties in specialty breads (like high fiber bread, rolls and buns) making it possible to increase the ingredients in bread other than flour, ingredients like fibers, rye-flour etc. This also increases the nutritive value of bread.

Gluten is normally accepted as a similar source of protein to bread. If wheat gluten is used as an ingredient to increase the content of utilizable protein, it must be fortified with lysine, minerals and vitamins before it is acceptable. SWP is more suitable in this respect.

In the developed world where most protein products are used, people consume more protein than they need for nutritional adequacy. In a normal balanced diet therefore wheat protein products can be regarded as containing good quality protein for incorporation in foods.

REFERENCES:

Amino Acid Content of Foods and Biological Data on Proteins /1970/ The Food Policy and Food Science Service, Nutrition Division, FAO Rome pp. 167, 228

Energy and Protein Requirements. Report of a Joint FAO/WHO Ad Hoc Expert Committee /1973/ FAO Nutrition Meetings Rep. Series 52. WHO Tech. Rep. Series 522.

Food and Nutrition Board: Recommended Dietary Allowances /1974/ 8th rev. Washingon, D.C., National Academy of Sciences - National Research Council

Hulse, J.H. and Lang E.M. /1974/ Nutritive Value of Triticale Protein, Monograph IDRC-021e, Canada

MacMaster, M.M., Hinton, J.J.C. & Bradbury, D. /1971/ Microscopic Structure and Composition of the Wheat Kernel Wheat Chemistry and Technology, ed. Pomeranz,Y. American Ass. Cereal Chem., Minnesota, p. 51

Private Study, John Labatt Limited, London, Ontario, Canada /1975/ adopted from J.Am. Oil Chemists Soc. /1979/ March. vol. 56, p. 478

Private Study, Raision Tehtaat, Raisio, Finland /1982/

Private Study, Raision Tehtaat, Raisio, Finland /1983/

Sanders, R.M., Walker, H.G. & Kohler, G.O. /1974/ Feed Uses of Wheat and its Products in Wheat Production and Utilization ed. Inglett, G.E. The AVI Publishing Company Inc. Westport, Connecticut, USA, p. 385

SF-patent No. 61988, The Process for Fractioning Grain-flour into Components of Food Quality

Woerman, J. H. & Safferbe, L.D. /1974/ Food Technology vol. 28, p. 50

Wookey, N. /1979/ Journal of the American Oil Chemists Society, vol. 56, No. 3, p. 307

PART 5
CEREALS IN FOOD AND FEED

Proc. Int. Assoc. Cereal Chem. Symp. Amino Acid Compn and Biol. Value of Cereal Proteins Budapest, Hungary 1983, R. Lásztity, M. Hidvégi, eds

AMINO ACID BIOAVAILABILITY FROM WHOLE-WHEAT FLOUR BREAD AND EXTRACTED WHEAT FLOUR BREAD BY HUMANS

CONSTANCE KIES

Department of Human Nutrition and Food Service Management
316 Ruth Leverton Hall, University of Nebraska, Lincoln,
Nebraska 68583-0807, USA

ABSTRACT

Lysine has been established as being the first limiting amino acid in wheat as it is for most cereal grains for meeting protein nutritional needs of humans. Therefore, it would seem reasonable that wheat cultivar providing grain containing lysine at highest levels per unit of protein would also be of highest protein nutritional quality. Amino acid proportionality patterns are not the same in all fractions of the wheat kernel and these fractions are not equally digestible by the human. Because of the poor digestibility of the bran-germ layers in comparison to the endosperm fraction, lysine contents of the endosperm layer are probably far more important in determining protein quality than are the bran-germ layers. Therefore, extracted wheat flour lysine content is a much better predictor of protein quality for the human than is the lysine content of whole wheat flour regardless of which type of flour is actually to be consumed. Data collected in this laboratory comparing protein quality evaluations of whole and extracted flours from several wheat cultivars using chemical, small animal, adult human and adolescent human assays support this conclusion.

INTRODUCTION

The enthusiasm generated by the discoveries of the nutritional effects of the opaque-2 and flourly-2 genes on the protein quality of maize awakened scientists to the possibilities of nutritional improvement of other cereals (Mertz et al., 1964; Nelson, 1965). It has been well established that lysine is the first limiting amino acid in wheat as well as the first limiting amino acid in several other grains (Kies and Fox, 1970a; Kies, 1972). Therefore, it is not surprising that massive efforts have been undertaken to identify gene materials in wheat and other cereals for protein and lysine differences which might lead to improvement in protein quality and quantity of the cereal species (Inglett, 1972). While increase in quantity of lysine is important in the improvement of wheat protein quality, a second question also has to be addressed. What is the protein and lysine bioavailability from theoretically improved products?

The terminology bioavailability of protein from cereals, or for that matter, from any food product, is really simply new terminology for a reawakening of interest in an old question - that of explaining why sometimes even if protein is present in desirable amounts with a desirable amino acid proportionality pattern the physiological/biochemical response is less than would be expected. Actually this question involves two separate, but related sets of problems: 1) problems associated with the actual digestion (the breaking down) of protein into absorbable units, the timing for absorption of this digestion product, and the absorption mechanism itself; and 2) problems with utilization and metabolism of amino constituents following absorption. Although these definitions are by no means universely accepted, bioavailability refers only to the first of these set of problems while the terminology bioutilization refers to the second set of problems.

In a series of studies conducted in this laboratory, various problems associated with bioavailability of protein from wheat have been conducted. Predictions of protein quality of ground whole wheat flours based on chemical analysis were verified in mouse bioassays; this was also true using human bioassays when the whole wheat flours were from cultivars of closely related genetic lines (Kies, 1975; Kies et al., 1978). However, predictions from chemical assays did not hold true when breads baked from ground whole wheat flours of widely different cultivar lines were evaluated by human bioassay techniques.

Results suggested that differences in digestiblity and bioavailability of protein from the different wheat materials for the human were the cause. When ground whole wheat flours and extracted wheat flours were compared by mouse bioassay, chemical assay values tended to accurately predict actual protein values as determined by this type of bioassay. In human bioassays, chemical assays did predict actual protein values of the extracted wheat flours but not of the ground whole wheat flours. Extracted wheat flours always were better digested in the human subjects than were their ground whole wheat flour counterparts. However, this was not true of the mice. The two types of bioassays were not identical since the flours were fed in the form of bread in the human bioassays while mice received the flours in a non-heat-treated form. Never-the-less, these results suggested that lysine from the bran and germ were probably not available to the human although they evidently were to the mouse.

The objective of the last study in this series was to compare the protein value of whole wheat flour, extracted wheat flour, and lysine enriched extracted flour from two lines of winter wheat for human adults.

EXPERIMENTAL PLAN

As shown in Table 1, the 35-day study was divided into a nitrogen depletion period, a nitrogen adjustment period, and 6 experimental periods of 5-days each. During the nitrogen depletion period, nitrogen intake was maintained at 1.12 g N/day in order to deplete subjects who customarily consume relatively high protein diets to the low protein content necessary for research evaluations. This technique in this laboratory has been found to reduce time required for subjects to reach a steady state of nitrogen excretion. The depletion period was followed by a nitrogen adjustment period during which the same level of nitrogen was fed from a mixture of all 6 flour types used in the following experimental periods.

During the six, 5-day experimental periods, bread made from six different flour types were fed. Grain from two wheat cultivars were whole ground or 72% extracted ground. The flours were analyzed for nitrogen and lysine contents. The extracted wheat flours were fed either alone or with lysine supplements added at a level to equalize the extracted wheat flours to the counterpart whole wheat flours. Thus, grain from each cultivar was fed in the form of whole wheat flour bread, 72% extracted wheat flour bread and 72% extracted wheat flour with added crystalline L-lysine bread. All were fed to provide 6.0 g N/subject/day. Since flours varied in protein content, this meant that various amounts of flour were fed. Wheat starch was used to equalize intake at 200 g flour + starch/subject/day.

The flours were incorporated into a yeast-risen bread product. The rest of the laboratory controlled diet provided 1.12 g N/subject/day and is described in Table 1. Vitamin and mineral supplements were fed so that recommended intakes for adult humans as set by the Food and Nutrition Board of the National Research Council were met.

Table 1

Experimental Plan

Period[1]	No. of Days	Flour Type[2]	N Intake, g/day		
			Diet[3]	Flour	Total
Depletion	2	Starch	1.12	--	1.12
Adjustment	3	Mixed flours	1.12	6.0	7.12
Expt. 1	5	Cultivar 1 - whole wheat	1.12	6.0	7.12
Expt. 2	5	Cultivar 1 - extracted	1.12	6.0	7.12
Expt. 3	5	Cultivar 1 - extracted + lysine	1.12	6.0	7.12
Expt. 4	5	Cultivar 2 - whole wheat	1.12	6.0	7.12
Expt. 5	5	Cultivar 2 - extracted	1.12	6.0	7.12
Expt. 6	5	Cultivar 2 - extracted + lysine	1.12	6.0	7.12

[1]Experimental periods randomized for each of the 10 adult human subjects.

[2]Flour and starch were incorporated into a yeast bread product.

[3]The low protein basal diet included in addition to the bread - sucrose; butter oil; applesauce, 100g; green beans, 100g; pears, 100g; peaches, 100g; stewed tomatoes; vitamin and mineral supplements. Calorie intake was maintained adequate to maintain weight for each subject by varying intakes of sucrose, hard candy, and soft drinks.

The eight women and two men who were subjects for this study ranged in age from 19 to 28 years and were in normal health as judged by health histories and/or physical examinations as evaluated by the medical staff of the University of Nebraska Health Center. All the volunteers (signing of consent forms required as a condition of participation) were students or employees of the University of Nebraska. All lived in their own housing accomodations but ate meals in the metabolism unit of this department. The project received University of Nebraska clearance for human subject participation.

Subjects made complete collections of urine and stools throughout the study. Urines were composited into 24-hour lots for each subject and were sampled for analyses. Feces were divided into period lots representing food eaten for each period on the basis of the appearance of fecal dye markers (carmine red and brilliant blue) given at the beginning and end of each experimental period. Feces were blended and sampled for analyses.

Creatinine contents of daily urine collections were used to determine accuracy of urine collections for each subject. Nitrogen content of feces, urine, breads, and food were determined by the Kjeldahl method (Scales and Harrison, 1920). This information was used to calculate nitrogen balances and protein digestibilities. Data was subjected to statistical analyses including analysis of variance and Duncan's Multiple Range Test.

RESULTS AND DISCUSSION

Mean results of this study are shown in Table 2. In the present study, nitrogen intake was maintained at a somewhat higher level than is customarily used in studies of this type. In order to assess protein quality, protein intake must be less than adequate. Otherwise, variations in quality cannot be determined. However, if diets are too severely deficient, changes in quality are also difficult to determine with accuracy. Since nitrogen balances were only slightly positive or actually negative, intakes could be classified as marginally negative in the present study.

Whole wheat flours from grain of cultivars 1 and 2 were considerably higher in lysine content than were their extracted flour counterparts on the basis of lysine content as a percentage of protein content. This would indicate that much of the improved lysine content provided by these two cultivars was due to changes in proteins in the germ and aleurone layers which were removed in the extraction milling of the bran. However, in cases of both cultivar grains, the crude digestibility of the extracted wheat flours were considerably better than were those for their whole wheat counterparts (79% versus 70% for cultivar 1 and 74% versus 62% for cultivar 2).

In both cases, the extracted wheat flour breads gave nitrogen balances which were equal to or slightly better (but not statistically significantly so) than their whole wheat counterparts. Feeding of the lysine supplemented extracted flours in both cases resulted in a statistically significant improvement in nitrogen balances of the subjects. These results suggest that protein including lysine is poorly available from the bran layer.

Results of this study are supported by results from other studies from this laboratory which indicate that nutrients from bran are poorly utilized or not utilized at all by the human (Kies, 1982; 1980; Kies et al., 1981; Mason et al., 1983; McEndree et al., 1983; Flewelling et al., 1983; Johnson et al., 1983; Downes et al., 1982; Bizem et al., 1983; Witte et al., 1982; Kies et al., 1979a; Kies et al., 1979b).

Thus, concern over loss of nutrients in the milling process probably have been overemphasized. This does not, of course, address the possible importance of fiber from wheat bran in human diets.

Another possible conclusion is in relationship to wheat breeding programs directly aimed at improving nutritional value of wheat grain for human consumption. Because of the poor availability of protein, lysine, vitamins and minerals from wheat bran, it is probably unwise to assume that an apparent increase in nutrient content of the whole wheat flour may or may not denote an increase in the actual nutritional value of the cereal for humans. A better index of this would probably be an analysis of the extracted milled flour. Obviously, a first step in nutritional improvement of cereals for human consumption is the increase in nutrient content. However, the question of whether or not these nutrients can be absorbed from the human gastrointestinal tract must not be ignored.

Table 2

Protein Quality of Whole Wheat Flour, Extracted Wheat Flour, and Lysine-Enriched Flour

Cultivar	Flour Type	Lysine Content	Crude Protein Digestibility	Nitrogen Balance[1]
		% Protein	%	g N/day
1	Whole wheat	2.9	70^{b}	-0.17^{bc}
	Extracted	2.1	79^{a}	-0.12^{b}
	Extracted + lysine	2.9	79^{a}	$+0.20^{a}$
2	Whole wheat	3.1	62^{c}	-0.33^{c}
	Extracted	2.2	74^{ab}	-0.21^{bc}
	Extracted + lysine	3.1	75^{ab}	$+0.12^{a}$

[1]Fed to provide 6.0 g N/day to human adults from wheat flour and 1.12 g N/day from the remainder of the diet.

REFERENCES

Bizem, H.R., Kies, C. and Fox, H.M. 1983. Vitamin B_6 bioavailability from wheat bran and iron supplemented diets. Fed. Proc. 42:1066. Abstract No. 4537.

DeBrie, K., Kies, C., McEndree, L. and Fox, H.M. 1984. Protein utilization from bran supplemented vegetarian and omnivore diets by vegetarian and omnivore subjects. Fed. Proc. 43(3): 470.

Downes, A., Ppapkyrikos, H., Kies, C. and Fox, H.M. 1982. Magnesium utilization of humans as affected by level and type of dietary wheat bran supplementation. Nebr. Acad. of Sci. annual meeting. Abstract No. 82-1694.

Drews, L.M., Kies, C. and Fox, H.M. 1979. Effect of dietary fiber on copper, zinc and magnesium utilization by adolescent boys. Am. J. Clin. Nutr. 32:1893.

Inglett, G.E. (ed.) 1972. Seed Proteins (Symposium). Westport, Conn.: AVI Press, 320 p.

Jank, J., Kies, C. and Fox, H.M. 1981. Protein nutritional status of human subjects fed wheat and rice bran supplemented diets. Nutr. Reports Int. 24:581.

Kies, C. 1972. Evaluation of the protein value of cereal/plant/oilseed products by human biological assay techniques. In: Seed Proteins (Symposium); ed. by G.E. Inglett. Westport, Conn: AVI Press, p. 256.

Kies, C. 1975. Comparative protein nutritive values of whole ground and white flours from five wheat varieties for humans. Milling and Baking Division, American Association of Cereal Chemists, Spring Conference, Fort Worth, Texas.

Kies, C. 1980. Bioavailability of proteins and fats. Institute of Food Technologists annual meeting; Symposium: Cereal Grain Products - Bioavailability of Nutrients.

Kies, C. 1981a. Edible fiber: practical problems. Contemporary Nutr. General Mills, Inc.

Kies, C. 1981b. Bioavailability: a factor in protein quality. J. Agric. Food Chem. 29:435-440.

Kies, C. 1982. Vitamin utilization by humans from bread. Amer. Bakers Association Technical Liason Committee, U.S.D.A. Western Regional Research Center, Albany, CA.

Kies, C. 1984. Calcium bioavailability in diets modified to meet U.S. Dietary Guidelines in fat and fiber content. In: Calcium Bioavailability: Effect of Selected Dietary Factors, ed. by C. Kies (in preparation).

Kies, C. and Fox, H.M. 1970a. Determination of first limiting amino acid of wheat and triticale grain for humans. Cereal Chem. 48:129.

Kies, C. and Fox, H.M. 1970b. Protein nutritive value of wheat and triticale grain for humans, studied at two levels of protein intake. Cereal Chem. 47:671.

Kies, C. and Fox, H.M. 1981. Iron utilization from AACC hard red spring wheat bran. American Assoc. of Cereal Chemists annual meeting.

Kies, C. and McEndree, L. 1982. Vegetarianism and the bioavailability of iron. In: Nutritional Bioavailability of Iron, ed. by C. Kies; American Chemical Society Symposium Series No. 203, p. 183.

Kies, C., Fox, H.M., Mattern, P.J., Johnson, V.A. and Schmidt, J.W. 1978. Comparative protein quality as measured by human and small animal bioassays of three lines of winter wheat. In: Nutritional Improvement of Food and Feed Proteins, ed. by M. Friedman, Plenum Press: Advances in Experimental Medicine and Biology. 105:91.

Kies, C., Drews, L. and Fox, H.M. 1979a. Copper, zinc, and magnesium nutritional status of adolescent boys as affected by dietary fiber. XI International Congress of Nutrition, Rio de Janeiro, Brazil.

Kies, C., Fox, H.M. and Vaughan, L. 1979b. Iron nutritional status of human adults as affected by dietary cellulose, hemicellulose and wheat bran. Proc. of annual meeting of Institute of Food Technologists p. 173.

Kies, C., Beshgetoor, C. and Fox, H.M. 1981. Dietary fiber and zinc bioavailability for humans. In: Antinutrients and Natural Toxicants in Foods, ed. by R.L. Ory; Food and Nutrition Press, Inc. p. 319.

Kies, C., Kan, S., and Fox, H.M. 1981. Vitamin B_6 availability from wheat, corn and rice brans for humans. Inst. of Food Technologists annual meeting.

Kies, C., Young, E. and McEndree, L. 1983. Zinc bioavailability from vegetarian diets: influence of dietary fiber, ascorbic acid and past dietary practices. In: Bioavailability of Zinc; ed. by G.E. Inglett, American Chemical Society Symposium Series No. 210, p. 115.

Lo, B.F., Kies, C. and Fox, H.M. 1979. Wheat, corn and rice bran supplementation of diets as factors in the zinc and copper nutritional status of humans. Proc. of The American Dietetic Association annual meeting.

Mason, K., Kan, S., Kies, C. and Fox, H.M. 1983. Vitamin B_6 utilization from extracted wheat flour bread with and without bran supplements. Proc. Nebr. Acad. of Sci., p. 26.

McCance, R.A. and Walsham. 1948. The digestibility and absorption of the calories, protein, fats and calcium in wholemeal wheaten bread. Brit. J. Nutr. 2:26.

McEndree, L.S., Kies, C. and Fox, H.M. 1983. Iron utilization from wheat bran by lacto-ovo-vegetarians and omnivores. Fed. Proc. 42: 1180. Abstract No. 5205.

Mertz, E.T., Bates, L.S. and Nelson, O.E. 1964. Mutant gene that changes protein composition and increases lysine content of maize endosperm. Science 145:279.

Nelson, O.E., Mertz, E.T. and Bates, L.S. 1965. Second mutant gene affecting amino acid pattern of maize endosperm proteins. Science 150:1469.

Nnakwe, N., Kies, C. and Fox, H.M. 1984. Calcium and phosphorus nutritional status of lacto-ovo-vegetarian and omnivore students consuming meals in a lacto-ovo-vegetarian food service. Nutr. Reports Int. (accepted, in press).

Scales, F.M. and Harrison, A.P. 1977. Boric acid modifications of the Kjeldahl method for crops and feeds. J. Eng. Chem. 12:356.

Trimbo, S., Kathman, J., Kies, C. and Fox, H.M. 1979. Pantothenic acid nutritional status of adolescent humans as affected by dietary fiber and bran. Fed. Proc. 38:556.

Unver, B., Kies, C. and Fox, H.M. 1981. Niacin/pantothenic acid/ protein interrelationships affecting the nutritive value of winter wheat for humans. Nutr. Reports Int. 23:841.

Witte, C., Kies, C., Fox, H.M. and McEndree, L. 1982. Pantothenic acid utilization from wheat bran by omnivore and lacto-ovo-vegetarians fed lacto-vegetarian, vegan and omnivore diets. Amer. Dietetic Assoc. annual meeting.

Supported by Nebr. Agricultural Experiment Station Project 91-024 and by U.S.D.A., C.S.R.S. Regional Research Project W-143.

Proc. Int. Assoc. Cereal Chem. Symp. Amino Acid Compn and Biol. Value of Cereal Proteins Budapest, Hungary 1983, R. Lásztity, M. Hidvégi, eds

AMINO ACID INDICES AND RAT BIODATA FOR COMPOSITE FLOUR BREADS FORTIFIED WITH LEGUME AND OILSEED PROTEINS AND LYSINE

F. W. SOSULSKI, S. E. FLEMING*

Department of Crop Science and Plant Ecology, University of Saskatchewan, Saskatoon, Sask. S7N OWO, Canada
*Department of Nutritional Sciences, University of California, Berkeley, California 94720, USA

ABSTRACT

The protein quality of breads fortified with sunflower protein concentrate (SFC) , soybean flour (SBF), fababean protein concentrate (FBC) and field pea protein concentrate (FPC) were investigated by amino acid analyses and rat growth assays. Compared to the value of 1.1 for the wheat flour bread, SBF, FBC and FPC breads gave high PER's of 1.7 to 1.8. Due to low lysine in SFC, the PER for the SFC bread diet was only 1.3. The bread diets were limiting in lysine and its supplementation at 4 g/100 g protein caused marked increases in protein nutritive value as evidenced by an increase in PER from 1.1 to 2.2 for the wheat control.

Based on human requirements, the amino acid scores of protein-supplemented breads were 50-66% as compared to 45% for the control bread. Lysine supplementation increased the amino acid scores of the control, SFC and SBF to 73-78% based on threonine deficiency but scores for FBC and FPC remained at 63-68% due to limitations in tryptophan.

Amino acid scores based on human requirements gave better prediction of rat assay data than scores based on the reference egg protein or rat requirements. The correlation coefficient between amino acid score and feed intake, weight gains, PER and NPR varied between r = 0.86** to 0.94**. It appeared that amino acid indices would be as useful as rat biodata in predicting the protein nutritive value of cereal-legume blends for human consumption.

INTRODUCTION

In previous studies, Sarwar (1973) determined that amino acid (chemical) scores as high as 60% could be obtained consistently by adjusting the proportions of cereals and grain legumes in composite flour blends. Maximum co-supplementation of wheat- and rice-based diets for weanling rats occurred when the ratios of cereal protein to legume protein were about 50:50 (Sarwar et al., 1975). To achieve the desired proportions of proteins in the diets, the ratios of grain legume to cereal were 1:2.5 in rice-based diets and 1:1.5 for the wheat-based diet. It appeared that the latter ratio of legume to wheat flour in the diet would be prohibitive from a functional and economic standpoint.

High proportions of supplementary protein could be incorporated into cereal-based diets more effectively by utilizing concentrated plant protein products. Certain oilseed flours and protein concentrates are available commercially. Also air classified protein concentrates are now being prepared from grain legumes after dehulling and pin milling of the seed (Sosulski and Youngs, 1979). In the present investigation, bread formulations were developed to contain high proportions of legume and oilseed protein supplements that were consistent with satisfactory loaf characteristics. Based on loaf volume, specific volume, crumb grain, crumb compressibility and loaf shape, breads with high protein content and satisfactory loaf properties were formulated with 15% soybean flour, fababean protein concentrate or field pea protein concentrate in the flour blends (Fleming and Sosulski, 1977). The same bread protein levels were obtained using 12% sunflower protein concentrate which had been processed to remove the chromogen, chlorogenic acid. The ratios of legume or oilseed protein to wheat protein in these breads were about 1:1.65.

In the present paper, the amino acid indices, amino acid (AA) score and essential amino acid index (EAAI), of the composite flour breads were calculated relative to egg protein, rat and human requirements. Protein efficiency ratios (PER) were determined in rat feeding trials in which the composite flour breads were the sole source of protein. Since lysine (lys) was the first limiting amino acid in all diets except the casein control, a second series of breads were prepared with 4% added L-lys in order to assess the effects of the second limiting amino acid in the bread diets.

MATERIALS AND METHODS

The wheat flour used in this study was commercially-milled from hard red spring wheat, 74% rate of extraction, with a high protein content (15.9%). Dehulled sunflower kernels were subjected to aqueous extraction (pH 4.5, 4 hr, 60°C) to remove chlorogenic acid, dried and defatted to produce a 76% protein concentrate. Soybeans were defatted with hexane to give a 50.5% protein flour. The fababean and field-pea protein concentrates were prepared by pin milling and air classification to yield fine fractions containing 61.1% and 56.5% protein, resp.

The breadmaking formula included 100 g flour (14% moisture basis), 4 g nonfat dry milk, 3 g sucrose, 1.75 g salt, 0.1 g ammonium phosphate monobasic, 10 ppm potassium bromate, 0.3 g malt syrup and water as required. For supplemented formulations, the wheat flour was replaced by the protein component(s) so that the total flour blend was 100 g. The dough was prepared by the straight dough procedure and baked at 220°C for 25 min.

Protein quality evaluations were conducted on blends of wheat flour: supplementary protein. gluten of 100:0:0 for the control wheat-flour bread (WF), 83:15:2 for soybean (SBF), fababean (FBC) and field-pea bread (FPC), and 86:12:2 for sunflower bread (SFC). In addition, the blends were baked with lys monohydrate (95% L-lys, 5% D-lys) in sufficient quantities to add 4.0 g L-lys/100 g protein. ANRC casein, with and without lys, was used as a control in the rat feeding trial.

The amino acid analyses were conducted on a Beckman Model 120C amino acid analyzer with separate hydrolyses for the sulfur-containing amino acid and tryptophan (try) determinations. Methionine and cystine (met + cys) were measured as methionine sulfone and cysteic acid, resp. AA scores and EAAI of the diets were calculated from the amino acid data. Reference proteins were based on either nine EAA values, namely histidine (his), isoleucine (ile), leucine (leu), lys, met + cys, phenylalanine + tyrosine (phe + tyr), threonine (thr), try and valine (val), or ten EAA values including arginine (arg). The amino acid compositions of the reference proteins and requirements are given in Table 1. The human requirement is based on the individual requirements of the infant, child and adult (NRC, 1980).

Table 1. EAA composition of the reference protein or species requirements (g amino acid/100 g protein)

EAA	Whole egg[1]	Rat requirements[2]	Human requirements[3]
Arg	6.1	5.0	-
His	2.4	2.5	1.7
Ile	6.3	4.6	4.2
Leu	8.8	6.2	7.0
Lys	7.0	7.5	5.1
Met + cys	5.8	5.0	2.6
Phe + tyr	9.9	6.7	7.3
Thr	5.1	4.2	3.5
Try	1.5	1.3	1.1
Val	6.9	5.0	4.8

[1]FAO (1970). [2]NAS (1972). [3]NRC (1980).

Diets for the rat growth study were formulated to contain 10% protein (N x 6.25) with corn oil, cellulose, vitamins, minerals and corn starch being added so that each diet contained 8% fat, 5% fiber, 1% vitamins and 5% ash. The isocaloric diets were fed to weanling male rats (40-50 g) in a seven-replicate factorial experiment during a 4-week period. In addition, one group of rats was fed a N-free diet, and the weights of both groups were recorded after 10 days for the calculation of net protein ratio (NPR) as well as the conventional 28-day PER assay. Weight gains were adjusted by regression to equal feed intake to determine the direct effects of protein quality on gains.

RESULTS AND DISCUSSION

Bread composition

The breads fortified with protein supplements had 21.9-23.3% protein compared to 15.9% for the control wheat-flour bread (Table 2). The lysine-supplemented breads were about 0.5% higher in protein content, based on Kjeldahl N x 6.25.

Compared to raw casein, the control and protein-supplemented breads were low in most EAA, especially lys, try and thr (Table 2). WF and SFC breads were particularly low in lys, and FBC and FPC breads contained less met + cys than the other breads.

Supplementation of the breads (and diets) with L-lys resulted in marked increases in lys, from 2.4-3.5 g to 5.7 - 6.3 g amino acid/100 g protein, which resulted in a slight decrease in the proportions of other EAA. Note that supplementation with 4.0 g L-lys per 100 g protein increased casein by 3.8% lys but the breads showed increases of only 2.8 to 3.3% lys due to partial destruction during baking.

Table 2. Protein (%), EAA (g amino acid/100 g protein) for casein and breads containing protein and lys supplements, dry basis

Protein ingredients	Protein[2]	Arg	His	Ile	Leu	Lys	Met + cys	Phe + tyr	Thr	Try	Val
Casein	90.7	3.5	2.9	5.2	9.6	8.2	3.1	11.3	4.3	2.6	7.1
WF (100:0:0)[1]	15.9	2.9	1.9	3.5	6.6	2.4	4.2	7.1	2.7	0.9	4.0
SFC (86:12:2)	23.2	4.7	2.1	3.7	6.5	2.6	3.7	6.9	2.9	0.9	4.3
SBF (83:15:2)	21.9	4.4	2.1	3.6	6.8	3.5	3.9	7.6	3.0	1.0	4.1
FBC (83:15:2)	23.3	5.1	2.1	3.5	6.6	3.4	3.3	7.3	2.9	0.9	4.1
FPC (83:15:2)	22.3	5.5	2.0	3.5	6.6	3.4	3.5	7.1	2.9	0.8	3.9
Casein + lys	89.8	2.6	2.4	4.6	8.5	10.3	2.9	7.9	3.9	2.5	5.7
WF + lys (100:0:0)	16.3	3.0	2.0	3.2	6.2	5.7	4.1	7.0	2.5	0.8	3.7
SFC + lys (86:12:2)	23.9	5.0	2.0	3.4	5.9	5.7	3.8	6.7	2.7	0.9	4.1
SBF + lys (83:15:2)	22.9	4.1	2.0	3.3	6.2	6.3	3.6	7.0	2.8	1.1	3.8
FBC + lys (83:15:2)	23.6	4.8	2.0	3.3	6.3	6.3	3.2	6.7	2.7	0.8	4.0
FPC + lys (83:15:2)	23.1	5.3	1.8	3.3	6.2	6.2	3.2	6.6	2.7	0.7	3.7

[1]Ratio of wheat flour: legume or oilseed: vital wheat gluten.

[2]N x 6.25

The values for AA score and first limiting amino acid for each protein source in the diets are presented in Table 3. The AA scores for the control WF bread, relative to egg protein and rat requirements, were only 32-34% but for human requirements was 45%. The supplemented breads were still deficient in lys and gave AA scores of 35-49% against egg and rat references and 50-66% relative to the human reference. Based on the three indices, the bread diets were ranked in the order of WF< SFC< SBF = FBC = FPC.

Supplementation with lys increased the AA scores for WF bread into the same range as the values for protein-supplemented breads containing added lys (Table 3). However, thr deficiency limited the scores based on egg and rat references to 50-67% except for the try-deficient FPC + lys bread (45-53%). Compared to human requirements, the lys supplementation increased the AA scores of WF, SFC and SBF to 73-78% while those of FBC and FPC were unchanged due to try deficiency.

Table 3. AA scores and EAAI for casein and bread diets based on the EAA in reference proteins

Protein source	Amino acid score, %			Essential amino acid index		
	Egg	Rat	Human	Egg	Rat	Human
Casein	52.6[S1]	61.0[S]	100.0[0]	85.7	91.7	100.0
WF	33.7[L]	31.5[L]	45.4[L]	58.6	70.3	82.5
SFC	37.6[L]	35.0[L]	50.6[L]	60.6	76.3	85.1
SBF	49.4[L]	46.1[L]	66.5[L]	66.6	79.2	90.1
FBC	48.1[L]	44.9[L]	64.8[L]	63.2	76.3	86.9
FPC	48.9[L]	45.6[L]	65.8[L]	63.1	67.3	85.4
Casein+lys	42.6[A]	52.0[A]	100.0[0]	77.2	87.5	100.0
WF + lys	49.8[Th]	60.4[Th]	72.5[Th]	62.3	75.3	86.7
SFC + lys	53.3[Th]	64.8[Th]	77.7[Th]	66.6	80.9	88.9
SBF + lys	54.9[Th]	66.6[Th]	78.1[V]	66.9	80.9	90.8
FBC + lys	52.9[Th]	58.6[Tr]	68.1[Tr]	63.9	78.1	86.9
FPC + lys	46.0[Tr]	53.1[Tr]	62.7[Tr]	62.8	76.6	85.1
Average	47.5	51.7	71.0	66.5	78.4	89.0

[1]Limiting amino acid designations: 0 = no limiting amino acid; A = arginine; L = lysine; S = methionine + cystine; Th = threonine; Tr = tryptophan; V = valine.

The EAAI demonstrated a narrow range of values among the breads and there was no clear distinction between the values for the control WF and protein-supplemented breads (Table 3). Also, lys-supplementation failed to increase the EAAI values more than a few units in most cases.

In the rat assays there were marked, significant differences in feed intake, weight gain, PER and NPR among the bread diets (Table 4). Considering all parameters measured, the bread diets could be ranked in the order of WF<SFC<SBF = FBC<FPC. After adjustment for feed intake, the weight gains of rats fed any of the three legume proteins which were rich in lys resulted in two times the gains obtained with the control WF. On the other hand, the SFC, with only intermediate lys content, failed to increase weight gains significantly above the control. The pattern of protein utilization was similar, with the adjusted PER for SFC of 1.3 being similar to that of WF at 1.1 while legume-supplemented breads had PER values of 1.7-1.8.

Table 4. Feed intake, weight gain and protein utilization by rats fed protein- and lys-supplemented breads for 28 days

Protein source	Feed intake (g)	Weight gain (g)	Adjusted wt. gain (g)	PER	Adjusted PER	NPR
Casein	398.1a[1]	114.6a	104.8a	2.60a	2.50	3.93a
WF	212.7g	24.9f	32.3f	1.13f	1.09	2.56d
SFC	235.1fg	32.0f	41.0ef	1.32e	1.27	2.80c
SBF	298.5cd	55.2e	66.3cd	1.76d	1.69	2.85c
FBC	297.1cde	56.1e	65.3cd	1.74d	1.67	2.91c
FPC	311.7cd	56.8e	71.0c	1.88c	1.81	3.05c
Casein+lys	356.5b	101.5b	88.5b	2.68a	2.58	3.91a
WF + lys	259.3ef	61.7de	50.5de	2.24b	2.15	3.54b
SFC + lys	286.3de	66.9d	61.1cd	2.23b	2.14	3.55b
SBF + lys	330.0bc	82.1c	78.1bc	2.30b	2.21	3.42b
FBC + lys	322.0bcd	80.0c	75.0bc	2.33b	2.24	3.62b
FPC + lys	302.1cd	69.5d	67.2cd	2.34b	2.25	3.51b

[1]Means with the same letter do not differ significantly ($P<0.05$).

AA scores based on egg ratios gave low significant correlations with rat performance data ($r = 0.56^*$ to 0.66^*)(Table 5). AA scores based on rat requirements gave better prediction of weight gain, PER and NPR ($r = 74^{**}$ to 0.84^{**}) but not feed intake or adjusted weight gain ($r = 0.60^*$). Surprisingly, the AA scores based on human requirements gave excellent prediction of rat feed intake, weight gains and protein utilization measurements ($r = 0.86^{**}$ to 0.94^{**}). The EAAI tended to be more highly correlated with feed intake than PER and NPR ($r = 0.68^*$ to 0.72^{**}) and represented no improvement over prediction by means of the first limiting amino acid. Generally the interrelationships among the rat assay values were highly significant. NPR measured on the 10th day of the feeding trial showed a correlation coefficient of 0.97^{**} with PER measured on the 28th day.

CONCLUSIONS

These results demonstrate that a shorter feeding period than the common 28-day test for PER may be sufficient for routine purposes. Also the number of parameters measured on the rat could be reduced because of the close relation of growth rate to feed intake and PER. However, the high correlation of AA score based on human requirements with rat assay values provides strong evidence for giving AA scores the same status as biodata for expressing the protein nutritive value of proteins in human diets.

Table 5. Correlation matrix for EAA indices and rat growth performance for protein- and lys- supplemented breads

Parameter	AA score			EAAI			Feed intake	Weight gain	Adj.wt. gain	PER
	Egg	Rat	Human	Egg	Rat	Human				
AA score										
-rat	0.87**									
-human	0.53	0.69*								
EAAI										
- egg	0.35	0.45	0.91**							
- rat	0.35	0.53	0.84**	0.89**						
- human	0.32	0.45	0.94**	0.96**	0.91**					
Feed intake	0.62*	0.60*	0.87**	0.86**	0.73**	0.83**				
Weight gain	0.61	0.74**	0.94**	0.87**	0.82**	0.86**	0.95**			
Adj. wt. gain	0.62*	0.60*	0.87**	0.86**	0.73**	0.83**	0.99**	0.94**		
PER	0.66*	0.84**	0.87**	0.69*	0.68*	0.70**	0.82**	0.94**	0.82**	
NPR	0.56*	0.81**	0.86**	0.71**	0.72**	0.71**	0.75**	0.91**	0.75**	0.97**

*Significant at P = 0.05. **Significant at P = 0.01.

REFERENCES

FAO. 1970. Amino acid contents of foods and biological data on proteins. FAO nutritional studies No. 24. Food and Agric. Organization of the United Nations. Rome.

Fleming, S.E. and Sosulski, F.W. 1977. Breadmaking properties of four concentrated plant proteins. Cereal Chem. 54: 1124-1140.

National Academy of Sciences (NAS). 1972. Nutrient Requirements of domestic animals. No. 10. Nutrient requirements of laboratory animals. 2nd Ed. Printing and Publishing Office, N.A.S., Washington, D.C.

NRC. 1980. Recommended dietary allowances. 9th ed. National Research Council, Nat. Acad. Sci., Washington, D.C.

Sarwar, G. 1973. Protein quality determinations of legumes and cereal-legume blends. Ph.D. thesis. Department of Crop Science, University of Saskatchewan, Saskatoon, Sask. Canada.

Sarwar, G., Sosulski, F.W. and Holt, N.W. 1975. Protein nutritive value of legume-cereal blends. Can. Inst. Food Sci. Technol. J. 8: 170-174.

Sosulski, F. and Youngs, C.G. 1979. Yield and functional properties of air-classified protein and starch fractions from eight legume flours. J. Amer. Oil Chem. Soc. 56: 292-295.

Proc. Int. Assoc. Cereal Chem. Symp. Amino Acid Compn and Biol. Value of Cereal Proteins Budapest, Hungary 1983, R. Lásztity, M. Hidvégi, eds

FORTIFICATION OF WHEAT FLOUR WITH POTATO PROTEIN

K. LINDNER

Nutrition Department, College of Commerce and Catering Trade, H-1054 Budapest, Alkotmány 9/11, Hungary

ABSTRACT

The biological value of the cereal proteins, the consumption rate of the cereal products and the factors influencing the cereal protein utilization have been investigated.

One of the purposes of the supplementation of the low quality protein is to avoid the unbalanced, monoton nutrition first of all by most "vulnerable" groups of population /e.g. children, pregnant and lactating women/. By menu planning it is required to take into consideration the consumed food complex and also the "time-factor" of supplementation. The protein supplementation with meals results in a better physiological effect which, in turn, should hardly be predicted from experiments with individual protein sources, because of the complementary patterns of amino acids.

INTRODUCTION

The cereal protein consumption in the developing countries is more than 50 % of the total protein, but actually, in the developed countries also reaches the 30 % as is shown in Table 1. The Hungarian consumption level is between these two values, about 40 %.

The reason of the high proportion of the cereal protein is its very low cost. In the point of view of the modern nutrition it is suitable to investigate the cereal proteins as definitive proteins of the future, too.

The proteins of cereals are considered to be incomplete for human beings because of the relative lack of two essential amino acids, namely lysine and tryptophan. The fact is that only twofold amount of bread protein is able to assure the nitrogen balance on the same level as egg protein. In the data of Fig. 1., a very big deviation of the nitrogen balance values existing in the literature /Sherman,1920/ is demonstrated.

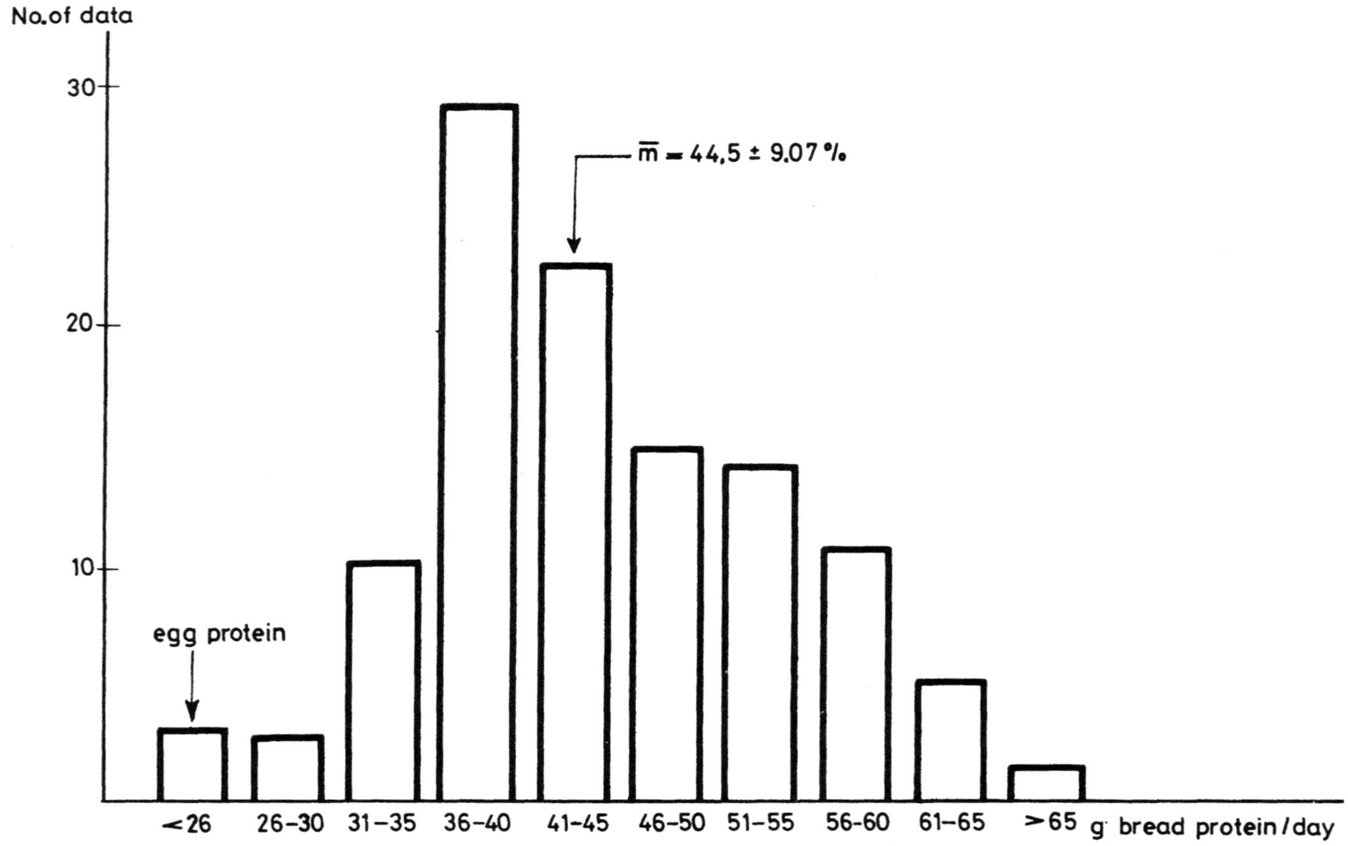

Fig.1. Different data concerning the protein requirement of a 70 kg weight man

Table 1. Food proteins in the daily diet /%/.

Protein source	Industrialized countries	Hungary	Developing countries
Cereals	32	43	52
Pulse, roots	9	3	26
Meat	25	29	8
Fish	4	1	4
Egg	4	5	1
Milk	21	13	6
Vegetables, fruits	5	6	3

Among others, for the different values, probably in the first place are responsible the wide variance of the investigated subjects, but in the second place exist, adjoining to the static factors, several dinamic factors,- as energy - protein ratio, adaptation fenomenon etc. -, too /Hegsted 1978/. /Table 2./

Table 2. Factors influencing protein requirement.

S T A T I C factors:
- body-weight,-composition,
- age,
- gravidity, lactation etc.,

D I N A M I C factors:
- food consumption structure,
- activity,
- adaptation,

In any case, the "vulnerable" groups of the population need the most serious attention on the incomplete amino acid patterns of the cereal proteins and the supplementation possibilities with high quality protein sources. It is well known, that in the case of bread the lysine and tryptophan fortification is a common application. But this method is expensive and in the case of healthy adults, at least, unnecessary. For the planification of the menu or meals, it is suitable to combine the cereals with protein sources with supplementation effects. This proteins are very expensive from the point of view of their protein-specific price /Table 3/.

Table 3. The protein-specific price of foods /price of food containing 100 g of protein/.

Food	Price in Ft	Food	Price in Ft
Wheat flour	5	Egg	40
Bread	6	Chicken meat	45
Milk	20	Beef meat /rumpst./	50
Cheese	25	Pork meat	60

But in Hungary there exists a cheaper source of high quality protein, too. This possibility is the combination of the cereal flour with mashed potatoes, in some traditionally consumed meals and cereal products.

METHODS FOR DETERMINING THE SUPPLEMENTATION EFFECTS

The supplementation experiments have been accomplished with experimental laboratory rats, in both sexes about 80-90 g of body weight. 8 male and 8 female rats have been enlisted in three experimental groups, in separate cages. The first group of rats has been fed only with wheat flour protein, the second with a mixture of potato protein and wheat flour protein, in ratio and form existing in the so-called potatonoodes. The third group of animals has been fed with casein as reference protein. Each group in the feedstuffs had the same proportion of nutrients, as shown in Table 4.

Table 4. The nutrient composition in the animal-experiments.

Nutrient	%
Carbohydrate	80.4
Fat	4.6
Protein	11.0
Salt mixture	2.0
Vitamin mixture	2.0

In contrary to the first experiment, in which the mashed potato and wheat flour ratio was 1:1, in the second experiment it was lower, 1:4, only.

The protein efficiency ratio /PER/ values, collected in Fig.2, show that the biological effects of the wheat products prepared with potato supplementation were considerably higher than suggested on basis of the amino acid pattern /Mitchell and Block, 1946/.

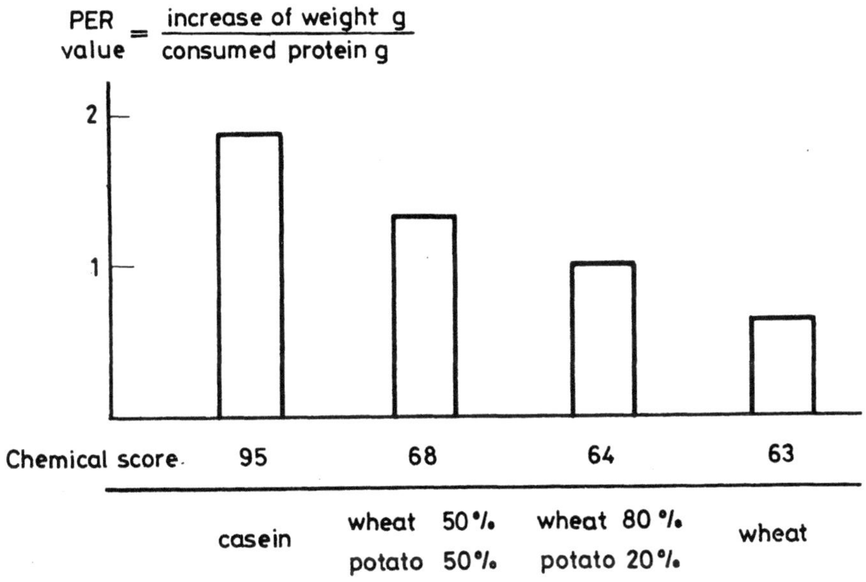

Fig. 2. PER and chemical score values

The PER value in the case of a diet of wheat flour supplemented with the same amount of potato /potato-noodles/ is very near to that of the casein diet. At the same time this combination duplicates the very low PER value of the wheat flour. On the other hand a bread produced with 20 percent of potatoes has a PER value 50 percent higher than the wheat basis alone.

From these data it is clear that in the case of the practical nutrition, products based on wheat flour combined with potato, give a more efficacious increase of the biological value, as it could be calculated from the data of the amino acid pattern /Lindner, 1964/.

For the investigation of the effect of the "time-factor" an experiment had been carried out, in the first period with a potato and wheat flour mixture, and after six weeks, in the second period the fodder was separately added. The time interval of the separate feeding with potatoes and wheat flour was 10 hours. The weight-gain curves in Fig.3. show a very characteristic breaking point in the curve when the fodder consumption was temporarily separated, while the body weight in this case decreased /Lindner and Bedő, 1956/.

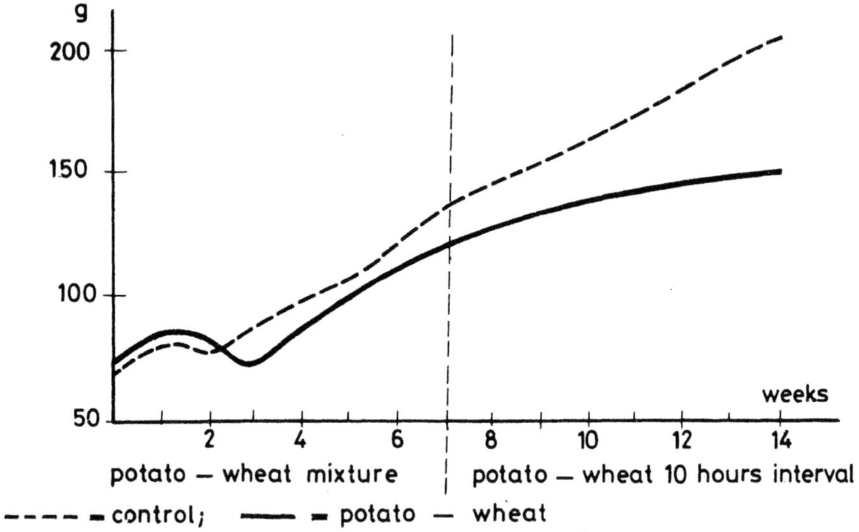

Fig. 3. Weight-gain curves with intermittent feeding

So, there is a good possibility to supplement the low quality protein of the wheat flour with potatoes in form of meals and bread. The biological supplementation effect is considerably higher than it is calculable from the amino acid pattern.

REFERENCES

Hegsted, D.M. /1978/.Assessment of nitrogen requirements. Am. J. Clin. Nutr. 31. 1669.

Lindner, K. /1964/. Aminosäurezusammensetzung und Nährwert der Weizeneiweiss-fraktionen. Qualitas Plant. 11. 31.

Lindner, K. and Bedő, M. /1956/. Adatok burgonyás buza-tésztáink biológiai értékéhez. Élelmezési Ipar. 10. 100.

Mitchell, H.H. and Block, R.J. /1946/. Some relationships between the amino acid contents of proteins and their nutritive values for rat. J. Biol. Chem. 163. 599.

Sherman, H.C. /1920/. Protein requirement of maintenance in man and the nutritive efficiency of bread protein. J.Biol. Chem. 41. 97.

Proc. Int. Assoc. Cereal Chem. Symp. Amino Acid Compn and Biol. Value of Cereal Proteins Budapest, Hungary 1983, R. Lásztity, M. Hidvégi, eds

CALCULATION OF THE AMINO ACID REQUIREMENTS OF GROWING BIRDS UNDER VARIABLE ENVIRONMENTAL CONDITIONS

SHMUEL HURWITZ

Institute of Animal Science, Agricultural Research Organization, The Volcani Center, Bet Dagan, Israel

ABSTRACT

A model which calculates protein and amino acid requirements in birds has been formulated. The model sums the requirements for maintenance, carcass growth and feathering, and calculates the energy intake. The resulting values are used to calculate the requirements in terms of the ratios of protein/energy and amino acids/energy, which are used for diet formulation. Parameters of amino acid needs, used in the model were obtained experimentally for chicks of different breeds and for turkeys. Parameters for the energy intake were determined in chickens and turkeys, kept at different environmental temperatures. Requirements could then be calculated for the different species, breeds and ages, under different environmental conditions. Some of the predicted requirements were validated by empirical approaches.

INTRODUCTION

The amount, quality and source of protein in the diet are determined by the amino acid requirements on the one hand, and the concentration and the amino acid profile of the feed ingredients, on the other. The amino acid requirements in farm animals are dependent on the type of product i.e. meat, eggs or milk, on the rate of production and on environmental factors such as temperature. Thus, in diets of growing turkeys the protein concentration decreases with age due to a reduced fractional growth. At the same time, the fraction of the protein supplied by grain increases (Table 1). Since the amount of feed consumed also increases with age, the market turkey consumes 2.8kg of cereal protein as compared with 5.8kg of protein from specific protein supplements.

In this presentation, the amino acid requirements of birds will be discussed. No attempt will be made to review the field exhaustively. Rather, the subject matter will be approached on a formal basis, according to which the requirements are represented by a series of equations. It is of interest to note that this approach was taken by classical nutritionists (Mitchell, 1962). Except for some studies such as that by Combs (1964) or Fisher and Morris (1970), in the last 20- 30 years this classical approach was replaced by the empirical one which is based on feeding of different concentrations of amino acids. The usefulness of system equations becomes clear if one

Table 1. The protein concentration and the fraction of cereal protein in total protein, in turkey diets*

Age, weeks	Dietary protein, %	Cereal protein % of total
0-4	28.0	12.0
5-8	26.0	13.7
9-12	22.0	22.0
13-16	18.4	30.0
17-20	16.5	36.0
21-24	13.8	48.6

*Calculated according to the recommendations of the National Research Council (1977).

realizes that amino acid requirements are different for each combination of genotype, age and environmental temperature. The multiple of these factors yields an almost infinite number of situations which, for practical considerations, cannot all be experimentally evaluated. The use of existing information to cover these situations by interpolation or extrapolation is difficult, since in most cases the behavior of the overall system is non-linear. This may also be one of the reasons why the solution of system-equations has been too difficult for popular use,in practice. At the present,however, the availability of computers with a marked computing ability and "friendly" software, provides the means to implement complex nutritional models for general use.

Models have been formulated by us also for laying hens (Hurwitz and Bornstein, 1973,1977,1978; Bornstein et al., 1979). However, only models for growing animals will be discussed in this chapter.

The construction of a useful nutritional model involves several steps:

(a) Modelling: The first step is the description of the system by the necessary equations. These may be set at different levels of detail, based on processes at the molecular level, the cellular level or the entire organism. Secondly, a model can describe in detail aspects which although exist may not be quantitatively important. To be useful, the model should be as simple as possible, avoiding details not necessary to achieve the goal of the model, but containing all the variables which are important quantitatively. The model does not have to be necessarily "correct". It should be looked upon rather as an approximation of reality. Obviously, the model should be powerful enough to predict closely the behavior of the system for the different conditions which may be encountered in practice.

(b) Parameter estimation: The equations describing metabolic processes contain various parameters and rate constants. In many cases these can be extracted from published experimental results. However, since such results would have been obtained without any exact definition in terms of the present model, parameters calculated from them may be not sufficiently accurate, in many cases. Such parameters could serve as first approximations, until replaced by data derived from direct experimentation. The parameters used in a model are usually determined in experiments aimed at a greater level of detail than the level of the target function. However, whenever a unique solution is possible, the behavior of the entire system can be used to extract parameters or to enable the final adjustments of the system.

(c) Validation: The ability of the model to predict the behavior of the system is evaluated in experiments designed independently of those which had been used in parameter estimation. Examples will be given to the validation of model-predicted amino acid requirements, by empirical means.

The model equations including parameters are incorporated into a computer program; the program includes a convenient interactive input part and an easily read output. This is followed by an examination of the usefulness of the model in practice.

THE MODEL

The model was orginally devised for chickens (Gallus domesticus) as described previously (Hurwitz et al., 1978), and more recently was investigated in greater detail with growing turkeys (Meleagris gallopavo; Hurwitz et al., 1983a). The protein requirement of the growing bird has been divided into three entities: maintenance, carcass and feathers. The reasons for this classification are that (a) each of the entities represents a large fraction of the total protein/amino acid requirements; (b) the variations in each are independent to some degree, and determined separately; and (c) large differences exist among these entities with regard to their amino acid profile.

In relative size, the maintenance requirement varies between 30% and 100% of the total protein and amino acid requirements, in the growing and adult animals, respectively. Of the carcass proteins, feather protein comprises 20-25% and, therefore, is quantitatively important. As will be formulated, the maintenance requirements are a function of metabolic body weight, while the requirements for carcass gain are a function of the rate of growth, and the requirements for feather protein are obviously dependent on the rate of feathering, which does not closely follow carcass growth. The amino acid profile of feathers and of the de-feathered carcass is illustrated in Table 2. Clearly, feathers are considerably lower in lysine, exceptionally high in cystine, and also higher in valine than the carcass. Since the rate of growth and feathering changes as a function of genetics, diet and environment, the proportions of the different entities making up the amino acid requirements change with these factors and therefore should be calculated separately.

Table 2. Amino acid profiles of selected proteins in birds

Amino acid	Carcass*	Feathers*	Egg**		
			Yolk	Albumen	Ovomucoid
			% of N x 6.25		
Arginine	6.9	7.2	7.3	6.0	5.4
Histidine	3.0	0.7	1.8	2.4	2.6
Lysine	8.0	1.9	5.5	7.2	7.3
Tryptophane	?	0.7	1.5	1.2	2.2
P.Alanine+ tyrosine	7.6	7.8	9.7	9.2	9.2
P.Alanine	4.6	5.1	4.6	5.3	5.0
Sulfur amino acids	3.0	9.1	4.8	7.2	7.9
Methionine	2.7	0.7	2.8	4.2	1.7
Threonine	4.6	4.6	5.3	5.0	6.7
Leucine	9.0	8.1	8.5	8.8	6.1
Isoleucine	4.4	5.0	6.8	6.5	7.7
Valine	5.4	7.7	7.3	7.5	7.3

*From Hurwitz et al. (1983a).
**From Block and Weiss (1956).

In the prediction of amino acid requirements, it is assumed that within the practical range, any interaction between the requirements (D'Mello and Lewis, 1970) is not of great importance. Thus, other than the methionine-cystine and phenylalanine-tyrosine relationships, the requirements are independent.

The maintenance requirements

For the chicken, Leveille and Fisher (1958) and Leveille et al. (1960) determined the amino acid requirements for maintenance by feeding decreasing amounts of protein or specific amino acids to adult roosters. They then selected the minimal level of the amino acid which supported a positive nitrogen balance. These results were the basis for obtaining the parameters needed for the model in the chicken (Hurwitz et al., 1978).

For the evaluation of the maintenance requirements in the turkey, a different experimental strategy was applied (Hurwitz et al., 1983a). It has been postulated that amino acids released into circulation by the "wear and tear" of carcass proteins are indistinguishable from those which appear in circulation as a result of intestinal absorption and are, therefore, effectively recycled.

However, some amino acids are catabolized by obligatory processes either related to synthesis of specialized carcass proteins, or converted to compounds which are not part of structural protein. Histidine is methylated irreversibly during synthesis of muscle protein, while proline is hydroxylated irreversibly to hydroxyproline during synthesis of collagen. Both are later excreted in the urine or catabolized by other means. Since these two amino acids are non-essential or partially essential, no specific allowance needs to be made for their catabolism. Arginine and methionine are used in equivalent amounts to synthesize creatine which is then excreted in the urine mainly as creatinine. This is part of the endogenous nitrogen metabolism (Mitchell, 1962). Thus, the loss of creatinine is nutritionally adjusted by the numerical addition of equivalent amounts to the arginine and methionine requirements. Amino acids are further lost through the gastrointestinal tract due to the secretion of digestive juices and to the loss of epithelial cells.

An important, although difficult to measure, route of loss of protein is that of skin integuments. Analysis revealed that the dust collected on the air-filters of the local experimental turkey facility, was composed of 80% protein, probably of skin origin. The heavy accumulation of this dust emphasized the magnitude of the loss of protein from the skin. An additional route of amino acid loss is synthesis of other nitrogen-containing compounds such as nucleic acids. This process is assumed to consume non-essential amino acids, and therefore, is neglected at the present.

On the basis of these considerations, the amino acid requirements for maintenance were assessed by determining of the endogenous amino acid losses from the intestine and the excretion of creatinine, and by the estimation of amino acid losses from the skin. In specifically designed experiments (Hurwitz et al., 1983a), adult turkeys were placed in metabolism cages, fed a nitrogen-free diet and their excreta were analyzed for amino acids and creatinine at steady state. For the measurements of the skin losses, the turkeys were fed a complete diet, and their excreta were collected. The nitrogen analyzed in this material represents only the loss through urine and feces. Furthermore, non-growing turkeys should have a nitrogen balance of zero. In these birds the value for the apparent nitrogen retention from the complete diet, which is obtained by the subtraction of the nitrogen loss in the excreta from the nitrogen intake, is taken as the nitrogen loss from the skin. Since most of this loss is made up of keratine, the amino acid profile of the skin loss was taken as equal to that of feathers.

The values obtained in this study for the turkey, as well as those of Leveillẹ et al. (1960) for the chicken, were expressed on a metabolic body weight basis, which represents body surface. The validity of this approach was discussed in detail by Mitchell (1962). It is self-evident that skin losses must be proportional to body surface. The same is true for creatinine excretion, which is related to energy metabolism. Furthermore, the size of the intestine of turkeys appears to be proportional to body surface (Y. Frisch, unpublished), and therefore the intestinal losses may also be related to body surface.

Nitrogen retention of the 17 kg adult turkeys consuming a complete diet was thus estimated at 2.3 g/day. For the same birds, creatinine excretion was estimated at 123 mg/day. When a 16.5 kg adult turkey was fed the nitrogen-free diet, the total excretion of amino acids was 3.5 g/day. The protein requirements for maintenance in the adult turkey are then calculated by dividing the sum of nitrogen in these losses by metabolic body weight ($BW^{2/3}$) and by 0.85, which is the nitrogen absorption from a diet containing natural ingredients (Hurwitz et al.,1972,1979; Bielorai et al., 1973; Sklan and Hurwitz, 1980). The coefficient of protein requirement for maintenance in the turkey (PRM) thus calculated in terms of an ideal amino acid mixture, was 32 $mg/g^{2/3}$, as compared with the corresponding coefficient of 23 $mg/g^{2/3}$ for the adult rooster, calculated from the results of Leveille and Fisher (1958). The protein requirements, in g/day are then calculated by

$$PRM = 0.023 \cdot BW^{2/3} \qquad (1)$$

for the chicken, and

$$PRM = 0.032 \cdot BW^{2/3} \qquad (2)$$

for the turkey, where BW is the body weight in g.

The amino acid requirements were obtained by totalling the needs for each amino acid for endogenous fecal excretion and for skin losses. In addition, the requirements for arginine and methionine were adjusted in order to account for the creatinine excretion. This sum was divided by the protein requirement. The resulting fractions of the amino acid requirements for maintenance in the turkey are given in Table 3, in comparison with the respective fractions for the chicken, as calculated from the results of Leveille et al. (1960).

In general, as proportions, the amino acid requirements are slightly higher in the turkey than in the chicken, except for methionine, for which the determined value in the turkey was considerably lower than that determined in the chicken by Leveille et al. (1960). Furthermore, for a protein with an ideal composition, about one half of the amino acid requirements for maintenance in turkeys is made up by essential amino acids. The value for the chicken is somewhat lower at 37%.

The amino acid requirements for maintenance (AAM_i) may be obtained by multiplying the protein requirements as obtained in Eqs. (1) or (2) by the amino acid profiles as given in Table 3 ($\%AM_i$):

$$AAM_i = PRM_i \cdot \%AM_i / 100 \qquad (3)$$

The requirements for growth and feathering

The protein requirement for carcass growth (PRC) and for feather growth (PRF) is given by,

$$PRC = [BW(t) \cdot \%PC(t) - BW(t-1) \cdot \%PC(t-1)]/0.85 \quad (4)$$

$$PRF = [BW(t) \cdot \%PF(t) - Bw(t-1) \cdot \%PF(t-1)]/0.85 \quad (5)$$

where, BW designates body weight, %PC and %PF are the percentages of protein from body weight, contained in the carcass and feathers, respectively, and t is the age in days. Since body weight and composition data are usually not available on a daily basis, values are obtained for the intervals between measurements, by interpolation.

Table 3. The amino acid profile of the protein requirements for maintenance in the turkey and in the chicken

Amino acid	Chicken*	Turkey**
	% of N x 6.25	
Arginine	6.8	7.3
Lysine	1.7	2.4
Tryptophane	1.1	?
Phenylalanine +tyrosine	3.4	7.4
Phenylalanine	1.5	4.6
Methionine + cystine	5.1	8.1
Methionine	4.1	1.7
Threonine	4.2	4.6
Leucine	7.1	7.4
Isoleucine	4.1	5.0
Valine	3.5	6.7
Total essential	37.0	50.0

*Calculated from the results of Leveille et al.(1960).
**From Hurwitz et al. (1983a).

Parameters for these equations were obtained by evaluating carcass composition in male and female broilers (White Rock), in male and female chicks of a layer strain (Leghorn x Rhode Island Red) and in male and female BUT (British United Turkeys) turkeys (Plavnik and Hurwitz, 1983; Hurwitz et al., 1983a). The results for chicks, (Table 4), show that the percentage of carcass protein was in most cases higher in males than in females, and in the layer as compared with the broiler strain. In all cases, the percentage of carcass protein increased with age. The percentage of feather protein increased to reach a plateau at the age of 4-6 weeks. Females were slighly higher in feather protein than males, and the layer strain was markedly higher in feather protein than the broiler at any time.

Table 4. The protein concentration in carcass and feathers of chickens*

Age,	Carcass				Feathers			
	White Rock		Leghorn x RIR		White Rock		Leghorn x RIR	
Weeks	Males	Females	Males	Females	Males	Females	Males	Females
	% of body weight							
1	15.8	15.4	16.1	16.6	1.05	1.27	1.63	2.82
2	15.9	15.5	16.4	16.7	1.25	1.23	1.97	3.17
3	16.1	15.7	16.7	16.9	2.74	3.15	4.24	4.97
4	16.2	15.8	16.9	17.0	3.99	4.42	5.72	5.26
5	16.3	15.9	17.2	17.1	4.08	4.26	5.76	5.76
6	16.5	16.1	17.5	17.3	3.73	4.59	5.78	5.99
7	16.6	16.2	17.7	17.4	4.03	4.12	6.67	6.47
8	16.7	16.3	18.0	17.6	4.25	4.52	6.67	6.80
9	16.9	16.5	18.3	17.7	4.23	4.87	6.53	7.12
10	17.0	16.6	18.6	17.8	4.18	4.86	6.10	7.56

* From Plavnik and Hurwitz (1983).

Only random variation could be found in the protein contents of turkey carcass (Table 5). Therefore, for the calculation of the requirements, a single value of 19.77% was taken for %PC in the turkey. Feather protein in this bird (Table 5) increased with age reaching a peak at the age of about 100 days, followed by a decline. There were no significant differences in feather protein between the sexes.

The requirements for the ith amino acid for carcass (AAC_i) and feathers (AAf_i) growth in actual intake (g/day) are given by

$$AAC_i = PRC \cdot \%AC_i/100 \quad (6)$$

$$AAF_i = PRF \cdot \%AF_i/100 \quad (7)$$

where $\%AC_i$ and $\%AF_i$, are the amino acid concentrations in the carcass and feather protein, respectively (Table 2).

The total protein (PRT) and the ith amino acid requirement (AAT_i), in g/day are given by

$$PRT = PRM + PRC + PRF \quad (8)$$

$$AAT_i = AAM_i + AAC_i + AAF_i \quad (9)$$

Table 5. Protein content in carcass and feathers of BUT turkeys*

Age,	Carcass		Feathers	
Days	Males	Females	Males	Females
	% of body weight			
8	19.7	18.6	2.18	2.39
15	18.7	18.5	2.68	3.13
23	18.6	19.9	2.71	3.25
37	20.0	21.4	3.78	3.69
51	20.0	19.6	4.33	3.89
72	21.5	20.8	5.45	4.12
99	22.1	16.1	4.56	4.74
133	20.0	19.8	4.03	4.38
154	20.4	-	3.56	-
168	20.0	-	3.28	-

*Calculated from Hurwitz et al. (1983a).

Protein-energy relationships

The protein and amino acid requirements, as calculated by Eqs. (8) and (9), respectively, are obtained in absolute terms and therefore cannot be used as such in feed formulation , where values are needed in units of concentration. Furthermore, within the practical range, the dietary energy concentration is determined mainly by economic considerations. Therefore, the requirements for protein and amino acids, as calculated, are divided by the daily energy intake and expressed in g/kcal. The requirements in terms of dietary concentrations are then obtained by multiplying the amino acid/calorie ratio by the energy concentration of the diet. This procedure can be included in the linear programs used for feed formulation.

Prediction of energy intake

Energy intake varies with the metabolic body weight, with the rate and composition of the weight gain, as normally determined by age and genotype, and with environmental factors such as temperature.

The model which predicts energy intake and the estimation of the necessary parameters were detailed in previous communications (Hurwitz et al., 1978, 1980b, 1983c). Since this subject matter is beyond the scope of this communication, it will be discussed briefly.

The energy intake (EI) of growing birds can be described by

$$EI = M \cdot BW^{2/3} + D \cdot G \quad (10)$$

$$M = h(T) \quad (11)$$

$$D = 0.6 + 9.3\ F \quad (12)$$

where EI is the energy intake (kcal/day); BW is the body weight (g); G is the weight gain (g/day); M is the coefficient of the energy requirement for maintenance ($kcal/g^{2/3}$); D is the requirement for weight gain (kcal/g); F is the fraction of fat in the weight gained; and T is the environmental temperature (°C).

Table 6. The energy requirement for maintenance of the 6-9 week old broiler chick*

Temperature	Requirement, kcal/g
12	2.55
19	2.20
27	1.90
34	2.10

*From Hurwitz et al. (1980b).

The estimated coefficients of energy requirements for maintenance have been related to metabolic body weight ($BW^{2/3}$) as discussed by Brody (1945). The values for young chicks (5-8 weeks) and turkeys are given in Tables 6 and 7, respectively. The energy use appears to be similar in chicks and young turkeys. In the old turkey the energy requirements were somewhat lower than in the young one. Also, unlike the young turkey, the older birds did not increase their energy expenditure at high environmental temperatures (Hurwitz et al., 1983c). In Eq. (10), actual and interpolated energy coefficients are used for any tested temperature. Furthermore, experimental results (Hurwitz and Bengal, 1982) suggest that with cycling ambient temperatures, as encountered under natural conditions, the average temperature can be used, provided that the maximal temperature does not exceed 30°.

The fraction of carcass fat as a function of age is given in Table 8 for the broiler strain (White Rock) and the layer strain (Leghorn x Rhode Island Red) of chickens, and for BUT turkeys of both sexes in Table 9. In chickens, fractional fat increased with age, was higher in females than in males, and higher in the broiler strain than in the layer strain. In the turkey, body fat remained rather constant until the age of 10-12 weeks, after which it started to increase. Moreover, there was little difference between males and females. In general, the fat content of the carcass of the chicken was considerably higher than that of the turkey. These values of carcass

Table 7. The energy requirements for maintenance in the 6-10 week and the 20-24 week-old turkey*

Temperature, °C	Requirement, kcal/g	
	6-10 weeks	20-24 weeks
12	2.59	2.30
18	2.48	2.10
24	2.00	1.85
28	2.22	1.60
32	2.42	1.55

*From Hurwitz et al. (1980b, 1983c).

Table 8. The fat content of the carcass of the chicken*

Age, weeks	White Rock		Leghorn x RIR	
	Males	Females	Males	Females
	% of body weight			
1	10.2	9.6	7.0	8.1
2	10.6	10.5	7.2	8.2
3	11.1	11.3	7.4	8.4
4	11.6	12.2	7.5	8.5
5	12.1	13.0	7.7	8.7
6	12.6	13.4	7.9	8.8
7	13.1	14.7	8.1	8.9
8	13.6	15.6	8.3	9.1
9	14.1	16.7	8.4	9.2
10	14.5	17.3	8.6	9.4

*From Plavnik and Hurwitz (1983).

fat supplied the data needed for use in Eq.(12), which calculated parameter D describing growth requirement in Eq.(10).The energy intake can be calculated for a combination of species, age and environmental temperature, when given the appropriate growth curve.

Calculation of the amino acid : energy ratios

For each condition, the required daily intake of the protein and i^{th} amino acid as calculated by Eqs. (8) and (9), respectively,

Table 9. Carcass fat in BUT turkeys*

Age, days	Males	Females
	% of body weight	
8	2.7	2.8
15	2.1	2.3
23	1.6	2.4
72	1.9	2.6
99	2.8	5.0
133	7.5	9.8
154	8.3	-
168	9.9	-

*From Hurwitz et al. (1983a).

was divided by the daily energy intake as calculated by Eq. (10). The resulting values, as used in feed formulation, were calculated for the species, breeds and sexes described in this paper, at different ages and environmental temperature. Table 10 gives the requirements for all amino acids in turkeys expressed in terms of g/kcal. The

Table 10. The predicted amino acid requirements of BUT* male turkeys

Amino acid	Age, days 22-28	50-56	78-84	106-112	134-140
			mg/kcal		
Arginine	5.74	4.48	4.43	3.24	2.61
Histidine	1.92	1.43	1.38	0.99	0.78
Lysine	5.11	3.80	3.66	2.61	2.03
Tryptophane	0.77	0.59	0.58	0.43	0.35
P.alanine+tyrosine	6.21	4.83	4.77	3.47	2.77
Phenylalanine	3.82	2.98	2.94	2.14	1.70
Sulfur amino acids	3.81	3.14	3.18	2.37	1.94
Methionine	1.85	1.40	1.37	1.00	0.83
Threonine	3.77	2.94	2.90	2.11	1.70
Leucine	7.09	5.49	5.38	3.89	3.07
Isoleucine	7.09	5.49	5.38	3.89	3.07
Valine	4.83	3.82	3.79	2.77	2.21

*Official BUT "Big 6" growth curve was used. Temperature is constant at 20°, from 5 weeks of age.

values are the result of calculations using actual body weight values and are therefore not "smooth". Thus, they cannot be taken as recommendations. The results illustrate the decrease in the requirements of all amino acids with age which is not uniform. Furthermore, the rate of decline is not parallel for the different amino acids, due to the differences in the fraction of the amino acid needed for growth, maintenance or feathering.

As an example of breed and sex differences, the lysine requirements for chickens are given in Table 11. In both breeds, the requirements of males were higher than those of females. This sex difference expanded with age, due to the greater decrease in the rate of weight gain and the increased fat deposition with age, in the females. There were no consistent differences between the breeds in lysine requirements in g/kcal, despite the large difference in the rate of growth in favor of the White Rock birds. The latter difference was, however, counteracted by the lower energy requirements of the light birds (Hurwitz et al., 1978).

Environmental temperature influences the amino acid requirements by affecting both rate of growth and energy intake. Furthermore, an interaction was observed between temperature and age (Hurwitz et al., 1983c) in their effect on both parameters. Growth rate of the older turkeys was depressed by environmental temperature to a greater extent than that of the younger birds. Furthermore, as shown in Table 7, the coefficient of energy requirement was also influenced by age. Therefore, as shown in Table 12, the effect of temperature on the amino acid requirements was not the same for all ages. In the younger

Table 11. Calculated lysine requirements of two strains of chickens at different ages*

	White Rock		Leghorn x RIR	
Age,days	Males	Females	Males	Females
		mg/kcal		
8-14	3.73	3.72	4.00	3.85
15-21	3.26	3.40	3.71	3.31
22-28	3.28	3.03	3.08	2.97
29-35	2.84	2.84	2.92	2.66
36-42	2.52	2.29	2.66	2.36
43-49	2.46	2.15	2.56	2.31
50-56	2.18	1.99	2.46	2.08
57-63	2.05	1.84	2.22	2.08
64-70	2.26	1.79	2.16	2.03

*For 20°, starting at the age of 5 weeks. Calculated on the basis of the growth curve given previously (Plavnik and Hurwitz, 1983).

bird the lysine requirement increased when the temperature was raised from 15 to 25°, but decreased when the temperature was further raised to 30°. In the older bird, on the other hand, the requirements increased constantly with increasing temperature.

VALIDATION

The validity of the model-calculated requirements was examined in two ways. In chicks (Hurwitz et al., 1980a), practical-type diets were designed by linear programs, based on the minimal requirements given by the model for male broiler chicks. These diets were fed to

Table 12. The effect of environmental temperature on the lysine requirements of turkeys*

Age, days	Temperature, °C			
	15	20	25	30
		mg/kcal		
36-42	3.88	4.19	4.32	3.59
43-49	3.73	4.02	4.20	3.53
50-56	3.53	3.81	4.01	3.34
57-63	3.98	4.29	4.53	3.88
64-70	3.78	4.01	4.21	3.74
71-77	3.18	3.43	3.66	3.14
78-84	3.40	3.66	3.86	4.18
85-91	3.13	3.36	3.50	3.83
92-98	2.99	3.21	3.31	3.68
99-105	2.64	2.82	2.87	3.22
106-112	2.44	2.61	2.63	2.99
113-119	2.19	2.34	2.34	2.72
120-126	1.98	2.12	2.10	2.50
127-133	1.80	1.92	1.89	2.29
134-140	1.90	2.04	2.00	2.64

* Calculated for BUT "Big 6", from the official growth curve.

chicks in comparison with controls fed diets based on National Research Council (1977) recommendations. The results of one such trial with the dietary regimes applied from 1 to 9 weeks of age are shown in Table 13. In the computation of the model diets, the most limiting amino acids determined the total dietary protein concentration. Thus, the model diets were considerably lower in protein than those based on the NRC recommendations. However, growth rate and feed efficiency were remarkably similar for both regimes. The only difference in performance was the lower abdominal fat in the NRC birds than in the model birds. This is probably the result of the difference in dietary protein concentration (Bartov et al., 1974).The model-predicted

Table 13. Validation of model-predicted requirements in chicks*

Dietary regime	NRC	Model
Body weight, 9 weeks,g	2523±34**	2535±34
Feed intake, g/7 weeks	5352±83	5399±60
Feed efficiency	.417±.005	.415±.003
Abdominal fat,%	2.2±.28	3.1±.27

*Dietary protein of NRC(1977) diets averaged 20.9%; the model diets averaged 16.4% protein. The energy concentration was 3100 kcal/kg in all diets. From Hurwitz et al. (1980a).
**Mean ±standard error.

requirements for laying hens were similarly validated (Hurwitz and Bornstein, 1977, 1978; Bornstein et al., 1979).

A different strategy was applied in validating the predicted amino acid requirements in turkeys. Here, the amino acid requirements were determined using the empirical approach and compared to the corresponding predicted value. According to the empirical approach, birds are fed graded levels of the respective amino acid and the requirement is defined as the minimal level which supported maximal growth and feed efficiency. In the study of Hurwitz et al. (1983b), the requirements for lysine and methionine were evaluated in turkeys of different ages. The calculated requirements were based on the growth curve and standard temperature prevailing at the Bet Dagan

Table 14. Validation of model-predicted requirements in turkeys*

Amino acid	Age, wks	Requirements	
		Predicted	Experimental
		mg/kcal	
Sulfur amino acids	1-3	3.6	3.4
Sulfur amino acids	5-7	3.3	3.2
Lysine	1-3	5.5	5.1
Lysine	12-15	2.6	2.7
Lysine	16-19	2.0	2.2

*From Hurwitz et al. (1983b).

turkey research center. The results given in Table 14 show a remarkable agreement between the empirical and calculated amino acid requirements, supporting the validity of the model for turkeys.

Contribution from The Agricultural Research Organization, Bet Dagan, No. 974E, 1984 series. Supported by a grant from The Israeli-American Binational Agricultural Research and Development Fund.

REFERENCES

Bartov, I., S. Bornstein and B. Lipstein (1974). Effect of calorie to protein ratio on the degree of fatness in broilers fed on practical diets. Brit. Poult. Sci. 15, 107-117.

Bielorai, R., M. Tamir, E. Alumot, A. Bar and S. Hurwitz (1973). Digestion and absorption of protein along the gastrointestinal tract of chicks fed raw and toasted soybean meal. J. Nutr. 103, 1291-1298.

Block, R.S. and K.W. Weiss (1956). Amino Acid Handbook. C.C. Thomas Publ., Springfield, Mass.

Bornstein, S. , S. Hurwitz and Y. Lev (1979). The amino acid and energy requirements of broiler-breeder hens. Poult. Sci. 58, 104-116.

Brody, S. (1945). Bioenergetics and Growth. Reinhold Publ. Corp. New York, N.Y.

Combs, G.F. (1964). Predicting amino acid requirements of chicks, based on growth rate, body size and body composition. Fed. Proc. 23, 46-51.

D'Mello, T.P.F. and D. Lewis (1970). Amino acid interactions in chick nutrition. 3. Interdependence in amino acid requirements. Brit. Poult. Sci. 11, 367-385.

Fisher, C. and T.R. Morris (1970). The determination of the methionine requirements of laying pullets by a diet-dilution technique. Brit. Poult. Sci. 11: 67-82.

Hurwitz, S. and I. Bengal (1982). Energy use and performance of young turkeys kept under various constant and cycling environmental temperatures. Poult. Sci. 61, 1082-1086.

Hurwitz, S. and S. Bornstein (1973). The protein and amino acid requirements of laying hens: suggested models for calculation. Poult. Sci. 52, 1124-1134.

Hurwitz, S. and S. Bornstein (1977). The protein and amino acid requirements of laying hens: experimental validation of the models for calculation.1. Application of two models under various conditions. Poult. Sci. 56, 969-978.

Hurwitz, S. and S. Bornstein (1978). The protein and amino acid requirements of laying hens: experimental validation of models of calculation. 2. Valine requirements and layer-starter diets. Poult. Sci. 57, 711-718.

Hurwitz, S. U. Eisner, D. Dubrov, D. Sklan, G. Riesenfeld and A. Bar, (1979). Protein, fatty acids, calcium and phosphate absorption along the gastrointestinal tract of the young turkey. Comp. Biochem. Physiol. 62A, 847-850.

Hurwitz, S., Y. Frisch, A. Bar, U. Eisner, I. Bengal and M. Pines, (1983a). The amino acid requirements of growing turkeys. 1. Model construction and parameter estimation. Poult. Sci. 62,2208-2217.

Hurwitz, S., I. Plavnik, I. Bartov and S. Bornstein (1980a). The amino acid requirements for chicks: experimental validation of model-calculated requirements. Poult. Sci. 59, 2490-2497.

Hurwitz, S., I. Plavnik, I. Bengal, H. Talpaz and I. Bartov (1983b). The amino acid requirements of growing turkeys. 2.Experimental validation of model-calculated requirements for sulfur amino acids and lysine. Poult. Sci., in press.

Hurwitz, S., N. Shamir and A. Bar (1972). Protein digestion and absorption in the chick: effect of Ascaridia galli. Am. J. Clin. Nutr. 25, 311-316.

Hurwitz, S., D. Sklan and I. Bartov (1978). New formal approaches to the determination of protein and amino acid requirements of chickens. Poult. Sci. 57, 197-205.

Hurwitz, S., E. Wax and I. Bengal (1983c). Performance and energy needs of 20-week old male turkeys at different environmental temperatures. Poult. Sci. 62, 1327-1329.

Hurwitz, S., M. Weisselberg, U. Eizner, I. Bartov, G. Riesenfeld, M. Sharvit, A. Niv and S. Bornstein (1980b). The energy requirements and performance of growing chicks and turkeys as affected by environmental temperature. Poult. Sci. 59, 2290-2299.

Leveille, G.A. and H. Fisher (1958). The amino acid requirements for maintenance in the adult rooster. I. Nitrogen and energy requirements in normal and protein-depleted animals receiving whole egg protein and amino acid diets. J. Nutr. 66,441-453.

Leveille, G.A., R. Shapiro and H. Fisher (1960). Amino acid requirements for maintenance in the adult rooster. IV. The requirements for methionine, cystine, phenylalanine, tyrosine, and tryptophane: the adequacy of the determined requirements. J. Nutr. 72, 8-15.

Mitchell, H.H. (1962). Comparative Nutrition of Man and Domestic Animals, Vol 1. Academic Press, New York, N.Y.

National Research Council (1977). Nutrient Requirements of Poultry. 7 ed., Natl. Acad. Sci., Washington, D.C.

Plavnik, I. and S. Hurwitz (1983). Organ weights and body composition in chicks as related to the energy and amino acid requirements: effect of strain, sex and age. Poult. Sci. 62, 152-163.

Sklan, D. and S. Hurwitz (1980). Protein digestion and absorption in young chicks and turkeys. J. Nutr. 110, 139-144.

Proc. Int. Assoc. Cereal Chem. Symp. Amino Acid Compn and Biol. Value of Cereal Proteins Budapest, Hungary 1983, R. Lásztity, M. Hidvégi, eds

REMARKS ON THE IMPORTANCE OF PROTEIN QUALITY IN MIXED FEEDS

LAJOS FEKETE

Department of Animal Feeding, University of Agriculture
Gödöllő, H-2103 Gödöllő, Hungary

Farm animals are usually divided into two major groups on the basis of their requirements for feed proteins of different biological values. One group contains the omnivorous, single-stomach pig and the various poultry species and the other group is made up of the ruminants. It is interesting that the physiological demands of both groups are, essentially, satisfied by protein of the same quality. The main difference between the groups, which is of vital importance for the economics of animal production, lies in the fact that for pigs, for instance, the protein in the feed must be of high biological value, while cattle accept foodstuffs containing protein of lower quality, or even some non-protein nitrogen. This is because in the cow the microorganisms in the rumen, this powerful fermenting vat, effect a radical change and, improve the biological value of the protein taken up in the feed. I have made a rough calculation, based on data on the microflora and microfauna of the rumen available in the literature, and found that at about halfway between two feeds, the protein in a cow's rumen has a biological value corresponding to the standard requirements of a 50 kg pig.

This contribution is concerned with protein supply in pigs and poultries, i.e. the so-called concentrate-eating animals.
These animals will only produce valuable animal protein when given feed protein of high biological value.

Previously, the science of nutrition tried to ensure the desired quality of protein for pigs by prescribing the proportions of vegetable and animal proteins in the concentrate mixture. This approach was based on the idea that vegetable protein is of no biological value while animal protein is. Learning the hard way, our experience since suggests that many foodstuffs of animal origin contain protein of poor quality, mainly as a result of the technology used in processing: excessive heat treatment, use of denaturing preservatives, etc.

When the role played by amino acids had been discovered, but neither the set of amino acids in feeds, nor the exact amino acid requirements of livestock were known, the rule of thumb followed in practice was to make up the concentrate mixture with as many components as possible, thereby enhancing the likelihood of a "complete" set of amino acids being present in the feed. When plans were made to build feed compounding plants, so-called "feed factories", one of the arguments in their favour was that such large factory-like plants would be in a much better position to secure a large number of concentrates and other components than would individual farms.

Since then, the set of essential amino acids has come to be used as a firm though rather biased criterion for the evaluation of feed proteins and the qualitative characterisation of the protein requirements of livestock.

This information on essential amino acids has opened a new and more advanced stage in pig and poultry feeding. It has enabled a considerable reduction in transformational losses of feed proteins in the processes involved in producing livestock feeds. However, I do not agree with claims made by some researchers, which I consider exaggerated, that economic pig feeding is possible using maize and extracted soybean meal alone, with the possible addition of some artificial amino acid supplement. Acceptable fattening and other results have been achieved in this way, but undoubtedly the standard energy: amino acid ratio is not the only possible qualitative criterion for concentrate mixtures. From this point of view /many other views are possible/ there is some advantage in the increased utilization of by-products and wastes which has been dictated by economic necessity in recent years.

I do not wish to be misunderstood on this point. I am referring to the palatability, structure and other physical properties, the so-called specific effects, such as bulk /crude fibre/ content, dietary effect, etc. of the concentrate mixtures. In other words my concern here is not only, or not primarily, the fact that the protein content of maize-soybean meal is of vegetable origin.

I should like to emphasize that in my opinion it is still justified to retain the distinction between vegetable and animal origin in the practice of protein feeding. However, I should also like to point out that the distinction based on origin is no longer valid in many important respects. The idea that protein of animal origin is valuable while that of vegetable origin is not, is not only wrong, but also misleading and consequently harmful. Here I do not refer to possible denaturing of proteins during feed processing, but to the fact that the differences in the sets of amino acids present in protein, of plant and animal origin do not justify such a distinction.

Before discussing this subject further, it should be noted that the quantities of lysine, methionine and cystine required by pigs and poultry are now prescribed and feed compounders are required to guarantee the level of these amino acids in their products. Although triptophan and treonine requirements have also been recorded, feed compounders are not yet obliged to supplement their products with these amino acids.

For practical purposes, therefore, it will suffice to concentrate on three components of the set of amino acids present in feeds of animal and plant origin, neamly lysine and the two sulphur-containing amino acids. Table 1.shows the relationship between these amino acids in various foodstuffs. Each figure is the quantity of methionine plus the quantity of cystine expressed as a percentage of the quantity of lysine.

If it is accepted that optimum weight gain in pigs is best ensured by protein in which the quantity of sulphur-containing amino acids equals two thirds of the quantity of lysine, and if this is regarded as a requirement for pig rations, it will be seen from the table that foods of neither vegetable nor animal origin meet this requirement.

Table 1.
Total amount of methionine and cystine as a percentage of the amount of lysine

/Based on data collected from tables/

Barley	115	Beans	33
Wheat	115	Peas	32
Sorghum	105	Lupin	52
Millet	150	Horse beans	25
Maize	135	Extr.soybean meal	45
Rye	75	Fish meal	55
Oats	105	Meat meal	46
Bran	90	Casein	50
Extracted sunflower meal	95	Whey	48
Crackling meal	100	Milk	54
		Blood	35

/Average requirement of growing pig: 66 %./

The statement that cereal proteins are deficient in lysine while feeds of animal origin contain an excess can be reversed by saying that animal proteins are deficient in sulphur-containing amino acids while cereal proteins contain an excess of such amino acids. The superiority of animal proteins does not appear so great in this light. Needless to say, both views are somewhat extreme. However, both from the point of view of nutrition physiology and from the point of view of practical feeding, it is correct to regard both types of protein as requiring complementation and as capable of complementing each other.

However true all this may be, it is also risky to equate the proteins found in cereal feeds with those in feeds of animal origin, for the following reasons:

- Feeds of animal origin contain a much higher proportion of protein than feeds of plant origin, and the total proportion of lysine, methionine and cystine in the protein is somewhat higher.

- Feeds of animal origin are rich in lysine and this is exactly what is needed because our domestic protein base is poor in lysine /as it is, incidentally, in most feed protein throughout the world/.

- Methionine + cystine deficiency in proteins of animal origin is smaller than lysine deficiency in cereals.

- High quality feeds of animal origin contain a special substance which has a beneficial effect on protein conversion. This fact was recognised by livestock farmers quite a long time ago.
Though the process was not understood, the supposed beneficial substance was called animal protein factor.

This brings us to the yield-increasing feed supplements in common use in modern feed compounding. It has been demonstrated under controlled conditions that these supplements are capable of raising the conversion rate of less valuable proteins to the level usually achieved with proteins containing a more complete set of amino acids.

The first group of yield-increasing supplements in the Hungarian foodstuffs code are the antibiotics. There is a strictly enforced principle that antibiotics used in animal and human medicine should not be applied for the purposes of nutrition, since such a practice might give rise to resistant strains of bacteria which would endanger the reliability of medication. Of the enormous number of antibiotics, only the following six are allowed in Hungary: - Zn-Bacitracin, Flavomycin, Monensin, Spiramycin, Tylosin and Virginiamycin. There are some so-called "other" yield-increasers of which only two, Carbadox and Nitrovin, are named in our foodstuffs code. Application of Carbadox is only allowed if prescribed and supervised by a vet.

Many aspects of the yield-increasing substances have yet to be clarified. It has already been proved that they have a beneficial effect on the microbial population of the digestive tract. In this connection, the frequently cited "selective effect" means that harmful organisms in the digestive tract are checked, thus improving conditions for beneficial organisms.

Here, we can content ourselves by stating that increased meat, milk and egg production involves a more efficient conversion of the same feed protein. Thus the effect of the yield-increasing supplements is the same as increasing the biological value of the feed protein.

Yield-increasing supplements achieve spectacular improvements. Similar though less dramatic effects on animal production can be recorded when concentrate mixtures are supplemented with major and minor elements, vitamins etc.

In summary, it can be concluded /and this conclusion is borne out in practical livestock husbandry/ that the biological value of the protein in the ration is determined, essentially, by the set of amino acids it contains, but the efficiency of protein conversion is not determined by the amino acids alone.

Finally I should like to raise a methodological problem encountered in experimental determinations of the biological value of proteins.

One of the most widely accepted methods for determining the biological value of protein in a farm or laboratory animal is to set up a nitrogen balance according to Thomas and Mitchell. This can be used to determine the proportion of the total protein intake which the animal builds into its own body and the proportion it builds into its product /offspring, milk, eggs/, i.e. the proportion that is considered biologically valuable.

In the nitrogen balance referred to above a distinction should be made between endogenous nitrogen in the urine and faeces, which has once been "built in", i.e. which is biologically valuable, and that exogenous nitrogen, which cannot be absorbed and built in and which is not biologically valuable.

On this principle, the biologically valuable protein in the food is calculated by subtracting the nitrogen voided in urine and faeces, minus the endogenous nitrogen fractions, from total nitrogen intake.

From this relationship it follows that if for some reason the endogenous faeces N changes, the experimentally determined biologically valuable proportion of the feed protein /its biological value/ will change.

This procedure is formulated as follows:-

$$\begin{matrix}\text{biologically}\\ \text{valuable N}\\ \text{in feed}\end{matrix} = \begin{matrix}\text{total}\\ \text{N}\\ \text{intake}\end{matrix} - \left(\begin{matrix}\text{N voided}\\ \text{in}\\ \text{faeces}\end{matrix} \quad \begin{matrix}\text{endogen-}\\ \text{ous}\\ \text{faeces}\\ \text{N}\end{matrix}\right) - \left(\begin{matrix}\text{N voided}\\ \text{in}\\ \text{urine}\end{matrix} \quad \begin{matrix}\text{endogen-}\\ \text{ous}\\ \text{urine}\\ \text{N}\end{matrix}\right)$$

From a detailed study of the role of crude fibre in pig rations I have found that crude fibre /which, histologically and in the present context can be equated with cell wall/ reduces digestibility of proteins, fats etc., not only by enclosing plasm which is rich in valuable nutrients by reducing its accessibility to digestive juices, but also by its very presence.

This latter point was demonstrated experimentally by adding an inert fibre carrier /e.g. wheat straw/ to a given concentrate mixture, which excluded the possibility of the crude fibre isolating nutrients from the digestive enzymes.

I called this crude fibre additional fibre and sought to explore the mechanism by which it brought about depression of the coefficients of digestion. The theory that feed protein combines with lignin from crude fibre to form an indigestible ligno-protein complex in the digestive tract, which has gained wide currency in the literature.

My own investigations provided proof that the increase in the faeces protein due to additional fibre, or at least most of the increase, is due to endogenous protein, that is, it originates from the highly worn cell walls of the internal mucous membrane, increased production of mucus and gastric juices.

Studies of metabolism based on full-value natural and protein-deficient semi-synthetic diets were carried out at Gödöllő, while those involving isotope techniques and fatty acid analyses were conducted at the Institute of Animal Physiology and Nutrition at the University of Göttingen.

If the above observations are correct, then the crude fibre intake may effect determinations of the biological value of food proteins made by measuring endogenous faeces nitrogen in nitrogen balance experiments. Consequently, if accuracy and comparability of results is to be attained, such studies of metabolism should only be made with feeds of standard crude fibre content. I think that this point may be especially important in cereals which have a highly variable crude fibre content.

Proc. Int. Assoc. Cereal Chem. Symp. Amino Acid Compn and Biol. Value of Cereal Proteins Budapest, Hungary 1983, R. Lásztity, M. Hidvégi, eds

THE IMPROVEMENT OF PROTEIN UTILIZATION IN INDUSTRIAL FEEDS AND CEREALS

ÁRPÁD TÓTH, ANDRÁS HERENDI, DÉLIA RÉTHER

Research Institute for Milling and Baking Industry,
H-1024 Budapest, Kis Rókus 15/b, Hungary

INTRODUCTION

Animal breeding and the production of animal products have been gradually transformed into production branches that consume growing quantities of materials, as their industrial character was strengthening and, consequently, they became heavily influenced by soaring raw material and energy prices.

Naturally, the fall of feeding costs always had its economic function, but it has never seemed so important as it does nowadays. To cut feeding costs is a complex task, in the performance of which several special fields must cooperate. Skipping the evaluation of their share in coping with this task we will, on our part, deal with possibilities primarily in the production technology and the process techniques.

Well known are the achievements of the discipline of feeding animals in the field of specifying and potently satisfying the animals' biological needs, for which one of the best examples is the optimization of the amino acid levels at calculating formulae, and the replacement of limiting amino acids by custom-blended formulae. Similarly, the performance boosters controlling absorption or tackling veterinary problems are also very important. The significance of these materials, requiring so much care and bringing good results, is not in the least diminished if we deal with other possibilities of improving performance which may seem, after all, simpler and more natural.

Generally speaking, biological needs are usually classified in simplified terms of nutritive matter, macro- and micro-element levels, and vitamin supplement, but it is obvious that the biological needs include the form and size of fodder, in one word the physical structure thereof.

The physical structure can be modified with simple methods and it can be proven that these processes are often accompanied by changes that imply favourable possibilities. The processes have, to a certain extent, combined effects, and in addition to the modification of the physical structure changes have been observed in the composition as well.

Energy saving cannot be separated from the saving of material: a practicable way of saving energy is the saving of material in which the solar energy involved in photosynthesis is accumulated along with the energy requirement of soil tilling, soil strength replacement, sowing and harvesting, dryjng, storage, transportation, etc.

All the processes, we intend to discuss, are energy consuming from the point of view of production technology. However, the energy consumed by processing is of small volume compared to the volume of energy embodied in the material, and in numerous cases the increased energy consumption, compared to that of the traditional processes, is not a prerequisite of achieving better utilization results.

OPTIMIZATION OF GRAIN SIZE

Considering quality assurance, the grain size is a feature of complex effect. A wide range of grain sizes is characteristic of the coarse mixed feeds produced in the traditional single-phase crushing, due to the fact that

- certain components, available in small quantities, have to be finely dispersed in order to ensure even distribution;

- ground materials to be added to them /such as shorts, meat meal, fish meal, etc./ display the characteristics of their own production methods;

- grain products and other materials can be crushed by the hammer grinder in a single-phase process so that the ratio of particles of flour-fineness is big, and the ratio of coarse particles, in line with the grid size of the applied screen, is big enough within the overall variety of grain sizes.

Controversial requirements must be satisfied in the following instances:

- grain size influences consumability, the accessibility through specific surface, and the enzyme activity in the alimentary canal /e.g. saliva production/;

- grain size affects loss through crush and dispersion, and it can be directly or indirectly related to veterinary problems /e.g. humidity content, ulcer, the blockage of the omasum, etc./;

- besides the relationship between grain size and the related production energy requirement, the average grain size and the variety are a prime function of separation and the development of susceptibility to grading.

On the basis of findings obtained via tests conducted with broilers of various kinds, their management and feeding technologies, it can be postulated that there is a pronounced biological sensitivity towards average grain size in coarse meal feeds and grain size range in general, and a rather definite optimum can be set.

The most favourable breeding results have been attained with 0.9 - 1.1 mm average grain-sized coarse meal feeds, while in the case of finer grits the sults deteriorated on account of losses via consumability and dispersion, and in the case of more coarse grits separation and selection led to the same phenomenon.

After several repetitions, the measurable fluctuation exceeded 5 % expressed in terms of the specific feed utilization fluctuation, which is rather large considering the number and nature of these fluctuations.

Grain size has been monitored at feeding crumbled and granulated mixed feeds, when only the preparation /grain size/ of the coarse meal feeds differed, and the composition and the consistency of feed at the time of distribution to animals and the method of distribution were identical /0.7 kg of crumbled starter feed, followed by breeding and finishing feeds with 3 mm grain sizes/.

The way the coarse meal feeds were prepared /the grid size of the screen used at the grinder/ and the results attained are shown in Table 1. The 3 % improvement in feed utilization observable at the switching point from grade 3 screen to grade 2 screen is highly significant if measured in value and the related energy increment consumed in the grinding process is negligible, all the more so since it is compensated by an output increment and the saving of energy at granulation. Skipping the details, similar results have been achieved with pigs, too.

Ruminants are capable of affecting the results depending on the quality and quantity of the structural fibres, since their effects can cancel out the impact of grain size of fodder given as forage.

SELECTIVE CRUSHING

Cereals and other types of seeds have retained the fundamental structure that facilitated the maintenance of their respective kinds which is not necessarily in line with the requirements of further use. By using various kinds of grains, mixed feeds of favourable formulae can be produced

Table 1. Group results

Preparation of grain products	unit	on grade 2 screen	on grade 3 screen	on grade 3.6 screen
initial stock	pieces	2400	2400	2400
loss through perishing	"	229	271	460
closing stock	"	2171	2129	1940
initial weight	kg	76.6	76.7	76.4
measured weight at changing feed				
- starter	kg	878.8	829.5	743.7
- breeding	kg	2195.2	2105.1	1910.84
- fattening	kg	3287.6	3177.9	2903.60
fodder consumption				
- starter	kg	1600	1600	1600
- breeding	kg	3428	3327	3024
- fattening	kg	1638	1669	1526
- total	kg	6666	6602	6150
average stock	pieces	2286	2265	2170
loss through perishing	%	9.5	11.2	19.2
average weight at the conclusion of experiment	kg/piece	1.51	1.49	1.49
average fodder consumption	kg/piece	2.91	2.91	2.83
fodder utilization	kg/kg	2.02	2.08	2.12

with certain limitations, but if these limitations are to be differed the most practicable trick is to disintegrate the grains into their main components. In order to reduce the limitations of application, the chemical structure may have to be modified, too.

A classic example of selective crushing is the old Hungarian technology of high grinding with its numerous types of finished products. Processes of this kind have fallen prey to rationalization, although their comeback, with new levels of quality, can be expected even for the purposes of human consumption.

Predictably, very simple process technologies will prevail in /or be developed for/ the processing of cereals, while the variety of finished products will approach the wide variety that existed in the past.

The utilization of defect points by using minimum quantities of energy is a new trend in selective crushing. In the case of the majority of the cereals the controlled energy collision facilitates a good separation of the hull from the inside of the grain and, very often, that of the germ as well.

By using an appropriate combination of hammer grinder and grader, a fraction of the inside of the grain can be obtained even in the case of barley which is not rich in fibre. The fraction containing a bigger portion of hull can be used for making feeds for ruminants; the fibre content does not limit the utilization of the inside of the barley grains for feeding young animals.

Several procedures are used for the selective crushing of maize, as well. With the traditional dry process the separation of maize germ, shorts and the inside of the grain is rather investment intensive, and the process cannot be fitted economically to the technologies utilized in minor mixing plants.

A simple process has been developed in the Research Institute for Milling and Baking Industry, which is perfectly satisfactory to satisfy feeding purposes, although the fractional purity usually required for human consumption cannot be achieved by it, but the fractions of shorts, germs and the inside of grain can be used rationally.

Tables 2, 3 and 4 contain the results of the amino acid analysis of products obtained when treating various hybrides. It can be seen that fractioning, comprising only three phases of operations, could result in considerable changes in composition. Broad bean, peas, sorghum, millet and blue peas can be hulled similarly easily. In their cases this process is more favourable than the traditional procedures, since the inside of the seed is not damaged and little valuable matter is mixed with the hull.

Table 2.

The results of the amino acid analysis of fractions obtained from hybride maize, PAU 340 TC

Amino acid %	Germ fraction	Fractions still containing germs	Fractions not containing germs
Lysine	0.58	0.42	0.25
Methionine	0.14	0.08	0.13
Cystine	-	-	-
Alanine	0.80	0.64	0.49
Arginine	0.60	0.30	0.21
Aspartic acid	1.07	0.44	0.53
Glutamic acid	2.26	1.70	1.33
Glycine	0.40	0.22	0.15
Histidine	0.34	0.56	0.18
Leucine	0.94	1.46	0.80
Isoleucine	0.66	0.34	0.29
Phenylalanine	0.60	0.58	0.33
Proline	0.82	1.48	0.36
Serine	0.33	0.34	0.28
Threonine	0.39	0.24	0.18
Tyrosine	0.25	0.26	0.17
Valine	0.64	0.54	0.88
Sum	10.82	9.60	6.56

Table 3.

The results of the amino acid analysis of fractions obtained from hybride maize, P3965 AMTC

Amino acid %	Germ fraction	Fractions still containing germs	Fractions not containing germs
Lysine	0.71	0.19	0.21
Methionine	0.08	0.11	0.06
Cystine	0.03	-	-
Alanine	0.85	0.75	0.41
Arginine	0.62	0.36	0.46
Aspartic acid	1.18	1.20	0.48
Glutamic acid	2.20	2.65	1.31
Glycine	0.53	0.41	0.25
Histidine	0.31	0.29	0.19
Leucine	0.96	1.24	0.76
Isoleucine	0.70	0.34	0.20
Phenylalanine	0.62	0.57	0.39
Proline	0.93	0.72	0.49
Serine	0.54	0.67	0.25
Threonine	0.37	0.63	0.16
Tyrosine	0.21	0.18	0.15
Valine	0.69	0.61	0.28
Sum	11.53	10.92	6.05

Table 4.

The results of the amino acid analysis of fractions obtained from hybride maize, P 3906 SC

Amino acid %	Germ fraction	Fractions still containing germs	Fractions not containing germs
Lysine	0.62	0.39	0.25
Methionine	0.10	0.08	0.06
Cystine	0.05	-	-
Alanine	0.95	0.80	0.70
Arginine	0.53	0.47	0.41
Aspartic acid	1.42	1.03	0.88
Glutamic acid	2.57	2.19	1.95
Glycine	0.56	0.42	0.31
Histidine	0.40	0.32	0.27
Leucine	0.96	1.33	1.08
Isoleucine	0.84	0.43	0.37
Phenylalanine	0.63	0.61	0.48
Proline	0.92	0.66	0.64
Serine	0.32	0.44	0.39
Threonine	0.47	0.33	0.27
Tyrosine	0.34	0.27	0.21
Valine	0.65	0.65	0.52
Sum	12.33	10.42	8.79

Tables 5 and 6 contain the crude protein and crude fibre contents of fractions obtained after hulling soy and broad beans.

In case of refill grinding, the fine shorts are derived from the hull that sticks to the grain and the layers under the hull, and are separated in the form of tips produced during the grinding procedures.

Naturally, other kinds of grinding procedures can also be introduced, and in the process of gradual crushing and grading individual fractions can be produced in optimal volumes.

Table 5.

Values of some chemical parameters in different fractions of broad bean

Fractions	Crude protein /% of dry matter/	Digestible protein /% of dry matter/	Digestibility /%/	Crude fibre /% of dry matter/
1	34.74	32.87	94.6	1.00
2	34.26	33.39	97.5	1.10
3	35.25	34.14	96.8	1.80
4	29.29	27.02	92.2	11.60
5	5.84	3.02	51.7	42.50

Table 6.

Values of some chemical parameters in different fractions of soy meal

Fractions	Crude protein /% of dry matter/	Crude fibre /% of dry matter/
1	35.1	4.5
2	33.0	10.7
3	29.6	13.5
4	17.3	34.1

As an extreme case, results obtained during the crushing and grading of bad quality extracted sunflower grits with high shell content can be shown. For selective crushing, a machine should be used which pérforms some sort of grading as early as in the crushing phase, and the effects leading to the increase of surface can also produce separation. Controllable crushers with self-adjusting port sizes are excellent for this purpose /e.g. the roller mill/, but the flyer crushers can also be used very well that provide variable collision work. The machines which cannot sense small physical differences, or have been constructed with the aim to produce equilized finished product despite diverse physical properties, cannot be used for this purpose. /They are excellent for other purposes though and can be used as first class homogenizing equipment./

Naturally, it is much simpler to remove the hull pieces from the extracted sunflower grits directly after toasting than separate the product by digestion after it has solidified. Subsequent fractionining may, however, become necessary in several cases, and not only in the case of sunflower grits.

It must be noted from Table 7 that the flyer grinder is better at drying than the hammer grinder. It must be obvious too that the digestion it performs is gentler and facilitates a better "offset". The transition of the screen with a characteristic size of 1.6 mm also deserves attention: it shows that the little crumbs that would persist without the intensive crushing effect strongly recall the internal properties representing the whole lot. On balance it can be noted that by using very simple facilities,fractions of small fibre content and fractions of high protein content can be produced that not only modifies the effects of applicability but can serve as the preparatory operation for the production of a much more complicated protein concentrate, as well. Although the mechanical processes are combined with a dust removing function of considerable impact,this is much simpler from the point of view of environmental protection than the digestive operations which produce big quantities of sevage as by-product.

Another special instant of selective crushing is the production of green plant meals. Stems with their different composition lend themselves differently to crushing than leaves do. A batch prepared by chaffing can be transformed into a substance by collision work that can be spilt into a fraction rich in fibres and another one devoid of fibres. The grading can be done with an air current separator. Although this operation would ensure better circumstances for setting only the optimum fibre level, it must not be underestimated at calculating formulae. /Of course, usefulness may be greater if the fraction devoid of fibres is to be transported for use to a great distance, because smaller specific costs would be attached to the utilization of the alfalfa leaf meal to be transported without ballast./

Table 7.

The fractioning of extracted sunflower grits after digestion with hammer grinder and flyer grinder

Description	Humidity content %	Crude protein %	Crude fibre %
Hammer grinder			
- particles smaller than 0.4 mm	8.8	42.2	9.8
- fraction between 0.4-0.8 mm	8.8	37.8	16.0
- fraction between 0.8-1.6 mm	8.9	32.8	19.6
- particles bigger than 1.6 mm	9.2	32.7	19.8
Flyer grinder			
- particles smaller than 0.4 mm	8.6	43.3	9.0
- fraction between 0.4-0.8 mm	8.5	37.8	15.7
- fraction between 0.8-1.6 mm	8.6	33.1	21.0
- particles bigger than 1.6 mm	8.8	36.5	16.0

Fractions rich in germs obtained by selective crushing, or fractions derived from the valuable layers between the hull and the inside of the grain facilitate the extensive /or exclusive/ application of natural vitamin and mineral carriers at the end of the broiler breeding process.

GRANULATION

Despite the fact that granulation has proved to be effective, scientific papers keep cropping up that deem its application unnecessary in creatine cases and in general.

Results related to granulation can be presented by the following data: 7-10 % of material can be saved, while the excess energy consumption, depending on quality, composition, technological standard, etc., is 15-20 kWh/t; by using excessive simplification 80 kg of material = 20 kWh.

Conversion to heat equivalent is not necessary: it is obvious that the material saved may contain more energy even if burnt than the expenditure. For the purposes of a more sophisticated analysis, it should be mentioned that a considerable portion of the energy contained in the material is highly limited liquid energy source, while the electric energy required for granulation can be obtained from coal, atomic power stations, or regenerating energy sources.

Granulation, as a form of value-improving treatment, has not acquired sufficient scope in the formula calculation. The general practice is that components are calculated as coarse meal feeds and the value improving effect of the procedure is not usually taken into consideration to a satisfactory extent. /There are, however, several examples to show that the negative effects of granulation, e.g. the damage done to vitamins, are reckoned with even if the products are not subjected to granulation./

Considerations given to the results of the value-improving treatment can be an important factor in saving material that may facilitate the distribution of granulated feeds to laying hens, without any detrimental effect. Granulation can be considered as the transition towards the group of real hydrothermic operations and other value-improving treatments.

There are no new types of digestive operations to limit their general application, since they imitate the physical properties of cereals in the form of operations that shape and condense materials, and it falls in line with the biological needs of the animals.

HYDROTHERMIC OPERATIONS

The hydrothermic operations have disinfecting and starch digestive effects. Additionally, they can be used effectively to break up enzyme inhibitors and other anti-nutritive substances, to produce protected proteins, etc. Their disadvantage is that they damage the heat sensitive amino acids, especially the limiting lysine and methionine suffer damages, which are in short supply anyway. /Of course, this applies to granulation, as well, but their extent is different./

Our experiments conducted with opaque-type maize led to very interesting results. One bath of maize was allowed to dry out under natural conditions, while others were dried out with 70-90 °C and 130 °C temperature air. The crude protein, digestible protein, and the water-soluble protein content of the batches and their dissolvability in rumen liquid were tested first in vitro then in vivo. It was found that the positive results of the in vivo experiments with ruminants, exceeding the forecasts of chemical methods that reflect the actual feeding values with varying accuracy only, supported the strongly protected protein effect.

The wide variety of the hydrothermic operations /i.e. flaking, swelling, micronizing, extruding, microwave treatment, etc./ requires careful application in view of the energy requirement of the operations. In order to exploit the advantages and to improve the results, substances obtained by selective crushing must be treated fraction by fraction, in addition to the treatment of the whole grains. The stabilization of fractions rich in germs must have due importance too, and different treatments must be specified as required by further processing.

In addition to the field of application of the by-pass proteins, the products obtained with the hydrothermic operations can be especially useful in the feeds intended for young animals, or for feeding broilers as per sex.

CLOSING REMARKS

It must be obvious from the paper that, in our opinion, the improvement of feed utilization is a highly realistic way of saving proteins and that very simple methods could bring good results towards this end.

We wish to reiterate that this does not mean that the importance of other methods would be underestimated.

The optimization of grain sizes, the widening range of the application of selective crushing and the exploitation of possibilities in granulation and the other hydrothermic operations represent considerable reserves as the results, confirmed via the feeding experiments, have proven.

They must not be applied without performing actual economic calculations, but obviously, they must be utilized if any progress is to be made in the field of meat production.

LIST OF CONTRIBUTORS

BARÁTH,Á., Central Food Research Institute, H-1525 Budapest, P.O.B. 76, Hungary

BARBER,S., Laboratorio de Cereales y Proteaginosas, Instituto de Agroquimica y Tecnologia de Alimentos, CSIC, Jaime Roig 11, Valencia-10, Spain

BAUDET,J., Laboratorie d'Etude des Protéines, Départment de Physiologie et Biochimie Végétales, INRA, 78000 Versailles, France

BÉKÉS,F., Department of Biochemistry and Food Technology, Technical University of Budapest, H-1111 Budapest, Müegyetem rkp. 3, Hungary

BENEDITO de BARBER,C., Laboratorio de Cereales y Proteaginosas, Instituto de Agroquimica y Tecnologia de Alimentos, CSIC, Jaime Roig 11, Valencia-10, Spain

CERLETTI,P., Department of General Biochemistry, University of Milan, Via Celoria, 2, I-20133 Milano, Italy

DAKO,D.Y., Department of Nutrition and Food Science, University of Ghana, Legon, Ghana

DODDS,S.J., Department of Biochemistry, School of Medicine, Oral Roberts University, Tulsa, OK. 74133, USA

FEKETE,L., Department of Animal Feeding, University of Agriculture Gödöllő, H-2103 Gödöllő, Hungary

FLEMING,S.E., Department of Nutritional Sciences, University of California, Berkeley, California 94720, USA

GANZLER,K., Institute of Enzymology, Biological Research Center, Hungarian Academy of Sciences, H-1113 Budapest, Karolina 29, Hungary

GEERVANI,P., Department of Foods and Nutrition, College of Home Science, Andhra Pradesh Agricultural University, Hyderabad 500004, India

GOLENKOV,V.F., All-Union Research Institute for Grain and Grain Products, Dmitrovskoe Chaussee 11, Moscow 127434, USSR

GUSTAFSON,J.M., Department of Biochemistry, School of Medicine, Oral Roberts University, Tulsa, OK. 74133, USA

HACKLER L.R., Department of Home Economics, State University of New York College, Oneonta, New York 13820, USA

HALÁSZ,A., Central Food Research Institute, H-1525 Budapest, P.O.B. 76, Hungary

HERENDI,A., Grain Trust, H-1053 Budapest, Dorottya 1, Hungary

HESSER,J.M., International Wheat Gluten Association, 10100 Santa Fe Drive, Suite 206, Overland Park, Kansas 66212, USA

HIDVÉGI,M., Department of Biochemistry and Food Technology, Technical University of Budapest, H-1111 Budapest, Müegyetem rkp. 3, Hungary, and Grain Trust, H-1053 Budapest, Dorottya 1, Hungary

HUET,J.-C., Laboratoire d'Etude des Protéines, Départment de Physiologie et Biochimie Végétales, INRA, 78000 Versailles, France

HURWITZ,S., Institute of Animal Science, Agricultural Research Organization, The Volcani Center, Bet Dagan, Israel

JÉCSAI,J., Department of Physiology, Institute for Animal Nutrition, Research-Center for Animal Production, H-2053 Herceghalom, Hungary

JUHÁSZ,B., Department of Physiology, Institute for Animal Nutrition, Research-Center for Animal Production, H-2053 Herceghalom, Hungary

KACZKOWSKI,J., Department of Biochemistry, Institute of Plant Biology, University of Agriculture, P-02-528 Warsaw, Poland

KÁRPÁTI,Gy., Faculty of Agriculture, University of Agricultural Sciences, H-9200 Mosonmagyaróvár, Lucsony 15-17, Hungary

KIES,C., Department of Human Nutrition and Food Service Management, 316 Ruth Leverton Hall, University of Nebraska, Lincoln, Nebraska 68583-0807, USA

KUROWSKA,E., Department of Biochemistry, Institute of Plant Biology, University of Agriculture, P-02-528 Warsaw, Poland

LÁSZTITY,R., Department of Biochemistry and Food Technology, Technical University of Budapest, H-1111 Budapest, Müegyetem rkp. 3, Hungary

LINDNER,K., Nutrition Department, College of Commerce and Catering Trade, H-1054 Budapest, Alkotmány 9/11, Hungary

MERCER,P.L., Department of Biochemistry, School of Medicine, Oral Roberts University, Tulsa, OK. 74133, USA

MOSKAL,M., Department of Biochemistry, Institute of Plant Biology, University of Agriculture, P-02-528 Warsaw, Poland

MOSSÉ,J., Laboratoire d'Etude des Protéines, Département de Physiologie et Biochimie Végétales, INRA, 78000 Versailles, France

MUNCK,L., Carlsberg Research Laboratory, Department of Biotechnology, Gamle Carlsberg Vej 10, DK-2500 Copenhagen Valby, Denmark

NEHÉZ,R., Cereal Research Institute, H-6701 Szeged, Alsókikötő-sor 9, Hungary

NÉMETH,I., Department of Crop Cultivation, Agricultural University, H-8361 Keszthely, Hungary

NIERLE,W., Institut für Biochemie und Analytik, Bundesforschungsanstalt für Getreide- und Kartoffelverarbeitung, Postfach 23, D-4930 Detmold, FRG

ÖRSI,F., Department of Biochemistry and Food Technology, Technical University of Budapest, H-1111 Budapest, Müegyetem rkp. 3, Hungary

PELLETT,P.L., Department of Food Science and Nutrition, University of Massachusetts, Amherst, Massachusetts 01003, USA

RESTANI,P., Department of General Biochemistry, University of Milan, Via Celoria, 2, I-20133 Milano, Italy

RÉTHER,D., Research Institute for Milling and Baking Industry, H-1024 Budapest, Kis Rókus 15/b, Hungary

RIGÓ,J., National Institute of Dietetics, H-1085 Budapest, Makarenko 24, Hungary

SAARINEN,E.-R., Raision Tehtaat, SF-21200 Raisio, Finland

SAEED,B.M., Central Food Research Institute, H-1022 Budapest, Herman Ottó 15, Hungary; permanent address: University of Erbil, Erbil, Iraque

SALGÓ,A., Department of Biochemistry and Food Technology, Technical University of Budapest, H-1111 Budapest, Müegyetem rkp. 3, Hungary

SARKKI,M.-L., Raision Tehtaat, SF-21200 Raisio, Finland

SARWAR,G., Bureau of Nutritional Sciences, Food Directorate, Health Protection Branch, National Health and Welfare, Tunney's Pasture, Ottawa, Ontario, K1A OL2., Canada

SHAROBEEM,S.F., Department of Biochemistry and Food Technology, Technical University of Budapest, H-1111 Budapest, Müegyetem rkp. 3, Hungary; permanent address: Department of Biochemistry, Faculty of Agriculture, Zagazig University, Zagazig, Egypt

SIMON-SARKADI,L., Department of Biochemistry and Food Technology, Technical University of Budapest, H-1111 Budapest, Müegyetem rkp. 3, Hungary

SOMSSICH,I., Institute of Plant Cultivation and Control, H-1024 Budapest, Kis Rókus 15/a, Hungary

SOSULSKI,F.W., Department of Crop Science and Plant Ecology, University of Saskatchewan, Saskatoon, Sask. S7N OWO, Canada

SZELÉNYI-GALÁNTAI,M., Department of Physiology, Institute for Animal Nutrition, Research-Center for Animal Production, H-2053 Herceghalom, Hungary

TÓTH,Á., Research Institute for Milling and Baking Industry, H-1024 Budapest, Kis Rókus 15/b, Hungary

TÖRÖK,E., College of Food Industry, H-6724 Szeged, Hungary

TSEN,C.C., Department of Grain Science and Industry, Kansas State University, Manhattan, KS. 66506, USA

TUREK,B., Regional Centre of Hygiene, Skrétova St. 15, 303 22 Plzeň, Czechoslovakia

VANIČEK F., Regional Centre of Hygiene, Skrétova St. 15, 303 22 Plzeň, Czechoslovakia

WALGER-KUNZE,B., Research Laboratory, College of Agriculture, H-7400 Kaposvár, Hungary

YOSHIDA,A., Department of Agricultural Chemistry, Nagoya University, Nagoya 464, Japan

SUBJECT INDEX

GPSR Compliance

The European Union's (EU) General Product Safety Regulation (GPSR) is a set of rules that requires consumer products to be safe and our obligations to ensure this.

If you have any concerns about our products, you can contact us on ProductSafety@springernature.com

In case Publisher is established outside the EU, the EU authorized representative is:

Springer Nature Customer Service Center GmbH
Europaplatz 3
69115 Heidelberg, Germany

Batch number: 10823769

Printed by Printforce, the Netherlands